# Exclusive Papers of the Editorial Board Members of the Organic Chemistry Section of Molecules

# Exclusive Papers of the Editorial Board Members of the Organic Chemistry Section of Molecules

Guest Editor

**Maged Henary**

MDPI

Basel • Beijing • Wuhan • Barcelona • Belgrade • Novi Sad • Cluj • Manchester

*Guest Editor*
Maged Henary
Department of Chemistry
Georgia State University
Atlanta
USA

*Editorial Office*
MDPI AG
Grosspeteranlage 5
4052 Basel, Switzerland

This is a reprint of the Special Issue, published open access by the journal *Molecules* (ISSN 1420-3049), freely accessible at: https://www.mdpi.com/journal/molecules/special_issues/EBM_OC.

For citation purposes, cite each article independently as indicated on the article page online and as indicated below:

| Lastname, A.A.; Lastname, B.B. Article Title. *Journal Name* **Year**, *Volume Number*, Page Range. |
|---|

**ISBN 978-3-7258-7022-6 (Hbk)**
**ISBN 978-3-7258-7023-3 (PDF)**
**https://doi.org/10.3390/books978-3-7258-7023-3**

# Contents

# About the Editor

**Maged Henary**

Maged Henary is currently a Professor and the Associate Chair of the Department of Chemistry at Georgia State University. Maged received his B.Sc. in Chemistry from Alexandria University, Egypt in 1990. He continued his graduate studies at Cairo University, Egypt, where he earned his M.Sc. in Organic Chemistry in 1996. Shortly thereafter, he moved to the United States and completed his Ph.D. in Organic/Medicinal Chemistry at Georgia State University (GSU) in 2000. He then pursued postdoctoral training at the Georgia Institute of Technology, focusing on the development of fluorescent sensors for imaging labile zinc and copper pools in live cells.

Dr. Henary also serves as the Editor-in-Chief of *Heterocyclic Communications* and has been a member of the Biological Staining Commission Board of Trustees since 2019. His research centers on the synthesis of novel heterocyclic small molecules as potential anticancer agents, as well as the design and development of advanced near-infrared (NIR) dyes for use in image-guided surgery. Dr. Henary has published more than 150 peers-reviewed articles in high-impact journals, accumulating over 8,572 citations with H-index 48. Dr. Henary is also the inventor on ten patents related to NIR imaging technologies and recently he has been elected as a Senior Member of National Academy of Inventors. His research program is supported by multiple funding sources, including NIH R01 grants, a Health Innovation Grant, and a Venture Lab Grant from the State of Georgia.

# Preface

Organic chemistry is, at its heart, a science of purposeful invention. We design transformations that did not exist yesterday; we orchestrate selectivity where none seemed possible; and, increasingly, we connect molecular structure to measurable function—optical, biological, and material. This volume, developed from the Special Issue Exclusive Papers of the Editorial Board Members of the Organic Chemistry Section of Molecules, gathers fourteen invited contributions into a single, homogeneous whole. My goal as editor has been to present not a loose anthology, but a coherent arc that moves from insight to implementation to impact.

The Reprint focuses on contemporary organic chemistry viewed through three complementary lenses: (i) foundational perspectives that re-examine known scaffolds and reactions with modern understanding; (ii) enabling methodologies that unlock chemo-, regio-, and stereocontrol in demanding settings; and (iii) application-oriented design, where molecules are built to deliver photochemical, therapeutic, or biological effects.

The chapters span chromophoric natural products (aurones), macrocyclic systems (phthalocyanines and porpholactones), carbohydrate–phenylpropanoid chemistry, practical oxidation and fluorination reagents, selective amination of heteroarenes, computation-guided annulations, and a suite of medicinally relevant chemotypes—tryptamines, quinoline–sulfonamide hybrids, natural-product-inspired anti-inflammatory scaffolds, and halogen-engineered bipyridines aimed at protein misfolding diseases.

We aim to provide readers with a usable map: why certain strategies matter, how they were realized, and where they can lead. The emphasis throughout is on decisions—choice of protecting groups, reagent selection, catalyst/solvent pairing, late-stage editing—because these are the levers that turn elegant concepts into robust practice.

The purpose is twofold: first, to serve as a ready reference for researchers who need reliable methods and design principles they can adopt immediately; second, to spark new directions by juxtaposing classical motifs with current tools, demonstrating how "old dogs" still learn "new tricks" when illuminated by modern analysis and instrumentation.

The motivation for assembling this collection is the conviction that progress often depends on connections. Safer preparation of a hypervalent iodine oxidant frees a synthesis from avoidable hazards and impurities; improved electrophilic fluorination expands physicochemical space in drug-like molecules; orthogonal protection on a disaccharide enables truly targeted acylation; precise editing of a porphyrinoid ring reopens photophysical territory; and judicious halogen placement in a bipyridine scaffold tunes protein engagement against amyloidogenesis. Each advance is meaningful on its own; taken together, they form a common language of selectivity, efficiency, and function—the language working chemists speak every day at the bench.

This Reprint is written for research chemists across academia, industry, and national labs—synthetic and medicinal chemists, chemical biologists, and materials-oriented organic chemists—who design, make, and evaluate molecules. It should also serve graduate students and advanced undergraduates, providing a compact survey of strategies that work in practice and the mechanistic thinking behind them. Finally, colleagues at disciplinary interfaces—computational chemists, biophysicists, and pharmacologists—will find clear chemical foundations for translating hypotheses into molecular probes, leads, and functional materials.

We open with Reviews & Perspectives that set the conceptual stage: the reappraisal of aurones as versatile polyphenolic scaffolds; the enduring adaptability of phthalocyanines in photochemistry; and a decade-scale synthesis perspective on α-aminophosphonates. The second section, Carbohydrate–Phenylpropanoid Chemistry, pairs orthogonal-protection–driven acylation of sucrose with the biological rationale of α-glucosidase inhibition. The third section, Methods, Reagents, and Selective Functionalization, provides the working toolkit—safer IBA synthesis, HF-based electrophilic fluorination, computation-guided annulations, adamantane-assisted amination of aza-arenes, and site-specific porpholactone editing. We close with medicinal and biological applications, where deliberate scaffold engineering yields antitumor, antimicrobial, anti-inflammatory, and anti-amyloid activities. Read linearly, the sections trace a path from context to capability to consequence; dipped into selectively, each chapter stands as a complete resource.

**Maged Henary**
*Guest Editor*

molecules

MDPI

*Review*

# Aurones: A Golden Resource for Active Compounds

**Ilaria Mazziotti, Giovanni Petrarolo and Concettina La Motta ***

Department of Pharmacy, University of Pisa, 56126 Pisa, Italy; i.mazziotti@studenti.unipi.it (I.M.); giovanni.petrarolo@phd.unipi.it (G.P.)
* Correspondence: concettina.lamotta@unipi.it; Tel.: +39-050-221-9593

**Abstract:** Deemed as poorly represented in nature, aurones have been often overlooked by researchers compared to other members of the flavonoid superfamily. However, over the past two decades, they have been reassessed by the scientific community, who are increasingly appreciating their ability to modulate several biological pathways. This review summarizes the recent literature on this class of compounds, which has been analyzed from both a chemical and a functional point of view. Original articles, reviews and editorials featured in Pubmed and Scifinder over the last twenty years have been taken into account to provide the readers with a view of the chemical strategies to obtain them, their functional properties, and their potential of technological use. The resulting comprehensive picture aims at raising the awareness of these natural derivatives as effective drug candidates, fostering the development of novel synthetic analogues.

**Keywords:** aurones; polyphenols; flavonoids; synthesis; functional activity

## 1. Introduction

In the early twentieth century, Gustav Klein coined the term *anthochlor* (*anthos* = flower, *chlōrós* = yellowish) to define a class of water-soluble pigments conferring color to plants able to synthesize them as secondary metabolites [1]. It included a restricted group of derivatives known as aurones (*aurum* = gold), due to the bright yellow/gold color that these compounds give to plants in which they are located.

Aurones (**1**, Figure 1) are part of the wide family of polyphenols. More specifically, they may be acknowledged as the lower structural counterparts of the best-known flavones (**2**, Figure 1), a subclass of flavonoids. Actually, as has been observed in detail, the basic structure of an aurone consists of a main 6:5 benzofuranone core, instead of the 6:6 chromane ring of flavones, but shares a 2-aryl decoration with the higher homologues [2].

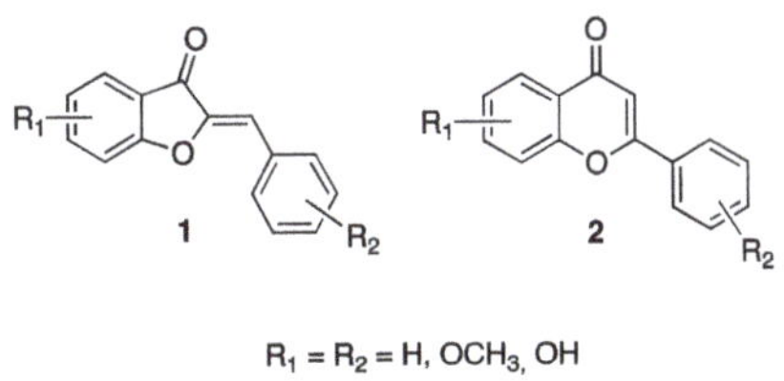


**Figure 1.** General structures of aurones **1**, and flavones, **2**.

Deemed as poorly represented in nature, aurones have been often overlooked by researchers compared to the other members of the flavonoid superfamily. However, in recent decades, they have been reassessed and more and more chemists, biologists, and practitioners are taking an interest in their structural and functional peculiarities. Actually, to date, the chemical structures of more than 100 different aurones have been identified, characterized by distinctive hydroxylated, methoxylated, and glycosylated substitution patterns. Moreover, their effective potential to predict viable therapeutic uses has begun to be unveiled [3–6]. Therefore, they represent a worth deepening class of natural compounds intended to provide bioactive compounds in the near future.

The first examples of aurones were characterized in 1940 in Asteraceae [7], the family of sunflowers, which synthesize the most common 4-deoxy-derivatives of the family including sulfuretin (**3**, Figure 2), maritimetin (**4**, Figure 2), leptosidin (**5**, Figure 2), and their corresponding glycosides. The species *variabilis* and *sulphureus* mainly express sulfuretin (Figure 2) and its glycosylated counterparts in leaves and petals. In the *bidens* species, maritimetin has been isolated while, in the genus Coreopsis, compounds such as sulfuretin, maritimetin, but also leptosidin may be found.

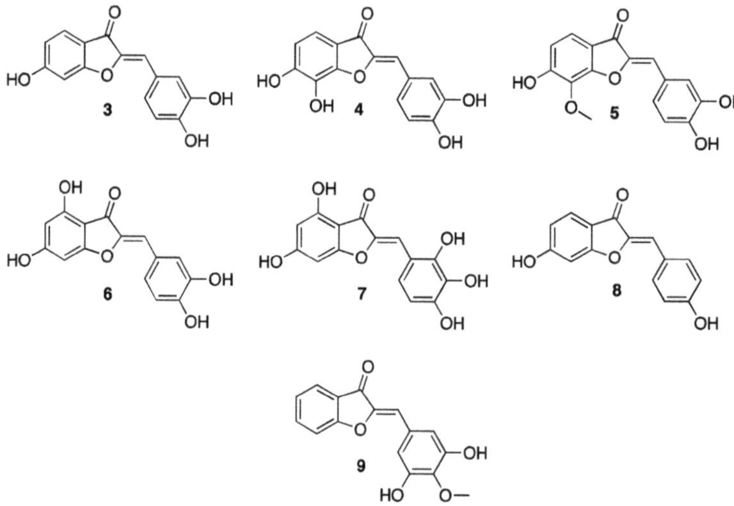


**Figure 2.** Chemical structures of 4-deoxy- and 4-hydroxy-aurones.

In addition to Asteraceae, aurones are synthesized as the secondary metabolites of many dicotyledons including Anacardiaceae, Cactaceae, Fabaceae, Gesneriaceae, Moraceae, Oxalidaceae, Plumbaginaceae, Rubiaceae, Rhamnaceae, Rosaceae, and Plantaginaceae [4]. Moreover, they have been found in some species of monocotyledons as well as in Bryophytes, as reported by recent studies [8].

While the 4-deoxy-aurones are mainly found in the flowers of the Asteraceae, the 4-hydroxylated derivatives, such as aureusidin (**6**, Figure 2) and bracteatin (**7**, Figure 2), are more common in other plant families, such as in Plantaginaceae, and particularly in the genera Misopates and Linaria, as well as in Rubiaceae and Plumbaginaceae. The flower of the snapdragon plant, defined by the scientific name of *Antirrhinum majus*, is probably the reference natural source of aurones, as high concentrations of the glycosilated form of aureusidin, but also bracteatin, may be found in the vacuoles of the epidermal cells of the petals [9].

Aurones are generally detected in petals or leaves but have also been found in different parts of plants such as leaves, nectar, seeds, wood, and also bark. Hispidol (**8**, Figure 2) and leptosidin, with their glycosylated derivatives, have been found in the seeds of plants such as *Retama raetam* and *Psophocarpus tetragonolobus*, both belonging to the Fabaceae family [4]. Sulfuretin is in charge for the yellow color of the young stems of the deciduous shrub *Cotinus coggygria*, belonging to the Anacardiaceae family, so much so that since ancient times it has been extracted as a pigment to be used as a textile dye [10].

The presence of aurones in primitive bodies such as bryophytes suggests their importance for the vital economy of plants; they pass on the genetic information for the synthesis of these compounds from generation to generation, preserving their expression. In addition to an undoubted natural relevance, due to their role as dyes, aurones are also emerging as possible functional agents, being able to modulate the activity of several biological pathways. Accordingly, they represent an intriguing reservoir of compounds waiting to be fully investigated and used by the scientific community.

## 2. Aurones as Natural Dyes

The color of flowers is the keystone of the evolutionary process that marked the transition from a random pollination, mediated exclusively by the wind, to the use of a vector, that is, insects, birds, and lizards. Being attracted from the nectar of flowers, vectors confer an advantage to the plant world, which may benefit from a greater chance of survival thanks to the passage of pollen from one plant to another and from one place to another. This is why, over the course of time, flowers and plants in general have equipped themselves to attract more and more vectors, in particular by expressing pigments that match the perceptions of these animals [11].

When walking in nature, the characteristic that most catches the eye is a bright yellow color. This is due to aurones and turns out to be more attractive than other shades of yellow given by other parent compounds such as flavonols. Actually, overall, aurones can be acknowledged as the brightest polyphenol pigments in the yellow color range, like anthocyanins are for the red/purple spectrum. The visual contrast that is perceived is the result of different UV absorption spectra. Flavones, isoflavones, and flavanones exhibit UV absorption at 350 nm and, for this reason, they are not characterized by any visible color. Instead, aurones have an absorption spectrum in the 390–430 nm range, thus resulting in a more intense colors than the parent chalcones, showing UV absorption in the 365–390 nm range, and flavonols, having 350–390 nm as the reference range [12].

Being characterized by a brilliant color, aurones play a key role in pollination, attracting vectors towards the flowers and to the pollen. Their distribution in the petals of flowers is generally unique. For example, in the case of *A. majus*, the production of aurones is limited to the upper side of the petal, but also affects two additional stripes at the level of the throat, mainly surrounded by a magenta or pink color due to the presence of anthocyanins. The brilliant stripes have the crucial role of warning the insect on the place of nectar [13]. There is also the case where the flowers appear completely yellow, but they this is not so: the contrast is perceived as two-tone by UV-sensitive insects, and these different colors act as a guide for nectar, as was observed in *Bidens ferulifolia* and *Coreopsis gigantea*. This is an example of the evolutionary adaptation of flowers, to better attract pollinating insects such as bees [14].

However, as ever, there is always the exception that proves the rule: a particular aurone does exist, 3′,5′-dihydroxy-4′-methoxyaurone (**9**, Figure 2), inducing a red/scarlet color in the nectar of the flowers of specific plants such as the Mauritian *Nesocodon mauritianus*. This is an almost unique exception as this compound provides a color that is not bright yellow. However, the special shade is thought to be due to the particularly alkaline pH of the nectar, which causes the deprotonation of the hydroxyl group of the aurone, leading to a different electronic delocalization [15].

From a commercial point of view, the color of the flowers is of great interest. In this regard, the use of aurones has been thought of to create transgenic plants endowed with bright yellow flowers through genetic engineering approaches. By investigating the natural biosynthetic pathways of *Torenia hybrida*, belonging to the Scrophulariaceae family, Tanaka and co-workers demonstrated that the *A. majus* aureusidin synthase (AmAS1) is the key enzyme catalyzing aurone biosynthesis from chalcones. However, to accomplish aurone biosynthesis and produce yellow-colored flowers in vivo, AmAS1 must work in tandem with chalcone 4′-*O*-glucosyltransferase (4′CGT). Actually, the co-expression of both the *AmAS1* and the *4′CGT* genes turned out to be sufficient for the accumulation of aureusidin-6-*O*-glucoside in the flowers of transgenic plants, thus opening up the obtainment of novel bright-yellow flowers for plant species lacking this color variant [16].

## 3. Aurones as Functional Agents

By virtue of their poly-hydroxylated nature, aurones are able to quench reactive oxygen species (ROS), thus showing antioxidant properties. In analogy with the higher homologous flavones, the main mechanism by which aurones exert their protective role is by transferring an H atom to ROS, thus becoming radical species [17]. In addition, they may also transfer a single electron, giving rise to a radical cation. The H atoms of the hydroxy groups in both positions 3′ and 4′ of the benzylidene residue are considered to be the first shield to the attack of ROS. Once formed, the phenoxy radical may be easily stabilized thanks to the assistance of the carbon atoms in positions 2 and 3 of the nucleus, and also by the exocyclic oxygen atom in position 3, thus allowing the radical to be less prone to act as a pro-oxidant [18]. Accordingly, a high potential for ROS scavenger activity has been acknowledged for all the aurones showing a 4′-hydroxy-, as well as a 3′,4′-dihydroxy- and also a 3′,4′,5′-trihydroxy- substitution patterns. Thanks to a quantum chemical investigation, Senthil Kumar and co-workers demonstrated the high antioxidant properties of bracteatin (**7**, Figure 2), whose poly-substitution pattern on the pendant benzylidene residue allows the lowest energy for both the H-atom and electron transfer mechanism [19].

Aurones have proved to be effective against *Escherichia coli, Bacillus subtilis, Staphylococcus aureus, Klebsiella pneumoniae, Proteus vulgaris,* and *Mycobacterium tuberculosis*, thus showing a broad-spectrum antibacterial activity. In addition to natural derivatives, a number of synthetic aurones were also developed as active agents, highlighting the importance of a diversified 2-substitution pattern to achieve a relevant efficacy. In particular, enlargement of the aromatic area in this position, as in derivatives **10** and **11** (Figure 3), provided the most performing compounds, showing minimal inhibitory concentrations (MICs) in the micromolar/submicromolar range against several pathogen bacteria. Similar functional results were also achieved when the benzofuranone core was replaced with the bioisosteric indolone, as in derivative **12** (Figure 3) [20–22].

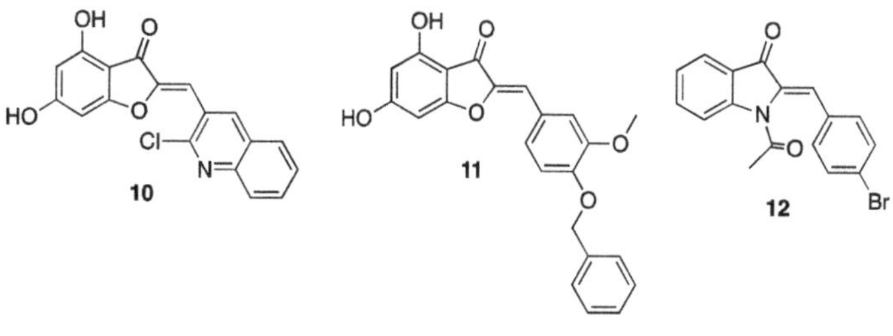


**Figure 3.** Representative synthetic antibacterial aurones.

As for the antifungal properties, aurones are mainly effective against *Aspergillus fumigatus, Aspergillus niger, Trichoderma virdie,* and *Penicillium chrysogenum*. Investigations into *Candida albicans* have demonstrated once more the importance of the 2-arylidene moiety for the antifungal activity. Derivatives **13** and **14** counteracted *Candida* spp., also displaying anti-biofilm activity for mid-maturation growth [23]. Aurones demonstrated insecticidal activity when tested against the larvae of *Spodoptera litura* [24]. In this case, the best activity was obtained in the presence of methoxylated derivatives. In particular, the 3′,4,4′,6 tetramethoxy-aurone **15** (Figure 4) is the compound that displayed the strongest insecticidal activity among the tested ones, thus highlighting positions 4, 6, 3′, and 6′ of the nucleus as those worth substituting with a view to implementing the activity. On the contrary, when the methoxy substituents were inserted in position 5 or 5′ the activity proved to decrease. Interestingly, the 3′,4,4′,6 tetramethoxy-aurone is also one of the main constituents isolated from the extract of *Cyperus radians*, an example of the Cyperaceae family that produce poly-methylated aurones as part of the body's chemical defense system.

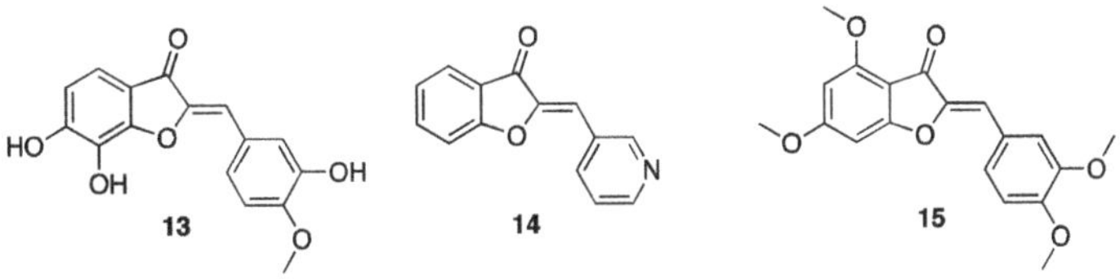

**Figure 4.** Representative natural and synthetic antifungal aurones.

The anti-malarian activity of a number of aurone derivatives has been demonstrated by several authors, who investigated both natural derivatives and synthetic analogues [25–27]. Analyses of structure–activity relationships have highlighted the importance of the substitution patterns in positions 4 and 6 of the benzofurane ring. In particular, the best in vitro anti-malarian efficacy was obtained in the presence of a halogen atom in position 4 of the nucleus and/or an amino group in position 6. Significantly, all the compounds turned out to be non-cytotoxic when tested in human cells. However, when the best performing derivative was tested in vivo in laboratory animals stricken by Plasmodium falciparum, the results were rather disappointing. Actually, as often occurs in the case of natural poly-hydroxylated derivatives, the functional efficacy observed in in vitro tests is hardly replicated in in vivo models, due to bioavailability limits that characterize this kind of compound.

Many aurones have also been evaluated for their inhibitory activity against the glycoprotein neuraminidase, which is involved in the infection processes of the most common influenza viruses. In this case, the analysis of the structure–activity relationship showed that the key structural elements of the natural compounds, represented by a hydroxyl group in position 4 or 6 of the nucleus and a double bond in position 2, are essential for the activity [28].

In 2011, some aurones were identified as inhibitors of the RNA polymerase RdRp, exploited by hepatitis C virus (HCV) for replication. Due to the extreme heterogeneity of the viral genome of the causative agent of hepatitis C, to date it has not yet been possible to develop a vaccine. Indeed, eight genotypes of HCV are currently known, each differing by 30% in nucleotide sequence [29]. For many years, the weak points of HCV have been found to make the infection, if not inert, at least less dangerous. In this regard, the research community has recently been focusing on RdRp, which is a key enzyme for viral replication [30]. Nucleoside and nucleotide analogues have been shown to target the active site of RdRp, but also non-nucleoside derivatives have been disclosed as allosteric inhibitors. Regarding aurones, aureusidin **6** proved to inhibit RdRp potently, showing an $IC_{50}$ value of 5.2 μM. Thanks to the use of a classical medicinal chemistry approach, it has been possible to identify both substitutes and ring positions conferring to aurones the best inhibitory potency. The presence of hydroxy groups in positions 4 and 6 of the nucleus turned out to be crucial for the activity. On the contrary, replacement of the hydroxy groups with methoxy substituents in the same positions resulted in a loss of activity. Different aromatic substituents were also investigated in position 2 of the benzofuran ring, demonstrating that the insertion of an indole nucleus in this position, as in compound **16** ($IC_{50}$ 2.2 μM, Figure 5), significantly ameliorated the antiviral activity of the natural **6** [31]. Remarkable efficacy was also seen in the case of pseudodimeric compounds such as derivative **17** ($IC_{50}$ 1.3 μM, Figure 5) [32]. Aurones displaying the most promising RdRp inhibitory activity did not show any cytotoxic effect on human cells, thus showing that they are prominent candidates for the obtainment of anti-HCV agents.

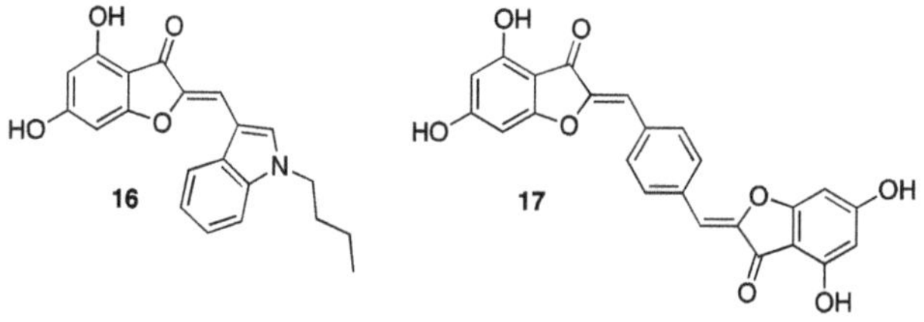

**Figure 5.** Representative examples of synthetic anti-HCV aurones.

Aurones and their derivatives have also been described as effective anti-inflammatory agents [6]. Actually, they are reported to inhibit the production of key cytokines such as TNF-α (tumor necrosis factor-alpha) and IL-6 (interleukin-6), released in most inflammatory processes and involved in many diseases such as autoimmune ones, diabetes, atherosclerosis, and cancer. Sulfuretin counteracts the activities of nitric oxide (NO) and prostaglandin $E_2$ (PGE2), both pro-inflammatory molecules [32]. The presence of a hydroxy group in position 6 of the nucleus boosts the inhibition of $PGE_2$ production, while its replacement with a methoxy group potentiates the inhibition of NO production. In any case, both substituents are crucial to combine the highest anti-inflammatory activity with the lowest toxicity. A number of sulfuretin derivatives have also been described, produced by modifying either the benzo-fused ring or the 2-benzylidene residue, or even both, which proved to be better in fighting inflammation. For example, the insertion of the 6-hydroxy substituent into a dihydropyran residue, as in compound **18** (Figure 6) [33], or the replacement of the 2-benzylidene residue with an heteroaryl moiety, as in compound **19** (Figure 6) [34].

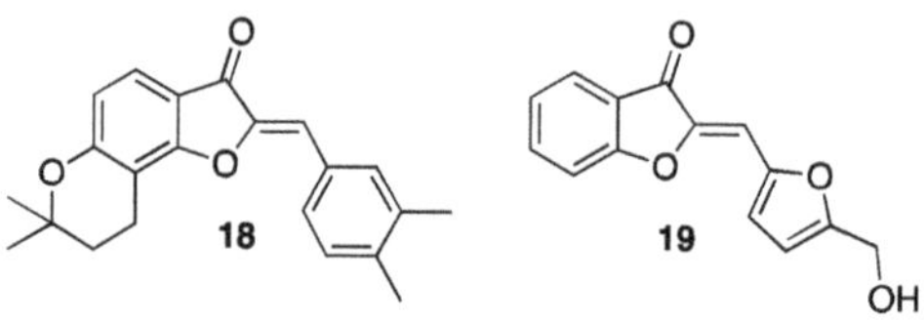

**Figure 6.** Representative examples of synthetic anti-inflammatory aurones.

However, most of the functional studies described by the literature aim at demonstrating the anti-cancer potential of aurones. Chemotherapy has always been the most powerful weapon at our disposal in the fight against cancer. Nevertheless, due to its high toxicity and the severe implications of resistance to the known anti-cancer drugs, the development of *magic bullets* for molecular targeted therapy has been progressing more and more. This is where aurones and their potential as anti-cancer agents come into play. The versatility of these natural compounds lies in the simplicity of their structure, which enables them to interact with key enzymes involved in tumor development. The first ever recorded antitumor activity of aurones has been described by Huang and co-workers, who demonstrated the ability of hamiltrone **20** (Figure 7), the 4,5,6-trimethoxy-substituted aurone obtained from the shrub *Uvaria hamiltonii*, to modulate the scissoring activity against the double-stranded DNA, thus damaging the DNA of proliferating cells [35]. From then on, a number of scientific reports have been published, thoroughly reviewed by Alsayari and co-workers, testifying to the ability of both aurones and their regioisomes isoaurones to interact with several key cancer targets.

Suzuki and co-workers demonstrated the anti-tumor efficacy of isoaurostatin **21** (Figure 7), the fungal metabolite of *Thermomonospora alba*, as the result of its inhibitory activity against Topoisomerase I [36], while Priyadarshani and co-workers reported on the ability of (Z)-2-(4-methoxybenzylidene)benzofuran-3(2*H*)-one **22** (Figure 7) to inhibit Topoisomerase II [37]. Overall, the benzofuran-3(2*H*)-one scaffold gave evidence these key enzymes regulating DNA replication and transcription, once decorated with appropriate substituents on the pendant phenyl ring. In any case, the reference pharmacophoric structure of both aurones and isoaurones, characterized by two main aromatic areas connected by a double bond having Z geometry, has been deemed by several authors to overlap the one of combrestatin A-4 **23** (Figure 7), a well-known tubulin polymerization inhibitor. This would explain the anti-cancer activity shown by several natural and synthetic aurones, which proved to interact at the colchicine binding site of tubulin, thus arresting cell cycle at the G2/M level.

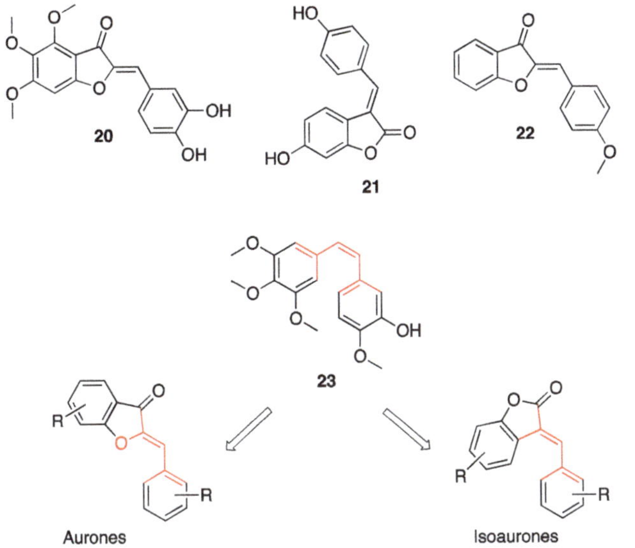


**Figure 7.** Representative examples of aurones endowed with anti-tumor efficacy.

Both aurones and isoaurones, as well as the synthetic benzofuranone derivatives closely related to them, have also been reported to interact with additional anti-tumor targets. These include the serine/threonine cyclin-dependent kinases CDK 1 and 2, playing a key role in cell cycle regulation [38], the Hypoxia-inducible Factor-1 (HIF-1), a marker reflecting angiogenesic activity in cancer cells [39,40], but also protein kinases such as fibroblast growth factor receptor, FGFR, which is involved in cancer development and progression [41], and sphingosine kinase, whose overexpression has been associated with tumor angiogenesis and resistance to radiation and chemotherapy [42]. Examples of synthetic aurones have also been described for their ability to dissipate the hyperpolarization of mitochondrial membranes of cancer cells, arresting cell cycle [43]. Instead, contrasting results were obtained against histone deacetylases (HDACs), a family of enzymes that, once mutated or overexpressed, induce the aberrant expression of genes involved in cell proliferation and apoptosis. Indeed, while Zwick and co-workers claimed an HDAC inhibitory activity in the micromolar range for a number of poly-hydroxylated aurones [44], Itoh and co-workers warned against the activity displayed by those aurones bearing a catechol fragment on the 2-benzylidene residue [45]. Actually, according to the authors, this structural motif proved to interfere with the proper functioning of the in vitro assay components, thus causing false positives.

The development of the ideal anti-tumor agent cannot ignore the multi-drug resistance that cancer cells are able to put in place. The activation of repairing and detoxifying systems, as well as a reduced uptake of drugs due to cell adhesion barriers, are just a few examples of strategies in force to malignancies to protect themselves against the toxic effects of drugs. However, the most effective resistance mechanism is mainly due to the activity of the

ATP-dependent efflux pumps of the ABC family, such as the P-glycoprotein (P-gp/ABCB1), multidrug resistance-associated protein 2 (MRP2/ABCC2), and the breast cancer resistance protein (BCRP/ABCG2), whose overexpression limits the prolonged and effective activity of chemotherapeutic drugs [46]. Additionally, in this case, aurones come in handy to obtain effective ATP-binding cassette inhibitors. Moreover, by suitably modifying the substitution pattern on either the benzylidene moiety or the benzo-fused ring, a selectivity profile against the three different efflux pumps may be also obtained. Indeed, several halogenated aurones have been described as effective P-gp inhibitors able to increase daunorubicin cyctotoxicity when tested in vitro in the chronic myelocytic leukemia K562 cell line [47] and paclitaxel accumulation in the human breast MDA-MB-436 cell line [48]. Instead, when the benzylidene moiety was replaced with an indolylmethylene residue, the resulting compound turned out to be effective against the ABCC2 protein [49]. Poly-methoxylated derivatives proved to interact with the ABCG2 efflux pump, inducing a mitoxantrone accumulation in cell lines [50]. All things considered, suitably modified members of this class of natural compounds offer the opportunity to sum up the ability to interact with key molecular anti-cancer targets with the potential to modulate the activity of efflux pumps, thus embodying the ideal anti-cancer agents.

Finally, it is worth mentioning the fluorescent potentials of this class of natural compounds. Organic molecules having fluorescence properties in the visible region of the electromagnetic spectrum are very useful investigative tools in biological systems. However, to be used for this purpose, compounds should bring only minimal perturbations to the biological macromolecules under study, to highlight their characteristics as accurately as possible to the physiological situation. Therefore, they should be characterized by rather small dimensions. Unfortunately, the currently available fluorophores, including xanthenes such as fluorescein and eosin, BODIPY, and cyanines, do not fully comply with this criterium. Shanker and co-workers demonstrated the fluorescent potential of some aurone derivatives, suggesting their possible use for biomolecular investigations [51]. Significantly, even the largest example proposed by the authors is smaller than xanthene dyes, and this structural characteristic is particularly advantageous for the use of the compounds. Studies on the potential application of aurone derivatives in the field of fluorescence are still ongoing but are proving to be rather promising. Ono and co-workers reported the ability of a synthetic aurone, 2-[(4-dimethylaminophenyl)methylene]-5-iodo-3(2*H*)-benzofuranone **24** (Figure 8), to efficiently stain Alzheimer's mouse brain sections, thanks to the high binding affinity to the peptides of the A$\beta$ aggregates displayed by the compound. A concomitant good brain penetration and fast washout, demonstrated through biodistribution studies carried out on normal mice, make the compound the ideal prototype probe for detecting amyloid plaques in the brain of people affected by Alzheimer disease, thus opening up a further role for these compounds [52].

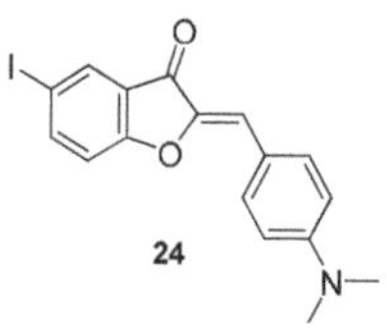


**Figure 8.** Synthetic aurone endowed with staining property.

The remarkable versatility of aurones, evidenced by an increasing amount of scientific evidence, makes these compounds worthy of consideration by the scientific community. However, the prospect of using them for both technological and functional purposes raises the problem of their availability. This is why, in addition to further clarifying their biological significance, it is crucial to develop synthetic strategies to obtain them in high amounts.

## 4. Synthetic Strategies to Obtain Aurones

A number of synthetic approaches have been proposed throughout years, to both replicate in the laboratory the natural aurones and obtain novel analogues. Attempts made by different researchers aimed at rebuilding the 2-functionalized benzofurane scaffold following different chemical strategies, all reviewed hereinafter.

### *4.1. Functionalization of the Benzofurane Nucleus*

Lawrence and co-workers investigated the natural biosynthesis of hamiltrone **20**, the aurone isolated from the *U. hamiltonii*, and putted in place a synthetic strategy that, in addition to the natural compound, allowed to get to a series of structural analogues [53]. As for hamiltrone, starting from the 3,4,5-trimethoxyphenol derivative **25**, the authors obtained the corresponding phenoxyacetic acid **26**, by reaction with chloroacetic acid, then cyclized the acid to the key intermediate benzofuranone **27**, by treatment with polyphosphoric acid, achieving a 51% yield of the target heterocycle. The reaction of **27** with the TBDMS-protected benzaldehyde **28**, in the presence of neutral alumina, allowed to obtain the protected aurone **29**, which lastly afforded the target hamiltrone **20** by reaction with tetra-butylammonium fluoride. The proposed synthetic pathway proved to work well using also differently substituted benzaldehydes, carrying either electron-withdrawing atoms, such as halogens, or electron-donating groups, such as the methoxy one. Altogether, the followed pathway only resulted in the (*Z*)-isomer, being more thermodynamically stable than the (*E*)-counterpart, as reported by the authors (Scheme 1).

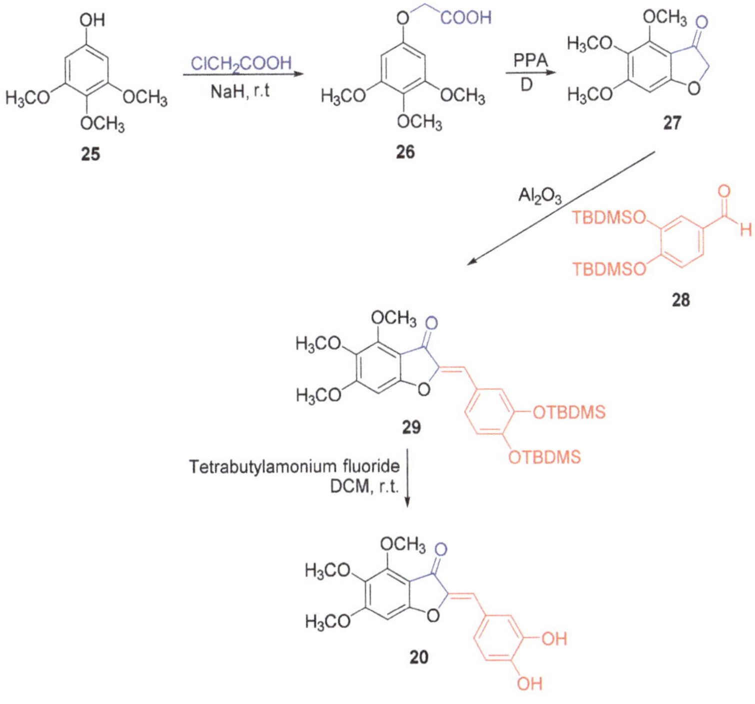


**Scheme 1.** Synthesis of hamiltrone according to Lawrence and co-workers [53].

A similar functionalization of the benzofurane ring was also carried out in 2013 by Hawkins and co-workers, who exploited a mixture of choline chloride and urea as the catalytic deep eutectic solvent to insert the benzylidene residue in position 2 of the benzofurane core **30** (Scheme 2) [54]. By heating at 80 °C equimolar amount of benzofurane and a suitably substituted arylaldehyde in a sealed vial, in the presence of the deep eutectic solvent, aurone derivatives were obtained in 40–78% yields within 12–48 h. The reaction proceeds under relatively mild conditions, without the need for basic and acid catalysts, thus proving to be invaluable for sensitive reactants. A few years later, Taylor and co-workers improved the procedure by pairing the use of the deep eutectic solvent with the highly performing microwave irradiation, thus maximizing both the yield of the obtained aurones and the time of reactions. Moreover, compounds not achievable with conventional heating were also obtained (Scheme 2) [55].

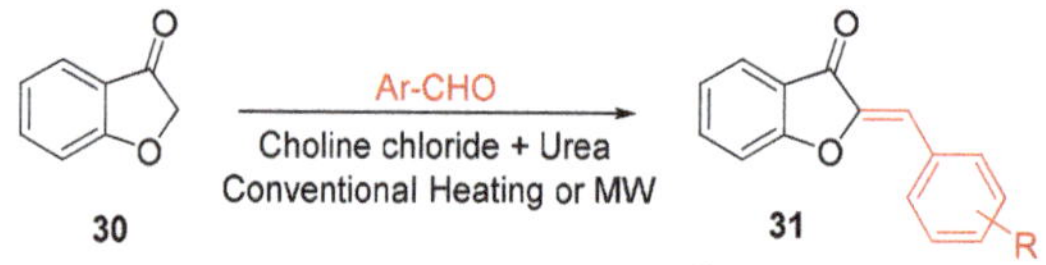


**Scheme 2.** Synthesis of (*Z*)-2-benzylidenebenzofuran-3(2*H*)-ones according to Hawkins and co-workers [54] and Taylor and co-workers [55].

Kraus and Gupta took advantage of a Steglich esterification [56], carried out in the presence of dicyclohexylcarbodiimide as the coupling reagent and 4-dimethylaminopiridine as the catalyst, to turn the phenol derivative **25** into the 3,4,5-trimethoxyphenyl-3,3-dibromoacrylate **32**, by reaction with 3,3-dibromoacrylic acid. A Fries rearrangement of the ester **32** into the ketone **33**, followed by its cyclization in dilute sodium hydroxide and THF, afforded the 2-bromomethylene benzofuran-3(2*H*)-one **34**. A conventional Suzuky–Miyaura coupling finally led to the aurone **35** (Scheme 3) [57].

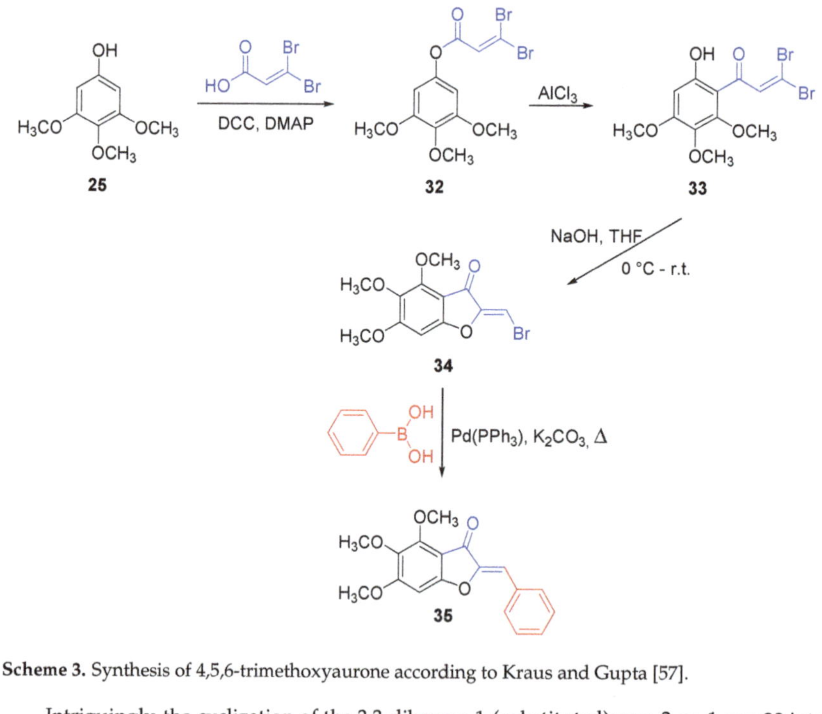


**Scheme 3.** Synthesis of 4,5,6-trimethoxyaurone according to Kraus and Gupta [57].

Intriguingly, the cyclization of the 3,3-dibromo-1-(substituted)prop-2-en-1-one **33** into the 6:5 aurone **34** turned out to be a surprising occurrence. Actually, the authors expected to obtain the higher homologous 6:6 chromone as, using the same procedure in the presence of 3,3-dichloroacrylic acid as the starting reactant, and treating the key intermediate **36** with dilute base, the corresponding 2-chloro-5,6,7-trimethoxy-4*H*-chromen-4-one **37** was obtained (Scheme 4).

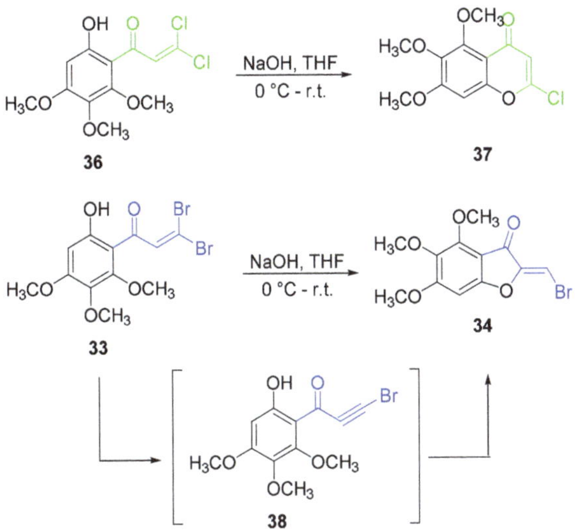


**Scheme 4.** Reactivity of α-dihalo-prop-2-en-1-ones in comparison.

However, in the case of the α-dibromo derivative **33**, two different and competing reaction may be assumed. Indeed, the cyclization reaction driven by the phenolic oxygen, and leading to the 6:6 nucleus, has to deal with the dehydrobromination reaction affording the bromo-acetylenic intermediate **38**, which in turn can cyclize to the 6:5 heterocycle. If the elimination reaction prevails, the aurone proves to be the predominant product (Scheme 4).

*4.2. Cyclization of Chalcones*

Agrawal and Soni focused on 2-hydroxycalcones **39**, achieving their cyclization to aurones **40** in oxidant conditions by means of $Hg(OAc)_2$ in the presence of pyridine. $CuBr_2$ in DMSO was also used to induce alternative cyclization conditions, leading to aurones in comparable yields [58] (Scheme 5). In both cases, the oxidant mixture promotes a *5-exo-trig* cyclization to the 6:5 nucleus deterring the also possible *6-endo-trig* cyclization to the 6:6 higher homologous. According to the authors, coordination between the oxygen atom of the hydroxy group and the metal species occurs, which prevents the six-member cyclization.

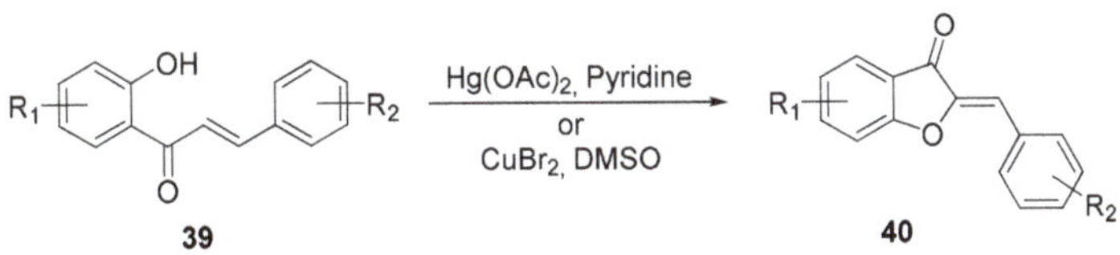


**Scheme 5.** Cyclization of chalcones according to Agrawal and Soni [58].

Additionally, Thanigaimalai and Yang pursued the cyclization of chalcones by exploiting thallium (III) nitrate in methanol solution followed by the addition of hydrochloric acid as the oxidant condition [59]. Using 1-(2-(cyclohexylmethoxy)-6-hydroxyphenyl)-3-phenylprop-2-en-1-one **41** as the starting material, they obtained either the aurone derivatives **42** or the isoflavone derivatives **43** depending on the substitution pattern on the B ring of the chalcone. In particular, the presence of electron-withdrawing substituents such as chloro, nitro, formyl, and methoxycarbonyl in the *para* position of the phenyl ring was mandatory to produce aurones, while their replacement with strong electron-donating groups such as hydroxy, methoxy, methoxymethoxy, and benzyloxy led to the obtainment of isoflavones. The presence of the weak electron-donating ethyl group allowed to obtain a 1:1 mixture of both isoflavones and aurones, while the presence of a carboxylic residue left the chalcone unreacted (Scheme 6).

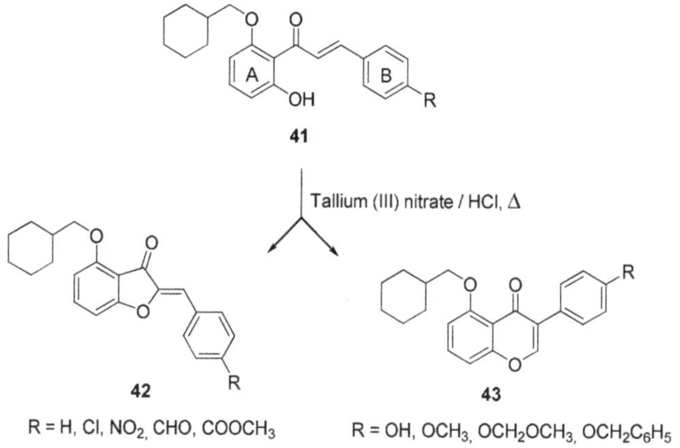


**Scheme 6.** Cyclization of chalcones according to Thanigaimalai and Yang [59].

A further example of chalcones cyclization has been provided by Yatabe and co-workers, who produced the expected aurones by treating the starting compounds with oxygen from air in the presence of an heterogeneous catalyst, made of Pd-on-Au nanoparticles supported on $CeO_2$ [60]. At first, the deprotonation of the hydroxy group of **44** occurs, which allows the coordination of chalcone with the heterogenous Pd catalyst as in **45**. Then, a six-membered palladacycle **46** is obtained, thanks to an intramolecular olefinic α-C-H activation promoted by the phenoxide residue. The following reductive elimination of Pd from the palladacycle leads to the desired aurone **47** in its (Z)-predominant isoform, while the resulting reduced Pd(0) is reoxidized by oxygen from air, thus maintaining the catalytic efficiency of the system (Scheme 7).

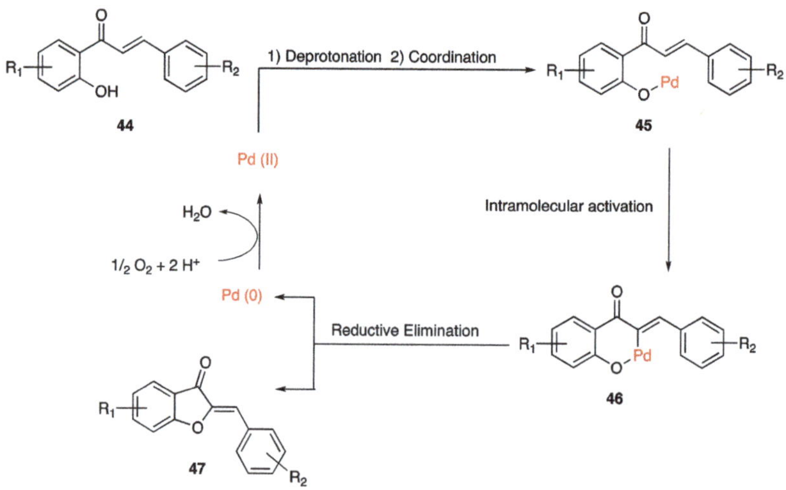


**Scheme 7.** Cyclization of chalcones according to Yatabe and co-workers [60].

### *4.3. Rearrangement of Six-Membered Cycles*

In 2015, Kandioller and co-workers succeeded in turning 3-tosilflavones **48** into five-membered benzofuranes **49**, by treating the six-membered heterocycles with suitably substituted alkylamines under mild reaction conditions. The rearrangement reactions proved to produce a high yield, but the resulting products were obtained as an *E-Z* mixture [61]. However, when the mixed isomers were treated with Lawesson's reagent, the thermodynamically favored *E*-isomers were isolated as the only 3(2*H*)-thioaurones **50** [61] (Scheme 8).

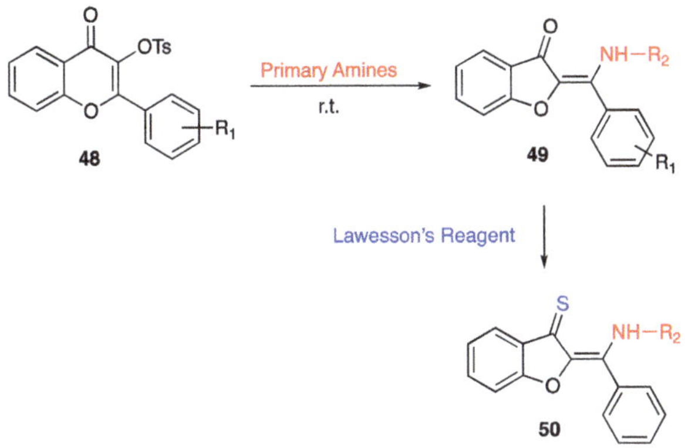


**Scheme 8.** Synthesis of thioaurones according to Kandioller and co-workers [61].

A few years later, Parveen and Ahmed yielded similar rearrangement results by using 3-bromoflavones **51** as the starting compounds [62]. Actually, by treatment with aniline derivatives in the presence of *t*-Bu-OK and CuI as the catalysts, the six-membered derivatives underwent a three-step cascade reaction including an Aza-Michael addition followed by ring opening and ring closing, leading to 2-aminated aurones **52** in their *trans*-conformation. The rearrangement took place under mild reaction conditions, proving to be effective in the presence of differently substituted aniline derivatives as well as N-phenylurea, but turned out to be unattainable when benzamide, 2-aminopyridine, and also piperidine were used as the key nucleophiles (Scheme 9).

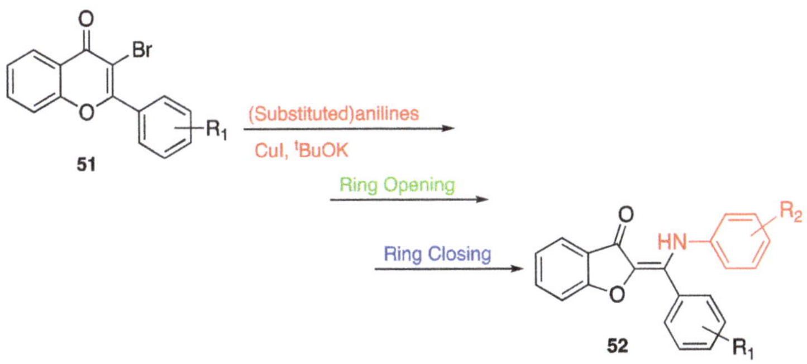


**Scheme 9.** Rearrangement of flavones according to Parveen and Ahmed [62].

As a whole, the rearrangement of flavones in the presence of nitrogen-based nucleophiles provides the insertion of an additional substituent in position 2 of the heterocyclic core, thus allowing to expand the structural variability of the benzofuran-3(2*H*)-ones and, accordingly, their usability in the most varied fields.

### 4.4. Reactions of Annulation

A number of annulation reactions has been proposed to obtain aurones, all starting from suitably substituted *ortho*-halo phenols. The carbonylative cyclization was carried out by using different types of catalysts, generally applying mild reaction conditions. In some cases, the target products were obtained as a mixture with the upper homologous flavones, thus forcing a further separation passage to obtain the pure aurones. Among the available catalysts, those made from palladium turned out to be the most effective ones, being used in most of the synthetic procedures described in the literature.

In 2013, Liu and co-workers described a $PdCl_2(PPhe_3)_2$–benzimidazolium complex as a viable catalyst to produce aurones by reacting suitably substituted *ortho*-bromo-phenols **53** and ethynylbenzenes **54** [63]. The target compounds **55** were obtained under mild conditions, although in a mixture with 20–40% of the parent flavones **56** (Scheme 10).

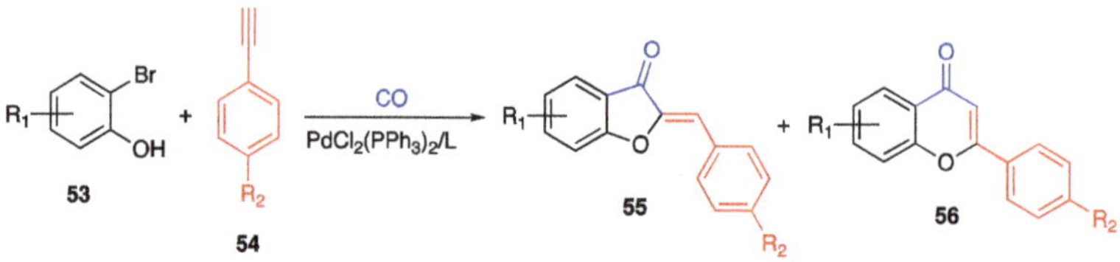


**Scheme 10.** Annulation of 2-bromo-phenols according to Liu and co-workers [63].

A similar reaction was described by Chavan and co-workers, who used $Pd^0$ complexed with 3-aminopropyl-triethoxysilane (APTES@K10) as the catalyst [64]. Additionally, in this case, the reaction of *ortho*-iodo-phenols **57** with terminal alkynes **54** resulted in the target 6:5 aurones **55**, which were eventually isolated with the upper 6:6 counterpart flavones **56**. However, the authors succeeded in ensuring the obtainment of a heterocycle rather than the other one by using different solvents. Actually, in the presence of 1,2-dimethoxyethane (DME), the regioselective 5-exo cyclization was predominant, leading to the desirable aurones as the reference reaction products. Instead, the 6-endo cyclization mainly took place when using DMF, thus producing the parent flavones (Scheme 11).

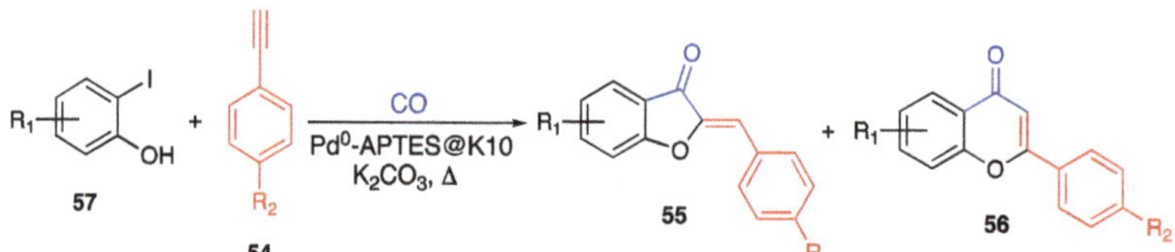


**Scheme 11.** Annulation of 2-iodo-phenols according to Chavan and co-workers [64].

An analogous example of solvent-driven regioselective carbonylative cyclization was given by Xu and co-workers, who obtained the 6:5 membered heterocycle and the 6:6 counterpart according to the solvent used [65]. In particular, triethylamine mainly led to the target aurones, managing a 5-exo cyclization, while piperazine preferentially pushed a 6-endo reaction, thus allowing us to obtain the corresponding flavones (Scheme 12).

However, when formic acid was used as the CO source, the annulation reaction proceeded to the target aurones as the reference products. Indeed, Qi and co-workers described the obtainment of differently substituted aurones **55** by reaction between *ortho*-iodo-phenols **57** and terminal alkynes **54**, carried out in the presence of tetrakis(triphenylphosphine)palladium as the catalyst [66] (Scheme 13).

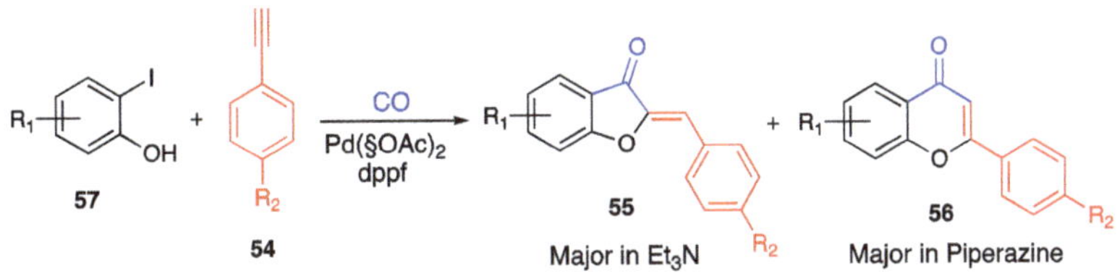


**Scheme 12.** Annulation of 2-iodo-phenols according to Xu and co-workers [65].

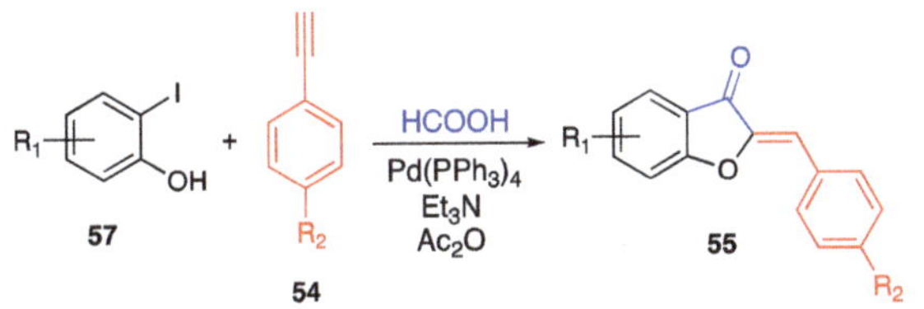


**Scheme 13.** Annulation of 2-iodo-phenols according to Qi and co-workers [66].

Regarding the Pd-catalyzed annulation reactions, a common mechanism may be assumed providing for the insertion of the carbonyl residue as the first step and the addition of the benzylidene moiety as the second one, both of them assisted by the metal catalyst. In particular, the *ortho*-iodo phenol **58** may be subjected to an oxidative addition of Pd(0), thus being converted into the arylpalladium derivative **59**, and this latter turns into the aroylpalladium derivative **60** due to the insertion of CO. The following sequentially alkyne attack and Pd(0) elimination give the key aryl-alkyn-one intermediate **62**, which is then complexed by Pd(0), to give **63**, cyclized to the palladacycle **64**, and finally transformed into the expected aurone **65** (Scheme 14).

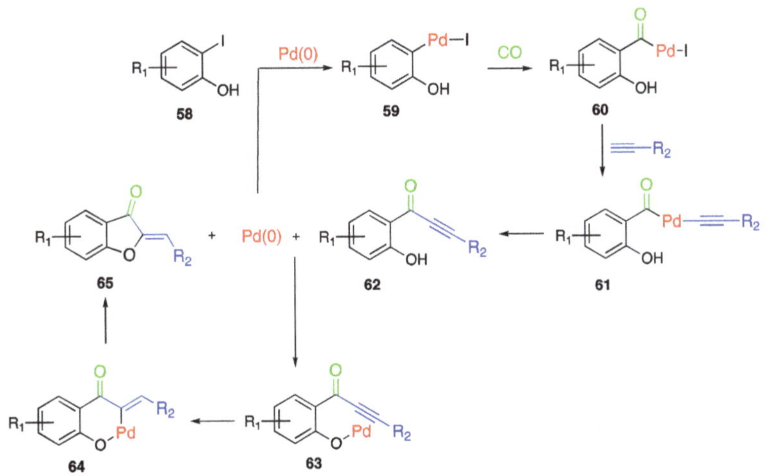


**Scheme 14.** Reaction mechanism proposed for the Pd-catalyzed annulation.

Although most researchers have focused on palladium-based compounds as the key catalysts to produce the target aurones, few examples have also been reported demonstrating the usefulness of additional metals such as rhodium, copper, and cesium.

Starting from *ortho*-alkynoylphenols **47**, Taylor and Bolshan obtained a series of aurones **44** by using cesium carbonate in acetone solution [67]. The adopted experimental conditions promoted an intramolecular 5-exo cyclization as the main reaction, thus leading to the benzofurane derivatives in good to high yields (Scheme 15).

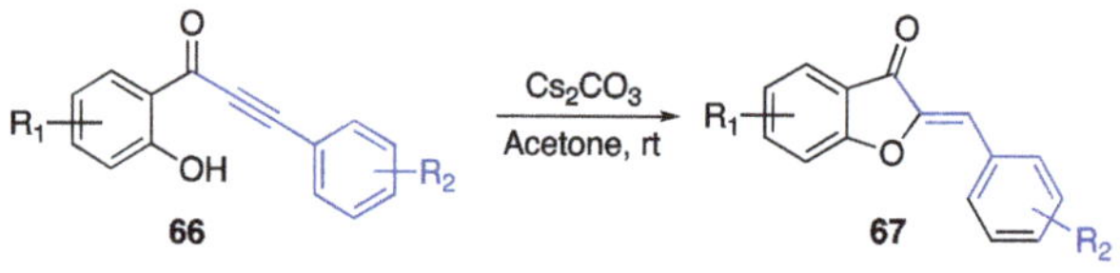

**Scheme 15.** Annulation of 2-alkynoylphenols according to Taylor and Bolshan [67].

A rhodium-based catalyst was used in basic medium by Rao and Ramakrishna to cyclize 1-bromo-alkynes, obtained in turn by the alkynylation of suitably substituted salicylaldehydes and 1,1-dibromoalkenes [68]. However, differently from the previously described strategy, the synthetic procedure adopted by Rao and Ramakrishna led mainly to the synthesis of the 6:6 heterocyles, with the 6:5 aurones being obtained in minor yields (Scheme 16).

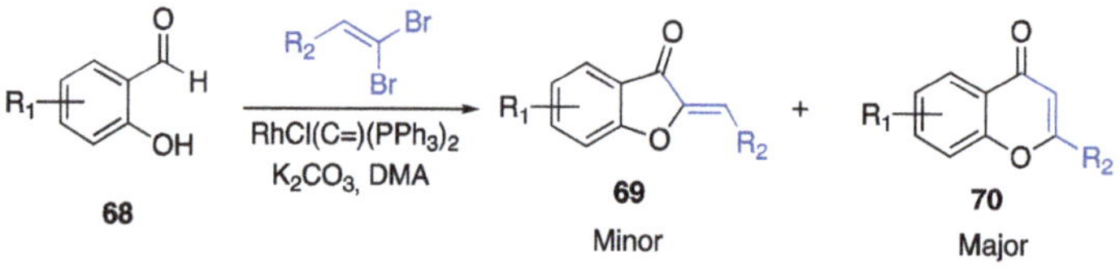

**Scheme 16.** Annulation of salicylaldehydes according to Rao and Ramakrishna [68].

## 5. Conclusions

Although having mentioned by the scientific literature since the beginning of the twentieth century, aurones have been long neglected by researchers to the benefit of the more homologous flavonoids. However, they are recently regaining interest, as their functional properties are unveiled. Being key determinants for color plants, these compounds have an undoubted technological role as natural dyes. At the same time, being acknowledged for their antioxidant, anti-inflammatory, antibacterial, antiviral, antimalarial, and anticancer properties, they may be claimed to be innovative drug candidates. Moreover, they may also be considered as viable diagnostic tools, due to their fluorescent properties. In addition to naturally occurring aurones, an increasing number of synthetic analogues have also been described, being similar though their improved functional properties, which further expands this class of compounds. The amount of scientific data collected so far clearly demonstrate the potential for the development of these natural derivatives and their synthetic analogues, yet we are only beginning to comprehend their real usability. Actually, a number of crucial matters still need to be clarified. The synthetic supply of the compounds provides an example: according to the literature, a straightforward, cost-effective, and environmentally friendly chemical procedure to achieve benzofuran derivatives on an industrial scale has yet to be finalized. Then, and more importantly, it is necessary to tidy up the information on both the biological activity and the bioavailability of these compounds. Indeed, as is often the case with natural products, aurones have a multi-functional profile. Although sometimes it may beneficial, depending on the disease in question, a redundancy of interactions with different targets often precludes the development of a compound as a real drug. Moreover, being characterized by polyphenolic structures, these derivatives are generally marked by unfavorable pharmacokinetic properties. Therefore, it is highly desirable to deepen the interactions of aurones with the identified molecular targets and the novel forthcoming ones, by using crystallographic and computations studies, to highlight the key structural discriminants for activity. In addition, a mathematical characterization of the time course of compounds' absorption, distribution, metabolism, and excretion is also necessary. These investigations will allow us to obtain compounds endowed with a clearly defined drug-like profile.

All things considered, even though it has already proven to be promising, research on aurones is just getting started.

**Author Contributions:** Conceptualization, C.L.M.; investigation, I.M. and G.P.; writing—original draft preparation, I.M.; writing—review and editing, C.L.M.; supervision, C.L.M. All authors have read and agreed to the published version of the manuscript.

**Funding:** The authors thank University of Pisa, Italy, for the financial support to their work. APC was sponsored by MDPI.

**Institutional Review Board Statement:** Not applicable.

**Informed Consent Statement:** Not applicable.

**Data Availability Statement:** Not applicable.

**Conflicts of Interest:** The authors declare no conflict of interest.

## References

1. Klein, G. Studien uber das Anthochlor. *Sitzb. Akad. Wiss. Wien.* **1920**, *129*, 341–395.
2. Abbas, M.; Saeed, F.; Anjum, F.M.; Afzaal, M.; Tufail, T.; Bashir, M.S.; Ishtiaq, A.; Hussain, S.; Suleria, H.A.R. Natural polyphenols: An overview. *Int. J. Food Prop.* **2017**, *20*, 1689–1699. [CrossRef]
3. Zwergel, C.; Gaascht, F.; Valente, S.; Diederich, M.; Bagrel, D.; Kirsch, G. Aurones: Interesting natural and synthetic compounds with emerging biological potential. *Nat. Prod. Commun.* **2012**, *7*, 389–394. [CrossRef] [PubMed]
4. Boucherle, B.; Peuchmaur, M.; Boumendjel, A.; Haudecoeur, R. Occurrences, biosynthesis and properties of aurones as high-end evolutionary products. *Phytochemistry* **2017**, *142*, 92–111. [CrossRef]
5. Alsayari, A.; Muhsinah, A.B.; Hassan, M.Z.; Ahsan, M.J.; Alshehri, J.A.; Begum, N. Aurone: A biologically attractive scaffold as anticancer agent. *Eur. J. Med. Chem.* **2019**, *166*, 417–431. [CrossRef]
6. Sui, G.; Li, T.; Zhang, B.; Wang, R.; Hao, H.; Zhou, W. Recent advances on synthesis and biological activities of aurones. *Bioorg. Med. Chem.* **2021**, *29*, 115895–115917. [CrossRef]
7. Geissman, T.A.; Heaton, C.D. Anthochlor pigments. IV. The pigments of *Coreopsis grandiflora*, Nutt. *J. Am. Chem. Soc.* **1943**, *65*, 677–683. [CrossRef]
8. Davies, K.M.; Jibran, R.; Zhou, Y.; Albert, N.W.; Brummell, D.A.; Jordan, B.R.; Bowman, J.L.; Schwinn, K.E. The evolution of flavonoid biosynthesis: A bryophyte perspective. *Front. Plant Sci.* **2020**, *11*, 7. [CrossRef] [PubMed]
9. Al-Snafi, A.E. The pharmacological importance of *Antirrhinum majus*—A review. *Asian J. Pharm. Sci. Technol.* **2015**, *5*, 313–320.
10. Valianou, L.; Stathopoulou, K.; Karapanagiotis, I.; Magiatis, P.; Pavlidou, E.; Skaltsounis, A.-L.; Chryssoulakis, Y. Phytochemical analysis of young fustic (*Cotinus coggygria* heartwood) and identification of isolated colourants in historical textiles. *Anal. Bioanal. Chem.* **2009**, *394*, 871–882. [CrossRef]
11. Ollerton, J. Pollinator Diversity: Distribution, Ecological Function, and Conservation. *Ann. Rev. Ecol. Evol. Syst.* **2017**, *48*, 353–376. [CrossRef]
12. Papiorek, S.; Junker, R.R.; Alves-dos-Santos, I.; Melo, G.A.R.; Amaral-Neto, L.P.; Sazima, M.; Wolowski, M.; Freitas, L.; Lunau, K. Bees, birds and yellow flowers: Pollinator-dependant convergent evolution of UV patterns. *Plant Biol.* **2016**, *18*, 46–55. [CrossRef] [PubMed]
13. Davies, K.M.; Marshall, G.B.; Bradley, J.M.; Schwinn, K.E.; Bloor, S.J.; Winefield, C.S.; Martin, C.R. Characterization of aurone biosynthesis in *Antirrhinum majus*. *Phys. Planta* **2006**, *128*, 593–603. [CrossRef]
14. Lunau, K.; Wacht, S.; Chittka, L. Colour choices of naive bumble bees and their implications for colour perception. *J. Comp. Physiol.* **1996**, *178*, 477–489. [CrossRef]
15. Hansen, D.M.; Beer, K.; Müller, C.B. Mauritian coloured nectar no longer a mystery: A visual signal for lizard pollinators. *Biol. Lett.* **2006**, *2*, 165–168. [CrossRef]
16. Ono, E.; Fukuchi-Mizutani, M.; Nakamura, N.; Fukui, Y.; Yonekura-Sakakibara, K.; Yamaguchi, M.; Nakayama, T.; Tanaka, T.; Kusumi, T.; Tanaka, Y. Yellow flowers generated by expression of the aurone biosynthetic pathway. *Proc. Natl. Acad. Sci. USA* **2006**, *103*, 11075–11080. [CrossRef]
17. Brewer, M.S. Natural antioxidants: Sources, compounds, mechanisms of action, and potential applications. *Compr. Rev. Food Sci. Food Saf.* **2011**, *10*, 221–247. [CrossRef]
18. Bowry, V.W.; Ingold, K.U. The unexpected role of vitamin E (α-Tocopherol) in the peroxidation of human low-density lipoprotein. *Acc. Chem. Res.* **1999**, *32*, 27–34. [CrossRef]
19. Senthil Kimar, K.; Kumaresan, R. A Quantum chemical study on the antioxidant properties of aureusidin and bracteatin. *Int. J. Quantum Chem.* **2011**, *111*, 4483–4496.

20. Olleik, H.; Yahiaoui, S.; Roulier, B.; Courvoisier-Dezord, E.; Perrier, J.; Pérès, B.; Hijazi, A.; Baydoun, E.; Raymond, J.; Boumendjel, A.; et al. Aurone derivatives as promising antibacterial agents against resistant Gram-positive pathogens. *Eur. J. Med. Chem.* **2019**, *165*, 133–141. [CrossRef]
21. Campanico, A.; Carrasco, M.P.; Njoroge, M.; Seldon, R.; Chibale, K.; Perdigão, J.; Portugal, I.; Warner, D.F.; Moreira, R.; Lopes, F. Azaaurones as potent antimycobacterial agents active against MDR- and XDR-TB. *ChemMedChem* **2019**, *20*, 1537–1546. [CrossRef] [PubMed]
22. Kumar, G.; Lathwal, E.; Saroha, B.; Kumar, S.; Chauhan, N.S.; Kumar, T. Synthesis and Biological Evaluation of Quinoline-Based Novel Aurones. *Chem. Sel.* **2020**, *5*, 3539–3543. [CrossRef]
23. Sutton, C.L.; Taylor, Z.E.; Farone, M.B.; Handy, S.T. Antifungal activity of substituted aurones. *Bioorg. Med. Chem. Lett.* **2017**, *27*, 901–903.
24. Morimoto, M.; Fukumoto, H.; Nozoe, T.; Hagiwara, A.; Komai, K. Synthesis and insect antifeedant activity of aurones against Spodoptera litura larvae. *J. Agric. Food Chem.* **2007**, *55*, 700–705. [CrossRef] [PubMed]
25. Carrasco, M.P.; Newton, A.S.; Goncalves, L.; Góis, A.; Machado, M.; Gut, J.; Nogueira, F.; Hänscheid, T.; Guedes, R.C.; dos Santos, D.J.V.A.; et al. Probing the aurone scaffold against Plasmodium falciparum: Design, synthesis and antimalarial activity. *Eur. J. Med. Chem.* **2014**, *80*, 523–534. [CrossRef] [PubMed]
26. Ramazani, A.; Hamidnezhad, R.; Foroumadi, A.; Mirzaei, S.A.; Maddahi, S.; Hassanzadeh, S.M. In Vitro antiplasmodial activity and cytotoxic effect of (*Z*)-2-benzylidene-4,6-dimethoxybenzofuran-3(2*H*)-one derivatives. *Iran J. Parasitol.* **2016**, *11*, 371–376.
27. Morimoto, M.; Cantrell, C.L.; Khan, S.; Tekwani, B.L.; Duke, S.O. Antimalarial and antileishmanial activities of phytophenolics and their synthetic analogues. *Chem. Biodivers.* **2017**, *14*, e1700324. [CrossRef]
28. Malbari, K.D.; Chintakrindi, A.S.; Ganji, L.R.; Gohil, D.J.; Kothari, S.T.; Joshi, M.W.; Kanyalkar, M.A. Structure-aided drug development of potential neuraminidase inhibitors against pandemic H1N1 exploring alternate binding mechanism. *Mol. Divers.* **2019**, *23*, 927–951. [CrossRef]
29. Zein, N.N. Clinical significance of Hepatitis C Virus genotypes. *Clin. Microbiol. Rev.* **2000**, *13*, 223–235. [CrossRef]
30. Waheed, Y.; Bhatti, A.; Ashraf, M. RNA dependent RNA polymerase of HCV: A potential target for the development of antiviral drugs. *Infect. Genet. Evol.* **2013**, *14*, 247–257. [CrossRef]
31. Meguellati, A.; Ahmed-Belkacem, A.; Yi, W.; Haudecoeur, R.; Crouillère, M.; Brillet, R.; Pawlotsky, J.-M.; Boumendjel, A.; Peuchmaur, M. B-ring modified aurones as promising allosteric inhibitors of hepatitis C virus RNA-dependent RNA polymerase. *Eur. J. Med. Chem.* **2014**, *80*, 579–592. [CrossRef] [PubMed]
32. Moon, J.E.; Kim, D.-K.; Kim, J.Y. Anti-inflammatory effect of *Rhus verniciflua* stokes extract in the murine macrophage cell line. *J. Korean Soc. Appl. Biol. Chem.* **2015**, *58*, 481–486. [CrossRef]
33. Wang, Z.; Bac, E.J.; Han, Y.T. Synthesis and anti-inflammatory activities of novel dihydropyranoaurone derivatives. *Arch. Pharm. Res.* **2017**, *40*, 695–703. [CrossRef] [PubMed]
34. Park, H.S.; Nelson, D.E.; Taylor, Z.E.; Hayes, J.B.; Cunningham, K.D.; Arivett, B.A.; Ghosh, R.; Wolf, L.C.; Taylor, K.M.; Farone, M.B.; et al. Suppression of LPS-induced NF-κB activity in macrophages by the synthetic aurone, (Z)-2-((5-(hydroxymethyl) furan-2-yl)methylene) benzofuran-3(2*H*)-one. *Int. Immunopharmacol.* **2017**, *43*, 116–128. [CrossRef] [PubMed]
35. Huang, L.; Wall, M.E.; Wani, M.C.; Navarro, H.; Santisuk, T.; Reutrakul, V.; Seo, E.K.; Farnsworth, N.R.; Kinghorn, A.D. New compounds with DNA strand-scission activity from the combined leaf and stem of *Uvaria hamiltonii*. *J. Nat. Prod.* **1998**, *61*, 446–450. [CrossRef]
36. Suzuki, K.; Yahara, S.; Maehata, K.; Uyeda, M. Isoaurostatin, a Novel Topoisomerase Inhibitor Produced by *Thermomonospora alba*. *J. Nat. Prod.* **2001**, *64*, 204–207. [CrossRef]
37. Priyadarshani, G.; Nayak, A.; Amrutkar, S.M.; Das, S.; Guchhait, S.K.; Kundu, C.N.; Banerjee, U.C. Scaffold-Hopping of Aurones: 2-Arylideneimidazo[1,2-*a*]pyridinones as Topoisomerase IIα-Inhibiting Anticancer Agents. *ACS Med. Chem. Lett.* **2016**, *7*, 1056–1061. [CrossRef] [PubMed]
38. Schoepfer, J.; Fretz, H.; Chaudhuri, B.; Muller, L.; Seeber, E.; Meijer, L.; Lozach, O.; Vangrevelinghe, E.; Furet, P. Structure-based design and synthesis of 2-benzylidene-benzofuran-3-ones as flavopiridol mimics. *J. Med. Chem.* **2002**, *45*, 1741–1747. [PubMed]
39. Dat, N.T.; Jin, X.; Hong, Y.S.; Lee, J.J. An isoaurone and other constituents from *Trichosanthes kirilowii* seeds inhibit hypoxia-inducible factor-1 and nuclear factor-kappa B. *J. Nat. Prod.* **2010**, *73*, 1167–1169. [CrossRef]
40. Mi, C.; Ma, J.; Shi, H.; Li, J.; Wang, F.; Lee, J.J.; Jin, X. 4′,6-dihydroxy-4-methoxyisoaurone inhibits the HIF-1a pathway through inhibition of Akt/mTOR/p70S6K/4E-BP1 phosphorylation. *J. Pharmacol. Sci.* **2014**, *125*, 193–201. [CrossRef] [PubMed]
41. Gerby, B.; Boumendjel, A.; Blanc, M.; Bringuier, P.P.; Champelovier, P.; Fortune, A.; Ronot, X.; Boutonnat, J. 2-Arylidenedihydroindole-3-ones: Design, synthesis, and biological activity on bladder carcinoma cell lines. *Bioorg. Med. Chem. Lett.* **2007**, *17*, 208–213. [CrossRef] [PubMed]
42. French, K.J.; Schrecengost, R.S.; Lee, B.D.; Zhuang, Y.; Smith, S.N.; Eberly, J.L.; Yun, J.K.; Smith, C.D. Discovery and evaluation of inhibitors of human sphingosine kinase 1. *Cancer Res.* **2003**, *63*, 5962–5969. [PubMed]
43. Chen, H.; Qi, X.D.; Qui, P. A novel synthesis of aurones: Their in vitro anticancer activity against breast cancer cell lines and effect on cell cycle, apoptosis and mitochondrial membrane potential. *Bangladesh J. Pharmacol.* **2014**, *9*, 501–510. [CrossRef]
44. Zwick, V.; Chatzivasileiou, A.O.; Deschamps, N.; Roussaki, M.; Simões-Pires, C.A.; Nurisso, A.; Denis, I.; Blanquart, C.; Martinet, N.; Carrupt, P.A.; et al. Aurones as histone deacetylase inhibitors: Identification of key features. *Bioorg. Med. Chem. Lett.* **2014**, *24*, 5497–5501. [CrossRef]

45. Itoh, Y.; Suzuki, M.; Matsui, T.; Ota, Y.; Hui, Z.; Tsubaki, K.; Suzuki, T. False HDAC inhibition by aurone compound. *Chem. Pharm. Bull.* **2016**, *64*, 1124–1128. [CrossRef]
46. Lee, C.A.; Cook, J.A.; Reyner, E.L.; Smith, D.A. P-glycoprotein related drug interactions: Clinical importance and a consideration of disease states. *Expert Opin. Drug Metab. Toxicol.* **2010**, *6*, 603–619. [CrossRef] [PubMed]
47. Hadjeri, M.; Barbier, M.; Ronot, X.; Mariotte, A.M.; Boumendjel, A.; Boutonnat, J. Modulation of P-glycoprotein-mediated multidrug resistance by flavonoid derivatives and analogues. *J. Med. Chem.* **2003**, *46*, 2125–2131. [CrossRef] [PubMed]
48. Vaclavíkova, R.; Boumendjel, A.; Ehrlichova, M.; Kovar, J.; Gut, I. Modulation of paclitaxel transport by flavonoid derivatives in human breast cancer cells. Is there a correlation between binding affinity to NBD of P-gp and modulation of transport? *Bioorg. Med. Chem.* **2006**, *14*, 4519–4525. [CrossRef] [PubMed]
49. Baiceanu, E.; Nguyen, K.A.; Gonzalez-Lobato, L.; Nasr, R.; Baubichon-Cortay, H.; Loghin, F.; Le Borgne, M.; Chow, L.; Boumendjel, A.; Peuchmaur, M.; et al. 2-Indolylmethylenebenzofuranones as first effective inhibitors of ABCC2. *Eur. J. Med. Chem.* **2016**, *122*, 408–418. [CrossRef] [PubMed]
50. Sim, H.M.; Wu, C.P.; Ambudkar, S.V.; Go, M.L. In vitro and in vivo modulation ofABCG2 by functionalized aurones and structurally related analogs. *Biochem. Pharmacol.* **2011**, *82*, 1562–1571. [CrossRef] [PubMed]
51. Shanker, N.; Dilek, O.; Mukherjee, K.; McGee, D.W.; Bane, S.L. Aurones: Small molecule visible range fluorescent probes suitable for biomacromolecules. *J. Fluoresc.* **2011**, *21*, 2173. [CrossRef]
52. Ono, M.; Maya, Y.; Haratake, M.; Ito, K.; Mori, H.; Nakayama, M. Aurones serve as probes of beta-amyloid plaques in Alzheimer's disease. *Biochem. Biophys. Res. Commun.* **2007**, *361*, 116–121. [CrossRef]
53. Lawrence, N.J.; Rennison, D.; McGown, A.T.; Hadfield, J.A. The total synthesis of an aurone isolated from *Uvaria hamiltonii*: Aurones and flavones as anticancer agents. *Bioorg. Med. Chem. Lett.* **2003**, *13*, 3759–3763. [CrossRef] [PubMed]
54. Hawkins, I.; Handy, S.T. Synthesis of aurones under neutral conditions using a deep eutectic solvent. *Tetrahedron* **2013**, *69*, 9200–9204. [CrossRef]
55. Taylor, K.M.; Taylor, Z.E.; Handy, S.T. Rapid synthesis of aurones under mild conditions using a combination of microwaves and deep eutectic solvents. *Tetrahedron Lett.* **2017**, *58*, 240–241. [CrossRef]
56. Neises, B.; Steglich, W. Simple method for the esterification of carboxylic acids. *Angew. Chem. Int. Ed.* **1978**, *17*, 522–524. [CrossRef]
57. Kraus, G.A.; Gupta, V. Divergent approach to flavones and aurones via dihaloacrylic acids. Unexpected dependence on the halogen atom. *Org. Lett.* **2010**, *12*, 5278–5280. [CrossRef] [PubMed]
58. Agrawal, N.N.; Soni, P.A. A new process for the synthesis of aurones by using mercury (II) acetate in pyridine and cupric bromide in dimethyl sulfoxide. *Indian J. Chem.* **2006**, *45B*, 1301–1303. [CrossRef]
59. Thanigaimalai, P.; Yang, H.M. The scope of thallium nitrate oxidative cyclization of chalcones: Synthesis and evaluation of isoflavone and aurone analogs for their inhibitory activity against interleukin-5. *Bioorg. Med. Chem.* **2010**, *18*, 4441–4445. [CrossRef] [PubMed]
60. Yatabe, T.; Jin, X.J.; Mizuno, N.; Yamaguchi, K. Usual olefinic C-H functionalization of simple chalcones toward aurones enabled by the rational design of a function-integrated heterogeneous catalyst. *ACS Catal.* **2018**, *8*, 4969–4978. [CrossRef]
61. Kandioller, W.; Kubanik, M.; Bytzek, A.K.; Jakupec, M.A.; Roller, A.; Keppler, B.K.; Hartinge, C.G. The rearrangement of tosylated flavones to 1′-(alkylamino)aurones with primary amines. *Tetrahedron* **2015**, *71*, 8953–8959. [CrossRef]
62. Parveen, I.; Ahmed, N. A route to highly functionalized stereospecific *trans*-aminated aurones from 3-bromoflavones with aniline and *N*-phenylurea via a domino aza-Michael ring opening and cyclization reactions. *Synthesis* **2019**, *51*, 960–970. [CrossRef]
63. Liu, J.M.; Liu, M.W.; Yue, Y.Y.; Zhang, N.F.; Zhang, Y.I.; Zhuo, K.I. Construction of the flavones and aurones through regioselective carbonylative annulation of 2-bromophenols and terminal alkynes. *Tetrahedron Lett.* **2013**, *54*, 1802–1807. [CrossRef]
64. Chavan, S.P.; Varadwaj, G.B.B.; Parida, K.M.; Bhanage, B.M. Solvent-switchable regioselective synthesis of aurones and flavones using Palladium-supported amine functionalized Montmorillonite as a heterogeneous catalyst. *ChemCatChem* **2016**, *8*, 2649–2658. [CrossRef]
65. Xu, S.; Sun, H.; Zhuang, M.; Zheng, S.; Jian, Y.; Zhang, W.; Gao, Z. Divergent synthesis of flavones and aurones via base-controlled regioselective palladium catalyzed carbonylative cyclization. *Mol. Catal.* **2018**, *452*, 264–270. [CrossRef]
66. Qi, X.X.; Li, R.; Wu, X.F. Selective Palladium-catalyzed carbonylative synthesis of aurones with formic acid as the CO source. *RSC Adv.* **2016**, *6*, 2810–62813. [CrossRef]
67. Taylor, C.; Bolshan, Y. Metal-free methodology for the preparation of sterically hindered alkynoylphenols and its application to the synthesis of flavones and aurones. *Tetrahedron Lett.* **2015**, *56*, 4392–4396. [CrossRef]
68. Rao, M.L.N.; Ramakrishna, R.S. Rh-catalyzed aldehydic C-H alkynylation and annulation. *Org. Biomol. Chem.* **2020**, *18*, 1402–1411. [CrossRef]

molecules

MDPI

*Review*

# Phthalocyanines: An Old Dog Can Still Have New (Photo)Tricks!

**Andrea M. Schmidt [1] and Mário J. F. Calvete [2,*]**

[1] LifeEstetika, Laser Solutions, Universitätstadt Tübingen, Maria-von-Linden Strasse, 72076 Tübingen, Germany; andrea.m.schmidt.dls@gmail.com

[2] University of Coimbra, CQC, Department of Chemistry, Rua Larga, 3004-535 Coimbra, Portugal

* Correspondence: mcalvete@qui.uc.pt

**Abstract:** Phthalocyanines have enjoyed throughout the years the benefits of being exquisite compounds with many favorable properties arising from the straightforward and diverse possibilities of their structural modulation. Last decades appreciated a steady growth in applications for phthalocyanines, particularly those dependent on their great photophysical properties, now used in several cutting-edge technologies, particularly in photonic applications. Judging by the vivid reports currently provided by many researchers around the world, the spotlight remains assured. This review deals with the use of phthalocyanine molecules in innovative materials in photo-applications. Beyond a comprehensive view on the recent discoveries, a critical review of the most acclaimed/considered reports is the driving force, providing a brief and direct insight on the latest milestones in phthalocyanine photonic-based science.

**Keywords:** phthalocyanine; photonics; photoelectronics; photovoltaics; photocatalysis; charge transfer; nonlinear optics

## 1. Introduction

Phthalocyanines (Pcs) are highly conjugated and essentially planar aromatic macrocycles, consisting of four iminoisoindoline units, containing 18 delocalized $\pi$-electrons and widely praised for their thermal and chemical stability. Such electronic delocalization permits Pcs to display intense absorption bands in the near infrared region of the electronic spectrum, reaching very high extinction coefficients (~$10^5$ $M^{-1}$ $cm^{-1}$), accompanied by high fluorescence quantum yields, concomitantly with favorable redox activity and rich electrochemistry [1–5].

Phthalocyanines display great structural flexibility, existing both as free bases (metal-free) and in the form of metal complexes, hosting ca. 70 different elements in the central cavity, some of them allowing structural modulation via functionalization with metal-axial ligands. In addition, a substantial variety of substituents can be incorporated into the phthalocyanine core at positions designated as $\alpha$ (non-peripheral) and as $\beta$ (peripheral) (Figure 1), allowing for the design of desired electronic and/or solubilizing properties, depending upon the application [5,6].

Beyond their absorption features, many other recognized properties arose from the preparation of Pcs, allowing these macrocycles to be considered leading chemical entities, applied in several technologies over the years, including as catalysts [7–10], sensors [11–13], thin films [14–17], liquid crystals [18–20], semi-conductors [21–23], textile dyes [24,25], light-harvesting dyes in solar cells/organic photovoltaics [26–29], absorbers in nonlinear optics [30–36], photocatalysts [37,38], photosensitizers in phototherapies [39, 40], photosensitizers photodynamic inactivation of bacteria [41,42], and as contrast agents in medical imaging [43–46].

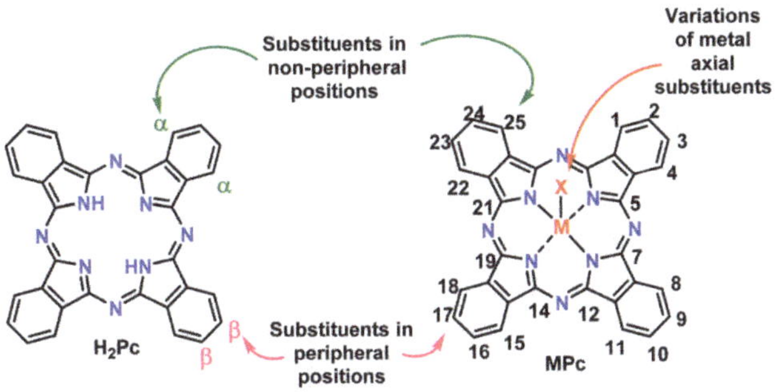


**Figure 1.** General structure of metal-free phthalocyanine (**left**) and metal phthalocyanine complex (**right**), with schematic representation of possible structural modulation sites and ring numbering.

Of the many applications found for phthalocyanines over the many decades after their discovery [47–49], recent years witnessed a solid growth in applications for phthalocyanines, particularly those relying on their excelling photophysical properties, and to the technological instrument development that permitted phthalocyanines to be used in several cutting-edge technologies, particularly in photonic applications. The intrinsic phthalocyanines photo-properties allowed this family of tetrapyrrolic macrocycles to emerge as prominent molecules, demonstrating how an "old" compound can still demonstrate groundbreaking applicability.

In this review, the focus is directed to the use of phthalocyanine molecules exclusively in innovative materials in photo-applications. Aware of the importance of phthalocyanine-related molecules, such as subphthalocyanines, naphthalocyanines, porphyrazines, and porphyrinoids, the recent discoveries (in the last five years) will solely consider the application of phthalocyanines in photonic-based materials technologies. Indeed, there are several highly cited review records in several sub-fields, e.g., photomedicine [50–60], photovoltaics [61–63], nonlinear optics [64–66], photocatalysis [67–69], among other photo-applications [70–72], portraying phthalocyanines among the therein discussed materials/molecules. Herein, more than a comprehensive view on the recent discoveries, a critical review of the most acclaimed/considered reports (i.e., most cited) was the driving force in this work, aiming to provide a brief and direct insight on the latest milestones in phthalocyanine science.

## 2. Bibliometric Analysis

To explore the research status on this area of study, a short bibliometric analysis was performed by assessing the publication trends from selected research area outputs [73,74]. The search strings (phthalocyanin*) and (phthalocyanin* AND photo*) present in the title and/or abstract and/or keywords were used in two well-known engines, Scopus collection and Web of Science Core Collection (WoS). Since the latter retrieved a larger number of records (Figure S1, Supplementary Materials), this was the data used to establish the conclusions regarding the production of new reports on the field.

Using the WoS search engine, the results were separated in five-year spans, in order to better establish possible trends (Figure 2). In a first look at the graphic, the sound increase in general publications in phthalocyanines stands out. Naturally, the photo-applications using these macrocycles accompany this trend, showing their prominence within the phthalocyanine field. The appearance of new equipment dedicated to study a vast array of photo-processes naturally boosted their applicability in the 1990s; nevertheless, the steady increase is remarkable. This demonstrates the lively interest that this sub-field brings into the phthalocyanine field.

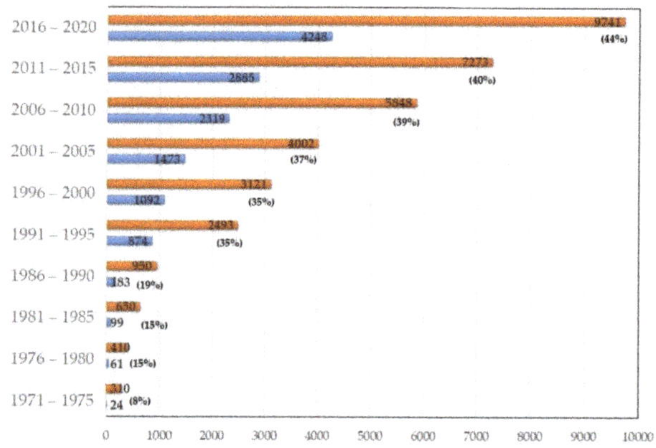


**Figure 2.** Relative weight of reports retrieved using the term "phthalocyanin*" (orange bars) vs. its refining with the term "photo*" (blue bars). In parentheses are the percentage weights of photo-applications over all others.

In the Web of Science retrieval of articles contained in title, abstract, or keywords, the term "phthalocyanin*" further refined with the term "photo*", from 1971 to 2020 (50 years), allowed the establishment of a tendency throughout the years. While increasing the number of publications on photo-applications of phthalocyanines (see Figure 2), the weight of each country in new reports has evolved (see Figure S2). The USSR weight in the beginning of the 1970s (continuing form earlier years) was replaced by North American countries (USA and Canada) in subsequent decades (until 1990). Until 2005, Japan also contributed largely to publication records, as well as European countries, such as England, Germany (including the extinct Federal Republic of Germany), and France. It was only at this time that the Peoples Republic of China claimed its prominent stand in the number of reports provided to the scientific community. In a relatively specialized field such as the synthesis and application of phthalocyanines, several countries stand out due to some prolific research groups, as was the case of Canada in the 1980s, or more recently Turkey and South Africa. Overall, favorable research policies and adequate funding opportunities represent what drive the success of the phthalocyanine field.

## 3. Materials Photo-Applications of Phthalocyanines

### 3.1. *Photovoltaics*

In light harvesting applications, Pcs hold a prominent position, acting first as antennas, since they absorb light very efficiently in the visible region of the solar spectrum, and, second, once photoexcited, they act as an electron donor for the acceptor moiety. Pcs are also good organic semiconducting chromophores, showing a prolonged photoresponse in the 600–800 nm range, where the photon flux is maximum, further displaying high charge-carrier mobilities and notable exciton diffusion lengths [75,76].

For instance, Leo and collaborators applied band structure engineering to tune the band gap and band-edge energies [77]. Empirically combining different inorganic semiconductors was a strategy to reach such purposes by blending materials with different energy levels [78], but this approach in organic semiconductors was prevented by the strong localization of the electronic states in these materials. The authors circumvented this issue by considering long-range Coulomb interactions, which enable continuous tuning in blends [79]. They studied a ternary bulk heterojunction of Pcs **1** and **2** (Figure 3) as donors with C60 as an acceptor and demonstrated by photoelectron spectroscopy the continuous tuning of the ionization energies of Pc thin films by blending Pc **1** with their halogenated derivatives, herein Pc **2**. The mixing ratio of Pc **2** and Pc **1** was varied from pure Pc **2** to pure Pc **1** while the C60 content was fixed at 60 weight percent. This in turn allows continued tuning of the photovoltaic gap and open-circuit voltage of organic solar cells.

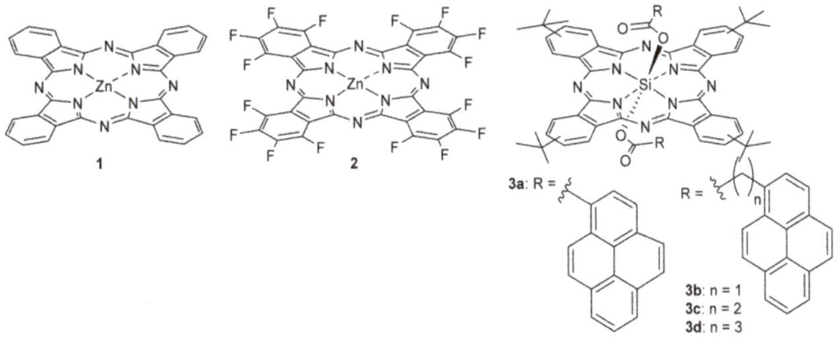

**Figure 3.** Pcs used in photovoltaic ternary systems.

Ke and Ameri reported a polymer/fullerene-based bulk heterojunction solar cell with extended absorption bandwidth by blending axially substituted silicon phthalocyanines (Pcs **3a–d**) (Figure 3 [80]. The authors used a system based on poly(3-hexylthiophene) (P3HT) and phenylC61-butyric acid methyl ester (PC61BM) as the electron donor and acceptor, respectively. The influence of the linker size on cell efficiency was studied, reaching a power conversion efficiency (PCE) of 4.14% bearing a 20% weight content of phthalocyanine when Pc **3d** was used. The authors attributed this higher efficiency of the solar cell containing the Pc dye with a longer linker to weaker intramolecular interactions as well as the higher solubility, which otherwise would cause aggregation.

Perovskite materials emerged recently, most prominently as components of solar cells. Synthetic perovskites are recognized as potential inexpensive base materials for high-efficiency commercial photovoltaics. These materials have unique photoelectric properties, being suitable for light harvesting in photovoltaics, e.g., appropriate and adjustable band gap [81], ambipolar charge transport [82], and long carrier diffusion length [83]. However, several issues remain to be addressed, namely the instability of Perovskite solar cells (PSC) [84–86]. One strategy is the use of improved hole-transporting materials (HTM), which may enhance both the long-time stability and performance of PSCs [87,88]. In this respect, phthalocyanines appeared as ideal partners due to their already highly suitable properties for solar cells. Figure 4 depicts a cross-sectional image of a typical perovskite solar cell device. It consists of a gold electrode, a HTM of a phthalocyanine, a light absorber of perovskite, and a compact (dense) $TiO_2$ ($dTiO_2$) layer, deposited with a FTO/glass.

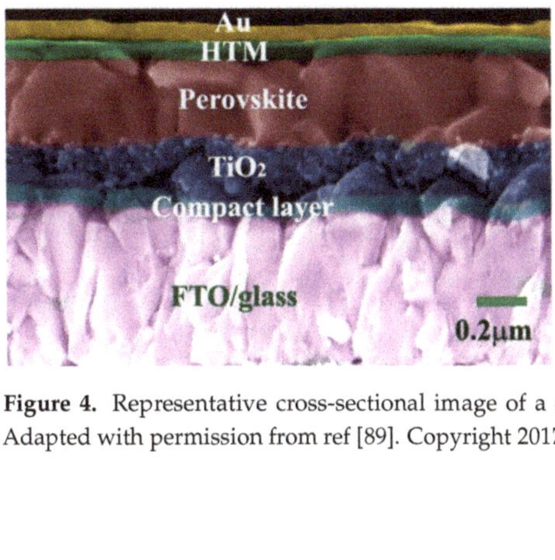


**Figure 4.** Representative cross-sectional image of a device based on phthalocyanine as HTM. Adapted with permission from ref [89]. Copyright 2017 Elsevier.

In recent years, several reports received merited attention, where some Pcs were used as HTMs in perovskite solar cells (Figure 5). Table 1 shows the photovoltaic parameters obtained for those PSCs employing Pcs as HTMs. The short-circuit current density $J_{SC}$, which can be obtained from the standard 100 mW/cm$^2$ solar spectrum (AM1. 5), is determined by optical losses, that is, by considering that photons from a part of the spectrum are either not absorbed in the solar cell or are absorbed without generating electron–hole pairs. The short-circuit current is the current through the solar cell when the voltage across the solar cell is zero (i.e., when the solar cell is short circuited). The open-circuit voltage, $V_{OC}$, is the maximum voltage available from a solar cell, and this occurs at zero current [63]. The open-circuit voltage corresponds to the amount of forward bias on the solar cell due to the bias of the solar cell junction with the light-generated current. The short-circuit current and the open-circuit voltage are the maximum current and voltage, respectively, from a solar cell. However, at both of these operating points, the power from the solar cell is zero. The "fill factor", "FF", is a parameter which, in conjunction with $V_{OC}$ and $J_{SC}$, determines the maximum power from a solar cell. Finally, the efficiency is the most commonly used parameter to compare the performance of one solar cell to another. Efficiency is defined as the ratio of energy output from the solar cell to input energy from the sun [63].

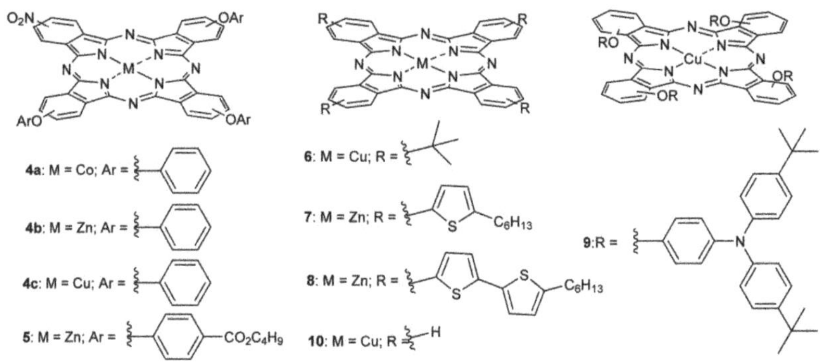


**Figure 5.** Pcs used in perovskite solar cells.

**Table 1.** Photovoltaic parameters obtained for perovskite solar cells employing phthalocyanines as hole-transporting materials.

| Entry | $J_{SC}$ (mA/cm$^2$) | $V_{OC}$ (V) | FF | PCE (%) | Cell Configuration [1] | Ref. |
|---|---|---|---|---|---|---|
| 1 | 11.79 | 1.04 | 0.64 | 8.24 | $dTiO_2$/$mpTiO_2$/perovskite/Pc **4a**/Au | [90] |
| 2 | 20.83 | 1.07 | 0.64 | 14.35 | $dTiO_2$/$mpTiO_2$/perovskite/Pc **4b**/Au | [89] |
| 3 | 20.46 | 1.06 | 0.58 | 12.72 | $dTiO_2$/$mpTiO_2$/perovskite/Pc **4c**/Au | [89] |
| 4 | 21.00 | 1.10 | 0.68 | 15.74 | $dTiO_2$/$mpTiO_2$/perovskite/Pc **3 4**/Au | [91] |
| 5 | 22.60 | 1.05 | 0.73 | 17.50 | $mpTiO_2$/m-perovskite/Pc **6**/Au | [92] |
| 6 | 20.28 | 1.05 | 0.80 | 17.10 | $mpTiO_2$/m-perovskite/Pc **7**/Au | [93] |
| 7 | 20.16 | 1.10 | 0.69 | 15.50 | $mpTiO_2$/m-perovskite/Pc **8**/Au | [93] |
| 8 | 21.00 | 0.98 | 0.63 | 13.5 | $mpTiO_2$/m-perovskite/Pc **9**/Carbon | [94] |
| 9 | 20.80 | 1.05 | 0.74 | 16.10 | $dTiO_2$/$mpTiO_2$/$MAPbI_3$-perovskite/Pc **10**/Carbon | [95] |
| 10 | 23.28 | 0.98 | 0.67 | 15.39 | $SnO_2$:$TiO_2$/m-perovskite/Pc **10**/Carbon [2] | [96] |
| 11 | 22.41 | 1.07 | 0.73 | 17.46 | Ni:$TiO_2$/m-perovskite/Pc **10**/Carbon [2] | [97] |
| 12 | 23.40 | 1.10 | 0.69 | 17.78 | FTO/Zn:$SnO_2$/m-perovskite/Pc **10**/Carbon [2,3] | [98] |

Performances were recorded under full Sun AM 1.5G light (solar simulator 100 mW/cm$^2$). $J_{SC}$ = short-circuit current density; $V_{OC}$ = open-circuit voltage; FF = fill factor; PCE = power conversion efficiency; $dTiO_2$ = dense $TiO_2$; $mpTiO_2$ = mesoporous $TiO_2$; m-perovskite = modified mixed-ion perovskite with ratio $(FAPbI_3)_{0.85}(MAPbBr_3)_{0.15}$; [1] all cells incorporate fluorine-doped tin oxide (FTO) as lower layer (not represented); [2] modified perovskite as $Cs_{0.05}(MA_{0.17}FA_{0.83})_{0.95}Pb(I_{0.83}Br_{0.17})_3$; [3] this cell is $TiO_2$ free.

For instance, Zhang and collaborators reported a small family of non-symmetrically substituted phthalocyanines (Pcs **4a–c** and **5**, Figure 5), synthesized to be used as HTM in PSCs [89–91]. Tetraphenoxy-substituted metallophthalocyanines **4a–c** were studied (entries 1–3, Table 1), and Zn as the central moiety was found to show higher performance with a PCE = 14.35%. Hence, having Zn as a central metal, the same authors additionally compared it with Pc **5** (entry 4, Table 1), a phthalocyanine bearing four peripheral oxyphenyl butylester groups, which further increased PCE to 15.74% [91].

Along with HTMs, the choice of suitable thermally stable electron-transport materials (ETMs) is essential to obtain highly efficient PSCs. Each material constituting the solar cells must have first-rate thermal stability. $TiO_2$ itself as an ETM is well-known to be thermally stable up to 500 °C, while standard perovskite is reported to have excellent thermal robustness up to 150 °C [99]. Additionally, light absorbers ought to be exceedingly thermally stable as well. To that end, Seok and Seo developed a new PSC using copper Pc **6** as HTM (Figure 5) [92], and organolead halide perovskite as a light absorber. The authors explored the thermal stability of PSCs prepared from a $PbI_2$-enriched mixed perovskite incorporating formaminium(FA)/methylaminium(MA) in the $(FAPbI_3)_{0.85}(MAPbBr_3)_{0.15}$ ratio. Besides reaching a very high value of average PCE = 17.50% (entry 5, Table 1 and Figure 6a), the PSC showed superior thermal stability. The cell's stability was compared to other cells, incorporating 2,2′,7,7′-tetrakis(*N*,*N*-di-*p*-methoxyphenylamine)-9,9′-spirobifluorene (spiro-OMeTAD) and poly(triaryl amine) (PTAA). Cells incorporating these HTMs are known to have high PCE values of ~20%; however, their presence reduces the stability of PSCs to thermal stress because of the relatively low glass transition temperature [100–105].

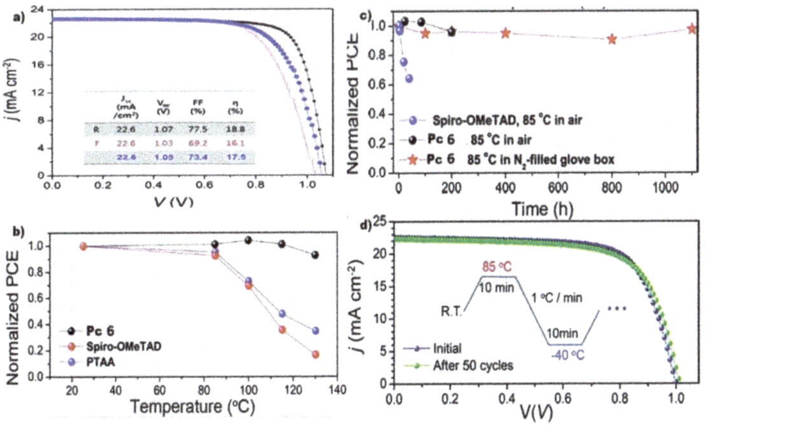


**Figure 6.** Cell performance and thermal stability. (**a**) J–V curves for the best cell using Pc **6** as HTM (in reverse (black) and forward (red) scans). The photovoltaic parameters of the best cell are shown in the inset table (average values in blue); (**b**) Stability of the devices tested at different temperatures (25, 85, 100, 115, and 130 °C, respectively) for 30 min, employing Pc **6** (black color), spiro-OMeTAD (red color), and PTAA (blue color); (**c**) Long-term stability of the devices stressed at 85 °C in air (25–30% humidity), using Pc **7** (black color) and spiro-OMeTAD (blue color) and 1100 h stability of the device utilizing Pc **6** at 85 °C in a nitrogen-filled glove box (red color); (**d**) J–V curves of a Pc **6** device before and after the thermal cycling test of 50 cycles within the temperature range between −40 °C and 85 °C. Adapted with permission from ref [92]. Copyright 2018 The Royal Society of Chemistry.

Changes in efficiency observed with heat treatments on a hot plate adjusted to several temperatures for 30 min are seen in Figure 6c, where the device incorporating Pc **6** exhibited no observable reduction in the PCE on moving from room temperature to 120 °C and a small decrease at 130 °C. Long-term thermal stability of Pc **6** based PSC, was also tested, and again much higher stability was displayed by this device against the spiro-OMeTAD containing device. Furthermore, even under exposure to ambient air (25 to 30% relative humidity) at 85 °C, the device without encapsulation was stable for 200 h. The device was also stable under thermal cycling tests for 50 cycles at temperatures ranging from −40 to 85 °C in dry air. Notwithstanding the absence of encapsulation, the device practically retained its initial PCE (98% of its initial PCE) [92].

Torres and Nazeeruddin reported a study using Pcs **7** and **8** (Figure 5) as HTMs in PSC devices [93]. The PSCs incorporating Pcs with four peripheral hexylthiophene (**7**) and hexylbisthiophene groups (**8**) were evaluated, and a crucial role of the molecular aggregation of Pcs in HTM layers in the charge transport properties was demonstrated. Using a combination of these Pcs with the mixed-ion modified perovskite light absorber $(FAPbI_3)_{0.85}(MAPbBr_3)_{0.15}$, PCEs of average 17.1% and 15.50% (entries 6 and 7, Table 1) for devices incorporating Pc **7** and Pc **8**, respectively, were obtained.

Wang and Sun also attempted to modulate the phthalocyanine structure to enhance its solubility in layer formation/deposition. They used Pc **9** (Figure 5) [94], bearing the widely well-known and widely used triphenylamine (TPA) as the electron donor. The other main change was the use of carbon as a cathode layer, a considerably cheaper option than using a noble metal as a counter-electrode [103,104]. Nevertheless, the authors could not improve the state of the art, reaching an average PCE of 13.50% (entry 8, Table 1). The same authors later managed to improve PCE values by using Pc **10** as a HTM (Figure 5) and a $MAPbI_3$ perovskite layer as an electron harvester, reaching a PCE = 16.10% (entry 9, Table 1) [95].

Liao, instead of using only $TiO_2$ as an electron transport layer (ETL), assembled a bilayer consisting of $SnO_2$ and $TiO_2$ [96]. The latter is, naturally, the most commonly used ETL [106,107] due to its suitable energy band matching and high transmittance toward visible light. However, the electron recombination rate for this ETL is very high due to low electron mobility, which is always an issue to overcome. Thus, Liao's research group developed a PSC incorporating copper Pc **10** (Figure 5) as a HTM, carbon as a counter-electrode, a modified perovskite layer as a light absorber with an increased amount of Br ions $[Cs_{0.05}(MA_{0.17}FA_{0.83})_{0.95}Pb(I_{0.83}Br_{0.17})_3]$, and a layered mixture of $SnO_2$ and $TiO_2$. The device displayed a PCE = 15.39% (entry 9, Table 1) and showed almost no decrease in PCE after 1200 h when stored in ambient air.

Pursuing their intents in improving the ETL capacity, the same authors produced a carbon-based planar heterojunction PSC using high-crystallinity Ni-doped $TiO_2$ as the ETL, using copper Pc **10** (Figure 5) as the HTM [97]. They found that 0.01 M Ni doping could cause an increase in the charge mobility of the $TiO_2$ film, thus enhancing the charge transport and extraction. An optimized PCE of 17.46% was therefore obtained (entry 10, Table 1), comparable to the best values obtained for Au containing PSCs.

The same authors, who completely replaced $TiO_2$ as the ETL and reported a low-temperature processed Zn-doped $SnO_2$ (below 200 °C) as the ETL [98], incorporating carbon as counter electrode and Pc **10** (Figure 5) as the HTM, delivered a further step forward in the research on PSCs. They observed improved conductivity for $SnO_2$ films doped with 2 mM Zn, resulting in efficient electron transfer and charge recombination suppression. An optimal efficiency of 17.78% was obtained, maintaining almost 100% of their initial efficiencies over 1200 h in ambient air.

### 3.2. Charge Transfer Materials

Transition metal dichalcogenides (TMDs) are layered two-dimensional (2D) materials that attracted much recent interest, mostly due to their capability to modulate materials' properties by the stacking of different compounds together [108].

This ability is enabled by the weak van der Waals bonding between layers and the absence of hanging bonds at the interface. Since organic molecules are also bonded by van der Waals forces, these readily combine with TMDs, providing synergized heterostructures. Hence, these materials are the most promising semiconductor platforms, with $MoS_2$ being the most prominent member [109,110]. As phthalocyanines are robust, chemically stable electron-rich systems with a high capability to generate charge-separated states, these are ideal candidates to produce excellent semiconducting charge transfer materials.

For instance, Choi studied the electronic charge transfer between several TMDs, such as $MoS_2$, $MoSe_2$, and $WSe_2$, with Pcs **11** and **12** (Figure 7) [111]. They demonstrated that the photoluminescence emission could be selectively and reversibly modulated through energetically favorable electron transfer from photo-excited TMDs to the metal-Pcs. Nickel Pc **12**, whose reduction potential is lower than the conduction band minima (CBM) of monolayers $MoSe_2$ and $WSe_2$, but is higher than that of $MoS_2$, acts as a photoluminescence quencher of $MoSe_2$ and $WSe_2$, but not $MoS_2$. Similarly, Mg Pc **12** quenches only $WSe_2$, as its reduction potential is lower than those of the CBM of $WSe_2$, but above those of $MoS_2$ and $MoSe_2$. The authors also found that photocurrents from TMDs increased more than two-fold, only when the PL was quenched by metalloPcs, further supporting the photoinduced charge transfer mechanism. The quenched PL emission could be fully recovered when the Pc molecules were removed from the TMD surfaces, allowing re-functionalization and recycling.

Other authors studied the influence of zinc Pc **13** (Figure 7) in the interface with $MoS_2$ [112–114]. Chan found that the optically excited singlet exciton in Pc **13** is able to transfer its electron to $MoS_2$ in 80 fs after photoexcitation to form a charge transfer exciton [112]. However, back electron transfer occurs on the time scale of ~1–100 ps, resulting in the formation of a triplet exciton in the Pc layer. The authors attributed this relatively fast singlet–triplet transition to the large singlet–triplet splitting in organic materials and the strong spin–orbit coupling in TMD crystal layers. Furthermore, the same authors demonstrated that the ZnPc **13**/monolyered $MoS_2$ behaves similar to typical donor–acceptor interfaces, in which charge transfer excitons dissociate into electron–hole pairs [113]. On the contrary, back electron transfer occurs at ZnPc/bulk-$MoS_2$, resulting in the formation of triplet excitons in the zinc Pc, due to the different amount of band bending found in the Zn Pc **13** film deposited on monolayered-$MoS_2$ and bulk-$MoS_2$.

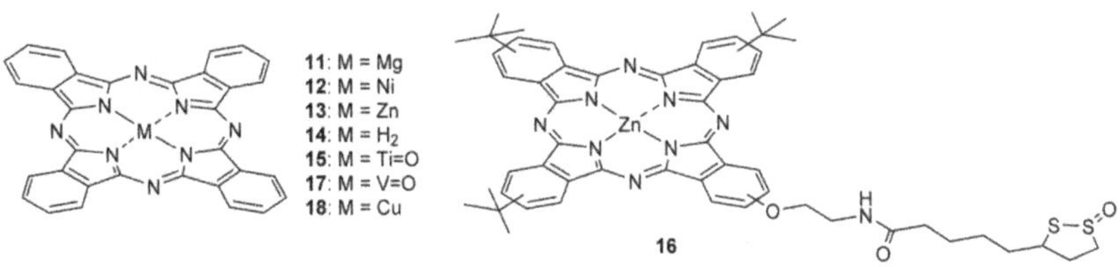


**Figure 7.** Phthalocyanines for application in semiconducting systems.

In addition, Zhai demonstrated the occurrence of ultrafast photoresponse dynamics in monolayered $MoS_2$ by using a charge transfer interface based on surface assembled zinc phthalocyanine molecules (Pc **13**, Figure 7) [114]. The formed Pc **13**/$MoS_2$ interface led to the separation of photogenerated holes to ZnPc **13** molecules [115], suppressing slow hole trapping in $MoS_2$, thus offering the significantly improved photoresponse dynamics in $MoS_2$ detectors by almost three orders (from > 20 s to <8 ms for the decay).

Other researchers developed $MoS_2$ nanosheets decorated with free base phthalocyanine (Pc **14**, Figure 7) [116]. The semiconducting heterostructure was then studied for its charge transfer properties. Using laterally confined $MoS_2$ nanosheets, the conduction band of the semiconductor was positioned between Pc's $S_1$ and $S_2$ states, causing bidirectional photoinduced electron transfer processes. On one side, excitation of Pc's $S_2$ state led to electron injection into the $MoS_2$ conduction band. However, charge transfer from the dye's $S_1$ transition to the $MoS_2$ nanosheet was found to be thermodynamically unfavorable, resulting in intense radiative recombination.

Kummel prepared a van der Waals interface between a monolayer (ML) of titanyl phthalocyanine (Pc **15**, Figure 7) and a ML of $MoS_2$ [117]. A strong negative charge transfer from $MoS_2$ to TiOPc molecules was observed and the $I_{ON}/I_{OFF}$ in backgated

$MoS_2$ transistors increased by more than two orders of magnitude, while the degradation in the photoluminescence signal was suppressed. The defect passivation methodology used permitted the demonstration that the defect states at low energy levels (near a conduction band edge) was observed with S vacancies, while defects at deep energy levels (in the middle of a band gap) were not observed. Because the Pc **15**/$MoS_2$ charge transfer van der Waals interface relied on the nonbonding interaction, it could present limitations in passivating deep-level defect states, which may be overcome by the introduction of a stronger interaction, perhaps a covalent one.

With that in mind, Sastre-Santos, D'Souza, and Tagmatarchis used zinc phthalocyanine Pc **16** (Figure 7) bearing an 1,2-dithiolane oxide linker to functionalize $MoS_2$ at defect sites located at the edges of the semiconducting surface [118]. The energy-level diagram depicted in Figure 8 shows different photochemical processes in Pc **16**-$MoS_2$, demonstrating a bidirectional electron transfer leading to a charge separated state of Pc **16** (ZnPc$\bullet^+$)-$MoS_2\bullet^-$. Marked evidence of the charge transfer in the hybrid material was demonstrated with involvement of excitons generated in $MoS_2$ in promoting the charge transfer while the transfer was also possible when Pc **16** was excited, suggesting their potential in light-energy-harvesting devices.

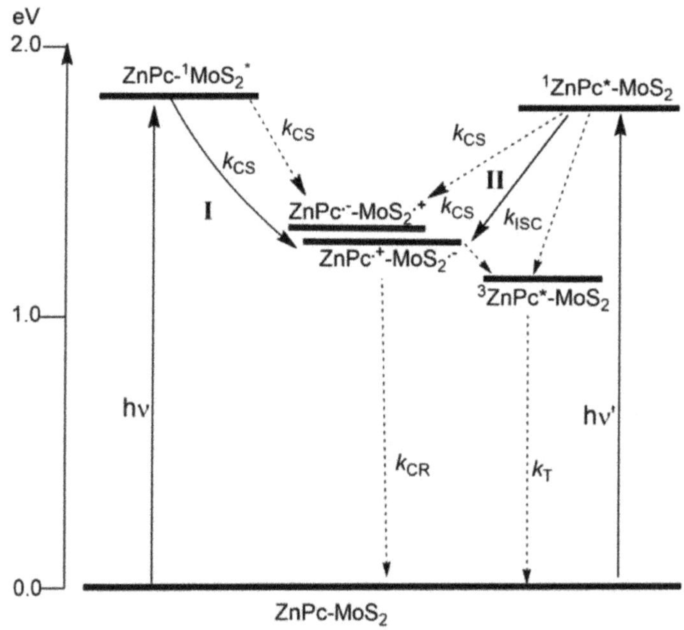


**Figure 8.** Energy-level diagram showing possible photochemical processes occurring in the Pc **16**-$MoS_2$ hybrid material. Solid arrows show major processes; dashed arrows show minor ones. Adapted with permission from ref [118]. Copyright 2019 John Wiley and Sons.

In addition to the charge carriers generated by charge transfer, organic phototransistors are devices that convert incident optical signals to electrical signals with amplification properties, and photomemory devices convert and also store the light information as an electrical signal, which is a building block for optical signal processing and photonic neuromorphic circuits [119]. Sun and Gao prepared organic heterojunction phototransistors based on phthalocyanine/*para*-sexiphenyl (Pc/p-6P) thin films [120,121]. In one case, they used vanadyl Pc **17** (Figure 7) [120]. Under 365 nm ultraviolet light irradiation, the ratio of photocurrent and dark current and photoresponsivity of the phototransistor were about $1.5 \times 10^5$ and 87 A/W, respectively. After applying a light pulse (4.2 mW/cm$^2$,

100 ms) on the device, the stored current level lasted for ~5000 s with only a 20% decrease, indicating a good photomemory behavior. In the other study, the authors used copper Pc **18** and managed to input an important role of the *para*-sexiphenyl thin film on the performance of CuPc **18**/p-6P heterojunction phototransistors [121]. It acted as a molecular template layer to induce the growth of highly ordered CuPc thin film, improving the charge transport and decreasing the grain boundaries. On the other hand, the p-6P thin film formed an effective heterojunction with Pc **18** thin film, enhancing the light absorption and photogenerated carriers. Under 365 nm ultraviolet light irradiation, the ratio of photocurrent to dark current and photoresponsivity of Pc **18**/p-6P heterojunction phototransistors reached ca. $2.2 \times 10^4$ and $4.3 \times 10^2$ A/W, respectively, which are much larger than that of Pc **18** phototransistors of ca. $2.7 \times 10^2$ and 7.3 A/W, respectively.

### 3.3. Photocatalysis

The use of phthalocyanines in photocatalysis is useful for light-triggered processes. Pcs are particularly applicable in composited photocatalytic materials that need visible light, deliberately inspired from photodynamic therapy in medical applications related to cancer treatment, or through the coupling of photosensitizing Pcs with semiconductor materials, intentionally inspired from cells in photovoltaic applications.

For instance, Tang and Jing reported the synthesis of an H-bond linked unsubstituted zinc phthalocyanine Pc **19**/$BiVO_4$ nanosheet composite (Figure 9) [122], which managed to function as a visible-light-driven photocatalyst for converting $CO_2$ into CO and $CH_4$ (under monochromatic beams at 520 and 660 nm), with the Pc presence as cause for a 16-fold increase over the BIVO4 performance (only at 520 nm).

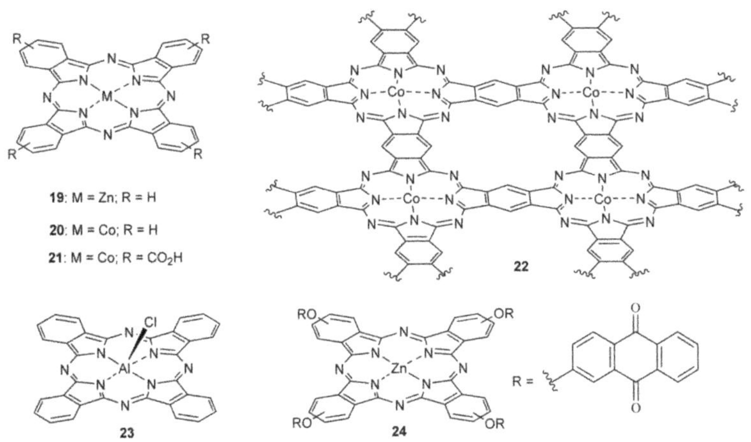


**Figure 9.** Pcs used in photocatalysis.

On the other hand, Jain prepared a nanoparticulated composite by the grafting of cobalt (II) Pc **19** (Figure 9) on the core-shell Ni/NiO semiconductor for the photocatalytic reduction of $CO_2$ to methanol under visible illumination [123]. The photocatalyst (10% Pc **19**) exhibited a remarkable enhancement in the yield of methanol as compared to the semiconductor Ni/NiO and Pc **19** for $CO_2$ reduction under identical conditions (a 12- and 8.5-fold increase, respectively). The maximum yield of methanol was found to be a ~3640 µmol/g catalyst with the conversion rate of ~152 µmol/g h, with reusability up to four times without loss of activity. The same group further reported another photocatalyst [124], which was prepared by intercalation of tetracarboxy-substituted Pc **20** (Figure 9) into graphitic carbon nitride g-$C_3N_4$. The best results were obtained with the photocatalyst containing 10% Pc **20**, with an 11- and a 7-fold increase in methanol production when compared to g-$C_3N_4$ and Pc **20** alone, respectively. The maximum methanol yields were 12,930 μmol/g catalyst after 24 h irradiation (rate = 540 μmol/g h).

Reisner prepared a photocatalyst based on mesoporous graphitic carbon nitride (mpg-CNx), incorporating the polymeric Co(II) Pc **21** (Figure 9) [125]. Under full solar spectrum irradiation, the photocatalyst mpg-CNx:Pc **22** (~12 mmol Co/g catalyst) generated a 1000 mmol CO/g catalyst after 48 h with 85% selectivity ($TON_{CO}$ = 85), a 65% increase in activity compared to that under visible light alone (607 mmol CO/g after 48 h, $TON_{CO}$ = 51). However, the catalyst only retained 85% of its activity after the second run.

Boyer used Pc **23** (Figure 9) in the radical polymerization of (meth)acrylate and (meth)acrylamide monomers [126], in combination with the solvent *N*-methyl-2-pyrrolidone (NMP), as a photoinitiation catalyst under visible and near-infrared light. The Pc reacted via a reductive quenching pathway to oxidize NMP to a NMP radical, which could directly initiate the polymerization of monomers. (Meth)acrylate and (meth)acrylamide monomers were initiated through a photoinduced electron/energy transfer process and subsequently controlled through reversible addition–fragmentation chain transfer equilibria. Thanks to the high molar extinction coefficients of Pc **23**, polymerization was accessible with an ultralow (5 ppm) catalyst concentration, besides tolerance to elemental oxygen.

Yilmaz and Versace reported Pc **24** (Figure 9) as a photoinitiator for free-radical and cationic photopolymerization reactions [127]. They combined the visible light-sensitive anthraquinone functionality with the phthalocyanine, further using a suitable electron acceptor for cationic polymerization (iodonium salt), and an electron donor (methyldiethanol amine, MDEA), or H-donor (thiol derivative, trithiol), for the free-radical polymerization. These combinations, carried out under visible light irradiation, promoted high acrylate and epoxy conversions with efficiency comparable to well-known camphorquinone-based photoinitiating systems [128,129].

Moth-Poulsen used Pc **20** (Figure 9) as a photocatalyst in a molecular photoswitching system [130], so-called molecular solar thermal energy storage (MOST). In this interesting concept, sunlight is collected and stored via photochemical reaction under flow conditions. When energy is required, a solution of the metastable molecule can be passed through a catalytic bed reactor to release the energy in the form of heat, which could be used for, in this instance, heating water or creating steam (Figure 10a). In the study, the authors used a norbornadiene derivative (**NBD1**), with improved absorptivity ($\lambda_{max}$ = 326 nm = $1.3 \times 10^4$ $M^{-1}$ $cm^{-1}$. Pc **20** was then used to promote the photoisomerization of **NBD1** into quadricyclane **QC1**, the couple isomer of the former compound, with high photoisomerization quantum yield (61%). **QC1** was characterized by its long half-life ($t_{1/2}$ = 30 days at 25 °C) and high solubility ($C_{max}$ = 1.52 M for **QC1** in toluene). Moreover, by using the small reaction center of the heterogeneous Pc **20** photocatalyst (Figure 10b), the stored energy could be efficiently released. A macroscopic heat release of up to ~63 °C using a 1.5 M solution of **QC1** was measured, with sustaining a reaction rate in toluene of $1.2 \times 10^4$ $s^{-1}$ $M^{-1}$ and a minimum TON of 482.

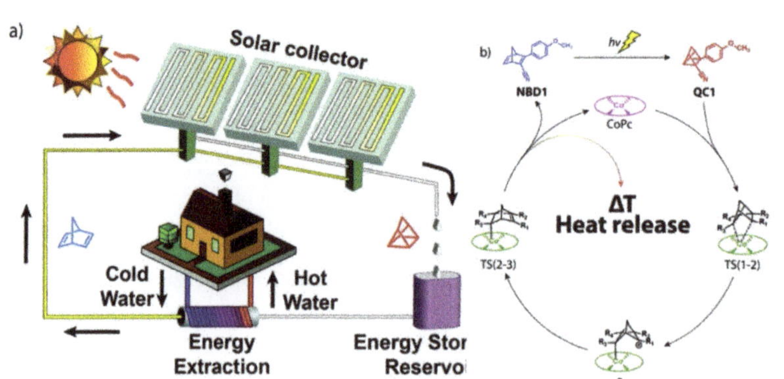


**Figure 10.** (**a**) Operating set up based on the MOST concept; (**b**) Catalytic cycle for the back-reaction. Adapted with permission from ref [130]. Copyright 2019 The Royal Society of Chemistry.

Degradation of pollutants present in the environment is crucial ensure continuity of life on Earth, since avoiding its pollution has been an impossible design. Among the many removal/degradation processes, advanced oxidation processes (AOPs) refer specifically to processes in which the oxidation of compounds occurs primarily through reactions with reactive oxygen species (ROS), and the reaction of these species with the target pollutants in water [67,69,131]. AOPs are considered as effective water treatment technologies. Particularly, semiconductor photocatalysis is one of the most effective technologies for the destruction of pollutants in water. As already pointed out, Pcs are photosensitizers that efficiently generate ROS and, hence, have been used in the photocatalytic degradation of many pollutants.

For instance, Lu's group reported the synthesis of photocatalysts Pc **25** and **26** (Figure 11) for the efficient and reusable photodegradation of pollutants rhodamine B (RhB) [132–134] and 4-chlorophenol (4-CP) [132,133] carbamazepine (CBZ) [133–135] and sulfaquinoxaline sodium (SQS) [134] under visible irradiation. In all cases, besides photogenerated holes, the presence of singlet oxygen ($^1O_2$), superoxide radical ($\bullet O_2^-$), and hydroxyl radical ($\bullet OH$) was evidenced in the visible light-responsive catalytic system.

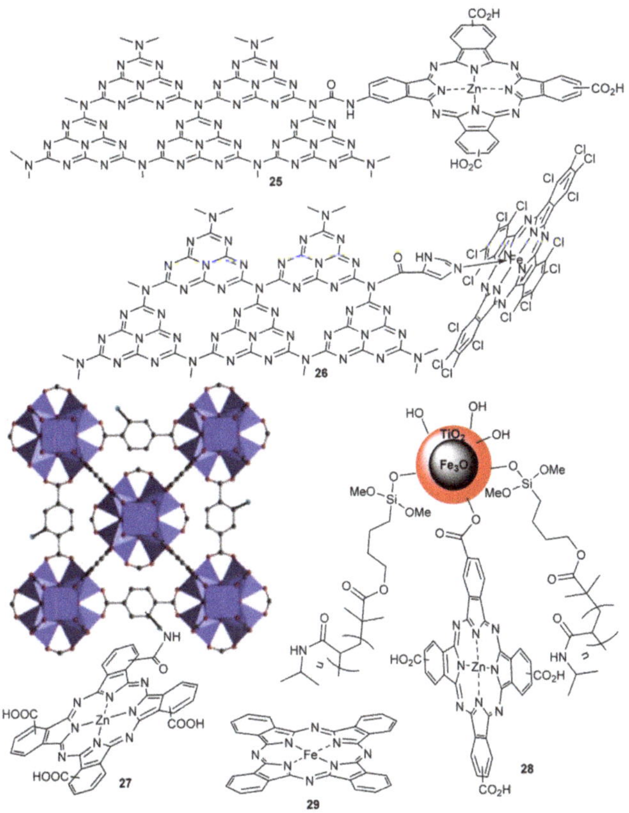


**Figure 11.** Immobilized phthalocyanine photocatalysts for degradation of pollutants. Structure of compound **27** was adapted with permission from ref [136]. Copyright 2017 Elsevier.

Liang and Li prepared photocatalyst **27** (Figure 11) [136], consisting of a zirconium-based metal organic framework [MOF UIO-66 ($NH_2$)], covalently coupled with α-tetracarboxy substituted Zn Pc, Which was prepared via a facile condensation process. Compared with the mixture of α-tetracarboxy Zn Pc and Zr-UIO-66 by impregnation, **27** presented an enhanced photocatalytic activity for the degradation of methylene blue (MB) under visible-light irradiation. The formation of strong covalent bonds and a synergistic interaction between α-tetracarboxy Zn Pc and UIO-66 ($NH_2$) proved more effective, retaining its stability after five recycles.

Duan promoted the covalent immobilization of β-tetracarboxy Zn Pc on the surface of $TiO_2$ coated magnetite, obtaining catalyst **28** (Figure 11) [137]. The absorption light range was effectively broadened from the ultraviolet to visible region, and photocatalytic studies revealed a high decomposition rate of RhB under visible and sun light, retaining its photocatalytic activity for four cycles.

Dong produced a visible-light-driven water-fueled micromotor based on iron Pc **29** (Figure 11) [138]. These micromotors are micrometer-sized machines, capable to undergo photoinduced self-propelling movement. In this case, the photocatalyst, prepared by emulsification of a gelatin solution of Pc **29** in olive oil, yielding the spherical micromotors, exhibited visible-light-driven self-propulsion behavior using water fuel based on the photocatalytic reaction and self-diffusiophoresis mechanism. The system showed good photocatalytic activity in the degradation of the RhB pollutant, with a normalized reaction rate constant of $2.49 \times 10^{-2}$ L/m$^2$ s.

We can generally observe that Pc's structure is not definite in providing adequate properties to any certain photocatalytic purpose. The most important issue regards the "to all cost" leaching prevention, since it hampers reusability to a large extent.

### 3.4. Nonlinear Optics

The control of the transmission of the energy transported by optical waves is of extreme importance for the realization of advanced technologies that require high speed of operation and fast switching. Nonlinear optics (NLO) are an example of such a technological application, where phthalocyanines may play a prominent role, motivated by the fact that the optical properties of such annulated systems can be finely modulated in a controlled fashion by changing the chemical structure of the complex. These changes involve the variation of the central metal, the extent of electronic conjugation of the ring, the nature and the number of peripheral ligands, and the eventual introduction of axial ligands coordinated by central metals with a valence higher than +2 [64,65,139,140]. The definition of NLO mechanisms can be seen in references [64,65].

For instance, Qi and Jiang reported Pcs **30** and **31** (Figure 12), bearing four and eight dibutylamino groups, respectively [141]. Electronic absorption spectroscopic studies revealed the more effective conjugation of the nitrogen lone pair of electrons in the dibutylamino side chains with the Pc π system in **30** than in **31**, which, in turn, resulted in superior third-order NLO properties. This was demonstrated by a larger effective imaginary third-order molecular susceptibility, a crucial parameter to define nonlinearity of a material (($\mathrm{Im}\{\chi^{(3)}\}$) of $6.5 \times 10^{-11}$ esu for the former and $3.4 \times 10^{-11}$ esu for the latter one).

The electronic absorption spectra of Pcs **30** and **31** were recorded in $CHCl_3$, where **30** shows a characteristic non-aggregated absorption spectrum of the metal-free phthalocyanines with a relatively broadened Soret absorption band appearing at 340 nm and a broad Q band at 765 nm. Of note, theoretical calculations revealed that, unlike typical metal-free Pcs [142,143], the Q band for **30** did not get split because of the more effective p-π conjugation between the peripheral nitrogen atoms and the central phthalocyanine chromophore, therefore extending the effective conjugation system for Pc **30** (Figure 13).

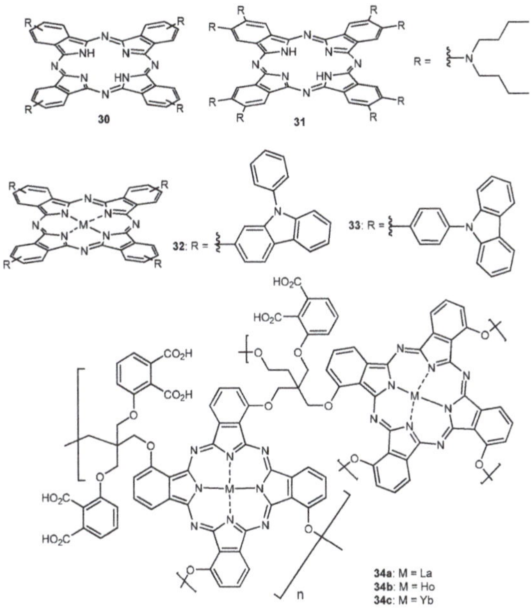


**Figure 12.** Phthalocyanines for nonlinear optics applications.

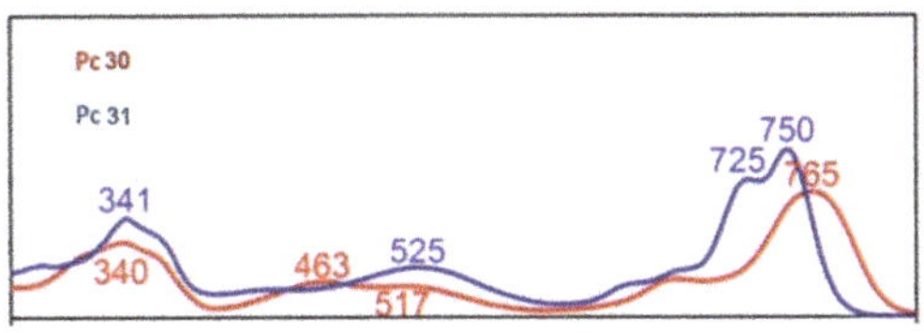


**Figure 13.** Comparison in the electronic absorption spectra between Pcs **30** and **31**, recorded in $CHCl_3$. Adapted with permission from ref [141]. Copyright 2016 American Chemical Society.

The nonlinear optical properties of carbazole substituted phthalocyanines were also reported by Giribabu and Rao Soma, having the carbazole units linked either through aromatic C-C bonds or C-N bonds (Figure 13, **32** and **33**, respectively) [144]. This particularity was revealed as crucial for the NLO properties of **32** and **33**, which were investigated using the Z-scan technique and femtosecond (fs) pulses, with kHz and MHz repetition rates, where two-photon absorption (TPA) was the dominant mechanism observed. At 800 nm under kHz pulses, Pc **32** displayed ($\mathrm{Im}\{\chi^{(3)}\}$) = $3.9 \times 10^{-15}$ esu while Pc **33** showed a ($\mathrm{Im}\{\chi^{(3)}\}$) = $7.9 \times 10^{-14}$ esu, 20 times higher.

The nonlinear optical properties of the polymeric carboxyl phthalocyanines with lanthanum (**34a**), holmium (**34b**), and ytterbium (**34c**) as central metals (Figure 12) were investigated using a by-scan method using a picosecond 532 nm laser [145]. NLO response was attributed to the reverse saturable absorption and self-focus refraction, decreasing in the order **34a** > **34b** > **34c** with $\mathrm{Im}\{\chi^{(3)}\}$ values of $4.86 \times 10^{-12}$ esu, $4.18 \times 10^{-12}$ esu and $3.60 \times 10^{-12}$ esu, respectively. Furthermore, **34a** showed a limiting threshold (that is, the incident fluence at which the transmittance drops to half) of 0.32 J/cm$^2$, while **34b** and **34c** displayed higher values of 0.5 J/cm$^2$ and 0.8 J/cm$^2$, respectively.

Figure 14 shows the nonlinear absorption of the three polymeric carboxyl phthalocyanines under open aperture conditions in the Z-scan test (left). All curves exhibit valleys, which indicate the reverse saturable absorption with a positive coefficient. Under closed aperture conditions (right), the valley-to-peak forms suggest a self-focus effect of nonlinear reflection [145].

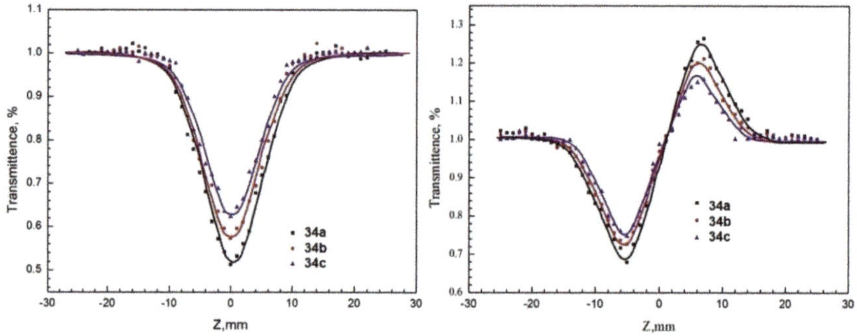


**Figure 14.** The nonlinear absorption and fitting curves (solid lines) of polymeric carboxyl phthalocyanines Z-scan (left: closed aperture; right: open aperture). Adapted with permission from ref [144]. Copyright 2017 American Chemical Society.

Prolifically, Nyokong's group reported the NLO properties of several phthalocyanine-based hybrid materials, of which we highlight compound **35–38** (Figure 15) [146–148]. For instance, double- and triple-decker phthalocyanines **35-QD** and **36-QD** were linked to mercaptosuccinic acid-capped ternary CdSeTe/CdTeS/ZnSeS quantum dots (QD), and their optical power limiting (OPL) properties were evaluated by the open-aperture Z-scan technique (532 nm laser and pulse rate of 10 ns) [146]. It was observed that both lowering of molecular symmetry and expansion of the $\pi$ electron system upon moving from double- to triple-decker complexes significantly improves the OPL characteristics, making the low-symmetry triple-decker complex **36-QD** the most efficient optical limiter, affording 50% lowering of light transmittance below 0.5 J/cm$^2$ input fluence, with a Im{$\chi^{(3)}$} value of 4.2 × $10^{-11}$ esu (Figure 16).

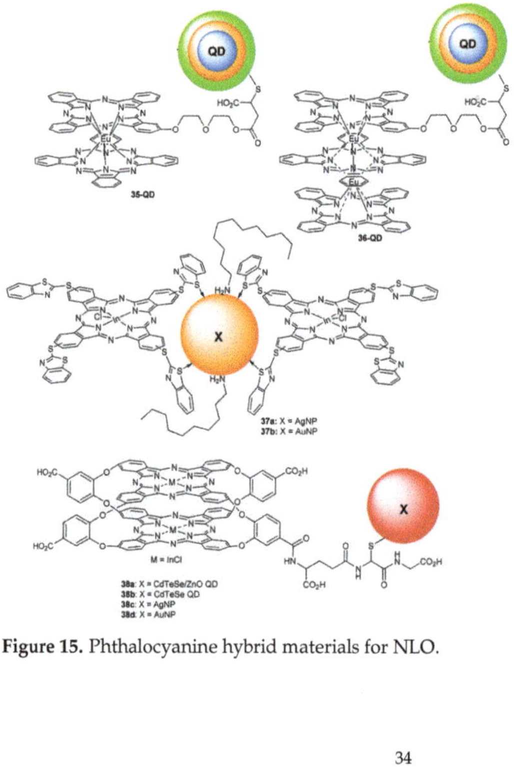


**Figure 15.** Phthalocyanine hybrid materials for NLO.

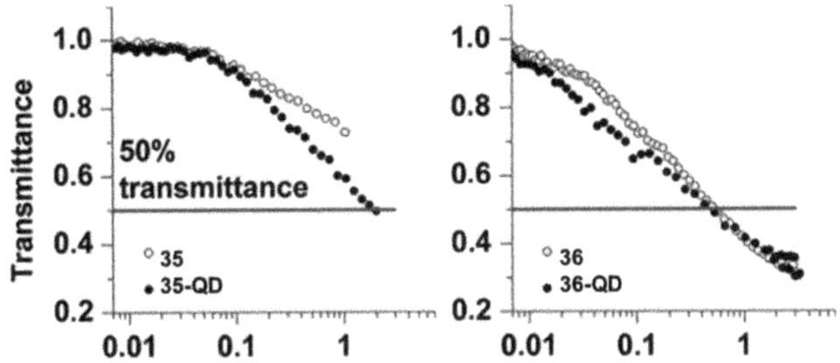


**Figure 16.** Transmittance of sandwich complexes and their conjugates with QDs depending on the incident fluence, performed at a pulse rate of 10 ns and $I_0 \approx 0.33$ GW/cm$^2$. The red solid line corresponds to 50% transmittance (limiting threshold). Adapted with permission from ref [146]. Copyright 2017 John Wiley and Sons.

The same authors measured the nonlinear absorption behavior of hybrids **36a–b** by using the open aperture z-scan technique with excitation pulses of 10 ns at a wavelength of 532 nm and a peak intensity of 50.0 MW/cm$^2$ [147]. A comparison with similar hybrid materials continuing other central moieties demonstrated that the In(III) containing complexes showed the best OPL performance, limiting thresholds of 0.14 and 0.12 for **36a** and **36b**, respectively. In sequence, the same group covalently attached a ball-type indium phthalocyanine to glutathione capped (Ag, Au, CdTeSe, CdTeSe/ZnO) nanoparticles [148]. The optical limiting threshold ranged from 0.40 to 0.78 J/cm$^2$, with the complex **37a** accounting for the most improved triplet state parameters and nonlinear optical behavior (0.40 J/cm$^2$).

## 4. Conclusions

Phthalocyanines find many photomaterial applications, where their photo-properties need to reach exquisite levels; the objectives are to modulate Pcs' photophysical properties, while ensuring their maneuverability in adequate media and ensuring stability for the macrocycle. Since Pcs usually act in combination with other materials, careful interfacial engineering should hold the key to enhance the applicability of phthalocyanine as photomaterials.

Many authors have been successful in their endeavors in recent years. Most of the applications require the utilization of previous knowledge, particularly regarding strategies to enhance Pcs' photophysical characteristics; nevertheless, a great deal of discoveries and milestones arise from empirical knowledge.

**Supplementary Materials:** The following are available online at, Figure S1: Results obtained using search strings (phthalocyanin*) and (phthalocyanin* AND photo*) present in the title and/or abstract and/or keywords in search engines Scopus and Web of Science (WoS), Figure S2: Country weight in publication of articles by five-year span, from 1971 to 2020. Articles were found by using search string "phthalocyanin*" followed by refining with term "photo*". (a) 1971–1975; (b) 1976–1980; (c) 1981–1985; (d) 1986–1990; (e) 1991–1995; (f) 1996–2000; (g) 2001–2005; (h) 2006–2010; (i) 2011–2015; (j) 2016–2020.

**Funding:** This research was partially funded by FCT—Foundation for Science and Technology, I.P., under project UIDB/00313/2020.

**Institutional Review Board Statement:** Not applicable.

**Informed Consent Statement:** Not applicable.

**Conflicts of Interest:** The authors declare no conflict of interest. The funders had no role in the design of the study; in the collection, analyses, or interpretation of data; in the writing of the manuscript; or in the decision to publish the results.

## References


1. Dini, D.; Hanack, M. Physical Properties of Phthalocyanine-based Materials. In *The Porphyrin Handbook, Phthalocyanines: Properties and Materials*; Kadish, K.M., Guilard, R., Smith, K.M., Eds.; Academic Press: San Diego, CA, USA, 2003; Volume 17, pp. 1–36.
2. L'Her, M.; Pondaven, A. Electrochemistry of Phthalocyanines. In *The Porphyrin Handbook, Phthalocyanines: Spectroscopic and Electrochemical Characterization*; Kadish, K.M., Guilard, R., Smith, K.M., Eds.; Academic Press: San Diego, CA, USA, 2003; Volume 16, pp. 117–170.
3. Nyokong, T.; Antunes, E. Photochemical and Photophysical Properties of Metallophthalocyanines. In *Handbook of Porphyrin Science, with Applications to Chemistry, Physics, Materials Science, Engineering, Biology and Medicine*; Kadish, K.M., Smith, K.M., Guilard, R., Eds.; World Scientific Publishing: Singapore, 2012; Volume 7, pp. 247–358.
4. Fukuda, T.; Kobayashi, N. UV-Visible Absorption Spectroscopic Properties of Phthalocyanines and Related Macrocycles. In *Handbook of Porphyrin Science, with Applications to Chemistry, Physics, Materials Science, Engineering, Biology and Medicine*; Kadish, K.M., Smith, K.M., Guilard, R., Eds.; World Scientific Publishing: Singapore, 2012; Volume 9, pp. 1–642.
5. Calvete, M.J.F. Phthalocyanines as top materials. In *Future Trends for Top Materials*; Bentham Science: Sarjah, United Arab Emirates, 2016; pp. 3–77.
6. Nemykin, V.N.; Lukyanets, E.A. The Key Role of Peripheral Substituents in the Chemistry of Phthalocyanines. In *Handbook of Porphyrin Science with Applications to Chemistry, Physics, Materials Science, Engineering, Biology and Medicine: Synthetic Methodology*; Kadish, K.M., Smith, K.M., Guilard, R., Eds.; World Scientific Publishing: Singapore, 2010; Volume 3, pp. 1–323.
7. Darwent, J.R.; Douglas, P.; Harriman, A.; Porter, G.; Richoux, M.C. Metal Phthalocyanines and Porphyrins as Photosensitizers for Reduction of Water to Hydrogen. *Coord. Chem. Rev.* **1982**, *44*, 83–126. [CrossRef]
8. Sorokin, A.B. Phthalocyanine Metal Complexes in Catalysis. *Chem. Rev.* **2013**, *113*, 8152–8191. [CrossRef]
9. Calvete, M.J.F.; Silva, M.; Pereira, M.M.; Burrows, H.D. Inorganic helping organic: Recent advances in catalytic heterogeneous oxidations by immobilised tetrapyrrolic macrocycles in micro and mesoporous supports. *RSC Adv.* **2013**, *3*, 22774–22789. [CrossRef]
10. Carrion, E.N.; Loas, A.; Patel, H.H.; Pelmus, M.; Ramji, K.; Gorun, S.M. Fluoroalkyl phthalocyanines: Bioinspired catalytic materials. *J. Porphyr. Phthalocyanine* **2018**, *22*, 371–397. [CrossRef]
11. Zhou, R.; Josse, F.; Gopel, W.; Ozturk, Z.Z.; Bekaroglu, O. Phthalocyanines as sensitive materials for chemical sensors. *Appl. Organomet. Chem.* **1996**, *10*, 557–577. [CrossRef]
12. Kumar, A.; Meunier-Prest, R.; Bouvet, M. Organic Heterojunction Devices Based on Phthalocyanines: A New Approach to Gas Chemosensing. *Sensors* **2020**, *20*, 4700. [CrossRef]
13. Stefanov, C.; van Staden, J.F.; Stefan-van Staden, R.I. Review-Enzymatic and Non-Enzymatic (bio)sensors Based on Phthalocyanines. A Minireview. *ECS J. Solid State Sci. Technol.* **2020**, *9*. [CrossRef]
14. Cook, M.J. Thin film formulations of substituted phthalocyanines. *J. Mater. Chem.* **1996**, *6*, 677–689. [CrossRef]
15. Papageorgiou, N.; Salomon, E.; Angot, T.; Layet, J.M.; Giovanelli, L.; Le Lay, G. Physics of ultra-thin phthalocyanine films on semiconductors. *Prog. Surf. Sci.* **2004**, *77*, 139–170. [CrossRef]
16. Valli, L. Phthalocyanine-based Langmuir-Blodgett films as chemical sensors. *Adv. Colloid Interface Sci.* **2005**, *116*, 13–44. [CrossRef]
17. Melville, O.A.; Lessard, B.H.; Bender, T.P. Phthalocyanine-Based Organic Thin-Film Transistors: A Review of Recent Advances. *ACS Appl. Mater. Interfaces* **2015**, *7*, 13105–13118. [CrossRef]
18. Giroudgodquin, A.M.; Maitlis, P.M. Metallomesogens—Metal-Complexes in Organized Fluid Phases. *Angew. Chem. Int. Ed.* **1991**, *30*, 375–402. [CrossRef]
19. Laschat, S.; Baro, A.; Steinke, N.; Giesselmann, F.; Hagele, C.; Scalia, G.; Judele, R.; Kapatsina, E.; Sauer, S.; Schreivogel, A.; et al. Discotic liquid crystals: From tailor-made synthesis to plastic electronics. *Angew. Chem. Int. Ed.* **2007**, *46*, 4832–4887. [CrossRef]
20. Basova, T.; Hassan, A.; Durmus, M.; Gurek, A.G.; Ahsen, V. Liquid crystalline metal phthalocyanines: Structural organization on the substrate surface. *Coord. Chem. Rev.* **2016**, *310*, 131–153. [CrossRef]
21. Hanack, M.; Lang, M. Conducting Stacked Metallophthalocyanines and Related-Compounds. *Adv. Mater.* **1994**, *6*, 819–833. [CrossRef]
22. Inabe, T.; Tajima, H. Phthalocyanines—Versatile components of molecular conductors. *Chem. Rev.* **2004**, *104*, 5503–5533. [CrossRef]
23. Gsanger, M.; Bialas, D.; Huang, L.Z.; Stolte, M.; Wurthner, F. Organic Semiconductors based on Dyes and Color Pigments. *Adv. Mater.* **2016**, *28*, 3615–3645. [CrossRef]
24. Ozdemir, P.S.; Ozguney, A.T. Chemical structures of phthalocyanine based dyestuffs and their useage in production of functional textiles. *PAJES* **2017**, *23*, 809–817. [CrossRef]
25. Benkhaya, S.; M'Rabet, S.; El Harfi, A. A review on classifications, recent synthesis and applications of textile dyes. *Inorg. Chem. Commun.* **2020**, *115*. [CrossRef]
26. Imahori, H.; Umeyama, T.; Ito, S. Large pi-Aromatic Molecules as Potential Sensitizers for Highly Efficient Dye-Sensitized Solar Cells. *Acc. Chem. Res.* **2009**, *42*, 1809–1818. [CrossRef]
27. Bottari, G.; de la Torre, G.; Guldi, D.M.; Torres, T. Covalent and Noncovalent Phthalocyanine-Carbon Nanostructure Systems: Synthesis, Photoinduced Electron Transfer, and Application to Molecular Photovoltaics. *Chem. Rev.* **2010**, *110*, 6768–6816. [CrossRef] [PubMed]
28. Li, X.Y.; Wang, H.X.; Wu, H.X. Phthalocyanines and Their Analogs Applied in Dye-Sensitized Solar Cell. In *Functional Phthalocyanine Molecular Materials*; Springer: Stuttgart, Germany, 2010; Volume 135, pp. 229–273.

29. Walter, M.G.; Rudine, A.B.; Wamser, C.C. Porphyrins and phthalocyanines in solar photovoltaic cells. *J. Porphyr. Phthalocyanine* **2010**, *14*, 759–792. [CrossRef]
30. Hanack, M.; Schneider, T.; Barthel, M.; Shirk, J.S.; Flom, S.R.; Pong, R.G.S. Indium phthalocyanines and naphthalocyanines for optical limiting. *Coord. Chem. Rev.* **2001**, *219*, 235–258. [CrossRef]
31. de la Torre, G.; Vaquez, P.; Agullo-Lopez, F.; Torres, T. Role of structural factors in the nonlinear optical properties of phthalocyanines and related compounds. *Chem. Rev.* **2004**, *104*, 3723–3750. [CrossRef] [PubMed]
32. Calvete, M.; Yang, G.Y.; Hanack, M. Porphyrins and phthalocyanines as materials for optical limiting. *Synth. Met.* **2004**, *141*, 231–243. [CrossRef]
33. Pereira, A.; Soares, A.R.M.; Calvete, M.J.F.; de la Torre, G. Recent developments in the synthesis of homo- and heteroarrays of porphyrins and phthalocyanines. *J. Porphyr. Phthalocyanine* **2009**, *13*, 419–428. [CrossRef]
34. Calvete, M.J.F. Near-infrared absorbing organic materials with nonlinear transmission properties. *Int. Rev. Phys. Chem.* **2012**, *31*, 319–366. [CrossRef]
35. Drobizhev, M.; Makarov, N.S.; Rebane, A.; de la Torre, G.; Torres, T. Strong two-photon absorption in push-pull phthalocyanines: Role of resonance enhancement and permanent dipole moment change upon excitation. *J. Phys. Chem. C* **2008**, *112*, 848–859. [CrossRef]
36. Drobizhev, M.; Makarov, N.S.; Stepanenko, Y.; Rebane, A. Near-infrared two-photon absorption in phthalocyanines: Enhancement of lowest gerade-gerade transition by symmetrical electron-accepting substitution. *J. Chem. Phys.* **2006**, *124*. [CrossRef]
37. Marin, M.L.; Santos-Juanes, L.; Arques, A.; Amat, A.M.; Miranda, M.A. Organic Photocatalysts for the Oxidation of Pollutants and Model Compounds. *Chem. Rev.* **2012**, *112*, 1710–1750. [CrossRef]
38. Das, S.; Daud, W. A review on advances in photocatalysts towards CO2 conversion. *RSC Adv.* **2014**, *4*, 20856–20893. [CrossRef]
39. Bonnett, R. Photosensitizers of the Porphyrin and Phthalocyanine Series for Photodynamic Therapy. *Chem. Soc. Rev.* **1995**, *24*, 19–33. [CrossRef]
40. Hamblin, M.R.; Hasan, T. Photodynamic therapy: A new antimicrobial approach to infectious disease? *Photochem. Photobiol. Sci.* **2004**, *3*, 436–450. [CrossRef]
41. Jori, G.; Fabris, C.; Soncin, M.; Ferro, S.; Coppellotti, O.; Dei, D.; Fantetti, L.; Chiti, G.; Roncucci, G. Photodynamic therapy in the treatment of microbial infections: Basic principles and perspective applications. *Lasers Surg. Med.* **2006**, *38*, 468–481. [CrossRef]
42. Maisch, T. A New Strategy to Destroy Antibiotic Resistant Microorganisms: Antimicrobial Photodynamic Treatment. *Mini-Rev. Med. Chem.* **2009**, *9*, 974–983. [CrossRef]
43. Lovell, J.F.; Liu, T.W.B.; Chen, J.; Zheng, G. Activatable Photosensitizers for Imaging and Therapy. *Chem. Rev.* **2010**, *110*, 2839–2857. [CrossRef]
44. Sekkat, N.; van den Bergh, H.; Nyokong, T.; Lange, N. Like a Bolt from the Blue: Phthalocyanines in Biomedical Optics. *Molecules* **2012**, *17*, 98–144. [CrossRef]
45. Josefsen, L.B.; Boyle, R.W. Unique Diagnostic and Therapeutic Roles of Porphyrins and Phthalocyanines in Photodynamic Therapy, Imaging and Theranostics. *Theranostics* **2012**, *2*, 916–966. [CrossRef]
46. Calvete, M.J.F.; Simoes, A.V.C.; Henriques, C.A.; Pinto, S.M.A.; Pereira, M.M. Tetrapyrrolic Macrocycles: Potentialities in Medical Imaging Technologies. *Curr. Org. Synth.* **2014**, *11*, 127–140. [CrossRef]
47. Braun, A.; Tcherniac, J. The products of the action of acetanhydride on phthalamide. *Ber. Dtsch. Chem. Ges.* **1907**, *40*, 2709–2714. [CrossRef]
48. de Diesbach, H.; von der Weid, E. Some salt complexes of o-dinitriles with copper and pyridine. *Helv. Chim. Acta* **1927**, *10*, 886–888. [CrossRef]
49. Linstead, R.P. Phthalocyanines part I A new type of synthetic colouring matters. *J. Chem. Soc.* **1934**, 1016–1017. [CrossRef]
50. Abrahamse, H.; Hamblin, M.R. New photosensitizers for photodynamic therapy. *Biochem. J.* **2016**, *473*, 347–364. [CrossRef]
51. Li, X.; Lee, S.; Yoon, J. Supramolecular photosensitizers rejuvenate photodynamic therapy. *Chem. Soc. Rev.* **2018**, *47*, 1174–1188. [CrossRef]
52. Roguin, L.P.; Chiarante, N.; Vior, M.C.G.; Marino, J. Zinc(II) phthalocyanines as photosensitizers for antitumor photodynamic therapy. *Int. J. Biochem. Cell Biol.* **2019**, *114*. [CrossRef]
53. Li, X.; Zheng, B.D.; Peng, X.H.; Li, S.Z.; Ying, J.W.; Zhao, Y.Y.; Huang, J.D.; Yoon, J. Phthalocyanines as medicinal photosensitizers: Developments in the last five years. *Coord. Chem. Rev.* **2019**, *379*, 147–160. [CrossRef]
54. Lo, P.C.; Rodriguez-Morgade, M.S.; Pandey, R.K.; Ng, D.K.P.; Torres, T.; Dumoulin, F. The Unique Features and Promises of Phthalocyanines as Advanced Photosensitisers for Photodynamic Therapy of Cancer. *Chem. Soc. Rev.* **2020**, *49*, 1041–1056. [CrossRef]
55. Zheng, B.D.; He, Q.X.; Li, X.S.; Yoon, J.; Huang, J.D. Phthalocyanines as contrast agents for photothermal therapy. *Coord. Chem. Rev.* **2021**, *426*. [CrossRef]
56. Zhang, Y.M.; Lovell, J.F. Recent applications of phthalocyanines and naphthalocyanines for imaging and therapy. *WIREs Nanomed. Nanobiotechnol.* **2017**, *9*. [CrossRef]
57. Calvete, M.J.F.; Pinto, S.M.A.; Pereira, M.M.; Geraldes, C. Metal coordinated pyrrole-based macrocycles as contrast agents for magnetic resonance imaging technologies: Synthesis and applications. *Coord. Chem. Rev.* **2017**, *333*, 82–107. [CrossRef]
58. Calvete, M.J.F.; Pinto, S.M. Synthesis of Pyrrole-Based Macrocycles as Molecular Probes for Multimodal Imaging Techniques: Recent Trends. *Curr. Org. Synth.* **2017**, *14*, 704–714. [CrossRef]

59. Merkes, J.M.; Zhu, L.M.; Bahukhandi, S.B.; Rueping, M.; Kiessling, F.; Banala, S. Photoacoustic Imaging Probes Based on Tetrapyrroles and Related Compounds. *Int. J. Mol. Sci.* **2020**, *21*, 3082. [CrossRef] [PubMed]
60. Dabrowski, J.M.; Pucelik, B.; Regiel-Futyra, A.; Brindell, M.; Mazuryk, O.; Kyziol, A.; Stochel, G.; Macyk, W.; Arnaut, L.G. Engineering of relevant photodynamic processes through structural modifications of metallotetrapyrrolic photosensitizers. *Coord. Chem. Rev.* **2016**, *325*, 67–101. [CrossRef]
61. de la Torre, G.; Bottari, G.; Torres, T. Phthalocyanines and Subphthalocyanines: Perfect Partners for Fullerenes and Carbon Nanotubes in Molecular Photovoltaics. *Adv. Energy Mater.* **2017**, *7*. [CrossRef]
62. Brogdon, P.; Cheema, H.; Delcamp, J.H. Near-Infrared-Absorbing Metal-Free Organic, Porphyrin, and Phthalocyanine Sensitizers for Panchromatic Dye-Sensitized Solar Cells. *ChemSusChem* **2018**, *11*, 86–103. [CrossRef] [PubMed]
63. Urbani, M.; de la Torre, G.; Nazeeruddin, M.K.; Torres, T. Phthalocyanines and porphyrinoid analogues as hole- and electron-transporting materials for perovskite solar cells. *Chem. Soc. Rev.* **2019**, *48*, 2738–2766. [CrossRef] [PubMed]
64. Dini, D.; Calvete, M.J.F.; Hanack, M. Nonlinear Optical Materials for the Smart Filtering of Optical Radiation. *Chem. Rev.* **2016**, *116*, 13043–13233. [CrossRef] [PubMed]
65. Calvete, M.J.F.; Dini, D. Conjugated macrocyclic materials with photoactivated optical absorption for the control of energy transmission delivered by pulsed radiations. *J. Photochem. Photobiol. C* **2018**, *35*, 56–73. [CrossRef]
66. Gounden, D.; Nombona, N.; van Zyl, W.E. Recent advances in phthalocyanines for chemical sensor, non-linear optics (NLO) and energy storage applications. *Coord. Chem. Rev.* **2020**, *420*. [CrossRef]
67. Fernandez, L.; Esteves, V.I.; Cunha, A.; Schneider, R.J.; Tome, J.P.C. Photodegradation of organic pollutants in water by immobilized porphyrins and phthalocyanines. *J. Porphyr. Phthalocyanine* **2016**, *20*, 150–166. [CrossRef]
68. Cecconi, B.; Manfredi, N.; Montini, T.; Fornasiero, P.; Abbotto, A. Dye-Sensitized Solar Hydrogen Production: The Emerging Role of Metal-Free Organic Sensitizers. *Eur. J. Org. Chem.* **2016**, *2016*, 5194–5215. [CrossRef]
69. Youssef, Z.; Colombeau, L.; Yesmurzayeva, N.; Baros, F.; Vanderesse, R.; Hamieh, T.; Toufaily, J.; Frochot, C.; Roques-Carmes, T.; Acherar, S. Dye-sensitized nanoparticles for heterogeneous photocatalysis: Cases studies with TiO2, ZnO, fullerene and graphene for water purification. *Dyes Pigments* **2018**, *159*, 49–71. [CrossRef]
70. Martynov, A.G.; Safonova, E.A.; Tsivadze, A.Y.; Gorbunova, Y.G. Functional molecular switches involving tetrapyrrolic macrocycles. *Coord. Chem. Rev.* **2019**, *387*, 325–347. [CrossRef]
71. Bettini, S.; Valli, L.; Giancane, G. Applications of Photoinduced Phenomena in Supramolecularly Arranged Phthalocyanine Derivatives: A Perspective. *Molecules* **2020**, *25*, 3742. [CrossRef]
72. Calmeiro, J.M.D.; Tome, J.P.C.; Lourenco, L.M.O. Supramolecular graphene-phthalocyanine assemblies for technological breakthroughs. *J. Mater. Chem. C* **2020**, *8*, 8344–8361. [CrossRef]
73. Mongeon, P.; Paul-Hus, A. The journal coverage of Web of Science and Scopus: A comparative analysis. *Scientometrics* **2016**, *106*, 213–228. [CrossRef]
74. Zhu, J.W.; Liu, W.S. A tale of two databases: The use of Web of Science and Scopus in academic papers. *Scientometrics* **2020**, *123*, 321–335. [CrossRef]
75. Imahori, H.; Umeyama, T.; Kurotobi, K.; Takano, Y. Self-assembling porphyrins and phthalocyanines for photoinduced charge separation and charge transport. *Chem. Commun.* **2012**, *48*, 4032–4045. [CrossRef]
76. Kerp, H.R.; Donker, H.; Koehorst, R.B.M.; Schaafsma, T.J.; van Faassen, E.E. Exciton transport in organic dye layers for photovoltaic applications. *Chem. Phys. Lett.* **1998**, *298*, 302–308. [CrossRef]
77. Schwarze, M.; Tress, W.; Beyer, B.; Gao, F.; Scholz, R.; Poelking, C.; Ortstein, K.; Gunther, A.A.; Kasemann, D.; Andrienko, D.; et al. Band structure engineering in organic semiconductors. *Science* **2016**, *352*, 1446–1449. [CrossRef]
78. Capasso, F. Band-Gap Engineering—From Physics and Materials to New Semiconductor-Devices. *Science* **1987**, *235*, 172–176. [CrossRef]
79. Poelking, C.; Andrienko, D. Design Rules for Organic Donor-Acceptor Heterojunctions: Pathway for Charge Splitting and Detrapping. *J. Am. Chem. Soc.* **2015**, *137*, 6320–6326. [CrossRef]
80. Ke, L.L.; Min, J.; Adam, M.; Gasparini, N.; Hou, Y.; Perea, J.D.; Chen, W.; Zhang, H.; Fladischer, S.; Sale, A.C.; et al. A Series of Pyrene-Substituted Silicon Phthalocyanines as Near-IR Sensitizers in Organic Ternary Solar Cells. *Adv. Energy Mater.* **2016**, *6*. [CrossRef]
81. Hu, M.; Bi, C.; Yuan, Y.B.; Bai, Y.; Huang, J.S. Stabilized Wide Bandgap MAPbBr(x)I(3-x) Perovskite by Enhanced Grain Size and Improved Crystallinity. *Adv. Sci.* **2016**, *3*. [CrossRef]
82. Aharon, S.; El Cohen, B.; Etgar, L. Hybrid Lead Halide Iodide and Lead Halide Bromide in Efficient Hole Conductor Free Perovskite Solar Cell. *J. Phys. Chem. C* **2014**, *118*, 17160–17165. [CrossRef]
83. Stranks, S.D.; Eperon, G.E.; Grancini, G.; Menelaou, C.; Alcocer, M.J.P.; Leijtens, T.; Herz, L.M.; Petrozza, A.; Snaith, H.J. Electron-Hole Diffusion Lengths Exceeding 1 Micrometer in an Organometal Trihalide Perovskite Absorber. *Science* **2013**, *342*, 341–344. [CrossRef]
84. Saliba, M. Perovskite solar cells must come of age. *Science* **2018**, *359*, 388–389. [CrossRef]
85. Berhe, T.A.; Su, W.N.; Chen, C.H.; Pan, C.J.; Cheng, J.H.; Chen, H.M.; Tsai, M.C.; Chen, L.Y.; Dubale, A.A.; Hwang, B.J. Organometal halide perovskite solar cells: Degradation and stability. *Energy Environ. Sci.* **2016**, *9*, 323–356. [CrossRef]
86. Divitini, G.; Cacovich, S.; Matteocci, F.; Cina, L.; Di Carlo, A.; Ducati, C. In situ observation of heat-induced degradation of perovskite solar cells. *Nat. Energy* **2016**, *1*. [CrossRef]

87. Suzuki, A.; Kida, T.; Takagi, T.; Oku, T. Effects of hole-transporting layers of perovskite-based solar cells. *Jpn. J. Appl. Phys.* **2016**, *55*. [CrossRef]
88. Swetha, T.; Singh, S.P. Perovskite solar cells based on small molecule hole transporting materials. *J. Mater. Chem. A* **2015**, *3*, 18329–18344. [CrossRef]
89. Guo, J.J.; Bai, Z.C.; Meng, X.F.; Sun, M.M.; Song, J.H.; Shen, Z.S.; Ma, N.; Chen, Z.L.; Zhang, F. Novel dopant-free metallophthalocyanines based hole transporting materials for perovskite solar cells: The effect of core metal on photovoltaic performance. *Sol. Energy* **2017**, *155*, 121–129. [CrossRef]
90. Guo, J.J.; Meng, X.F.; Niu, J.; Yin, Y.; Han, M.M.; Ma, X.H.; Song, G.S.; Zhang, F. A novel asymmetric phthalocyanine-based hole transporting material for perovskite solar cells with an open-circuit voltage above 1.0 V. *Synth. Met.* **2016**, *220*, 462–468. [CrossRef]
91. Guo, J.J.; Meng, X.F.; Zhu, H.W.; Sun, M.M.; Wang, Y.B.; Wang, W.N.; Xing, M.Y.; Zhang, F. Boosting the performance and stability of perovskite solar cells with phthalocyanine-based dopant-free hole transporting materials through core metal and peripheral groups engineering. *Org. Electron.* **2019**, *64*, 71–78. [CrossRef]
92. Kim, Y.C.; Yang, T.Y.; Jeon, N.J.; Im, J.; Jang, S.; Shin, T.J.; Shin, H.W.; Kim, S.; Lee, E.; Kim, S.; et al. Engineering interface structures between lead halide perovskite and copper phthalocyanine for efficient and stable perovskite solar cells. *Energy Environ. Sci.* **2017**, *10*, 2109–2116. [CrossRef]
93. Cho, K.T.; Trukhina, O.; Roldan-Carmona, C.; Ince, M.; Gratia, P.; Grancini, G.; Gao, P.; Marszalek, T.; Pisula, W.; Reddy, P.Y.; et al. Molecularly Engineered Phthalocyanines as Hole-Transporting Materials in Perovskite Solar Cells Reaching Power Conversion Efficiency of 17.5%. *Adv. Energy Mater.* **2017**, *7*. [CrossRef]
94. Jiang, X.Q.; Yu, Z.; Lai, J.B.; Zhang, Y.C.; Hu, M.W.; Lei, N.; Wang, D.P.; Yang, X.C.; Sun, L.C. Interfacial Engineering of Perovskite Solar Cells by Employing a Hydrophobic Copper Phthalocyanine Derivative as Hole-Transporting Material with Improved Performance and Stability. *ChemSusChem* **2017**, *10*, 1838–1845. [CrossRef]
95. Zhang, F.G.; Yang, X.C.; Cheng, M.; Wang, W.H.; Sun, L.C. Boosting the efficiency and the stability of low cost perovskite solar cells by using CuPc nanorods as hole transport material and carbon as counter electrode. *Nano Energy* **2016**, *20*, 108–116. [CrossRef]
96. Liu, Z.Y.; Sun, B.; Liu, X.Y.; Han, J.H.; Ye, H.B.; Tu, Y.X.; Chen, C.; Shi, T.L.; Tang, Z.R.; Liao, G.L. 15% efficient carbon based planar-heterojunction perovskite solar cells using a TiO2/SnO2 bilayer as the electron transport layer. *J. Mater. Chem. A* **2018**, *6*, 7409–7419. [CrossRef]
97. Liu, X.Y.; Liu, Z.Y.; Sun, B.; Tan, X.H.; Ye, H.B.; Tu, Y.X.; Shi, T.L.; Tang, Z.R.; Liao, G.L. 17.46% efficient and highly stable carbon-based planar perovskite solar cells employing Ni-doped rutile TiO2 as electron transport layer. *Nano Energy* **2018**, *50*, 201–211. [CrossRef]
98. Ye, H.B.; Liu, Z.Y.; Liu, X.Y.; Sun, B.; Tan, X.H.; Tu, Y.X.; Shi, T.L.; Tang, Z.R.; Liao, G.L. 17.78% efficient low-temperature carbon-based planar perovskite solar cells using Zn-doped SnO2 electron transport layer. *Appl. Surf. Sci.* **2019**, *478*, 417–425. [CrossRef]
99. Smecca, E.; Numata, Y.; Deretzis, I.; Pellegrino, G.; Boninelli, S.; Miyasaka, T.; La Magna, A.; Alberti, A. Stability of solution-processed MAPbI(3) and FAPbI(3) layers. *Phys. Chem. Chem. Phys.* **2016**, *18*, 13413–13422. [CrossRef]
100. Saliba, M.; Matsui, T.; Domanski, K.; Seo, J.Y.; Ummadisingu, A.; Zakeeruddin, S.M.; Correa-Baena, J.P.; Tress, W.R.; Abate, A.; Hagfeldt, A.; et al. Incorporation of rubidium cations into perovskite solar cells improves photovoltaic performance. *Science* **2016**, *354*, 206–209. [CrossRef]
101. Zhao, X.; Kim, H.S.; Seo, J.Y.; Park, N.G. Effect of Selective Contacts on the Thermal Stability of Perovskite Solar Cells. *ACS Appl. Mater. Interfaces* **2017**, *9*, 7148–7153. [CrossRef]
102. Malinauskas, T.; Tomkute-Luksiene, D.; Sens, R.; Daskeviciene, M.; Send, R.; Wonneberger, H.; Jankauskas, V.; Bruder, I.; Getautis, V. Enhancing Thermal Stability and Lifetime of Solid-State Dye-Sensitized Solar Cells via Molecular Engineering of the Hole-Transporting Material Spiro-OMeTAD. *ACS Appl. Mater. Interfaces* **2015**, *7*, 11107–11116. [CrossRef]
103. Molina-Ontoria, A.; Zimmermann, I.; Garcia-Benito, I.; Gratia, P.; Roldan-Carmona, C.; Aghazada, S.; Graetzel, M.; Nazeeruddin, M.K.; Martin, N. Benzotrithiophene-Based Hole-Transporting Materials for 18.2% Perovskite Solar Cells. *Angew. Chem. Int. Ed.* **2016**, *55*, 6270–6274. [CrossRef]
104. Huang, C.Y.; Fu, W.F.; Li, C.Z.; Zhang, Z.Q.; Qiu, W.M.; Shi, M.M.; Heremans, P.; Jen, A.K.Y.; Chen, H.Z. Dopant-Free Hole-Transporting Material with a C-3h Symmetrical Truxene Core for Highly Efficient Perovskite Solar Cells. *J. Am. Chem. Soc.* **2016**, *138*, 2528–2531. [CrossRef]
105. Zhang, J.B.; Hua, Y.; Xu, B.; Yang, L.; Liu, P.; Johansson, M.B.; Vlachopoulos, N.; Kloo, L.; Boschloo, G.; Johansson, E.M.J.; et al. The Role of 3D Molecular Structural Control in New Hole Transport Materials Outperforming Spiro-OMeTAD in Perovskite Solar Cells. *Adv. Energy Mater.* **2016**, *6*. [CrossRef]
106. Zhou, H.P.; Chen, Q.; Li, G.; Luo, S.; Song, T.B.; Duan, H.S.; Hong, Z.R.; You, J.B.; Liu, Y.S.; Yang, Y. Interface engineering of highly efficient perovskite solar cells. *Science* **2014**, *345*, 542–546. [CrossRef]
107. Gao, X.F.; Li, J.Y.; Baker, J.; Hou, Y.; Guan, D.S.; Chen, J.H.; Yuan, C. Enhanced photovoltaic performance of perovskite CH3NH3PbI3 solar cells with freestanding TiO2 nanotube array films. *Chem. Commun.* **2014**, *50*, 6368–6371. [CrossRef]
108. Novoselov, K.S.; Mishchenko, A.; Carvalho, A.; Neto, A.H.C. 2D materials and van der Waals heterostructures. *Science* **2016**, *353*. [CrossRef] [PubMed]

109. Huang, Y.L.; Zheng, Y.J.; Song, Z.B.; Chi, D.Z.; Wee, A.T.S.; Quek, S.Y. The organic-2D transition metal dichalcogenide heterointerface. *Chem. Soc. Rev.* **2018**, *47*, 3241–3264. [CrossRef] [PubMed]
110. Wang, H.M.; Li, C.H.; Fang, P.F.; Zhang, Z.L.; Zhang, J.Z. Synthesis, properties, and optoelectronic applications of two-dimensional $MoS_2$ and $MoS_2$-based heterostructures. *Chem. Soc. Rev.* **2018**, *47*, 6101–6127. [CrossRef] [PubMed]
111. Choi, J.; Zhang, H.Y.; Choi, J.H. Modulating Optoelectronic Properties of Two Dimensional Transition Metal Dichalcogenide Semiconductors by Photoinduced Charge Transfer. *ACS Nano* **2016**, *10*, 1671–1680. [CrossRef]
112. Kafle, T.R.; Kattel, B.; Lane, S.D.; Wang, T.; Zhao, H.; Chan, W.L. Charge Transfer Exciton and Spin Flipping at Organic Transition-Metal Dichalcogenide Interfaces. *ACS Nano* **2017**, *11*, 10184–10192. [CrossRef]
113. Kafle, T.R.; Kattel, B.; Yao, P.; Zereshki, P.; Zhao, H.; Chan, W.L. Effect of the Interfacial Energy Landscape on Photoinduced Charge Generation at the ZnPc/$MoS_2$ Interface. *J. Am. Chem. Soc.* **2019**, *141*, 11328–11336. [CrossRef]
114. Huang, Y.; Zhuge, F.W.; Hou, J.X.; Lv, L.; Luo, P.; Zhou, N.; Gan, L.; Zhai, T.Y. Van der Waals Coupled Organic Molecules with Monolayer $MoS_2$ for Fast Response Photodetectors with Gate-Tunable Responsivity. *ACS Nano* **2018**, *12*, 4062–4073. [CrossRef]
115. Lopez-Sanchez, O.; Lembke, D.; Kayci, M.; Radenovic, A.; Kis, A. Ultrasensitive photodetectors based on monolayer $MoS_2$. *Nat. Nanotechnol.* **2013**, *8*, 497–501. [CrossRef]
116. Nguyen, E.P.; Carey, B.J.; Harrison, C.J.; Atkin, P.; Berean, K.J.; Della Gaspera, E.; Ou, J.Z.; Kaner, R.B.; Kalantar-Zadeh, K.; Daeneke, T. Excitation dependent bidirectional electron transfer in phthalocyanine-functionalised $MoS_2$ nanosheets. *Nanoscale* **2016**, *8*, 16276–16283. [CrossRef]
117. Park, J.H.; Sanne, A.; Guo, Y.Z.; Amani, M.; Zhang, K.H.; Movva, H.C.P.; Robinson, J.A.; Javey, A.; Robertson, J.; Banerjee, S.K.; et al. Defect passivation of transition metal dichalcogenides via a charge transfer van der Waals interface. *Sci. Adv.* **2017**, *3*. [CrossRef]
118. Canton-Vitoria, R.; Gobeze, H.B.; Blas-Ferrando, V.M.; Ortiz, J.; Jang, Y.; Fernandez-Lazaro, F.; Sastre-Santos, A.; Nakanishi, Y.; Shinohara, H.; D'Souza, F.; et al. Excited-State Charge Transfer in Covalently Functionalized $MoS_2$ with a Zinc Phthalocyanine Donor-Acceptor Hybrid. *Angew. Chem. Int. Ed.* **2019**, *58*, 5712–5717. [CrossRef]
119. Baeg, K.J.; Binda, M.; Natali, D.; Caironi, M.; Noh, Y.Y. Organic Light Detectors: Photodiodes and Phototransistors. *Adv. Mater.* **2013**, *25*, 4267–4295. [CrossRef]
120. Qian, C.; Sun, J.; Kong, L.A.; Fu, Y.; Chen, Y.; Wang, J.X.; Wang, S.T.; Xie, H.P.; Huang, H.; Yang, J.L.; et al. Multilevel Nonvolatile Organic Photomemory Based on Vanadyl-Phthalocyanine/para-Sexiphenyl Heterojunctions. *ACS Photonics* **2017**, *4*, 2573–2579. [CrossRef]
121. Qian, C.; Sun, J.; Kong, L.A.; Gou, G.Y.; Zhu, M.L.; Yuan, Y.B.; Huang, H.; Gao, Y.L.; Yang, J.L. High-Performance Organic Heterojunction Phototransistors Based on Highly Ordered Copper Phthalocyanine/para-Sexiphenyl Thin Films. *Adv. Funct. Mater.* **2017**, *27*. [CrossRef]
122. Bian, J.; Feng, J.N.; Zhang, Z.Q.; Li, Z.J.; Zhang, Y.H.; Liu, Y.D.; Ali, S.; Qu, Y.; Bai, L.L.; Xie, J.J.; et al. Dimension-Matched Zinc Phthalocyanine/BiVO4 Ultrathin Nanocomposites for CO2 Reduction as Efficient Wide-Visible-Light-Driven Photocatalysts via a Cascade Charge Transfer. *Angew. Chem. Int. Ed.* **2019**, *58*, 10873–10878. [CrossRef]
123. Prajapati, P.K.; Singh, H.; Yadav, R.; Sinha, A.K.; Szunerits, S.; Boukherroub, R.; Jain, S.L. Core-shell Ni/NiO grafted cobalt (II) complex: An efficient inorganic nanocomposite for photocatalytic reduction of CO2 under visible light irradiation. *Appl. Surf. Sci.* **2019**, *467*, 370–381. [CrossRef]
124. Kumar, A.; Prajapati, P.K.; Aathira, M.S.; Bansiwal, A.; Boukherroub, R.; Jain, S.L. Highly improved photoreduction of carbon dioxide to methanol using cobalt phthalocyanine grafted to graphitic carbon nitride as photocatalyst under visible light irradiation. *J. Colloid Interface Sci.* **2019**, *543*, 201–213. [CrossRef]
125. Roy, S.; Reisner, E. Visible-Light-Driven CO2 Reduction by Mesoporous Carbon Nitride Modified with Polymeric Cobalt Phthalocyanine. *Angew. Chem. Int. Ed.* **2019**, *58*, 12180–12184. [CrossRef]
126. Corrigan, N.; Xu, J.T.; Boyer, C. A Photoinitiation System for Conventional and Controlled Radical Polymerization at Visible and NIR Wavelengths. *Macromolecules* **2016**, *49*, 3274–3285. [CrossRef]
127. Breloy, L.; Brezova, V.; Blacha-Grzechnik, A.; Presset, M.; Yildirim, M.S.; Yilmaz, I.; Yagci, Y.; Versace, D.L. Visible Light Anthraquinone Functional Phthalocyanine Photoinitiator for Free-Radical and Cationic Polymerizations. *Macromolecules* **2020**, *53*, 112–124. [CrossRef]
128. Xiao, P.; Dumur, F.; Graff, B.; Fouassier, J.P.; Gigmes, D.; Lalevee, J. Cationic and Thiol-Ene Photopolymerization upon Red Lights Using Anthraquinone Derivatives as Photoinitiators. *Macromolecules* **2013**, *46*, 6744–6750. [CrossRef]
129. Zhang, J.; Hill, N.; Lalevee, J.; Fouassier, J.P.; Zhao, J.C.; Graff, B.; Schmidt, T.W.; Kable, S.H.; Stenzel, M.H.; Coote, M.L.; et al. Multihydroxy-Anthraquinone Derivatives as Free Radical and Cationic Photoinitiators of Various Photopolymerizations under Green LED. *Macromol. Rapid Commun.* **2018**, *39*. [CrossRef] [PubMed]
130. Wang, Z.H.; Roffey, A.; Losantos, R.; Lennartson, A.; Jevric, M.; Petersen, A.U.; Quant, M.; Dreos, A.; Wen, X.; Sampedro, D.; et al. Macroscopic heat release in a molecular solar thermal energy storage system. *Energy Environ. Sci.* **2019**, *12*, 187–193. [CrossRef]
131. Calvete, M.J.F.; Piccirillo, G.; Vinagreiro, C.S.; Pereira, M.M. Hybrid materials for heterogeneous photocatalytic degradation of antibiotics. *Coord. Chem. Rev.* **2019**, *395*, 63–85. [CrossRef]
132. Lu, W.Y.; Xu, T.F.; Wang, Y.; Hu, H.G.; Li, N.; Jiang, X.M.; Chen, W.X. Synergistic photocatalytic properties and mechanism of g-C3N4 coupled with zinc phthalocyanine catalyst under visible light irradiation. *Appl. Catal. B Environ.* **2016**, *180*, 20–28. [CrossRef]

133. Xu, T.F.; Ni, D.J.; Chen, X.; Wu, F.; Ge, P.F.; Lu, W.Y.; Hu, H.G.; Zhu, Z.X.; Chen, W.X. Self-floating graphitic carbon nitride/zinc phthalocyanine nanofibers for photocatalytic degradation of contaminants. *J. Hazard. Mater.* **2016**, *317*, 17–26. [CrossRef] [PubMed]
134. Xu, T.F.; Wang, D.N.; Dong, L.L.; Shen, H.B.; Lu, W.Y.; Chen, W.X. Graphitic carbon nitride co-modified by zinc phthalocyanine and graphene quantum dots for the efficient photocatalytic degradation of refractory contaminants. *Appl. Catal. B Environ.* **2019**, *244*, 96–106. [CrossRef]
135. Dong, L.L.; Xu, T.F.; Chen, W.X.; Lu, W.Y. Synergistic multiple active species for the photocatalytic degradation of contaminants by imidazole-modified g-C3N4 coordination with iron phthalocyanine in the presence of peroxymonosulfate. *Chem. Eng. J.* **2019**, *357*, 198–208. [CrossRef]
136. Liang, Q.; Zhang, M.; Zhang, Z.H.; Liu, C.H.; Xu, S.; Li, Z.Y. Zinc phthalocyanine coupled with UIO-66 (NH2) via a facile condensation process for enhanced visible-light-driven photocatalysis. *J. Alloys Compd.* **2017**, *690*, 123–130. [CrossRef]
137. Liu, C.; Li, Y.H.; Duan, Q. Preparation of magnetic and thermal dual-responsive zinc-tetracarboxyl-phthalocyanine-g-Fe3O4@SiO2@TiO2-g-poly(N-isopropyl acrylamide) core-shell green photocatalyst. *Appl. Surf. Sci.* **2020**, *503*. [CrossRef]
138. Tong, J.T.; Wang, D.L.; Wang, D.C.; Xu, F.; Duan, R.M.; Zhang, D.F.; Fan, J.; Dong, B. Visible-Light-Driven Water-Fueled Ecofriendly Micromotors Based on Iron Phthalocyanine for Highly Efficient Organic Pollutant Degradation. *Langmuir* **2020**, *36*, 6930–6937. [CrossRef]
139. Dini, D.; Calvete, M.J.F.; Hanack, M.; Chen, W.Z.; Ji, W. Synthesis of axially substituted gallium, indium and thallium phthalocyanines with nonlinear optical properties. *Arkivoc* **2006**, 77–96. [CrossRef]
140. Carvalho, E.F.A.; Calvete, M.J.F.; Cavaleiro, J.A.S.; Dini, D.; Meneghetti, M.; Tome, A.C. Synthesis and high ranked NLT properties of new sulfonamide-substituted indium phthalocyanines. *Inorg. Chim. Acta* **2010**, *363*, 3945–3950. [CrossRef]
141. Chen, Y.X.; Cao, W.; Wang, C.M.; Qi, D.D.; Wang, K.; Jiang, J.Z. Four Dibutylamino Substituents Are Better Than Eight in Modulating the Electronic Structure and Third-Order Nonlinear-Optical Properties of Phthalocyanines. *Inorg. Chem.* **2016**, *55*, 3151–3160. [CrossRef]
142. Farinha, A.S.F.; Calvete, M.J.F.; Paz, F.A.A.; Tome, A.C.; Cavaleiro, J.A.S.; Sessler, J.L.; Tome, J.P.C. Octatosylaminophthalocyanine: A reusable chromogenic anion chemosensor. *Sens. Actuators B Chem.* **2014**, *201*, 387–394. [CrossRef]
143. Carvalho, E.F.A.; Calvete, M.J.F.; Tome, A.C.; Cavaleiro, J.A.S. Synthesis of sulfonamide-substituted phthalocyanines. *Tetrahedron Lett.* **2009**, *50*, 6882–6885. [CrossRef]
144. Bhattacharya, S.; Biswas, C.; Raavi, S.S.K.; Krishna, J.V.S.; Krishna, N.V.; Giribabu, L.; Soma, V.R. Synthesis, Optical, Electrochemical, DFT Studies, NLO Properties, and Ultrafast Excited State Dynamics of Carbazole-Induced Phthalocyanine Derivatives. *J. Phys. Chem. C* **2019**, *123*, 11118–11133. [CrossRef]
145. Zhao, P.; Wang, Z.H.; Chen, J.S.; Zhou, Y.; Zhang, F.S. Nonlinear optical and optical limiting properties of polymeric carboxyl phthalocyanine coordinated with rare earth atom. *Opt. Mater.* **2017**, *66*, 98–105. [CrossRef]
146. Oluwole, D.O.; Yagodin, A.V.; Mkhize, N.C.; Sekhosana, K.E.; Martynov, A.G.; Gorbunova, Y.G.; Tsivadze, A.Y.; Nyokong, T. First Example of Nonlinear Optical Materials Based on Nanoconjugates of Sandwich Phthalocyanines with Quantum Dots. *Chem. Eur. J.* **2017**, *23*, 2820–2830. [CrossRef]
147. Nwaji, N.; Jones, B.; Mack, J.; Oluwole, D.O.; Nyokong, T. Nonlinear optical dynamics of benzothiazole derivatized phthalocyanines in solution, thin films and when conjugated to nanoparticles. *J. Photochem. Photobiol. A* **2017**, *346*, 46–59. [CrossRef]
148. Nwaji, N.; Oluwole, D.O.; Mack, J.; Louzada, M.; Khene, S.; Britton, J.; Nyokong, T. Improved nonlinear optical behaviour of ball type indium(III) phthalocyanine linked to glutathione capped nanoparticles. *Dyes Pigments* **2017**, *140*, 417–430. [CrossRef]

*molecules* MDPI

*Review*

# Synthesis of α-Aminophosphonates and Related Derivatives; The Last Decade of the Kabachnik–Fields Reaction

**Petra R. Varga and György Keglevich ***

Department of Organic Chemistry and Technology, Budapest University of Technology and Economics, 1521 Budapest, Hungary; varga.petra.regina@vbk.bme.hu
* Correspondence: keglevich.gyorgy@vbk.bme.hu; Tel.: +36-1-463-1111 (ext. 5883)

**Abstract:** The Kabachnik–Fields reaction, comprising the condensation of an amine, oxo compound and a P-reagent (generally a >P(O)H species or trialkyl phosphite), still attracts interest due to the challenging synthetic procedures and the potential biological activity of the resulting α-aminophosphonic derivatives. Following the success of the first part (*Molecules* 2012, 17, 12821), here we summarize the synthetic developments in this field accumulated in the last decade. The procedures compiled include catalytic accomplishments as well as catalyst-free and/or solvent-free "greener" protocols. The products embrace α-aminophosphonates, α-aminophosphinates, and α-aminophosphine oxides along with different bis derivatives from the double phospha-Mannich approach. The newer developments of the aza-Pudovik reactions are also included.

**Keywords:** Kabachnik–Fields reaction; phospha-Mannich reaction; α-aminophosphonates; α-aminophosphine oxides; bis derivatives; catalysts; green methods; aza-Pudovik reaction

## 1. Introduction

The Kabachnik–Fields reaction involves the condensation of a primary or secondary amine, an oxo compound such as an aldehyde or ketone, and a >P(O)H-containing reagent, which is in most cases a dialkyl phosphite, but may also be an alkyl-*H*-phosphinate or a secondary phosphine oxide, to result in the formation of α-aminophosphonates, α-aminophosphinates, and α-aminophosphine oxides, respectively [1–5]. The classical version of the "phospha-Mannich" reaction was discovered independently by Kabachnik and Fields more than sixty years ago [6,7].

The α-aminophosphonic and α-aminophosphinic derivatives incorporating an N–C–P moiety are still a focus due to their real or potential biological activity. The acid derivatives of the species under discussion may be regarded as the analogues of their natural counterparts, carboxylic acids. As such, as a consequence of their different properties (tetrahedral P vs. planar C, different acidity, and steric bulk) they are recognized by receptors and enzymes as false substrates/inhibitors [8–12]. The bioactivity realized in this way may be manifested in applications as agrochemicals and medicines.

The mechanism of the phospha-Mannich reaction depends on the nature of the substrates applied. It has been said that the condensation may proceed via an imine (Schiff base) or α-hydroxyphosphonate intermediate (Scheme 1/route "A" and "B" respectively) [13–15].

The number of publications describing different variations of the Kabachnik–Fields reaction exceeds 450 papers. The usual phospha-Mannich protocol includes the condensation of equimolar quantities of the three components in organic solvents and the use of various catalysts, comprising in most cases Lewis and Brönsted acids. A wide range of catalysts have been described, such as metal perchlorates; Amberlysts; succinic-, sulfonic-, and oxalic- acids; zinc, iron, and niobium salt; lanthanide triflates; boron trifluoride etherate; titanium dioxide; etc. [16]. However, it has been found that catalyst-free methods may also be appropriate, especially under solvent-free and/or microwave-assisted conditions [17–23]. The latter protocols represent green chemical approaches that are the focus of this article.

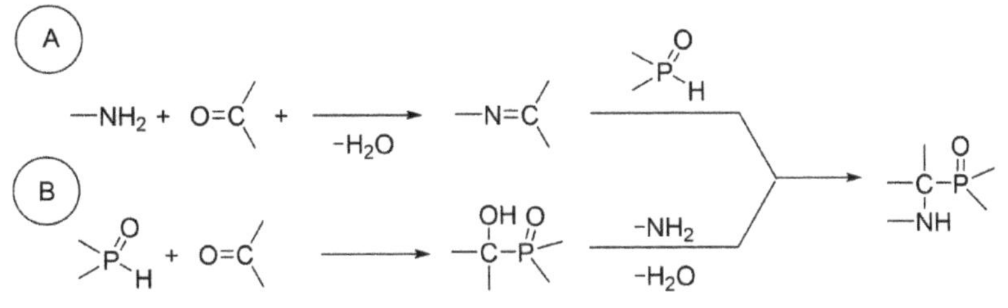

**Scheme 1.** The general mechanism of the phospha-Mannich reaction.

In this review, we summarize the new developments of the Kabachnik–Fields reaction accumulated in the last decade.

## 2. Kabachnik–Fields Reactions with Dialkyl Phosphites, Alkyl *H*-Phosphinates, and Secondary Phosphine Oxides

### *2.1. Metal-Catalyzed Kabachnik–Fields Reactions*

In the first block, metal-catalyzed condensations are summarized. Applying (tetra-tert-buthylphthalocyaninato)aluminum chloride, a series of amines, acetophenone, and diethyl phosphite were condensed to afford the corresponding α-aminophosphonates (**1**) in acceptable yields (Scheme 2(1)). The reaction of benzylamine, indanone (**2**), and ethyl phenyl-*H*-phosphinate led to the respective phosphinate (**3**) (Scheme 2(2)) [24].

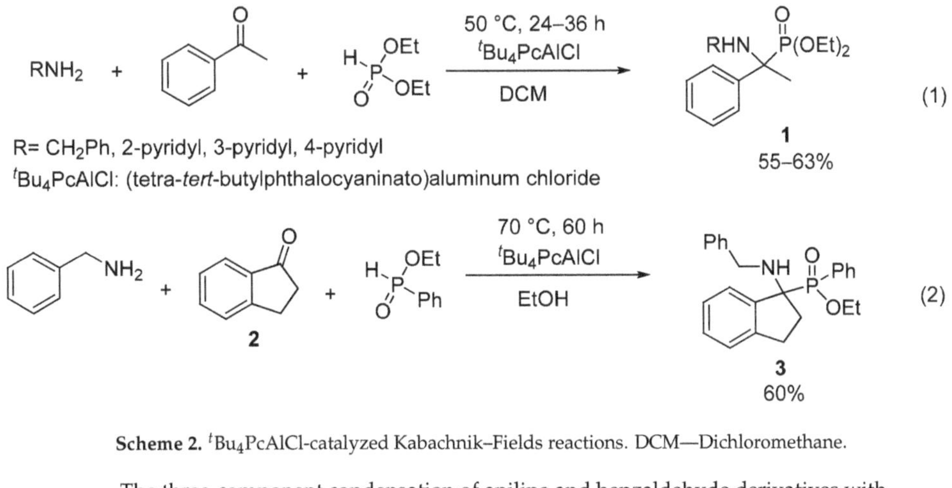

**Scheme 2.** $^{t}Bu_4PcAlCl$-catalyzed Kabachnik–Fields reactions. DCM—Dichloromethane.

The three-component condensation of aniline and benzaldehyde derivatives with dialkyl phosphite (or with diphenyl phosphite) was performed in the presence of a cyclopentadienyl ruthenium(II) complex at 80 °C in a solvent-free manner. The α-aminophosphonates (**4**) were obtained in good to excellent yields (Scheme 3) [25].

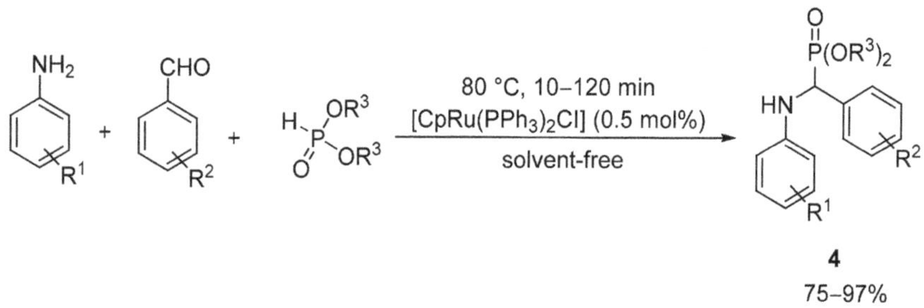

| R¹ | H | C₆H₅ | C₆H₅ | C₆H₅ | C₆H₅ | C₆H₅ | C₆H₅ |
|---|---|---|---|---|---|---|---|
| R² | 4-MeSC₆H₄ | H | 4-CF₃C₆H₄ | 4-BrC₆H₄ | 4-FC₆H₄ | 4-MeSC₆H₄ | 4-MeSC₆H₄ |
| R³ | Et | Et | Et | Et | Et | Et | Me |
| R¹ | C₆H₅ | C₆H₅ | C₆H₅ | 4-FC₆H₄ | 2-HOC₆H₄ | 2-MeOC₆H₄ | |
| R² | 4-MeSC₆H₄ | 4-MeSC₆H₄ | 4-MeOC₆H₄ | 4-MeSC₆H₄ | 4-MeSC₆H₄ | 4-MeSC₆H₄ | |
| R³ | Bu | Ph | Et | Et | Et | Et | |

**Scheme 3.** Ruthenium(II)-complex-catalyzed Kabachnik–Fields reactions.

Potentially biologically active α-aminophosphonates (**6**) were synthesized from quinazolinone-based hydrazides (**5**), aromatic aldehydes, and diphenyl phosphite using $ZnCl_2/PPh_3$ as the catalyst at room temperature (Scheme 4) [26]. The yields fell in the range of 75–84%.

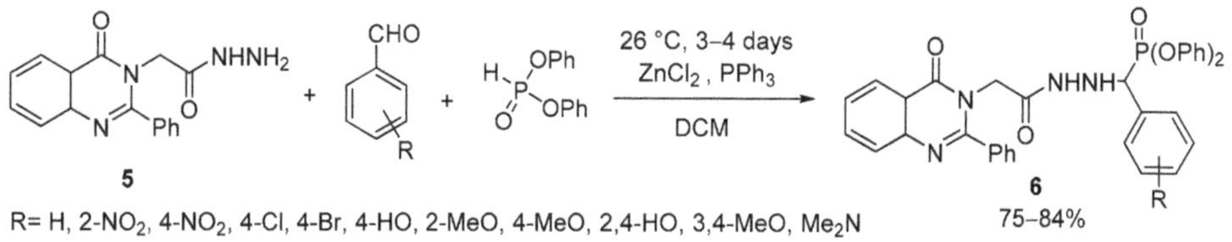

**Scheme 4.** Phospha-Mannich reactions applying quinazolinone-based hydrazides as the amine component.

A similar $ZnCl_2$·choline-chloride-catalyzed transformation of mostly aromatic amines, benzaldehyde derivatives, and diethyl phosphite led to α-amino-benzylphosphonates (**7**) in yields of 70–96% (Scheme 5) [27].

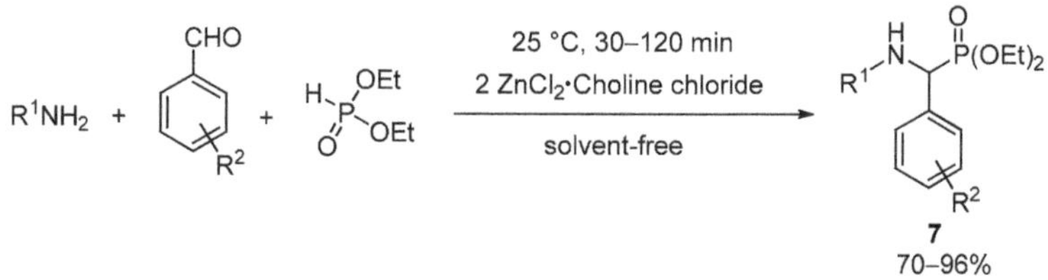

| R¹ | C₆H₅ | C₆H₅ | C₆H₅ | C₆H₅ | C₆H₅ | C₆H₅ | C₆H₅ | C₆H₅ |
|---|---|---|---|---|---|---|---|---|
| R² | C₆H₅ | 4-NO₂C₆H₄ | 2-ClC₆H₄ | 3-ClC₆H₄ | 4-BrC₆H₄ | 3-BrC₆H₄ | 4-HOC₆H₄ | 4-MeOC₆H₄ |
| R¹ | 4-ClC₆H₄ | 4-BrC₆H₄ | 4-FC₆H₄ | 4-ClC₆H₄ | 4-FC₆H₄ | 4-MeOC₆H₄ | C₆H₅CH₂ | |
| R² | C₆H₅ | C₆H₅ | C₆H₅ | 3-ClC₆H₄ | 4-BrC₆H₄ | 4-MeOC₆H₄ | C₆H₅ | |

**Scheme 5.** $ZnCl_2$·choline-chloride-catalyzed three-component condensation.

Zn di[bis(trifluoromethylsulfonyl)imide] (**11**) was also described as a catalyst in a similar condensation, and the product (**8**) was dearylated, suprisingly, by NBS; the intermediate (**9**) so formed was hydrolyzed (**10**) (Scheme 6) [28,29]. Application of an optically active additive (**12**, pybim) allowed an enantioselective synthesis.

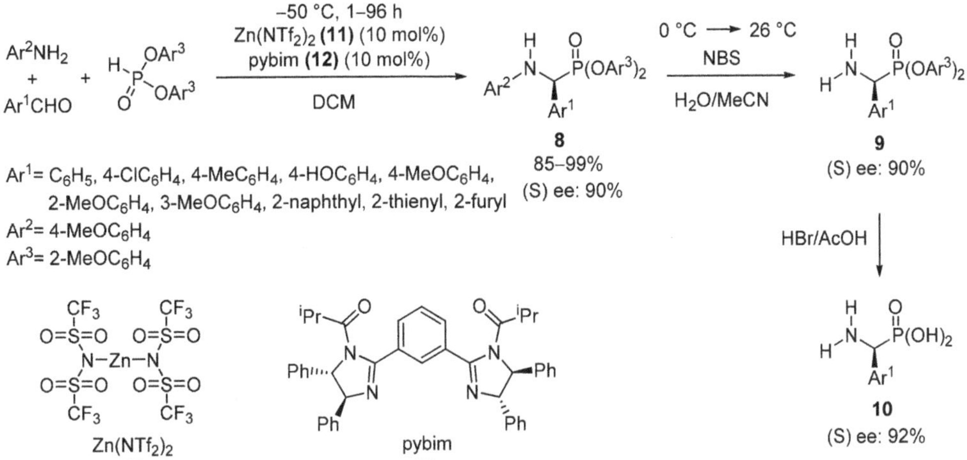


**Scheme 6.** Zn di[bis(trifluoromethylsulfonyl)imide]-catalyzed Kabachnik–Fields reaction. NBS—*N*-bromosuccinimide; pybim—pyridinebisimidazoline; ee—enantiomeric excess.

Zinc triflate and iron triflate also proved to be efficient catalysts in the three-component condensation when different substituted amines or an oxadiazole-related acid hydrazide (**14**) were reacted with benzaldehyde and diethyl phosphite. These reactions took place under mild conditions, mostly in good yields (Schemes 7 and 8) [30,31].

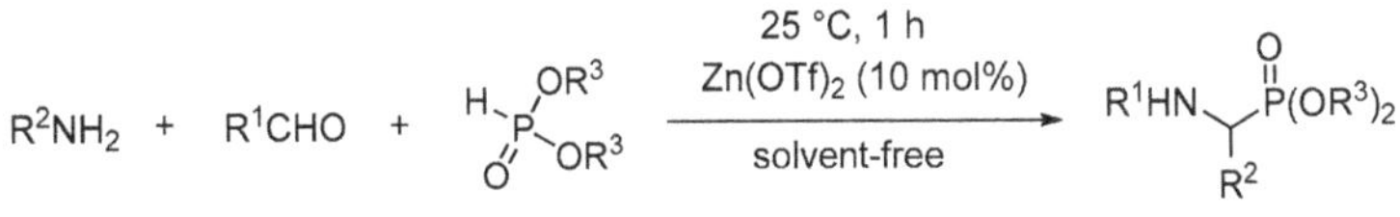


| | | | | | | | |
|---|---|---|---|---|---|---|---|
| **R¹** | $C_6H_5$ | $C_6H_5$ | 4-Cl$C_6H_5$ | 4-MeO$C_6H_5$ | 4-MeO$C_6H_5$ | Et | $^i$Bu |
| **R²** | $CH_2C_6H_5$ | $CH_2C_6H_5$ | $CH_2C_6H_5$ | $CH_2C_6H_5$ | $CH_2C_6H_5$ | $CH_2C_6H_5$ | $CH_2C_6H_5$ |
| **R³** | Et | Me | Et | Et | Me | Et | Et |
| **R¹** | $^i$Bu | 4-$NO_2C_6H_5$ | 4-Cl$C_6H_5$ | 4-Cl$C_6H_5$ | 4-Me$C_6H_5$ | 4-MeO$C_6H_5$ | 4-MeO$C_6H_5$ |
| **R²** | $CH_2C_6H_5$ | $C_6H_5$ | $C_6H_5$ | $C_6H_5$ | $C_6H_5$ | $C_6H_5$ | $C_6H_5$ |
| **R³** | Me | Et | Et | Me | Et | Et | Me |

**Scheme 7.** Zinc-triflate-catalyzed Kabachnik–Fields reaction.

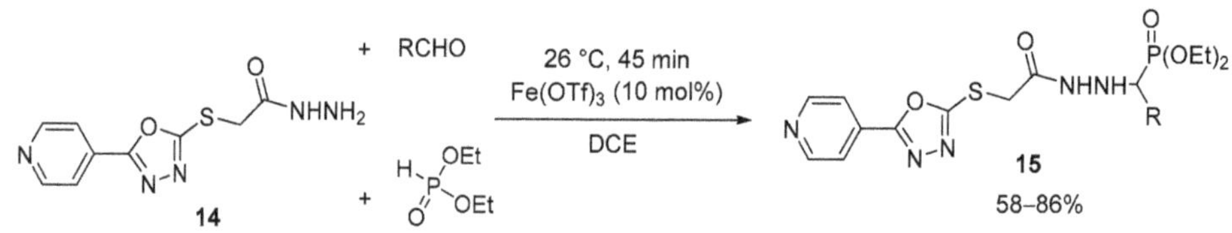

R= $C_6H_5$, 4-$NO_2C_6H_4$, 4-$CNC_6H_4$, 2-$ClC_6H_4$, 4-$BrC_6H_4$, 4-$FC_6H_4$, 4-$HOC_6H_4$, 3-$MeOC_6H_4$, 4-$MeC_6H_4$, 3,4-$HOC_6H_3$, 2,5-$MeOC_6H_3$, 2-thienyl, 2-naphthyl

**Scheme 8.** Oxadiazole-related (**14**) acid hydrazide as the amine component in the phospha-Mannich reaction. DCE—1,2-dichloroethane.

The indium(III)-complex-catalyzed (**17, 18**) methods allowed the efficient condensation of various aldehydes, amines, and >P(O)H reagents under neat conditions at room temperature to give the corresponding α-aminophosphonates or α-aminophosphine oxides (**16**) (Scheme 9) [32]. Theyields were 86–98%. The need for special indium catalysts presents a disadvantage.

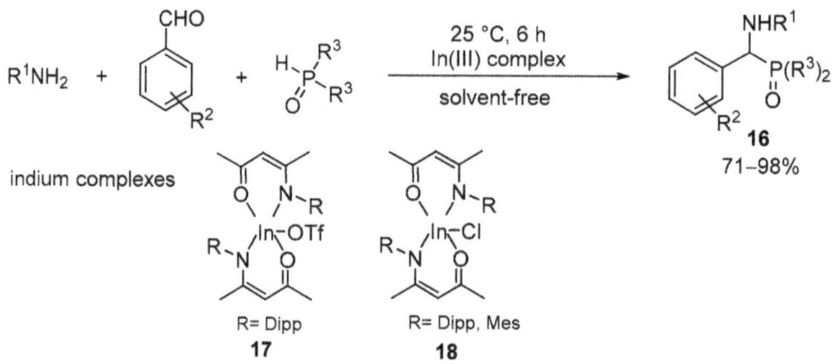

| | | | | | | | |
|---|---|---|---|---|---|---|---|
| **R¹** | $C_6H_5$ | $C_6H_5$ | $C_6H_5$ | $C_6H_5$ | $C_6H_5$ | $C_6H_5$ | $C_6H_5$ |
| **R²** | $C_6H_5$ | 4-$NO_2C_6H_5$ | 4-$CNC_6H_5$ | 4-$ClC_6H_5$ | 3-$ClC_6H_5$ | 4-$FC_6H_5$ | 2-$FC_6H_5$ |
| **R³** | $C_6H_5$ | $C_6H_5$ | $C_6H_5$ | $C_6H_5$ | $C_6H_5$ | $C_6H_5$ | $C_6H_5$ |
| **R¹** | $C_6H_5$ | $C_6H_5$ | $C_6H_5$ | 4-$MeC_6H_5$ | $C_6H_5$ | $CH_2C_6H_5$ | 4-$ClC_6H_5CH_2$ |
| **R²** | 4-$MeC_6H_5$ | 4-$^iPrC_6H_5$ | 4-$MeOC_6H_5$ | 4-$NMe_2C_6H_4$ | 4-$MeSC_6H_5$ | $C_6H_5$ | $C_6H_5$ |
| **R³** | $C_6H_5$ | $C_6H_5$ | $C_6H_5$ | $C_6H_5$ | $C_6H_5$ | $C_6H_5$ | $C_6H_5$ |
| **R¹** | 4-$MeOC_6H_5$ $CH_2$ | 4-$ClC_6H_5$ | 4-$BrC_6H_5$ | 4-$MeC_6H_4$ | 4-$MeOC_6H_4$ | $C_6H_4$ | $C_6H_4$ |
| **R²** | $C_6H_5$ | $C_6H_5$ | 4-$^iPrC_6H_5$ | 3,4-$MeOC_6H_5$ | 4-$PhOC_6H_5$ | 4-$ClC_6H_5$ | 4-$FC_6H_5$ |
| **R³** | $C_6H_5$ | $C_6H_5$ | $C_6H_5$ | $C_6H_5$ | $C_6H_5$ | PhO | PhO |
| **R¹** | $C_6H_4$ | $C_6H_4$ | $C_6H_5$ | $C_6H_5$ | 2-$MeC_6H_5$ | 2-$MeC_6H_5$ | 2-$MeC_6H_5$ |
| **R²** | 4-$^iPrC_6H_5$ | 4-$MeOC_6H_5$ | 4-$NMe_2C_6H_5$ | 3,4-$MeOC_6H_4$ | $C_6H_5$ | $C_6H_4$ | 3,4-$MeOC_6H_4$ |
| **R³** | PhO | PhO | PhO | PhO | PhO | EtO | PhO |
| **R¹** | $C_6H_4$ | $C_6H_5$ | $C_6H_5$ | $C_6H_5$ | $C_6H_5$ | $C_6H_5$ | |
| **R²** | $C_6H_5$ | 4-$BrC_6H_5$ | 4-$MeC_6H_5$ | 4-$^iPrC_6H_5$ | 4-$NMe_2C_6H_5$ | 3,4-$MeOC_6H_4$ | |
| **R³** | EtO | EtO | EtO | EtO | EtO | EtO | |

**Scheme 9.** In(III)-complex-catalyzed three-component condensation. Dipp—2,6-diisopropylphenyl; Mes—2,4,6-trimethylphenyl.

Nickel chloride and niobium chloride were efficient catalysts in the reaction of aniline derivatives, substituted benzaldehydes, and diethyl phosphite at a temperature of 82 °C (Schemes 10 and 11) [33,34]. The use of these catalysts gave the corresponding products (**19** and **4**) in similar yields.

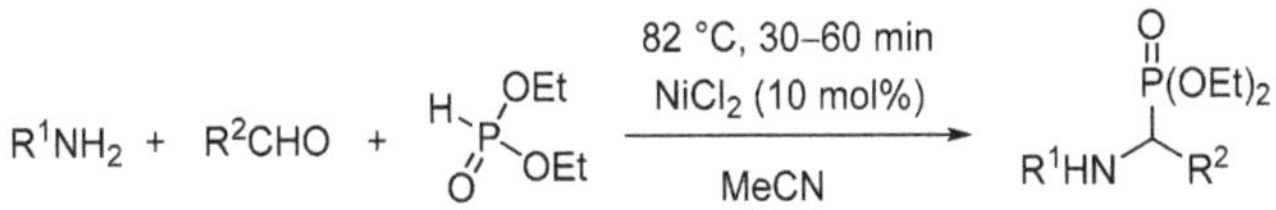

**19**
80–95%

| | | | | | |
|---|---|---|---|---|---|
| **R¹** | $C_6H_5$ | 4-$NO_2C_6H_5$ | 4-$ClC_6H_5$ | 4-$HOC_6H_5$ | 4-$MeC_6H_5$ |
| **R²** | $C_6H_5$ | $C_6H_5$ | $C_6H_5$ | $C_6H_5$ | $C_6H_5$ |
| **R¹** | 4-$MeOC_6H_5$ | $C_6H_5$ | $C_6H_5$ | $C_6H_5$ | $C_6H_5$ |
| **R²** | $C_6H_5$ | 4-$NO_2C_6H_5$ | 4-$ClC_6H_5$ | 4-$MeC_6H_5$ | 4-$MeOC_6H_5$ |

**Scheme 10.** Ni(II)-chloride-catalyzed Kabachnik–Fields reaction.

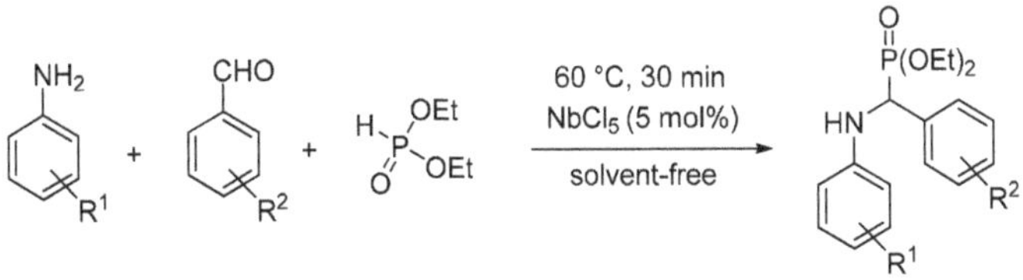

**4** ($R^3$= Et)
87–95%

| | | | | | | | |
|---|---|---|---|---|---|---|---|
| **R¹** | H | 2-$NO_2$ | 4-$NO_2$ | 4-Cl | 4-Br | 4-Me | 4-MeO |
| **R²** | H | H | H | H | H | H | H |
| **R¹** | H | H | H | H | 4-$NH_2$ | 4-$NO_2$ | 4-$NO_2$ |
| **R²** | 4-CHO | 4-Cl | 2-Cl | 4-Me | H | H | 4-CHO |
| **R¹** | 4-$NO_2$ | 4-Cl | 4-Cl | 4-Br | 4-Br | | |
| **R²** | 4-MeO | 4-$NO_2$ | 4-Cl | 4-$NO_2$ | 4-MeO | | |

**Scheme 11.** Niobium-chloride-catalyzed phospha-Mannich reaction.

A series of α-aminophosphonate derivatives (**21**) incorporating an uracil moiety was synthesized using $Mg(ClO_4)_2$ as the catalyst and acetonitrile as the solvent at 80 °C (Scheme 12) [35]. The products showed potential herbicidal activity.

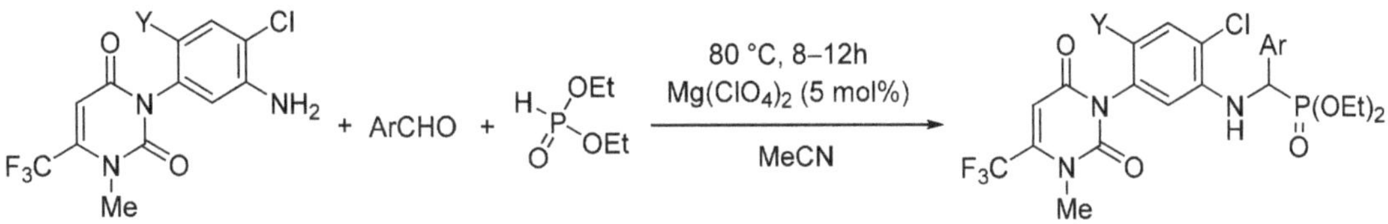

**20**

**21**
72–93%

| | | | | | | |
|---|---|---|---|---|---|---|
| **Ar** | $C_6H_5$ | $C_6H_5$ | 4-$NO_2C_6H_5$ | 4-$NO_2C_6H_5$ | 3-$NO_2C_6H_5$ | 3-$NO_2C_6H_5$ |
| **Y** | Cl | H | Cl | H | Cl | H |
| **Ar** | 4-$ClC_6H_5$ | 4-$ClC_6H_5$ | 4-$FC_6H_5$ | 4-$FC_6H_5$ | 4-$MeC_6H_5$ | 4-$MeC_6H_5$ |
| **Y** | Cl | H | Cl | H | Cl | H |

**Scheme 12.** $Mg(ClO_4)_2$-catalyzed Kabachnik–Fields reactions.

A series of substituted diethyl α-phenylamino-benzylphosphonates (**4** ($R^3$ = Et)) was prepared using cerium chloride or cerium oxide from aniline derivatives, substituted benzaldehydes, and diethyl phosphite under mild and solvent-free conditions (Schemes 13 and 14) [36,37]. The yields were 87–95%.

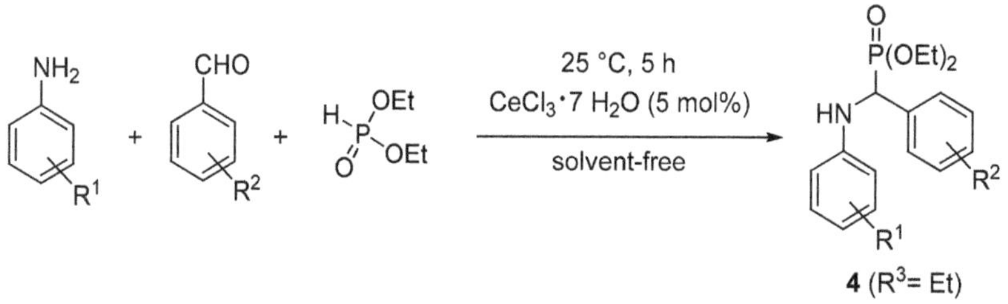


| | | | | | | |
|---|---|---|---|---|---|---|
| $R^1$ | H | H | H | H | H | H |
| $R^2$ | H | 4-$NO_2$ | 4-CN | 4-Cl | 2-Cl | 4-F |
| $R^1$ | H | H | H | H | 2-$NO_2$ | 4-CN |
| $R^2$ | 2-HO | 4-MeO | 3,4-MeO | 2,5-MeO | H | H |
| $R^1$ | 4-Cl | 3-Cl | 4-Br | 2-HO | 4-HO | 4-MeO |
| $R^2$ | H | H | H | H | H | H |

**Scheme 13.** Cerium-chloride-catalyzed condensations.

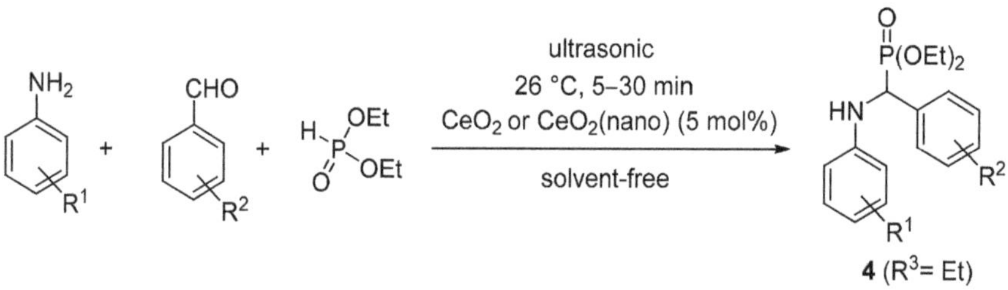


| | | | | | | |
|---|---|---|---|---|---|---|
| $R^1$ | H | 4-$NO_2$ | 4-Cl | 4-Me | 4-HO | 4-MeO |
| $R^2$ | H | H | H | H | H | H |
| $R^1$ | H | H | H | H | H | |
| $R^2$ | 4-$NO_2$ | 4-Cl | 4-Me | 4-HO | 4-MeO | |

**Scheme 14.** Cerium-oxide-catalyzed Kabachnik–Fields reaction.

Cu/Au and Gd oxide nanocatalysts allowed the efficient condensation of different amines, benzaldehyde derivatives, and dimethyl phosphite under conventional heating or under microwave (MW) irradiation (Schemes 15 and 16) [38,39]. The use of these catalysts gave the corresponding products (**22** and **24**) in similar yields.

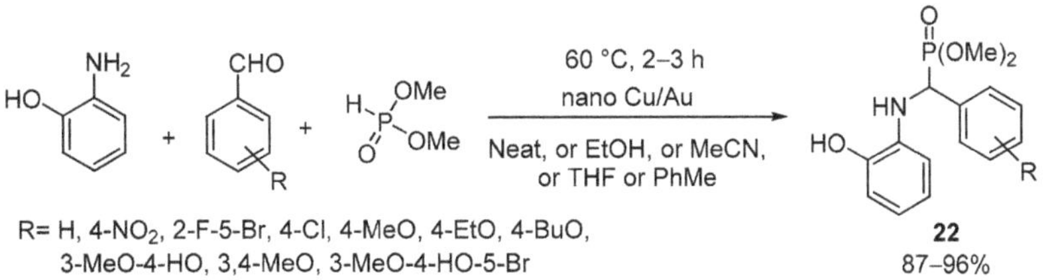

**Scheme 15.** Cu/Au nanocatalyst in the Kabachnik–Fields reaction. THF—tetrahydrofuran.

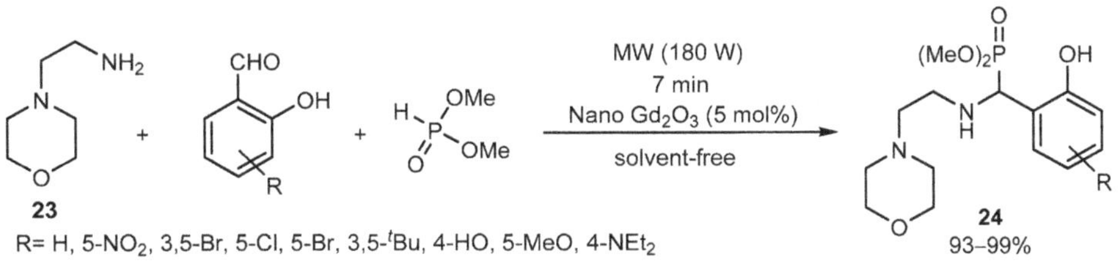

**Scheme 16.** Gadolinium oxide as a nanocatalyst in the phospha-Mannich reaction.

Dehydroascorbic acid (DHAA)-capped magnetite nanoparticles were successfully applied in the phospha-Mannich condensation of aromatic amines and aldehydes with dimethyl phosphite (Scheme 17) [40].

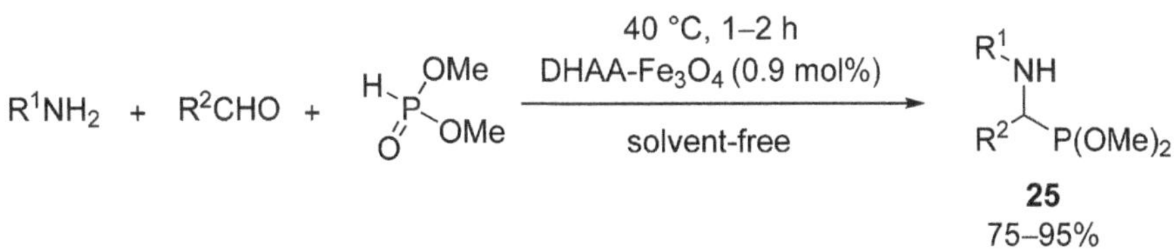

| | | | | | | | |
|---|---|---|---|---|---|---|---|
| **R¹** | $C_6H_5$ | $C_6H_5$ | $C_6H_5$ | $C_6H_5$ | $C_6H_5$ | 4-Br$C_6H_4$ | 4-Me$C_6H_4$ |
| **R²** | $C_6H_5$ | 4-Cl$C_6H_4$ | 4-Me$C_6H_4$ | 4-MeO$C_6H_4$ | thien-2-yl | $C_6H_5$ | $C_6H_5$ |

**Scheme 17.** Dehydroascorbic-acid-catalyzed Kabachnik–Fields reactions.

A deep eutectic solvent (DES) comprising $ZrOCl_2 \cdot 8H_2O$ and urea in a 1:5 ratio made possible the efficient condensation of aryl-(heteroaryl)aldehydes, aniline derivatives and dimethyl phosphite at room temperature. The role of the DES was to serve as a reaction medium and as a catalyst (Scheme 18) [41].

In the above discussion, metal-catalyzed reactions are summarized. The application of metal catalysts makes possible efficient condensations, most of which occur at room temperature; however, these methods, especially the ones applying Zn or Ni promoters, cannot be considered environmentally friendly. At the same time, MW-assisted and solvent-free approaches may be considered as green techniques.

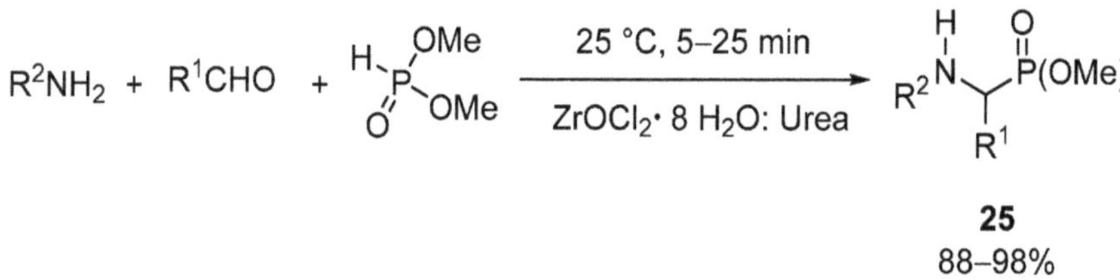

| | | | | | |
|---|---|---|---|---|---|
| **R¹** | $C_6H_5$ | $C_6H_5$ | $C_6H_5$ | 3-$NO_2C_6H_4$ | 4-$ClC_6H_4$ |
| **R²** | $C_6H_5$ | 4-$BrC_6H_4$ | 4-$MeOC_6H_4$ | $C_6H_5$ | $C_6H_5$ |
| **R¹** | 4-$ClC_6H_4$ | 4-$ClC_6H_4$ | 4-$MeOC_6H_4$ | 4-$MeOC_6H_4$ | 2-$MeOC_6H_4$ |
| **R²** | 3-$ClC_6H_4$ | 4-$MeOC_6H_4$ | $C_6H_5$ | 3-$ClC_6H_4$ | $C_6H_5$ |
| **R¹** | 2-$MeOC_6H_4$ | 2-$MeOC_6H_4$ | 2-$MeOC_6H_4$ | 3,4-$(MeO)_2C_6H_3$ | 3,4-$(MeO)_2C_6H_3$ |
| **R²** | 4-$BrC_6H_4$ | 3-$ClC_6H_4$ | 4-$MeOC_6H_4$ | $C_6H_5$ | 3-$ClC_6H_4$ |
| **R¹** | 3,4-$(MeO)_2C_6H_3$ | 3,4,5-$(MeO)_3C_6H_2$ | 3,4,5-$(MeO)_3C_6H_2$ | 1-furyl | 1-naphthyl |
| **R²** | 4-$BrC_6H_4$ | $C_6H_5$ | 3-$ClC_6H_4$ | $C_6H_5$ | $C_6H_5$ |

**Scheme 18.** Kabachnik–Fields reaction with a DES as the solvent and the catalyst.

## 2.2. *Acid-Catalyzed Kabachnik–Fields Reactions*

The Kabachnik–Fields condensations outlined in the next section are promoted by acidic catalysts. The reaction of aniline derivatives, substituted benzaldehydes, and dimethyl phosphite was performed using a bifunctional acid–base catalyst (IRMOF-3, where MOF is a metal organic framework: $Zn_4O(H_2N\text{-}TA)_3$ prepared from 2-aminoterephthalic acid ($H_2ATA$) and $Zn(NO_3)_2{\cdot}6H_2O$) (Scheme 19) [42]. The other option was to use a sulfated polyborate as the catalyst (Scheme 20) [43]. When applying IRMOF-3 and sulfated polyborate as the catalyst, the corresponding products were formed in similar yields.

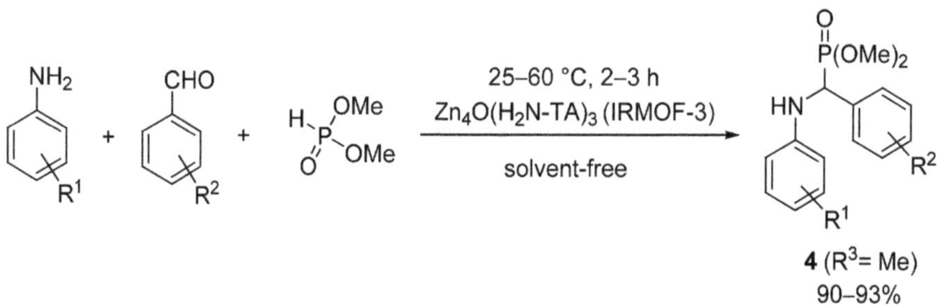

| | | | | | | |
|---|---|---|---|---|---|---|
| **R¹** | H | H | H | 4-Me | 4-Me | 4-Me |
| **R²** | H | 3-$NO_2$ | 4-Cl | 4-$NO_2$ | 2-Cl | 2-MeO |

**Scheme 19.** $Zn_4O(H_2N\text{-}TA)_3$ as the catalyst in three-component reactions.

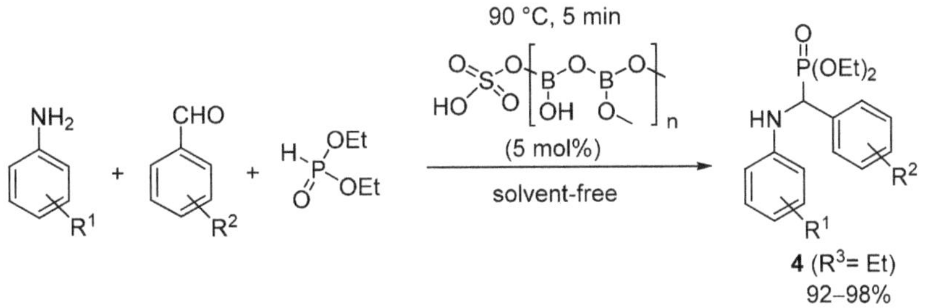

| R¹ | H | H | H | H | H | H | H | H |
|---|---|---|---|---|---|---|---|---|
| R² | H | 2-$NO_2$ | 3-$NO_2$ | 4-$NO_2$ | 2-Cl | 3-Cl | 4-Cl | 4-Br |
| R¹ | H | H | H | H | 4-$NO_2$ | 4-Cl | 4-Br | 4-Me |
| R² | 4-HO | 4-MeO | 2-MeO | 4-Me | H | H | H | H |

**Scheme 20.** Sulfated polyborate-catalyzed condensations.

An efficient method was developed for the preparation of α-aminophosphonates (**26**), which involved applying phenylboronic acid as the catalyst under solvent-free conditions at 50 °C (Scheme 21) [44].

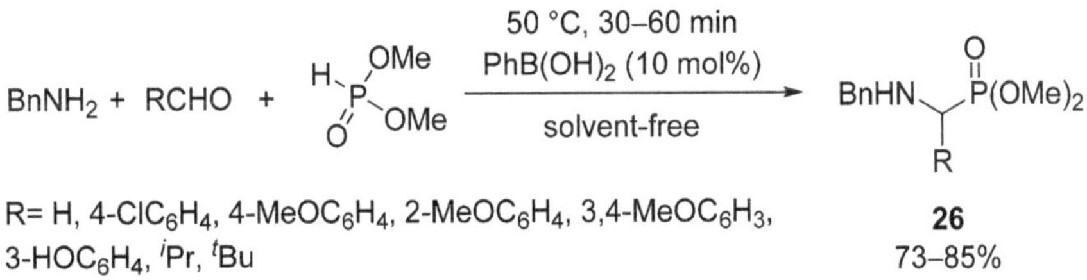

**Scheme 21.** Phenylboronic-acid-catalyzed phospha-Mannich reactions.

Phenylphosphonic acid was found to be an efficient reusable heterogeneous catalyst in the three-component phospha-Mannich reaction of benzylamine, aldehydes/ketones, and dimethyl phosphite (Scheme 22) [45].

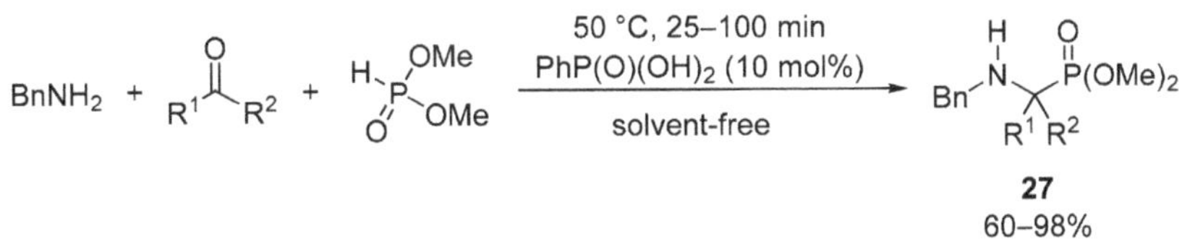

| R¹ | 4-Cl$C_6H_4$ | 4-F$C_6H_4$ | 4-Ph$C_6H_4$ | 3-MeO$C_6H_4$ | 2-MeO$C_6H_3$ | 3-HO$C_6H_4$ |
|---|---|---|---|---|---|---|
| R² | H | H | H | H | H | H |
| R¹ | 3,4-$(HO)_2C_6H_3$ | 3,4-$(MeO)_2C_6H_3$ | 3-indole | 2-pyrrole | 2-furyl | Pr |
| R² | H | H | H | H | H | H |
| R¹ | $^i$Bu | $^i$Pr | Me | Et | | |
| R² | H | H | Me | Et | | |

**Scheme 22.** Phenylphosphonic-acid-catalyzed condensations.

The condensation of aminophenols, benzaldehyde derivatives, and dimethyl phosphite was performed in an aqueous medium containing oxalic acid as the catalyst at 90 °C. No yields were achieved (Scheme 23) [46].

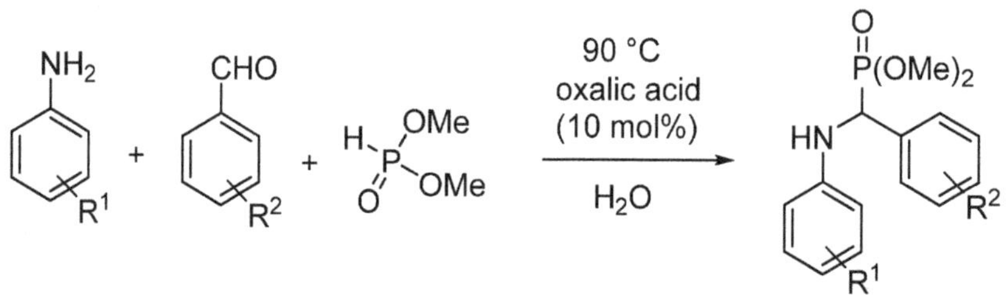


**4** ($R^3$= Me)

| **R¹** | 4-HO | 4-HO | 4-HO | 2-HO | 2-HO | 2-HO |
|---|---|---|---|---|---|---|
| **R²** | H | 4-$NO_2$ | 4-MeO | H | 4-$NO_2$ | 4-MeO |

**Scheme 23.** Oxalic-acid-catalyzed Kabachnik–Fields reactions.

The latter approach provided the α-aminophosphonates in almost quantitative yields.

In another, more general example, a highly efficient biodegradable supramolecular polymer-supported catalyst was applied (Scheme 24) [47]. The catalyst represents a green component.

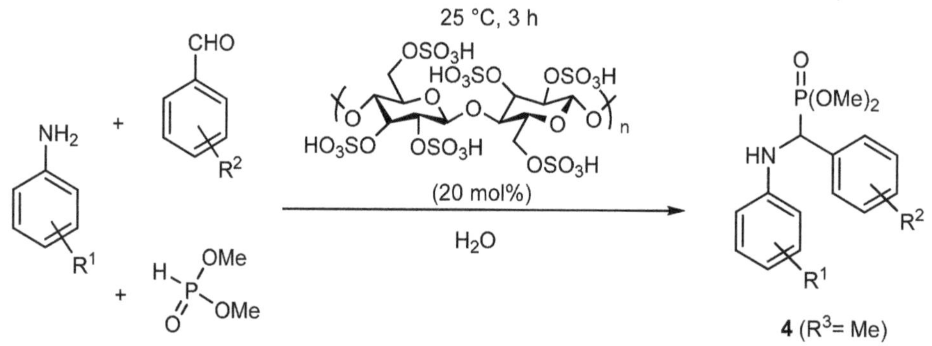


**4** ($R^3$= Me)
94–95%

| **R¹** | H | H | H | 4-Me | 4-Me | 4-Me |
|---|---|---|---|---|---|---|
| **R²** | H | 3-$NO_2$ | 4-Cl | 4-$NO_2$ | 2-Cl | 2-MeO |

**Scheme 24.** Application of biodegradable supramolecular polymer-supported catalyst in the Kabachnik–Fields reaction.

The readily available paratoluenesulfonic acid (PTSA) was found to be a suitable catalyst in a series of phospha-Mannich reactions. The thoroughly investigated model reaction is shown in Scheme 25 [48].

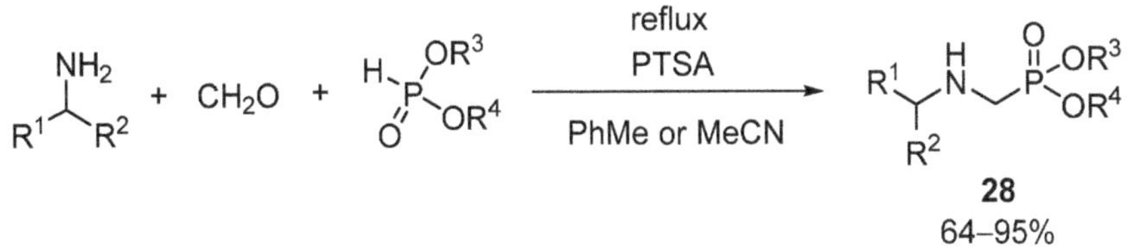

| | | | | | |
|---|---|---|---|---|---|
| **R¹** | Me | Me | Me | COOH | COOH |
| **R²** | $C_6H_5$ | $C_6H_5$ | $C_6H_5$ | Me | Me |
| **R³** | $^nC_8H_{17}$ | $^nC_{10}H_{21}$ | $^c$Hex | $^nC_{10}H_{21}$ | $^c$Hex |
| **R⁴** | $^nC_8H_{17}$ | $^nC_{10}H_{21}$ | $^c$Hex | $C_6H_5$ | $^c$Hex |

**Scheme 25.** PTSA-catalyzed Kabachnik–Fields reactions.

PTSA was also used in the condensation of different amines, formaldehyde, and secondary phosphine oxides in toluene at the boiling point (Scheme 26) [49]. The yields of products **29** and **30** were ≥90%.

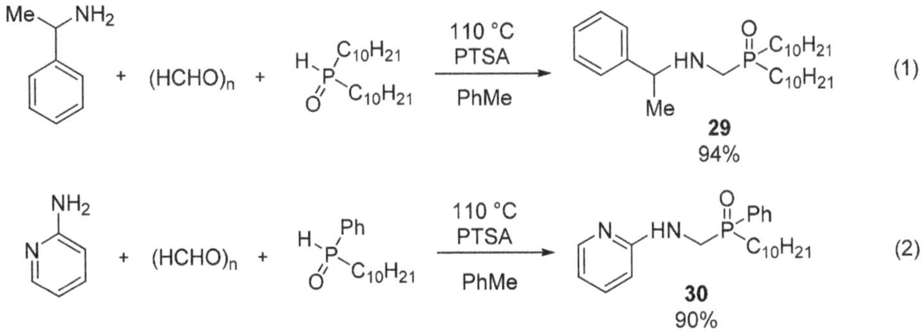

**Scheme 26.** Other PTSA-catalyzed condensations.

New α-aminophosphine oxides and α-aminophosphonates (**32**/**33**) were made available by the PTSA-catalyzed reaction of amines containing an acetal group (**31**), paraformaldehyde, and >P(O)H reagents (Schemes 27 and 28) [50,51]. No yields were achieved for the second series of reactions.

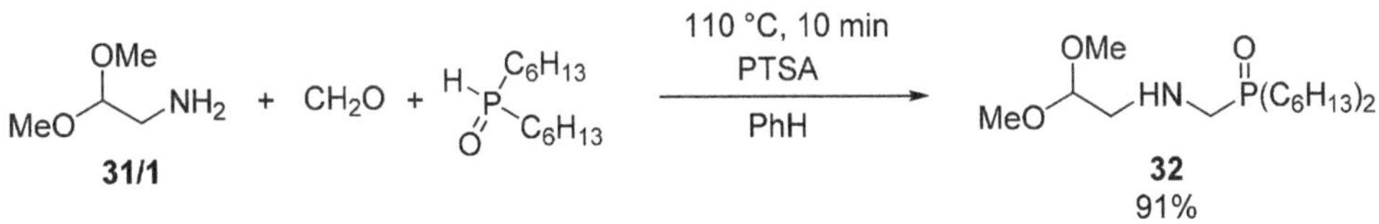

**Scheme 27.** Further application of the PTSA catalyst in phospha-Mannich condensations.

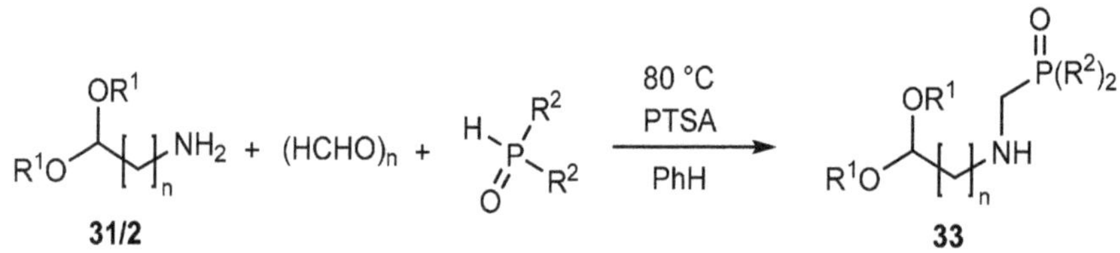

| $R^1$ | Me | Me | Me | Me | Me | Et | Et | Et |
|---|---|---|---|---|---|---|---|---|
| $R^2$ | EtO | $^i$PrO | $C_6H_{13}$ | $C_8H_{17}$ | $C_{10}H_{21}$ | $C_6H_{13}$ | $C_8H_{17}$ | $C_{10}H_{21}$ |
| n | 1 | 1 | 1 | 1 | 1 | 2 | 2 | 3 |

**Scheme 28.** Extension of the Kabachnik–Fields reactions outlined in Scheme 19.

Solvent-free realizations may be typically associated with MW irradiation. This was the case with the polystyrene-supported PTSA-catalyzed condensation of 2-aminofluorene (**34**), a number of aldehydes, and dimethyl phosphite (Scheme 29) [52].

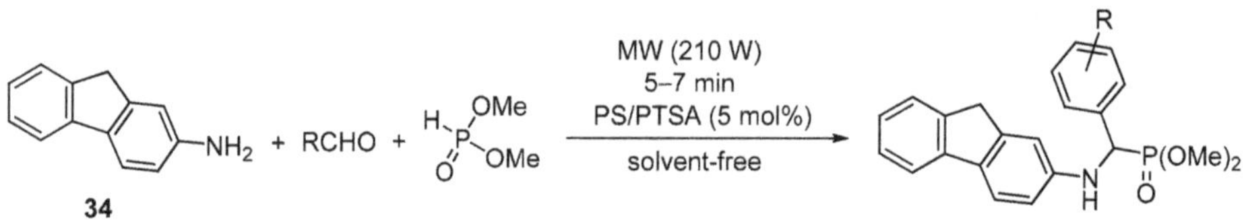

R= 4-$NO_2C_6H_4$, 2-$NO_2C_6H_4$, 4-$ClC_6H_4$, 2-$ClC_6H_4$, 4-$BrC_6H_4$, 4-$FC_6H_4$, 4-$MeC_6H_4$, 4-$HOC_6H_4$, 3-$HOC_6H_4$, 4-$MeOC_6H_4$, 3-$MeOC_6H_4$, Et, Pr, $^i$Pr, $^n$Bu, $^c$Hex

**Scheme 29.** Solvent-free, PTSA-catalyzed condensations involving 2-aminofluorene.

β-Cyclodextrin-supported sulfonic acid was also used as an efficient and reusable heterogeneous catalyst in the preparation of thiazolylaryl α-aminophosphonates (**37**) (Scheme 30) [53].

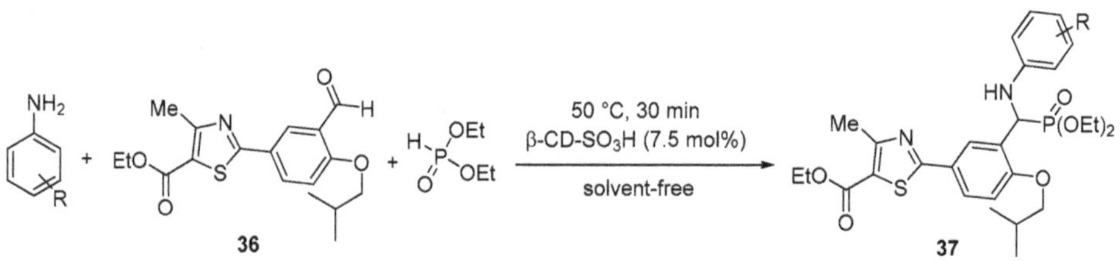

R= H, 4-$NO_2$, 4-$CF_3$, 4-F, 3-Cl, 4-Br, 2-I, 4-MeO

**Scheme 30.** β-Cyclodextrin-supported sulfonic-acid-catalyzed condensation.

6-Amino-1,3-dimethyluracil (**38**) was found to be a good starting material in condensation with benzaldehyde derivatives and diethyl phosphite. Phosphorus pentoxide in methanesulfonic acid (1:10), known as Eaton's reagent, was the catalyst (Scheme 31) [54].

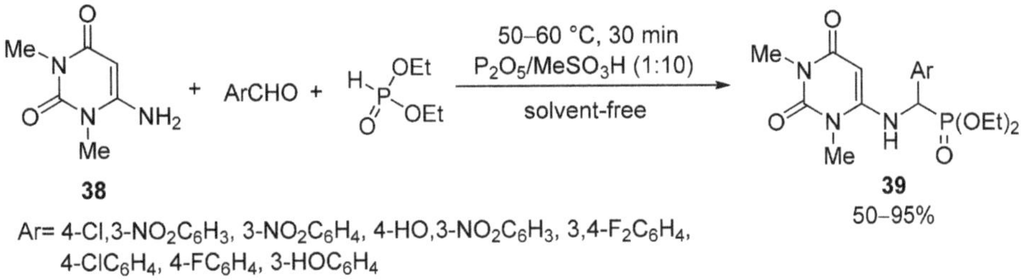

Scheme 31. Eaton's reagent used as a catalyst in the condensations.

The condensation of the basic model (aniline derivatives, substituted benzaldehydes, and diethyl phosphite) was also performed with water as the medium, using different organic acid catalysts (Scheme 32) [55]. The yields were variable.

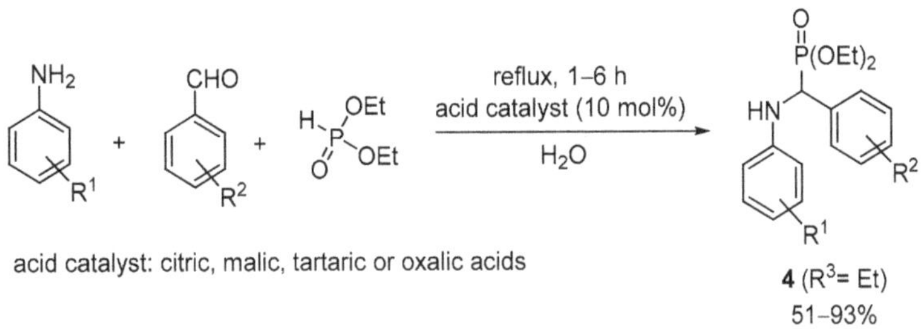

| | | | | | | | |
|---|---|---|---|---|---|---|---|
| $R^1$ | H | H | H | 2-HO, 4-$NO_2$ | 2-HO, 2-Cl | 4-HO | 2-HO |
| $R^2$ | H | 4-$NO_2$ | 4-MeO | H | H | H | H |
| $R^1$ | 2-HO, 4-Me | 2-HO, 4-$NO_2$ | 2-HO, 2-Cl | 4-HO | 2-HO | 2-HO, 4-Me | 2-HO, 4-MeO |
| $R^2$ | H | 4-$NO_2$ | 4-$NO_2$ | 4-$NO_2$ | 4-$NO_2$ | 4-$NO_2$ | 4-$NO_2$ |
| $R^1$ | 2-HO, 4-$NO_2$ | 2-HO, 2-Cl | 4-HO | 2-HO | 2-HO, 4-Me | 2-HO, 4-MeO | |
| $R^2$ | 4-MeO | 4-MeO | 4-MeO | 4-MeO | 4-MeO | 4-MeO | |

Scheme 32. Various organic-acid-catalyzed Kabachnik–Fields reactions.

Potassium hydrogen sulfate also proved to be a powerful catalyst in the above type of reaction (Scheme 33) [56].

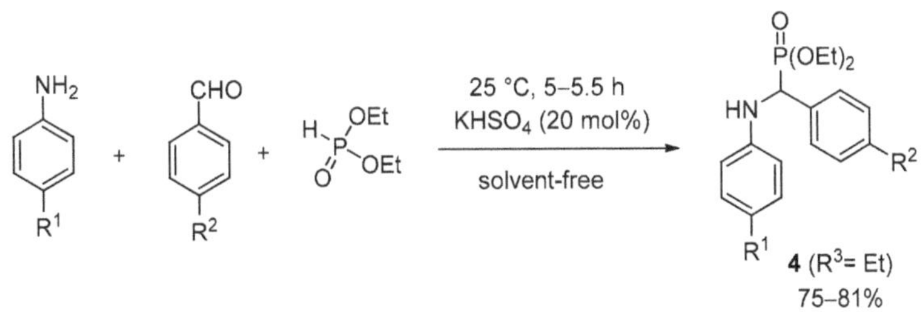

| | | | | | |
|---|---|---|---|---|---|
| $R^1$ | H | Br | H | Br | Br |
| $R^2$ | H | H | Me | Me | Br |

Scheme 33. Potassium-hydrogen-sulfate-catalyzed condensations.

2-Cyclopropylpyridimidine-4-carbaldehyde (**40**) was also used as the starting material in three-component condensations. In one case, phosphomolybdic acid was applied as the catalyst (Scheme 34) [57]; in another, camphor-derived thiourea organocatalysts (**42, 43**) were utilized (Scheme 35) [58]. The yields of products (**41**) were mostly high.

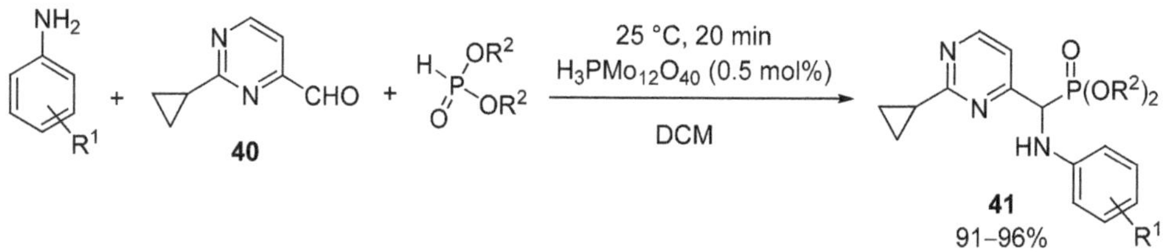


| R¹ | H | 4-Cl | 4-Br | 4-Me | H | 4-Cl | 4-Me |
|---|---|---|---|---|---|---|---|
| R² | $C_6H_5$ | $C_6H_5$ | $C_6H_5$ | $C_6H_5$ | Et | Et | Et |

**Scheme 34.** 2-Cyclopropylpyridimidine-4-carbaldehyde (**40**) as a special actor in the Kabachnik–Fields reactions.

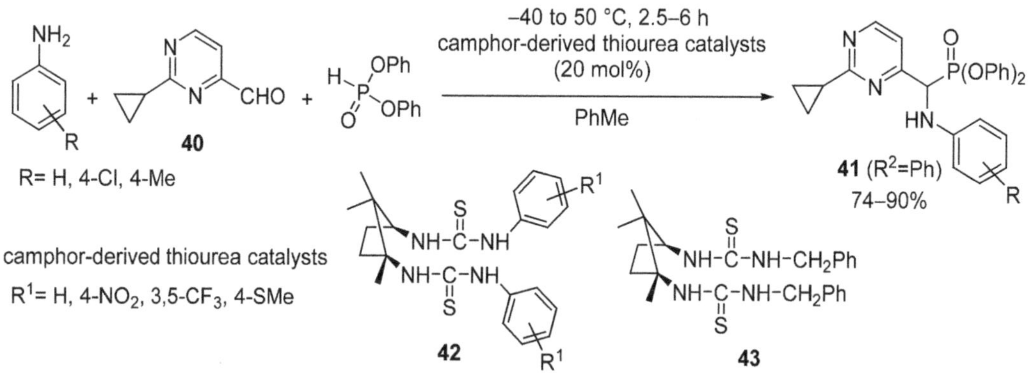


**Scheme 35.** Camphor-derived thiourea organocatalysts used in Kabachnik–Fields reactions.

Zeolite derivatives such as H-β zeolite and MCM-41 were applied as green catalysts in different kinds of three-component condensations under discussion (Schemes 36 and 37) [59,60]. In the second series, quinoline-4-carbaldehyde (**44**) was the oxo component.

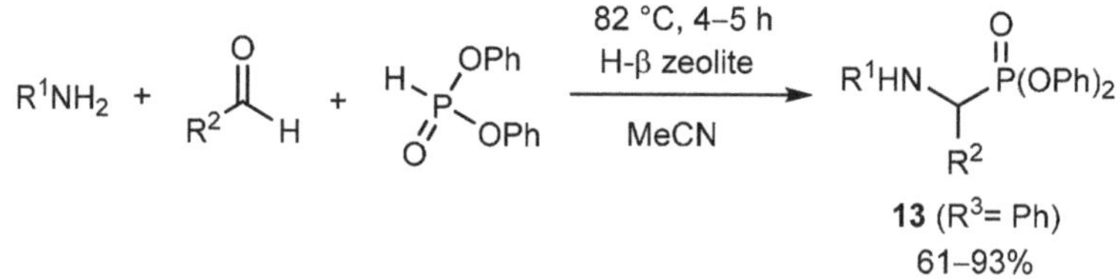


| R¹ | $C_6H_5$ | 4-$NO_2C_6H_4$ | 4-$MeOC_6H_4$ | 4-$MeOC_6H_4$ | Bu | ᶜHex |
|---|---|---|---|---|---|---|
| R² | $C_6H_5$ | 4-$NO_2C_6H_4$ | 4-$MeOC_6H_4$ | Bu | $CH_2C_6H_5$ | $CH_2C_6H_5$ |

**Scheme 36.** H-β zeolite as a green catalyst in the phospha-Mannich reaction.

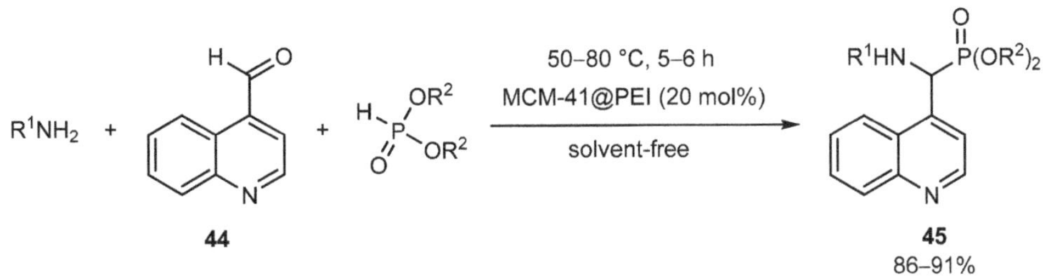


| | | | | | |
|---|---|---|---|---|---|
| **R¹** | $C_6H_5$ | 4-$FC_4H_6$ | $C_6H_4CH_2CH_2$ | $C_6H_5$ | 4-$FC_4H_6$ |
| **R²** | $C_6H_5$ | $C_6H_5$ | $C_6H_5$ | Et | Et |

**Scheme 37.** MCM-41 as a catalyst in the Kabachnik–Fields reaction.

Regarding the acid-catalyzed Kabachnik–Fields reactions, those applying water as the solvent or a biodegradable catalyst, or those that may be performed under solvent-free conditions, can be considered "green". PTSA has been used in various Kabachnik–Fields reactions as an efficient catalyst. The application of other acidic catalysts (camphor-derived thiourea catalysts, H-β zeolite, MCM-41) gave the corresponding products in variable yields.

The phospha-Mannich reaction of 5-hydroxymethyl-furan-1-carbaldehyde (**46**) with aniline and diethyl phosphite was catalyzed by elemental iodine, allowing the condensation under mild conditions (Scheme 38) [61]. It is noteworthy that 2-methyltetrahydrofuran was used as a green solvent. The yields of the α-aminophosphonates (**47**) were variable.

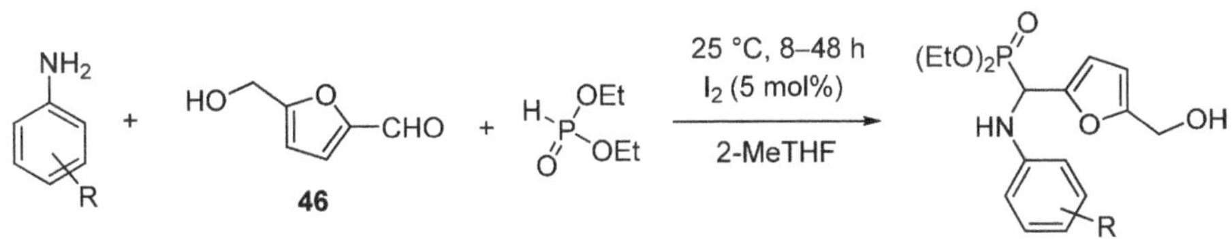


R= $C_6H_5$, 4-$NO_2C_6H_5$, 3-$CF_3C_6H_5$, 4-$ClC_6H_5$, 2-$ClC_6H_5$, 3-$ClC_6H_5$, 4-$BrC_6H_5$, 4-$IC_6H_5$, 4-$MeOC_6H_5$, Bu, $^c$Hex, $CH_2C_6H_5$

**47**
53–91%

**Scheme 38.** 5-Hydroxymethyl-furan-1-carbaldehyde applied as the oxo component in the Kabachnik–Fields reaction.

It was proven that the reaction proceeds via the imine pathway, which is followed by the nucleophilic attack of the diethyl phosphite to furnish the α-aminophosphonate. The role of iodine is to activate the imine(s) in the nucleophilic addition. Iodine may act as a Lewis acid [61].

α-(Furfurylamino)-alkylphosphonates (**49**) were synthesized by the Kabachnik–Fields reaction of furfurylamine (**48**), aromatic aldehydes, and dialkyl phosphites under MW irradiation. Silica-gel-supported iodine was used as the catalyst under solvent-free conditions. The plant growth regulatory activity of the products was investigated (Scheme 39) [62].

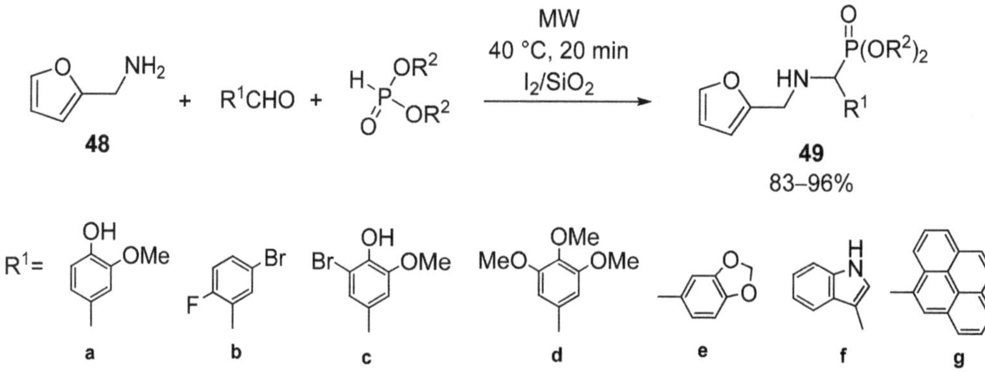

| R¹ | a | a | b | c | d | d | e | f | f | g |
|---|---|---|---|---|---|---|---|---|---|---|
| R² | Me | Et | Et | Et | Me | Et | Me | Me | Et | Et |

**Scheme 39.** Silica-gel-supported iodine-catalyzed condensations.

A Lewis-acid-type ionic liquid ([bmim][$AlCl_4$]) was a novel catalyst in the three-component condensations performed under sonochemical irradiation (Scheme 40) [63].

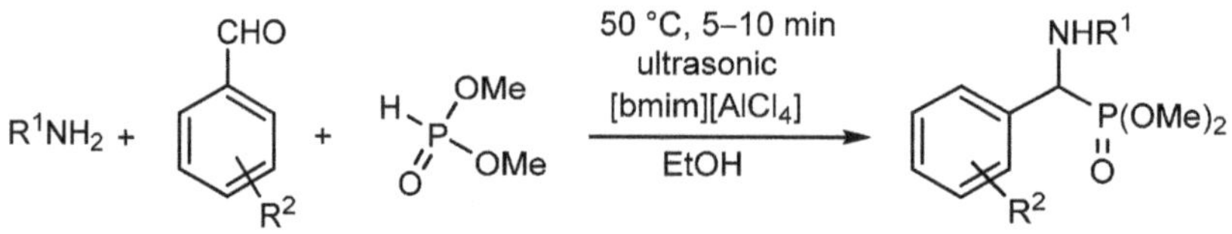

**16** ($R^3$= OMe)
88–93%

| R¹ | $C_6H_5$ | $C_6H_5$ | $C_6H_5$ | 4-Me$C_6H_4$ | 4-Me$C_6H_4$ | 4-Me$C_6H_4$ |
|---|---|---|---|---|---|---|
| R² | H | 3-$NO_2$ | 4-Cl | 4-$NO_2$ | 2-Cl | 2-MeO |

**Scheme 40.** Examples of the ionic-liquid-catalyzed Kabachnik–Fields reaction. [bmim]—butyl-methylimidazolyl.

### 2.3. *Catalyst-Free Kabachnik–Fields Reactions*

Having discussed the catalyst-promoted Kabachnik–Fields condensations, let us focus instead on the catalyst-free variations, which represent an environmentally friendly approach. The application of ionic liquids (**50** or **51**) as the solvent allowed the condensation of the three-components at room temperature (Scheme 41(1) and (2)) [64]. Both mono- (**4**) and bis products (**52**) were identified. The yields were variable, and fell in the range of 25–96%. There were no data provided on the recycling of the ionic liquids.

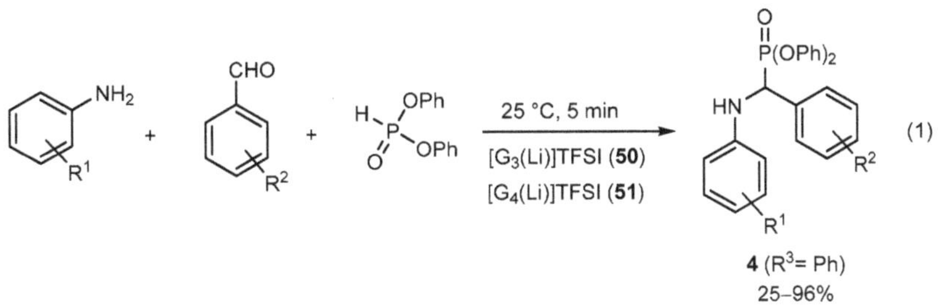


| | | | | | | | |
|---|---|---|---|---|---|---|---|
| R¹ | H | 4-NO₂ | 3-CF₃ | 4-Cl | 3-Cl | 4-F | 3,5-CF₃ |
| R² | H | H | H | H | H | H | H |
| R¹ | 4-OH | H | H | H | H | H | H |
| R² | H | 4-NO₂ | 4-F | 4-Br | 3,4-Cl | 2-OH | 4-Me |

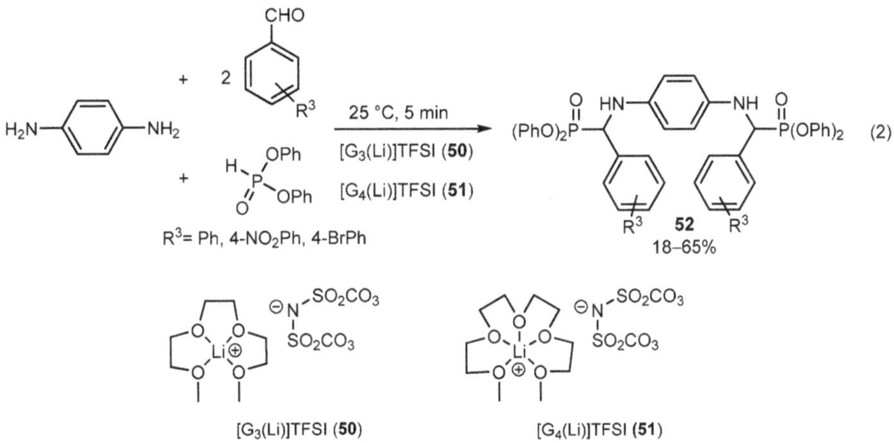


**Scheme 41.** Catalyst-free approaches towards α-aminophosphonates. (Li)TFSI—lithium bis(trifluoromethanesulfonyl)imide.

The expected reaction of alkylamines, 2-hydroxy-4-methoxyacetophenone (**53**), and a series of phosphites in boiling toluene followed an intramolecular cyclization to furnish heterocyclic α-aminophosphonates (**54**) (Scheme 42) [65].

In a somewhat analogous reaction, Bálint et al. reacted 2-formylbenzoic acid, primary amines, and dialkyl phosphites to afford, eventually, after an intramolecular cyclization, isoindolin-1-one-3-phosphonates [66].

The catalyst-free conversion of pyrene-1-carboxaldehyde (**56**) to the corresponding α-aminophosphonate (**57**) in reaction with amines (**55**) and dibenzyl phosphite is noteworthy (Scheme 43) [67]. It was observed that the corresponding α hydroxyphosphonate (**58**) was also present in the mixture formed as an intermediate in the Pudovik reaction.

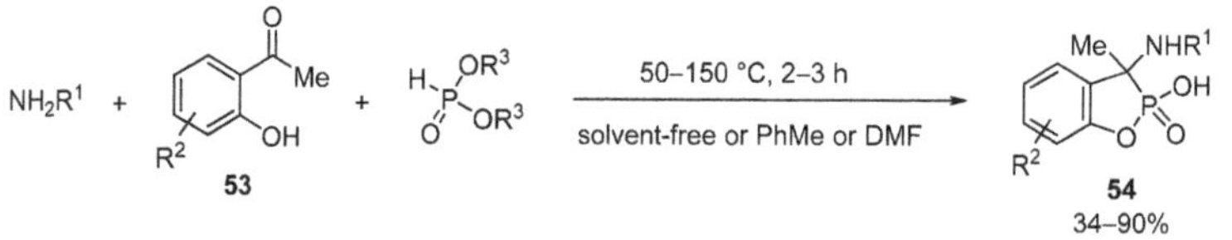

| | | | | | | | | | | |
|---|---|---|---|---|---|---|---|---|---|---|
| **R1** | $^n$Bu | $^n$Bu | $^n$Bu | $^n$Bu | $^n$Pr | Me | Et | $^n$Bu | $^n$Pr | $^n$Bu |
| **R2** | MeO | MeO | MeO | MeO | 6-MeO | 6-MeO | 6-MeO | 6-MeO | H | H |
| **R3** | $^i$Pr | Me | $CH_2C_6H_5$ | $C_6H_5$ | $^i$Pr | $^i$Pr | $^i$Pr | $^i$Pr | $^i$Pr | $^i$Pr |
| **R1** | $^n$Pr | $^n$Pr | $^n$Pr | $^n$Pr | $^n$Pr | $^n$Pr | $^n$Pr | Et | Et | Et |
| **R2** | H | H | H | H | H | H | H | H | H | H |
| **R3** | $^i$Pr | Et | Me | $^n$Bu | $^i$Bu | $C_6H_5$ | $CH_2C_6H_5$ | $C_6H_5$ | $CH_2C_6H_5$ | $C_6H_5$ |
| **R1** | $^n$Pr | $^n$Bu | $^n$Hex | $^n$Oct | Et | $^n$Pr | $^n$Bu | $^n$Hex | Et | $^n$Pr |
| **R2** | H | H | H | H | 5-$NO_2$ | 5-$NO_2$ | 5-$NO_2$ | 5-$NO_2$ | 3-$NO_2$ | 3-$NO_2$ |
| **R3** | $C_6H_5$ | $C_6H_5$ | $C_6H_5$ | $C_6H_5$ | $C_6H_5$ | $C_6H_5$ | $C_6H_5$ | $C_6H_5$ | $C_6H_5$ | $C_6H_5$ |
| **R1** | $^n$Bu | $^n$Hex | $^n$Pr | $^n$Pr | $^n$Pr | $^n$Bu | $^n$Pr | $^n$Bu | $EtNH_2$ | |
| **R2** | 3-$NO_2$ | 3-$NO_2$ | 5-Br | 3,5-Br | 3,5-I | 3,5-I | 5-I | 5-I | H | |
| **R3** | $C_6H_5$ | $C_6H_5$ | $C_6H_5$ | $C_6H_5$ | $C_6H_5$ | $C_6H_5$ | $C_6H_5$ | $C_6H_5$ | $C_6H_5$ | |

**Scheme 42.** 2-Hydroxy-acetophenones as the oxo components in a catalyst- and solvent-free Kabachnik–Fields reaction. DMF—dimethylformamide.

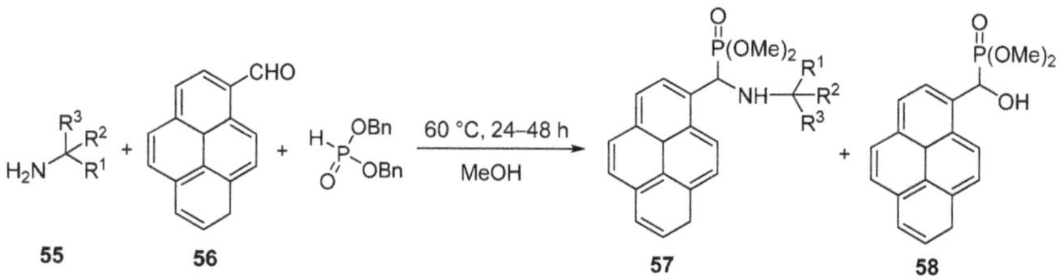

| | | | | |
|---|---|---|---|---|
| **R1** | H | H | Me | H |
| **R2** | H | H | Me | H |
| **R3** | Et | Pr | Me | $^c$Hex |

**Scheme 43.** Catalyst-free condensation of pyrene-1-carboxaldehyde with amines and dibenzyl phosphite.

A series of new α-aminophosphonates (**58**) was prepared applying aryl- or heteroarylaldehydes, aryl- or heteroarylamines, and diphenyl phosphite in three-component condensations using polyethylene glycol (PEG) as the solvent (Scheme 44) [68].

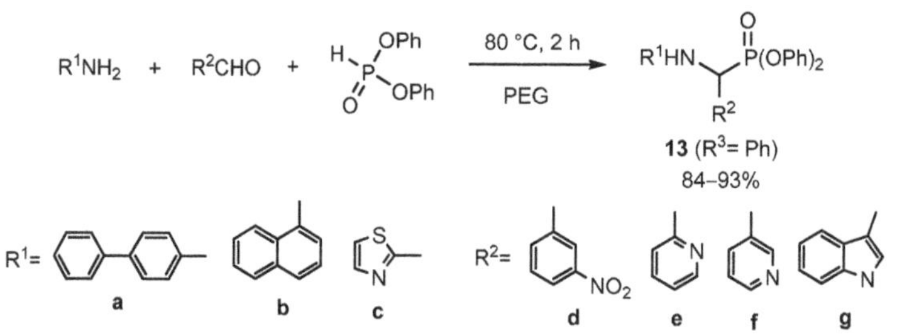

| | | | | | | | | | | |
|---|---|---|---|---|---|---|---|---|---|---|
| **R1** | a | a | a | b | b | b | c | c | c | c |
| **R2** | f | f | g | d | f | g | d | e | f | g |

**Scheme 44.** Catalyst-free Kabachnik–Fields reactions using polyethylene glycol (PEG) as the solvent.

A phenothiazine carbaldehyde (**59**) was converted to different α-aminophosphonates (**60**) in a similar way (Scheme 45) [69].

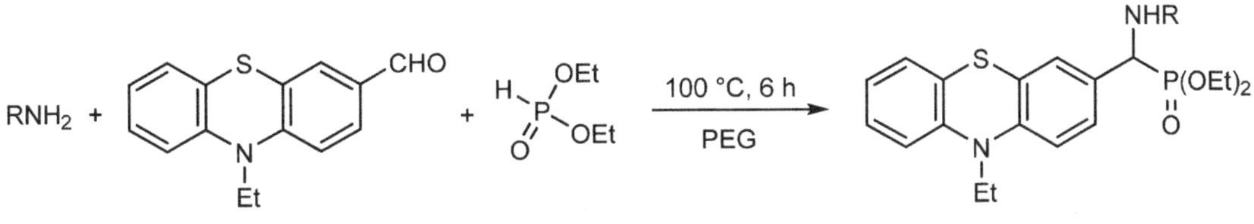


**59** **60** 80–93%

R= $C_6H_5$, 4-$NO_2C_6H_4$, 4-$BrC_6H_4$, 4-$FC_6H_4$, 4-$MeC_6H_4$, 4-$^iPrC_6H_4$, 4-$HOC_6H_4$, 4-$MeOC_6H_4$, $CH_2Ph$, $^cHex$

**Scheme 45.** Further examples of catalyst-free condensations performed using PEG as the solvent.

Glycerol could also be used as the solvent in the catalyst-free condensation of amines, arylaldehydes, and phosphites (Scheme 46) [70].

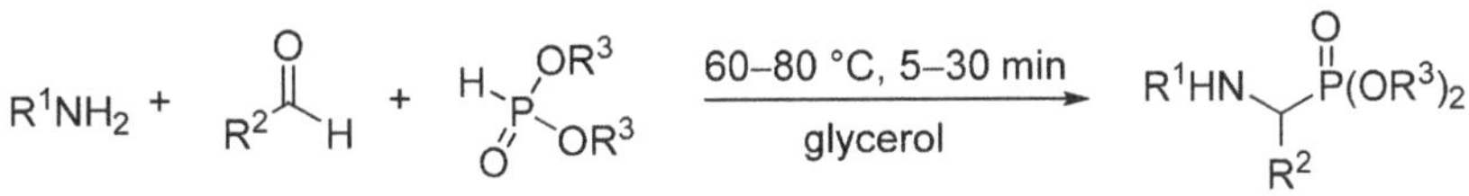


**13** 80–90%

| | | | | | | | |
|---|---|---|---|---|---|---|---|
| **R¹** | 4-$NO_2C_6H_5$ | 4-$NO_2C_6H_5$ | 4-$ClC_6H_5$ | 4-$BrC_6H_5$ | 4-$MeC_6H_5$ | 4-$MeC_6H_5$ | $C_6H_5$ |
| **R²** | 2-$ClC_6H_5$ | $C_6H_5$ | $C_6H_5$ | $C_6H_5$ | 4-$ClC_6H_5$ | $C_6H_5$ | 4-$ClC_6H_5$ |
| **R³** | $C_6H_5$ | Me | Me | Me | Me | Me | Me |
| **R¹** | $C_6H_5$ | $C_6H_5$ | $C_6H_5$ | $C_6H_5$ | $C_6H_5$ | Bu | |
| **R²** | 4-$MeOC_6H_5$ | 4-$MeOC_6H_5$ | $C_6H_5$ | $C_6H_5$ | $C_6H_5$ | $C_6H_5$ | |
| **R³** | Me | Me | Et | Me | $C_6H_5$ | Me | |

**Scheme 46.** Catalyst-free accomplishment of the phospha-Mannich condensation applying glycerol as the solvent.

A series of new α-sulfamidophosphonates and cyclosulfamidophosphonates incorporating quinoline or a quinolone moiety was synthesized by the Kabachnik–Fields reaction in the presence of a suitable ionic liquid under ultrasound irradiation [71].

A series of catalyst-free and MW-assisted Kabachnik–Fields reactions were elaborated by the Keglevich group. The first observation was that MW irradiation may substitute for the catalysts [17,72]. Among other examples, phospha-Mannich reactions with paraformaldehyde and ethyl phenyl-*H*-phosphinate were elaborated using primary and secondary amines (Scheme 47(1) and (2), respectively). Moreover, bis derivatives (**63**) were also prepared (Scheme 47(3)) [73]. The yields were variable.

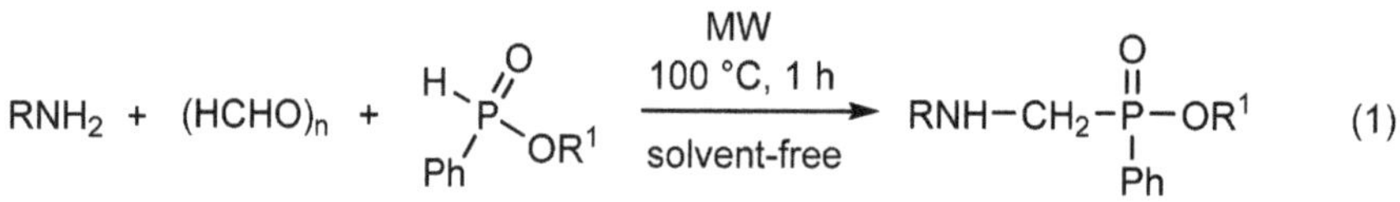

**61**
42–81%

| R | Pr | Bu | $^{c}$Hex | Bn | Pr | Bu | $^{c}$Hex | Bn | Pr | Bu | $^{c}$Hex | Bn |
|---|---|---|---|---|---|---|---|---|---|---|---|---|
| R[1] | Et | Et | Et | Et | Pr | Pr | Pr | Pr | Bu | Bu | Bu | Bu |

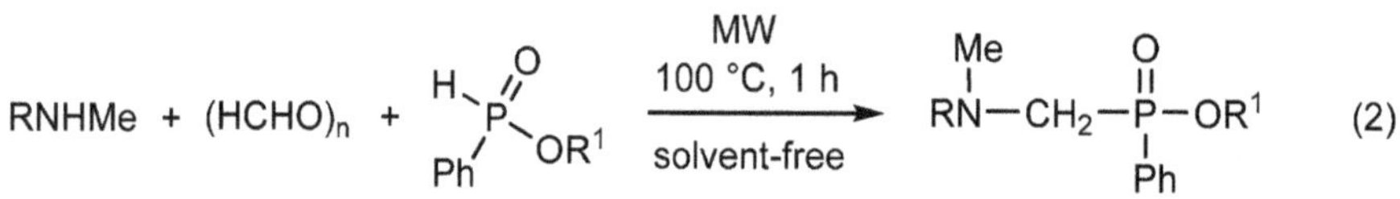

**62**
45–81%

| R | Bu | $^{c}$Hex | Bn | Bu | $^{c}$Hex | Bn | Bu | $^{c}$Hex | Bn |
|---|---|---|---|---|---|---|---|---|---|
| R[1] | Et | Et | Et | Pr | Pr | Pr | Bu | Bu | Bu |

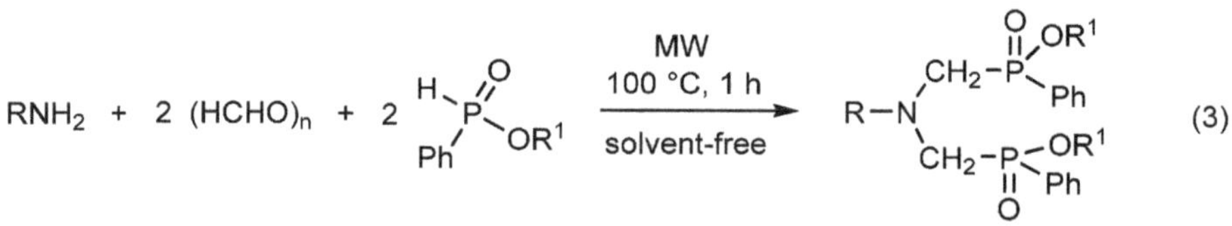

**63**
80–90%

| R | Pr | Bu | $^{c}$Hex | Bn | Pr | Bu | $^{c}$Hex | Bn | Pr | Bu | $^{c}$Hex | Bn |
|---|---|---|---|---|---|---|---|---|---|---|---|---|
| R[1] | Et | Et | Et | Et | Pr | Pr | Pr | Pr | Bu | Bu | Bu | Bu |

**Scheme 47.** Variations of the MW-assisted Kabachnik–Fields reactions.

A series of α-aminophosphonates (**64**, **66**, **68** and **70**) with sterically demanding α-aryl substituents was synthesized using a MW-assisted catalyst-free and solvent-free protocol (Scheme 48) [74].

A similar method was applied to the preparation of 6-methyl-2*H*-pyran-2-on (**71**)-based α-aminophosphonates and an α-aminophosphine oxide (**72**) (Scheme 49) [75].

Functionalized amines may also be used in the Kabachnik–Fields reaction. Amines with hydroxyalkyl substituents were condensed with paraformaldehyde and dialkyl phosphites or ethyl phenyl-*H*-phosphinate under MW irradiation (Scheme 50(1)). After measuring in the >P(O)H reagents and formaldehyde in a double amount, bis derivatives (**74**) were formed (Scheme 50(2)) [76].

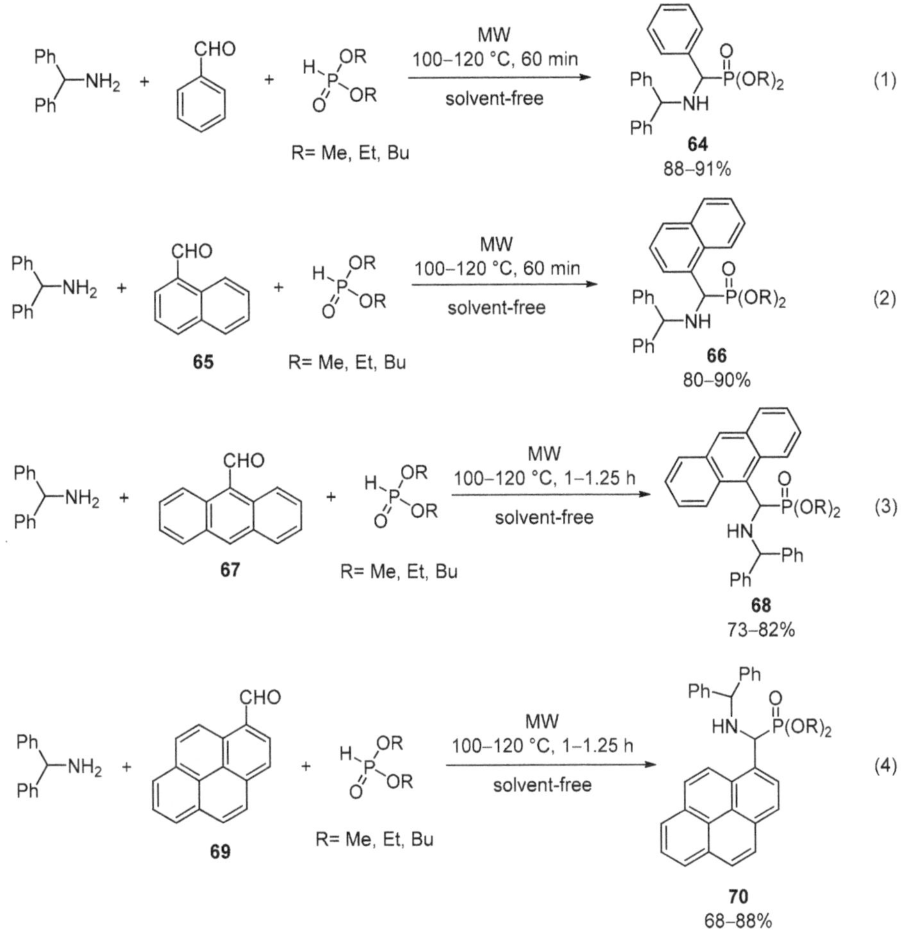

**Scheme 48.** Further variations of the MW-assisted catalyst-free and solvent-free phospha-Mannich reactions.

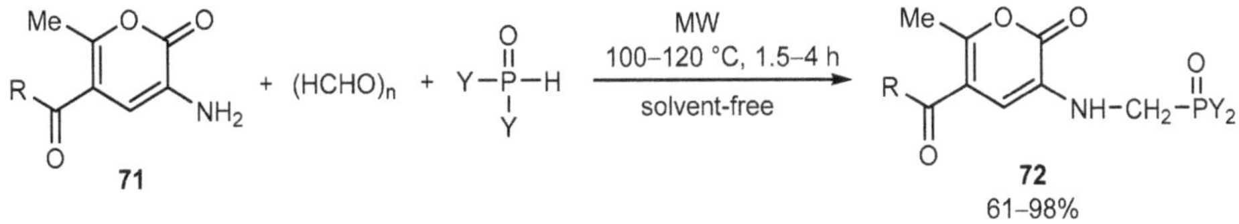

| R | $C_6H_5$ | $C_6H_5$ | Me | Me | Me | Me |
|---|---|---|---|---|---|---|
| Y | $C_6H_5$ | EtO | $C_6H_5$ | MeO | EtO | BuO |

**Scheme 49.** Synthesis of 6-methyl-2*H*-pyran-2-on-based α-aminophosphonic derivatives.

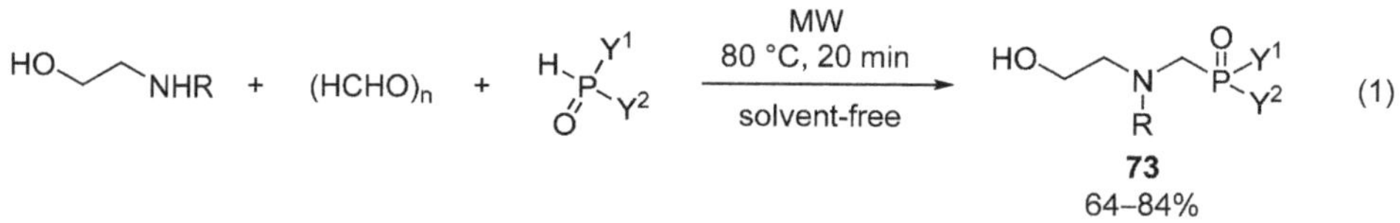

| R | Me | Me | Me | Et | Et | Et |
|---|---|---|---|---|---|---|
| Y[1] | EtO | BuO | EtO | EtO | BuO | EtO |
| Y[2] | EtO | BuO | $C_6H_5$ | EtO | BuO | $C_6H_5$ |

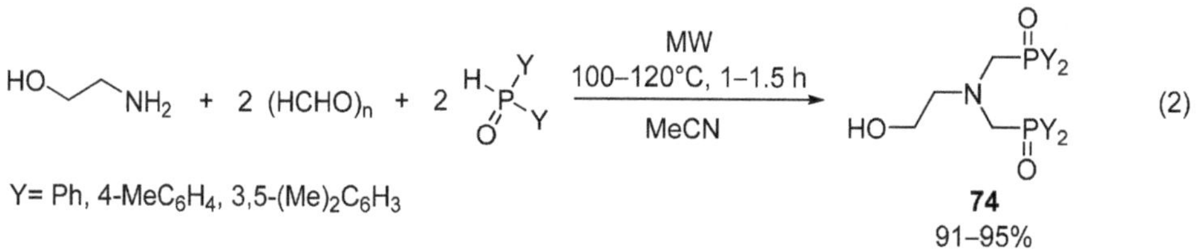

**Scheme 50.** The application of ethanolamines in Kabachnik–Fields condensation.

The esters of glycine were converted to the corresponding bis(phosphonoylmethyl) amines (**75**) by MW-promoted reaction with two equivalents of paraformaldehyde and dialkyl phosphites (Scheme 51(1)). The application of diphenylphosphine oxide resulted in bis(phosphinoylmethyl)amine derivatives (**76**) (Scheme 51(2)) [77].

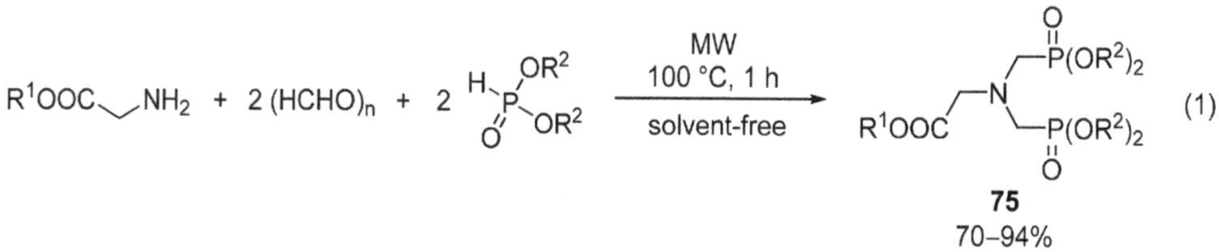

| R[1] | Me | Me | Et | Et | Et | Et |
|---|---|---|---|---|---|---|
| R[2] | Et | Bu | Me | Et | Bu | Bn |

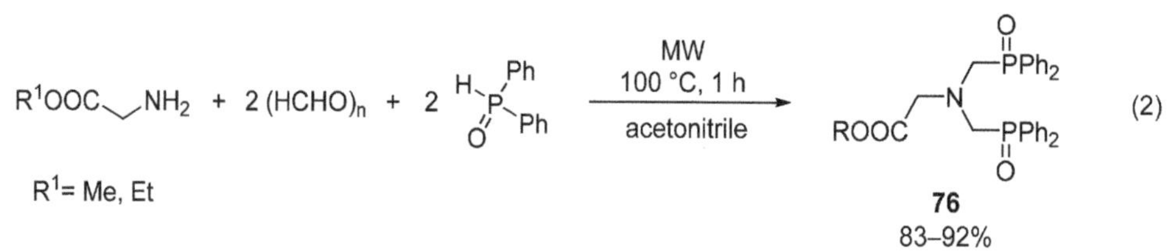

**Scheme 51.** Double Kabachnik–Fields reactions applying glycine esters as the amine component.

In a similar way, β-aminophosphonic derivatives (**77**) also served as starting materials for the respective bis(phosphonoylmethyl)amines (Scheme 52) [78].

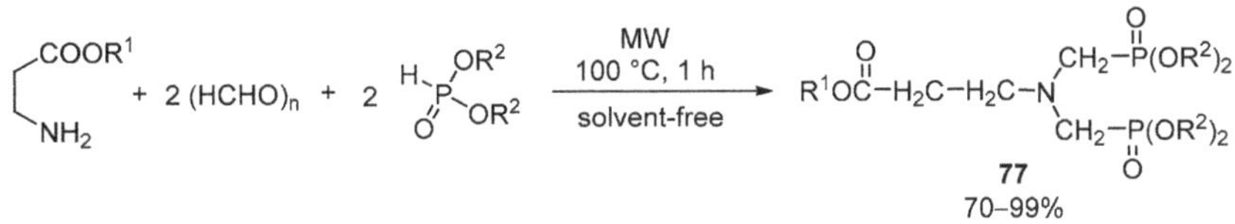

| $R^1$ | H | H | H | H | Me | Me | Me | Me | Et | Et | Et | Et |
|---|---|---|---|---|---|---|---|---|---|---|---|---|
| $R^2$ | Me | Et | Bu | Bn | Me | Et | Bu | Bn | Me | Et | Bu | Bn |

**Scheme 52.** Bis(phosphonoylmethyl)amines produced via the double Kabachnik–Fields reaction of β-aminoacid esters.

A series of amines was utilized in a tandem Kabachnik–Fields reaction to afford the corresponding nonsymmetric bis(phosphinoylmethyl)amines (**79**) after a two-step transformation (Scheme 53(1)). Subsequently, after debenzylation of intermediate **79** (R = Bn) to species **80** (the details were not reported), valuable tris derivatives (**81**) were prepared (Scheme 53(2)) [79].

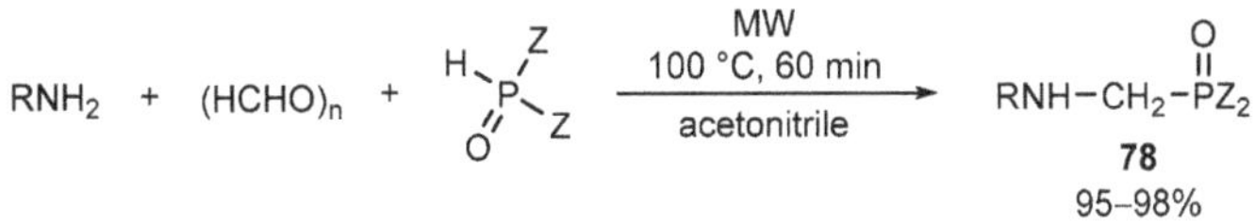

| R | Bu | Cy | Bn | Bu | Cy | Bn |
|---|---|---|---|---|---|---|
| Z | 4-$MeC_6H_4$ | 4-$MeC_6H_4$ | 4-$MeC_6H_4$ | Bn | Bn | Bn |

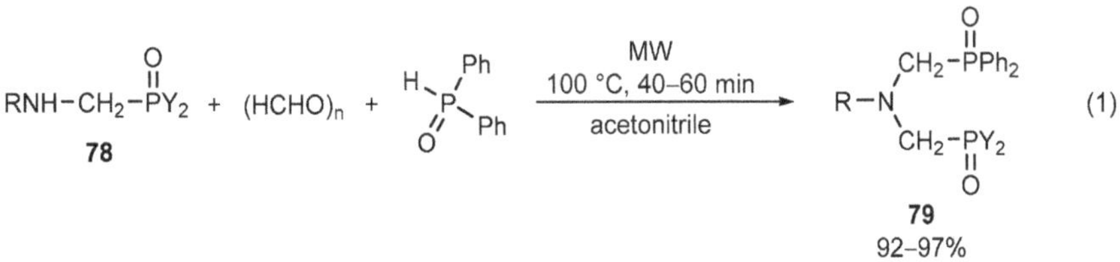

| R | Bu | Cy | Bn | Bu | Cy | Bn |
|---|---|---|---|---|---|---|
| Y | 4-$MeC_6H_4$ | 4-$MeC_6H_4$ | 4-$MeC_6H_4$ | Bn | Bn | Bn |

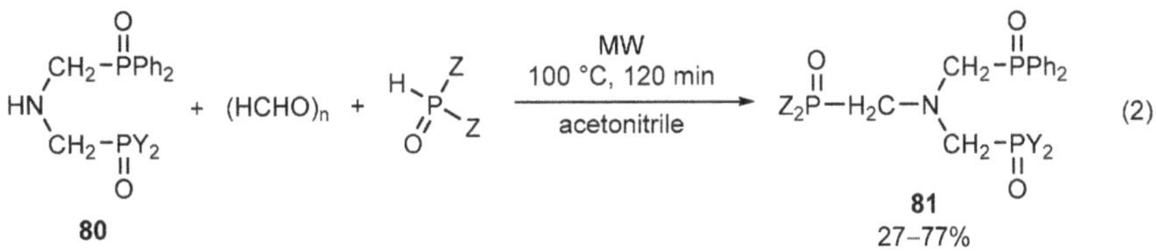

| Y | $C_6H_5$ | $C_6H_5$ | $C_6H_5$ | 4-$MeC_6H_4$ |
|---|---|---|---|---|
| Z | $C_6H_5$ | 4-$MeC_6H_4$ | Bn | Bn |

**Scheme 53.** Further extensions and variations of the Kabachnik–Fields reaction.

A dialkyl phosphite with an octyl and ethyl group was also utilized in the phospha-Mannich reaction, to give species **82** and the bis variation (**83**) (Scheme 54(1) and (2)) [80].

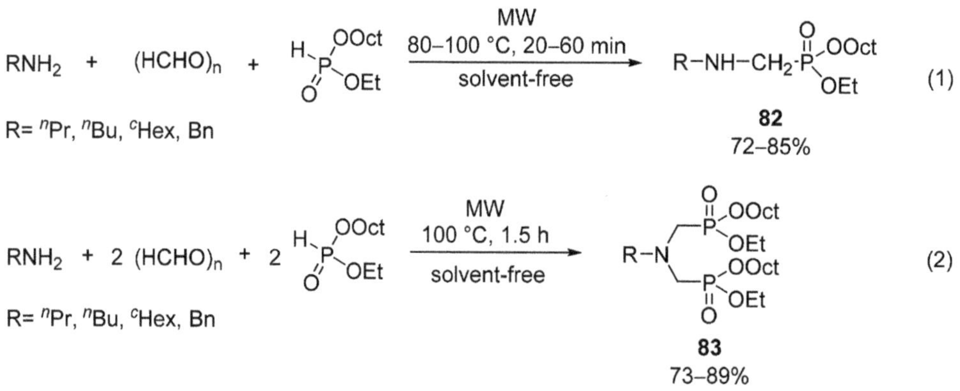

**Scheme 54.** The application of a phosphite with different alkyl groups in the phospha-Mannich reaction.

The results of the Keglevich group were summarized as conference proceedings [81]. The bis(phosphinoylmethyl)amine derivatives (**84**) were excellent precursors of the corresponding bisphosphines (**85**) and could be converted to ring Pt complexes (**86**) (Scheme 55) [82–84].

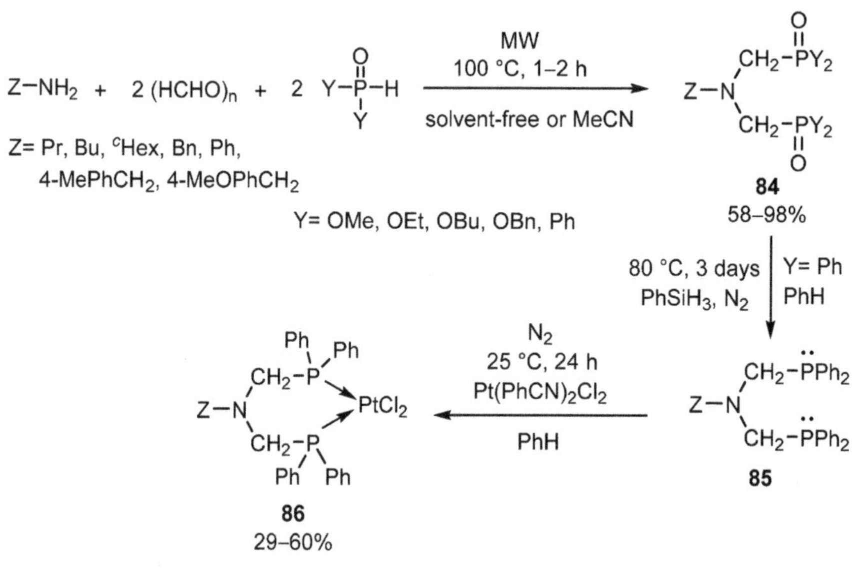

**Scheme 55.** Utilization of bis(phosphine oxides) in the synthesis of ring Pt complexes.

Optically active α-phenylethylamine (**87/1**) was applied in the preparation of chiral α-aminophosphonates (**88**, $Y^1$ and $Y^2$ = alkoxy), an α-aminophosphine oxide (**88**, $Y^1$ and $Y^2$ = Ph), and an α-aminophosphinate (**88**, $Y^1$ = EtO $Y^2$ = Ph), along with the corresponding bis derivatives (**89**) utilized in the synthesis of the corresponding ring Pt complex (**90**) (Scheme 56) [85].

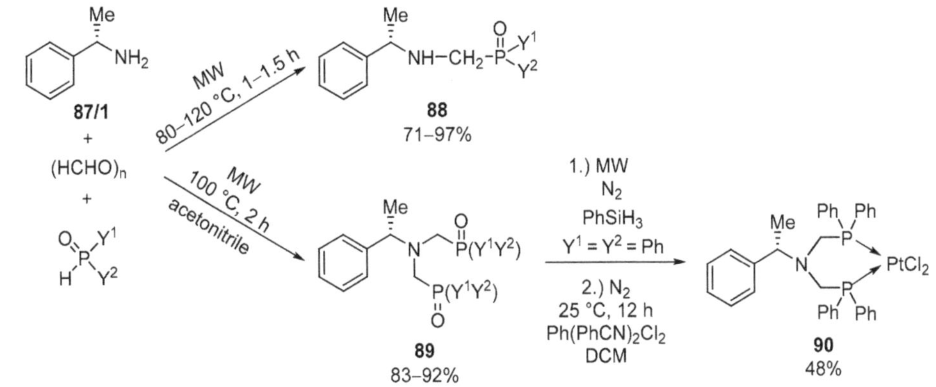


| $Y^1$ | $C_6H_5$ | EtO | MeO | EtO | BuO | EtO |
|---|---|---|---|---|---|---|
| $Y^2$ | $C_6H_5$ | $C_6H_5$ | MeO | EtO | BuO | OctO |

**Scheme 56.** Optically active α-phenylethylamine used as the amine component in the Kabachnik–Fields reaction; conversion of the product to a ring Pt complex.

α-Aminophosphines may be special ligands in platinum, palladium, and rhodium complexes [86].

It was rather surprising that carboxylic acid amides could also be utilized as starting materials in the Kabachnik–Fields reaction. However, the amides had to be applied in a 10-fold excess under practically solvolytic and forcing conditions (Scheme 57) [87].

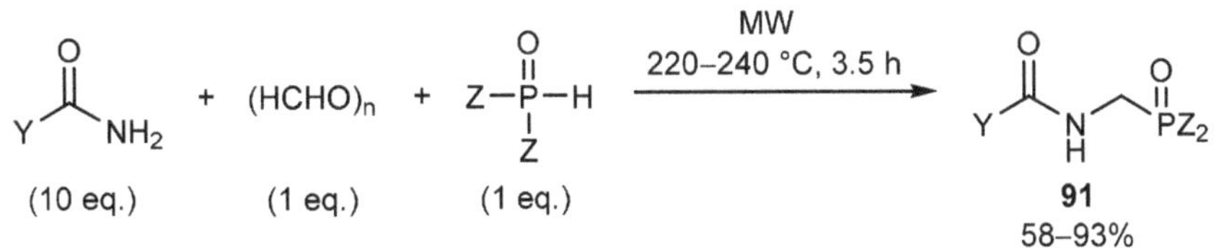


| Y | $C_6H_5$ | $C_6H_5$ | $C_6H_5$ | $C_6H_5$ | Me | Me |
|---|---|---|---|---|---|---|
| Z | $C_6H_5$ | 4-$MeC_6H_4$ | 3,5-$Me_2C_6H_3$ | Bn | $C_6H_5$ | 4-$MeC_6H_4$ |
| Y | Me | Me | Et | Et | Et | Et |
| Z | 3,5-$Me_2C_6H_3$ | Bn | $C_6H_5$ | 4-$MeC_6H_4$ | 3,5-$Me_2C_6H_3$ | Bn |

**Scheme 57.** Carboxylic acid amides as the amine component in the phospha-Mannich reaction.

Another series of bis(phosphine oxides) (**84**) was prepared via the double Kabachnik–Fields reaction (Scheme 58(1)). The precursors were converted to ring Pt complexes (**93**) (Scheme 58(2)). A few bisphosphines (**92**) were stabilized as bis(phosphine boranes) (**94**) (Scheme 58(3)). The catalytic activity of the Pt(II) complexes **93** was investigated in the hydroformylation of styrene. The advantages of applying Pt(II) complexes (**93**) include their high chemo- and regioselectivity at low temperatures [88].

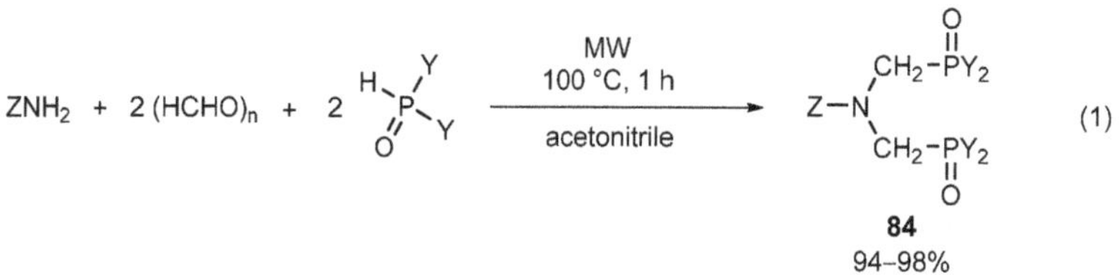

| Z | $C_6H_5$ | 4-$MeOC_6H_4$ | Bn | 4-$MeOC_6H_4CH_2$ | Pr | Bu | $^c$Hex |
|---|---|---|---|---|---|---|---|
| Y | Bn | Bn | Bn | Bn | Bn | Bn | Bn |
| Z | 4-$MeOC_6H_4$ | Bn | 4-$MeOC_6H_4CH_2$ | $C_6H_5$ | Pr | Bu | Pr |
| Y | 4-$MeC_6H_4$ | 4-$MeC_6H_4$ | 4-$MeC_6H_4$ | 4-$MeC_6H_4$ | 4-$MeC_6H_4$ | 4-$MeC_6H_4$ | 4-$MeC_6H_4$ |

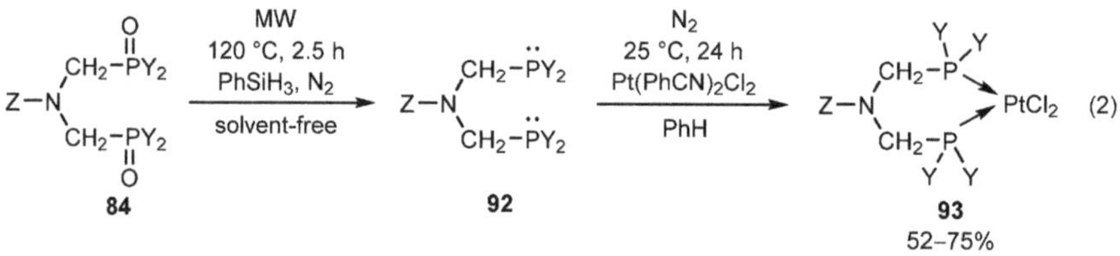

| Z | 4-$MeC_6H_4$ | 4-$MeC_6H_4$ | 4-$MeC_6H_4$ | Bn | Bn | Bn |
|---|---|---|---|---|---|---|
| Y | Bn | Bu | $^c$Hex | Bn | Bu | $^c$Hex |

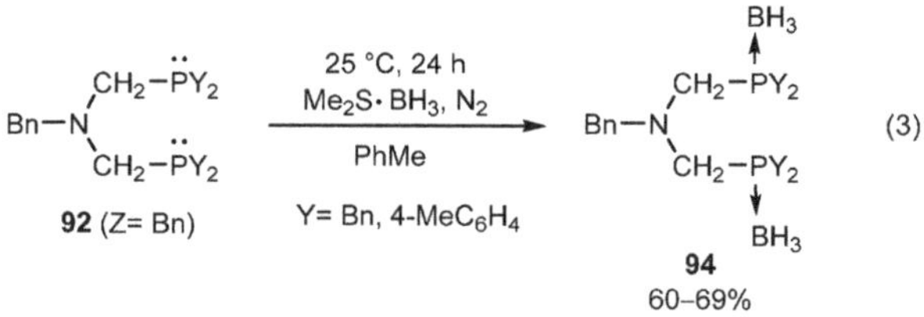

**Scheme 58.** Synthesis and derivatization of bis(phosphine oxides).

α-Hydroxyphosphonates formed reversibly from suitable ketones and dialkyl phosphites [89] may also be converted to α-aminophosphonates by substitution reaction with amines. This reaction is enhanced by an adjacent group effect [90,91].

Somewhat analogous compounds, (aminomethylene)bisphosphine oxides and (aminomethylene)bisphosphonates (**95**/**96**), were prepared via the three-component condensation of secondary or primary amines, triethyl orthoformate, and the corresponding >P(O)H reagent (Scheme 59(1) and (2)) [92].

In the third part of the first section, green methods utilizing MW irradiation were summarized. These solvent- and catalyst-free protocols produce α-aminophosphonates, α-aminophosphinates, and phosphine oxides, along with their bis and tris derivatives in good yields. The advantages of applying MW irradiation include the mild reaction conditions, selectivity, and high yields. To compare the methods described, it goes without saying that MW-assisted accomplishment is the most suitable method to synthesize α-aminophosphonates and their derivatives.

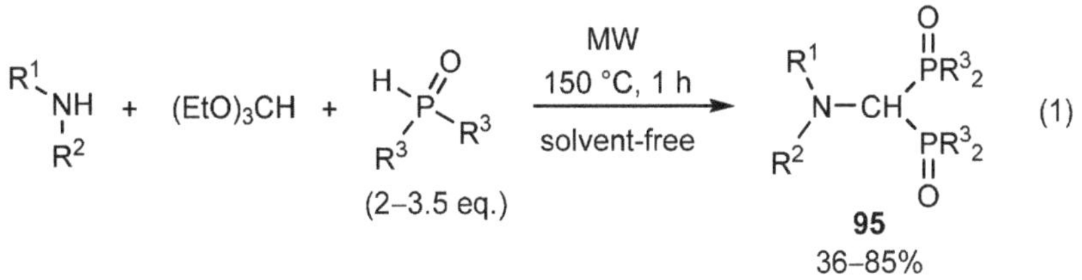

| $R^1$ | Et | Bu | Bu | $^c$Hex | Bn | $C_6H_5$ | Et | Bu | Bu | $^c$Hex | Bn | $C_6H_5$ |
|---|---|---|---|---|---|---|---|---|---|---|---|---|
| $R^2$ | Et | Bu | Me | Me | Me | Me | Et | Bu | Me | Me | Me | Me |
| $R^3$ | $C_6H_5$ | $C_6H_5$ | $C_6H_5$ | $C_6H_5$ | $C_6H_5$ | $C_6H_5$ | EtO | EtO | EtO | EtO | EtO | EtO |

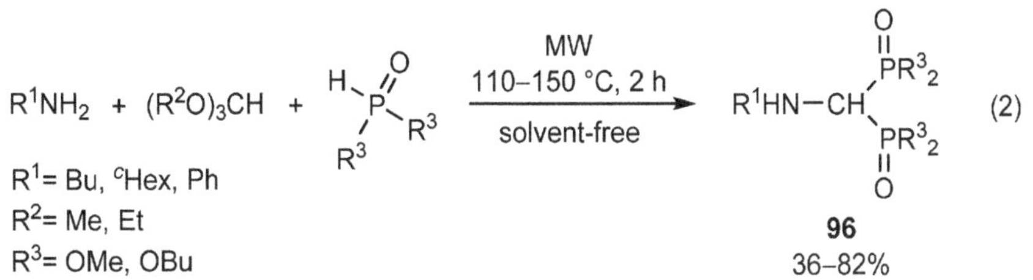

**Scheme 59.** Synthesis of (aminomethylene)bisphosphonates and bis(phosphinic oxides) via a three-component reaction..

### *2.4. Kabachnik–Fields Reactions Leading to Optically Active α-Aminophosphonates*

Optically active α-aminophosphine oxides (**98**) were synthesized from the ethyl ester of proline (**97**), benzaldehyde derivatives, and diphenylphosphine oxide in toluene at reflux (Scheme 60) [93]. The chiral center in the proline derivative influenced the enantioselectivity.

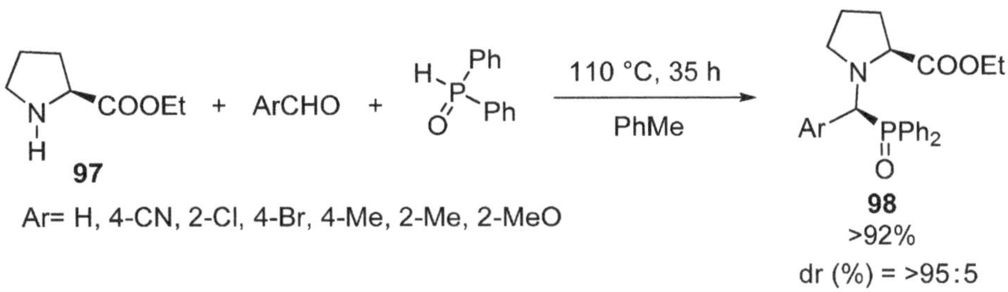

**Scheme 60.** Synthesis of optically active α-aminophosphine oxides.

Starting from the optically active forms of α-phenylethylamines (**87/2**), benzaldehyde, and dimethyl phosphite, the corresponding products (**99/1, 99/2**) were formed in a diastereoselective manner under MW-assisted solvent-free and catalyst-free conditions (Scheme 61) [94].

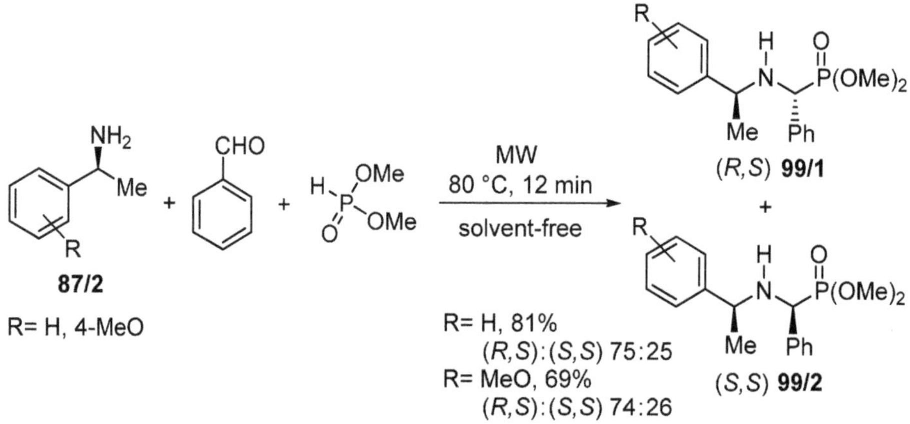

**Scheme 61.** MW-assisted catalyst-free diastereoselective synthesis of α-aminophosphonates.

In the above examples, the application of optically active amines as the starting materials allowed a diastereoselectivity of 74–92%.

## 3. Kabachnik–Fields Reactions Applying Trialkyl Phosphites or Related Derivatives as the P Reagent

In the next section, Kabachnik–Fields condensations applying trialkyl phosphites and related derivatives are discussed. Primary amines, 4-(4′-pyridyl)benzaldehyde (**100**), and triethyl phosphite were condensed in the presence of PEG–$SO_3H$ in toluene at 40–50 °C to give the corresponding aminophosphonates (**101**) (Scheme 62) [95].

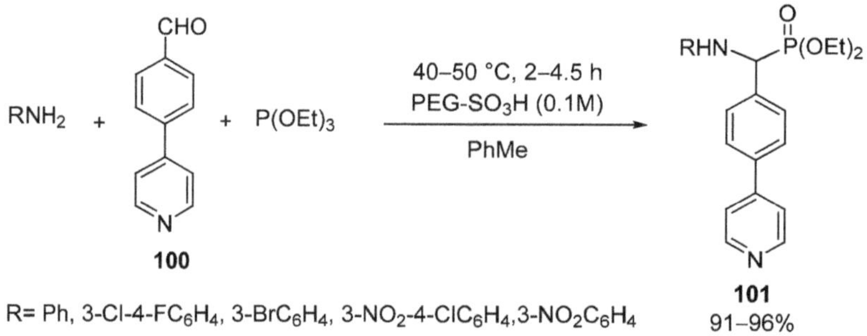

**Scheme 62.** The condensation of 4-(4′-pyridyl)benzaldehyde, triethyl phosphite and different aniline derivatives.

The reaction of substituted anilines, benzaldehyde derivatives, and triethyl phosphite was carried out in the presence of the HCl salt of DABCO at 26 °C in MeOH (Scheme 63) [96].

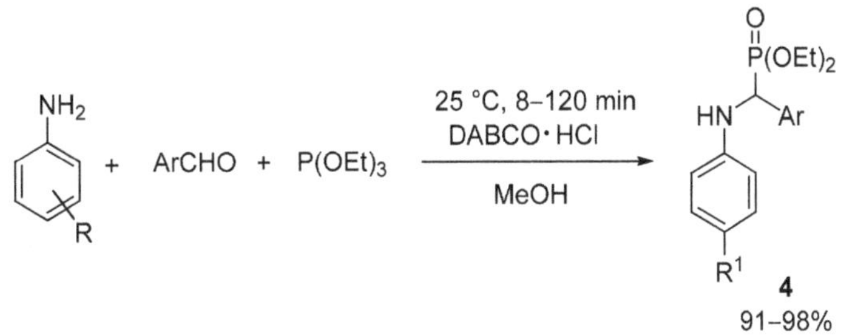


| **R** | H | 4-F | 4-MeO | 4-F | 4-F | 4-F | 4-F |
|---|---|---|---|---|---|---|---|
| **Ar** | $C_6H_5$ | $C_6H_5$ | $C_6H_5$ | 4-$NO_2C_6H_4$ | 2-$NO_2C_6H_4$ | 3-$NO_2C_6H_4$ | 4-$ClC_6H_4$ |
| **R** | 4-F | H | H | H | H | H | |
| **Ar** | 4-$MeOC_6H_4$ | 4-$NO_2C_6H_4$ | 4-$ClC_6H_4$ | 4-$MeOC_6H_4$ | 2-thienyl | 2-furyl | |

**Scheme 63.** The HCl salt of 1,4-diazabicyclo[2.2.2]octane (DABCO) as a catalyst in the three-component reaction.

Aniline derivatives and benzaldehyde, or aniline and benzaldehyde derivatives, were reacted in combination with triethyl phosphite in the presence of the T3P® reagent at 26° C in ethyl acetate. It is a disadvantage that 1 equivalent of the reagent is needed in these condensations. The products (**4**) were obtained in 80–96% yields (Scheme 64(1) and (2)) [97].

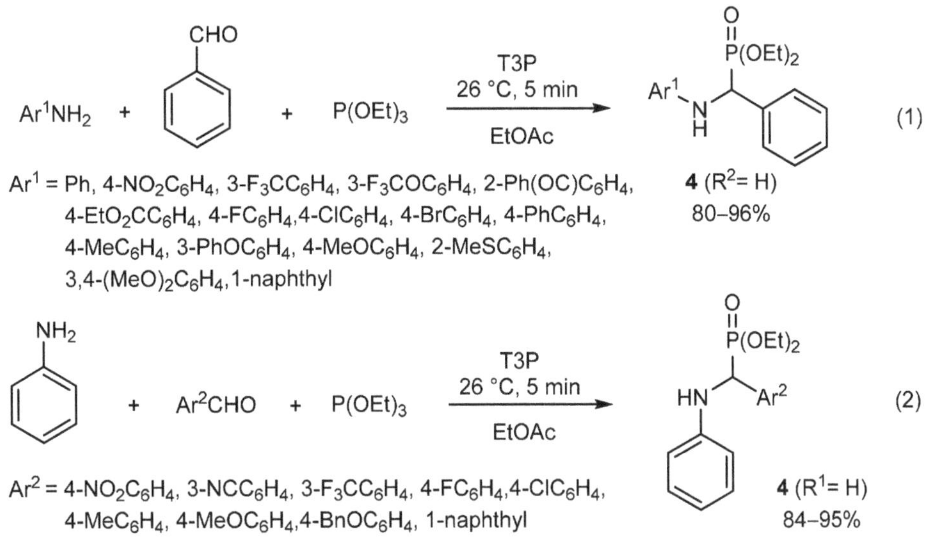


**Scheme 64.** T3P®-promoted Kabachnik–Fields reactions.

A possible mechanism is demonstrated via the reaction of benzaldehyde, aniline, and triethyl phosphite (Scheme 65). In the first stage, the corresponding imine (**102**) is formed along with P, P′, P″-tripropyl triphosphonic acid ("T3P·$H_2O$") as the byproduct. The imine then reacts with triethyl phosphite, and, after protonation with "T3P·$H_2O$", the phosphonium salt (**104**) so formed is converted to the final α-aminophosphonate (**4** ($R^3$ = Et)) via an Arbuzov fission. In this step T3P·EtOH is the byproduct [97].

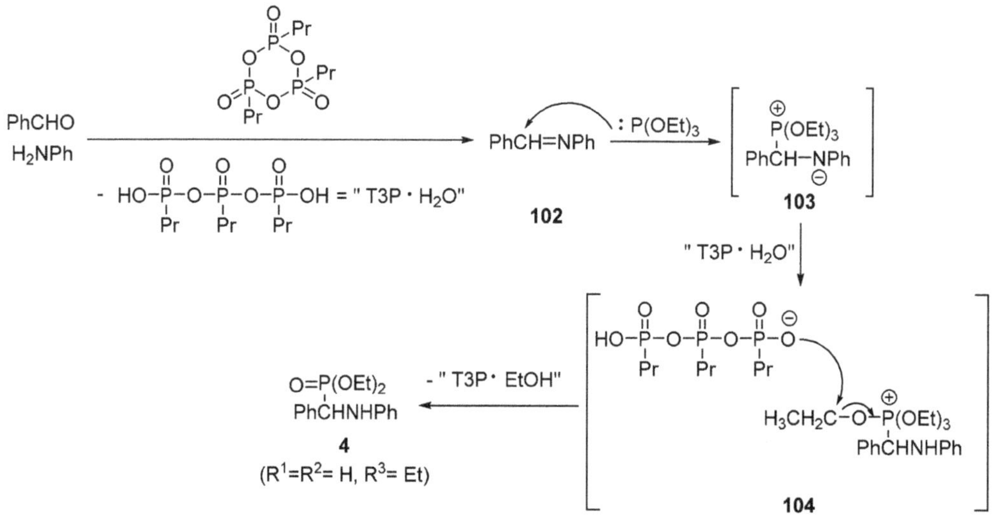

**Scheme 65.** The mechanism of the T3P-promoted Kabachnik–Fields reaction applying triethyl phosphite.

Although the triesters of phosphorous acid are hydrolyzable in water, still water was used as the medium in a few cases. The interaction of primary amines, salicylaldehydes, and triphenyl phosphite using *p*-toluenesulfonic acid (PTSA) as the catalyst in water at room temperature afforded the corresponding aminophosphonates (**105**) in good yields (Scheme 66) [98].

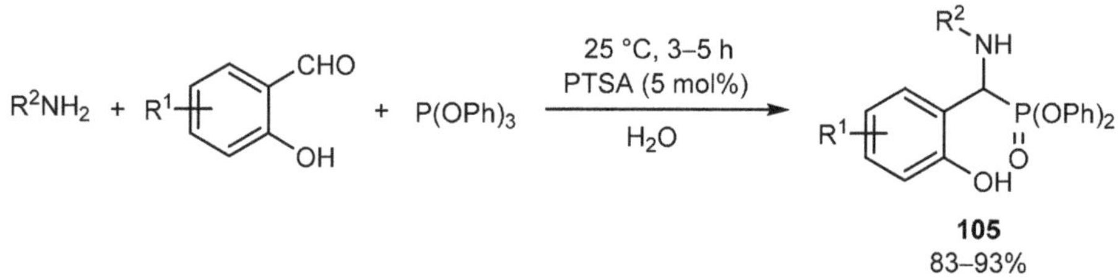

| | | | | | | |
|---|---|---|---|---|---|---|
| **R¹** | H | H | H | H | H | H |
| **R²** | $C_6H_5$ | $3\text{-}NO_2C_6H_4$ | $2,5\text{-}Cl_2C_6H_3$ | $4\text{-}ClC_6H_4$ | $4\text{-}BrC_6H_4$ | $2\text{-}MeC_6H_4$ |
| **R¹** | H | $5\text{-}NO_2$ | 5-Cl | 5-Cl | 5-Br | |
| **R²** | $2\text{-}MeOC_6H_4$ | $4\text{-}MeOC_6H_4$ | $2\text{-}MeOC_6H_4$ | $2\text{-}MeC_6H_4$ | $4\text{-}MeC_6H_4$ | |

**Scheme 66.** The use of water as a solvent in the Kabachnik–Fields condensation.

The condensation of aniline and benzaldehyde with triethyl phosphite was also performed in water, applying the salts of dodecyl sulfonic acid or dodecylbenzene sulfonic acid (Scheme 67) [99].

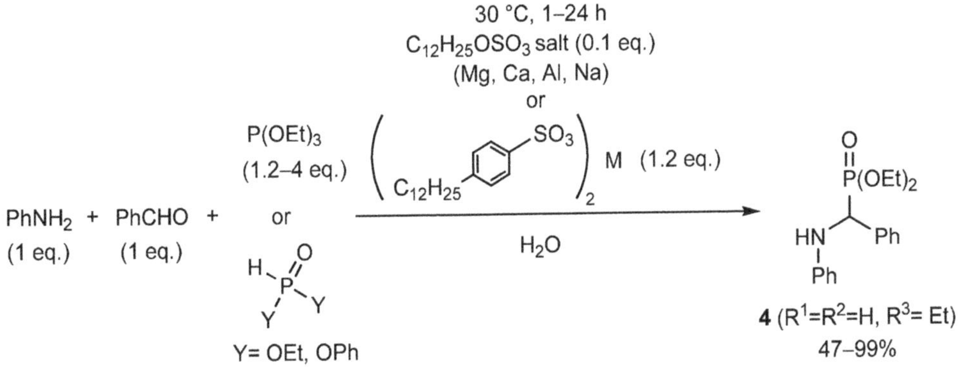

**Scheme 67.** The use of magnesium salts of dodecyl sulfonic or dodecylbenzene sulfonic acid as a catalyst.

Hafnium(IV) chloride was found to be an efficient catalyst in the condensation of amines/diamines, aldehydes, and trialkyl phosphites using ethanol as the solvent at 60 °C (Scheme 68) [100].

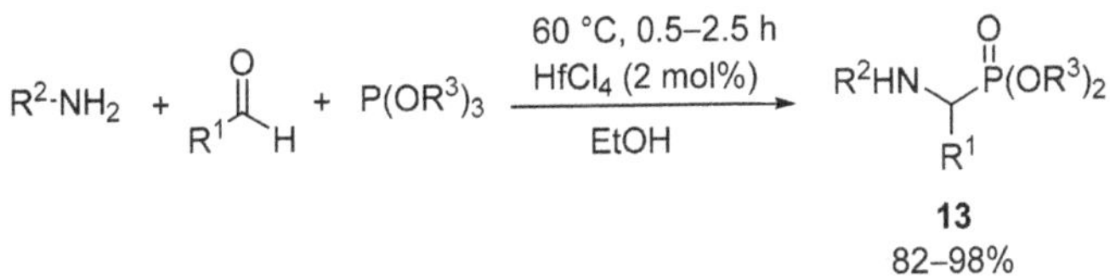

| | | | | | |
|---|---|---|---|---|---|
| **R¹** | $C_6H_5$ | $C_6H_5$ | $C_6H_5$ | 4-MeO$C_6H_4$ | 4-MeO$C_6H_4$ |
| **R²** | $C_6H_5$ | $C_6H_5$ | $C_6H_5$ | $C_6H_5$ | 4-NC$C_6H_5$ |
| **R³** | Me | Et | Ph | Me | Et |
| **R¹** | 4-Me$C_6H_4$ | 4-Me$C_6H_4$ | $C_6H_5$ | $C_6H_5$ | $C_6H_5$ |
| **R²** | $C_6H_5$ | 4-MeO$C_6H_4$ | 4-NC$C_6H_4$ | 4-MeO$C_6H_4$ | Bn |
| **R³** | Et | Et | Et | Et | Et |
| **R¹** | $C_6H_5$ | 2-Me$C_6H_4$ | 2-MeO$C_6H_4$ | $^c$Hex | Pr |
| **R²** | $^c$Hex | $^c$Hex | $^c$Hex | $^c$Hex | $C_6H_5$ |
| **R³** | Me | Me | Me | Et | Me |
| **R¹** | $^c$Hex | $^c$Hex | $^c$Hex | furyl | furyl |
| **R²** | $C_6H_5$ | 4-NC$C_6H_4$ | 4-MeO$C_6H_4$ | $C_6H_5$ | $CH_2C_6H_5$ |
| **R³** | Me | Me | Me | Et | Et |

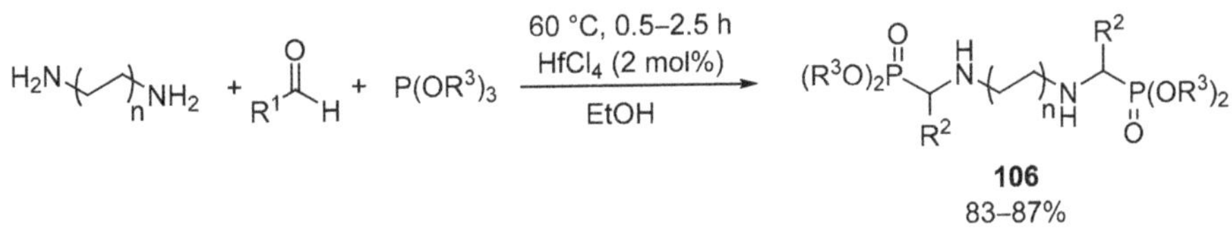

| **n** | 2 | 3 | 2 | 3 |
|---|---|---|---|---|
| **R¹** | $C_6H_5$ | $C_6H_5$ | $^c$Hex | $^i$Bu |
| **R³** | Me | Me | Me | Et |

**Scheme 68.** Hafnium(IV)-chloride-catalyzed Kabachnik–Fields reaction.

The following example for condensation in water involves the reaction of aniline and benzaldehyde derivatives with triethyl phosphite, utilizing a $SO_3H$-functionalized ionic liquid as the catalyst (Scheme 69) [101].

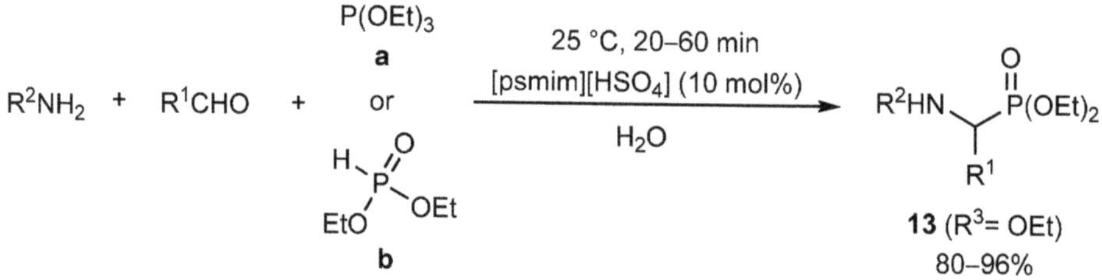

| R1 | 4-NO2C6H4 | 4-ClC6H4 | 2-ClC6H4 | 4-HOC6H4 | 4-MeOC6H4 | 4-MeOC6H4 |
|---|---|---|---|---|---|---|
| R2 | C6H5 | C6H5 | C6H5 | C6H5 | 4-NO2C6H4 | 4-ClC6H4 |
| P-reagent | a | a | a | a | b | b |
| R1 | 4-MeOC6H4 | 4-MeOC6H4 | C6H5 | C6H5 | 4-MeOC6H4 | 4-MeOC6H4 |
| R2 | 4-BrC6H4 | 4-FC6H4 | 4-NO2C6H4 | 3-NO2C6H4 | C6H5 | C6H5 |
| P-reagent | b | b | a | a | a | b |
| R1 | 4-MeOC6H4 | 4-MeC6H4 | C6H5 | C6H5 | Bu | cHex |
| R2 | 4-MeC6H4 | C6H5 | C6H5 | C6H5 | C6H5 | C6H5 |
| P-reagent | a | b | a | b | a | a |

**Scheme 69.** The use of a $SO_3H$-functionalized ionic liquid as a catalyst. [psmim]—propylsulfonyl-methyl-imidazolyl.

The three-component reactions were also realized under ultrasonic irradiation at 26 °C in an ethyl lactate–water mixture (Scheme 70) [102]. Under these conditions, the corresponding products were obtained in good yields.

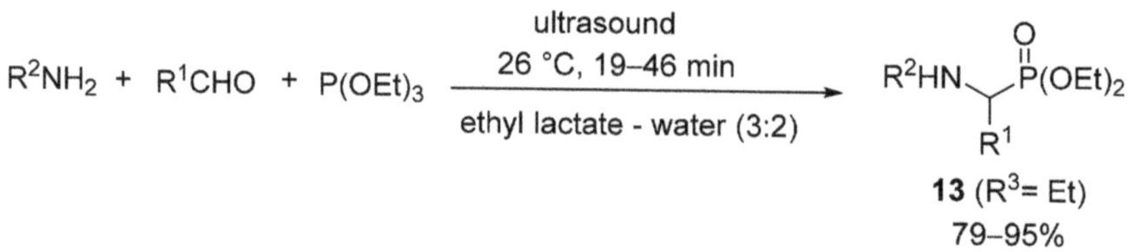

| R1 | C6H5 | 4-NO2C6H5 | 4-ClC6H4 | 3-ClC6H4 | 2-ClC6H4 | 4-BrC6H4 |
|---|---|---|---|---|---|---|
| R2 | C6H5 | C6H5 | C6H5 | C6H5 | C6H5 | C6H5 |
| R1 | 4-FC6H4 | 4-MeC6H4 | 4-MeOC6H5 | 3-MeOC6H4 | C6H5 | C6H5 |
| R2 | C6H5 | C6H5 | C6H5 | C6H5 | 4-NO2C6H5 | 4-ClC6H4 |
| R1 | C6H5 | C6H5 | C6H5 | 4-MeOC6H4 | 4-MeOC6H4 | 3-ClC6H4 |
| R2 | 3-ClC6H4 | 2-BrC6H5 | 4-MeC6H5 | 4-ClC6H4 | 3-MeC6H4 | 4-MeC6H4 |
| R1 | 4-BrC6H4 | 4-MeOC6H4 | 4-MeOC6H4 | 4-MeOC6H5 | | |
| R2 | 4-MeC6H4 | 4-MeC6H4 | 3-MeC6H4 | 4-MeOC6H4 | | |

**Scheme 70.** Kabachnik–Fields reaction under ultrasonic irradiation.

Ultrasound activation allowed a solvent- and catalyst-free condensation of aniline and benzaldehyde derivatives with triethyl phosphite (Scheme 71) [103].

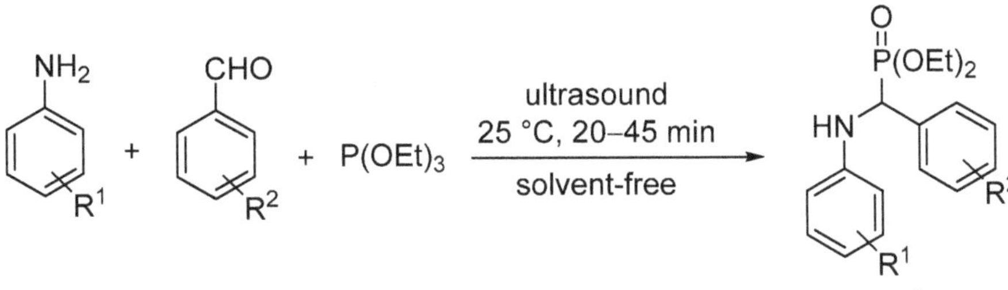


**4** ($R^3$= Et)
80–99%

| | | | | | | | |
|---|---|---|---|---|---|---|---|
| **$R^1$** | 2,6-Cl | 4-Cl | 4-Cl | 4-Cl | 4-Cl | 4-Cl | 4-Cl |
| **$R^2$** | 4-Cl | 4-Cl | 3,5-F | 2-MeO, 4-Br | 2-OH | 4-F | 2,4,5-MeO |
| **$R^1$** | 4-F | 4-F | 4-Me | 4-Me | 4-Me | 4-$CF_3$O | 4-$CF_3$O |
| **$R^2$** | H | 4-MeO | 4-Cl | H | 4-MeO | H | 4-MeO |

**Scheme 71.** Phospha-Mannich reaction under ultrasonic irradiation.

We now consider further solvent-free methods. [Emim][Br] was found to be an efficient catalyst in the neat condensation of different amines, aldehydes, and phosphites, allowing the use of temperatures as low as 26 °C (Scheme 72) [104].

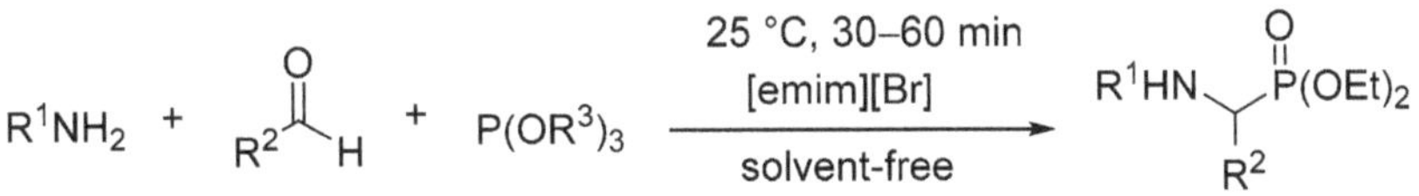


**13** ($R^3$= Et)
65–76%

| | | | | | | |
|---|---|---|---|---|---|---|
| **$R^1$** | $C_6H_5$ | $C_6H_5$ | $C_6H_5$ | Bu | $^c$Hex | $C_6H_5$ |
| **$R^2$** | $C_6H_5$ | 4-Cl$C_6H_4$ | $C_6H_5$ | $C_6H_5$ | $C_6H_5$ | Pr |
| **$R^3$** | $C_6H_5$ | $C_6H_5$ | Me | $C_6H_5$ | $C_6H_5$ | Me |

**Scheme 72.** An ionic-liquid-catalyzed Kabachnik–Fields reaction. [emim]—ethyl-methyl-imidazolyl.

A solvent-free sonochemical transformation utilized a magnetically recoverable composite catalyst (Scheme 73) [105].

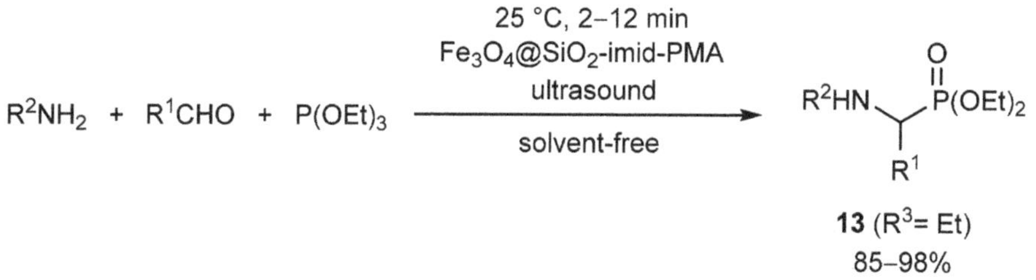

| | | | | | |
|---|---|---|---|---|---|
| R1 | $C_6H_5$ | 4-$NO_2C_6H_5$ | 3-$NO_2C_6H_5$ | 4-$ClC_6H_4$ | 2-$ClC_6H_4$ |
| R2 | $C_6H_5$ | $C_6H_5$ | $C_6H_5$ | $C_6H_5$ | $C_6H_5$ |
| R1 | 4-$BrC_6H_4$ | 4-$MeC_6H_4$ | 2-$MeC_6H_4$ | 4-$HOC_6H_4$ | 4-$MeOC_6H_4$ |
| R2 | $C_6H_5$ | $C_6H_5$ | $C_6H_5$ | $C_6H_5$ | $C_6H_5$ |
| R1 | $C_6H_5$ | $C_6H_5$ | 4-$NO_2C_6H_5$ | 4-$MeOrC_6H_5$ | 4-$BrC_6H_5$ |
| R2 | 4-$NO_2C_6H_5$ | 4-$MeC_6H_4$ | 4-$NO_2C_6H_5$ | 4-$NO_2C_6H_5$ | 4-$MeC_6H_5$ |
| R1 | 4-$MeC_6H_5$ | 4-$MeOC_6H_5$ | Pr | 4-$MeC_6H_5$ | $C_6H_5$ |
| R2 | 4-$MeC_6H_5$ | 4-$MeOC_6H_5$ | 4-$MeOC_6H_4$ | Bu | $CH_2C_6H_4$ |

**Scheme 73.** The use of a magnetically recoverable catalyst in the Kabachnik–Fields reaction. PMA—phosphor molybdic acid.

Boric acid was a suitable catalyst for the condensation of amines, benzaldehyde derivatives, and trimethyl phosphite (Scheme 74) [106].

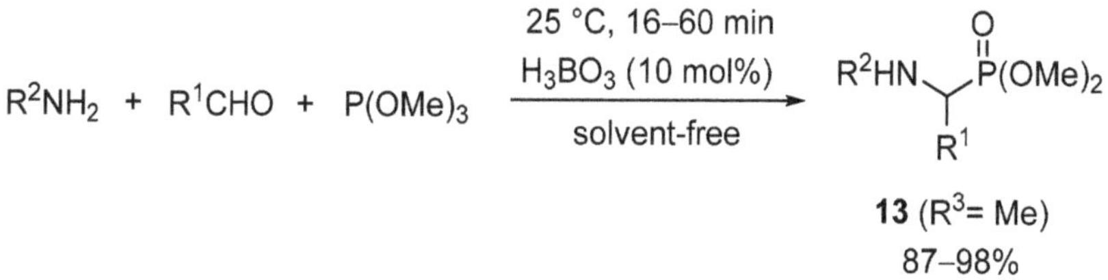

| | | | | | |
|---|---|---|---|---|---|
| R1 | $C_6H_5$ | 4-$NO_2C_6H_5$ | 4-$CNC_6H_4$ | 4-$ClC_6H_5$ | 4-$MeC_6H_4$ |
| R2 | $C_6H_5$ | $C_6H_5$ | $C_6H_5$ | $C_6H_5$ | $C_6H_5$ |
| R1 | 4-$HOC_6H_4$ | 2-$MeOC_6H_4$ | $C_6H_5$ | 4-$HOC_6H_4$ | |
| R2 | $C_6H_5$ | $C_6H_5$ | 4-$ClC_6H_5$ | 4-$ClC_6H_5$ | |

**Scheme 74.** Boric acid as the catalyst in a solvent-free reaction.

Dicationic ionic liquids were used as recyclable catalysts in the solvent-free synthesis of aminophosphonates starting from primary amines, benzaldehyde derivatives, and trimethyl phosphite (Scheme 75) [107].

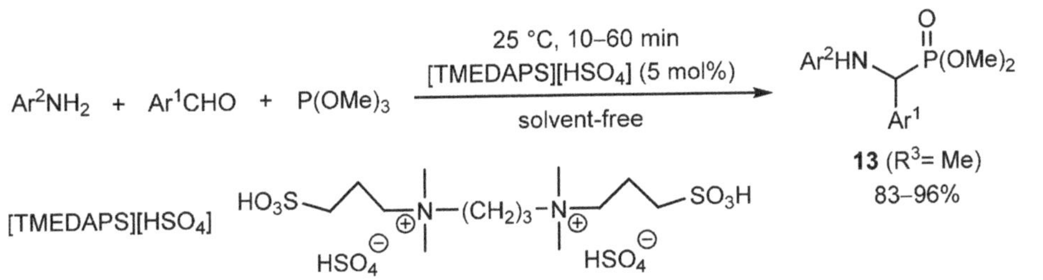


| | | | | | |
|---|---|---|---|---|---|
| **Ar¹** | $C_6H_5$ | 4-$NO_2C_6H_4$ | 2,6-$Cl_2C_6H_3$ | 4-$ClC_6H_4$ | 4-$MeC_6H_4$ |
| **Ar²** | $C_6H_5$ | $C_6H_5$ | $C_6H_5$ | $C_6H_5$ | $C_6H_5$ |
| **Ar¹** | 4-$MeOC_6H_4$ | 2,5-$(MeO)_2C_6H_3$ | 3,4,5-$(MeO)_3C_6H_2$ | 2-thiazolyl | $C_6H_5$ |
| **Ar²** | $C_6H_5$ | $C_6H_5$ | $C_6H_5$ | $C_6H_5$ | 4-$FC_6H_5$ |
| **Ar¹** | 4-$MeC_6H_4$ | 4-$MeOC_6H_4$ | 4-$MeOC_6H_4$ | | |
| **Ar²** | 4-$NO_2C_6H_4$ | $C_6H_5CH_2$ | 2-pyridyl | | |

**Scheme 75.** A dicationic ionic liquid as the catalyst in the three-component Kabachnik–Fields reaction. [TMEDAPS]—*N,N,N′,N′*-tetramethyl-*N,N′*-di(sulfonylpropyl)-1,3-propanediammonium bis(hydrogen sulfate).

When an ortho-ethoxycarbonylmethyl-benzaldehyde derivative (**107**) was the oxo component, the condensation was followed by an intramolecular cyclization to furnish the corresponding isoquinolone derivative (**108**) (Scheme 76) [108].

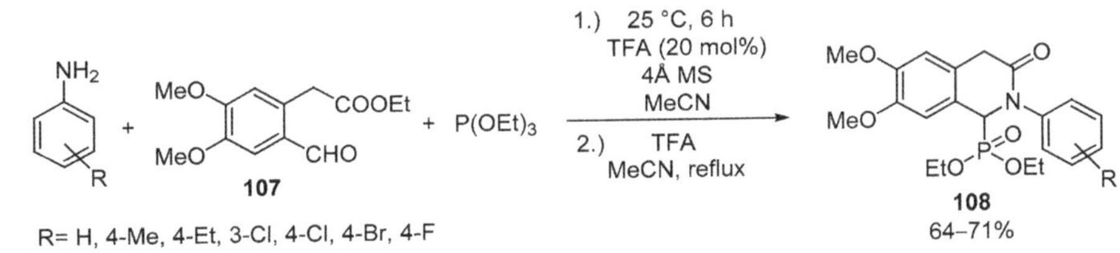


**Scheme 76.** Kabachnik–Fields reaction starting from ortho-ethoxycarbonylmethyl-benzaldehyde as the oxo component followed by cyclization. TFA—trifluoroacetic acid.

A few other Kabachnik–Fields reactions followed by intramolecular cyclization have also been described. Ordóñez et al. elaborated the MW-assisted condensation of 2-formylbenzoic acid, aromatic amines (including optically active ones), and dimethyl phosphite [109–111] or triethyl phosphite [112] to afford the corresponding isoindolin-1-one-phosphonates after a ring closure in the final step.

To compare the methods with each other, a few studies have been performed in solvents, like the protocol using T3P, which gives the products in good yields. On the other hand, a few other methods applying $Fe_3O_4$@$SiO_2$-imid PMA and $H_3BO_3$ as the catalysts in a solvent-free manner have been to give the corresponding products in good yields. The advantage of using dicationic ionic liquids is that the catalysts are recyclable. These issues are of importance from the point of view of green chemistry. These methods play an important role in allowing mild conditions, reducing the reaction times, and giving the products in high yields. However, if the Kabachnik–Fields reactions utilizing dialkyl phosphites and trialkyl phosphites are compared, the protocol applying dialkyl phosphites (see subchapter 3) is unambiguously the method of choice due to its atomic efficiency. Moreover, trialkyl phosphites have an unpleasant smell.

## 4. The aza-Pudovik Reaction

The aza-Pudovik reaction involving the addition of a dialkyl phosphite to an imine is another approach to synthesize α-aminophosphonates. A carbazole-related imine (**109**) was reacted with dialkyl phosphites and diphenylphosphine oxide in the presence of tetramethylguanidine as the catalyst in toluene to give the corresponding adducts (**110**) in good yields (Scheme 77) [113].

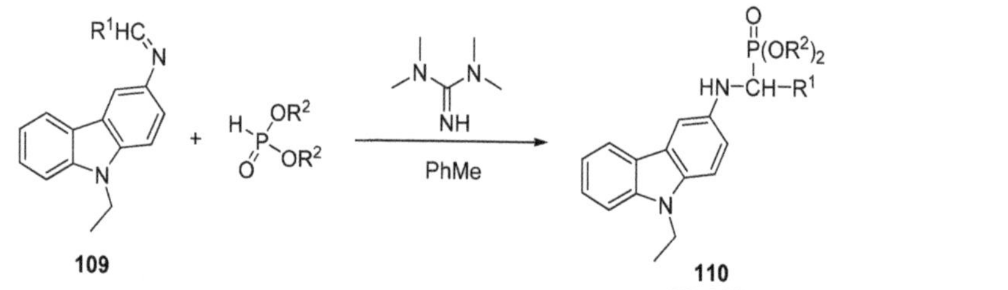


| | | | | | |
|---|---|---|---|---|---|
| $R^1$ | 3-$CH_3$-thiophene | 5-$CH_3$-thiophene | 2-HO-5-$ClC_6H_3$ | 3-$CH_3$-thiophene | 5-$CH_3$-thiophene |
| $R^2$ | Me | Me | Me | Et | Et |
| $R^1$ | 2-HO-5-$ClC_6H_3$ | 5-$CH_3$-thiophene | 3-$CH_3$-thiophene | 2-HO-5-$ClC_6H_3$ | |
| $R^2$ | Et | $C_6H_5$ | $C_6H_5$ | $C_6H_5$ | |

**Scheme 77.** Kabachnik–Fields reactions starting from imines and applying tetramethylguanidine as the catalyst.

In another case, the simple starting materials benzylideneimines were reacted with secondary phosphine oxides, where a guanidium salt (**112**) served as the catalyst (Scheme 78) [114].

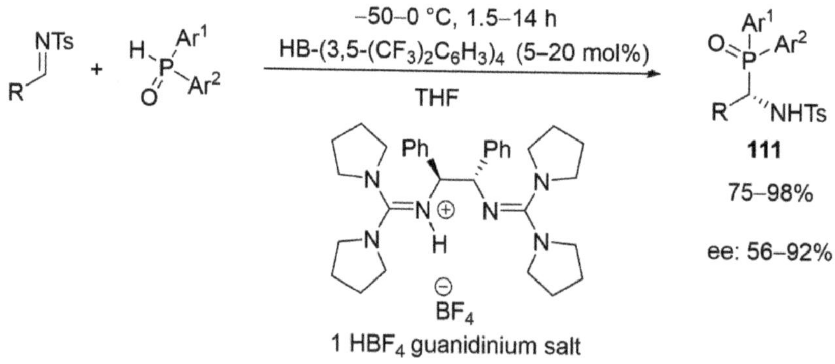


| | | | | | |
|---|---|---|---|---|---|
| **R** | 4-$FC_6H_4$ | 4-$MeC_6H_4$ | 2-naphthyl | 2-furyl | ${}^t$Bu |
| **Ar¹** | 1-naphthyl | 1-naphthyl | 1-naphthyl | 1-naphthyl | 1-naphthyl |
| **Ar²** | 1-naphthyl | 1-naphthyl | 1-naphthyl | 1-naphthyl | 1-naphthyl |
| **R** | ${}^c$Hex | $C_6H_5$ | $C_6H_5$ | $C_6H_5$ | |
| **Ar¹** | 1-naphthyl | $C_6H_5$ | 2-$CF_3C_5H_4$ | $C_6H_5$ | |
| **Ar²** | 1-naphthyl | $C_6H_5$ | 2-$CF_3C_5H_4$ | 1-naphthyl | |

**Scheme 78.** Guanidium salt as the catalyst in the aza-Pudovik reaction.

A cinchona-derived thiourea (**117–122**) was applied in the addition of diphenyl phosphite to ketimines (Scheme 79) [115]. The yields of products **114** and **116** varied within the range of 48–88%.

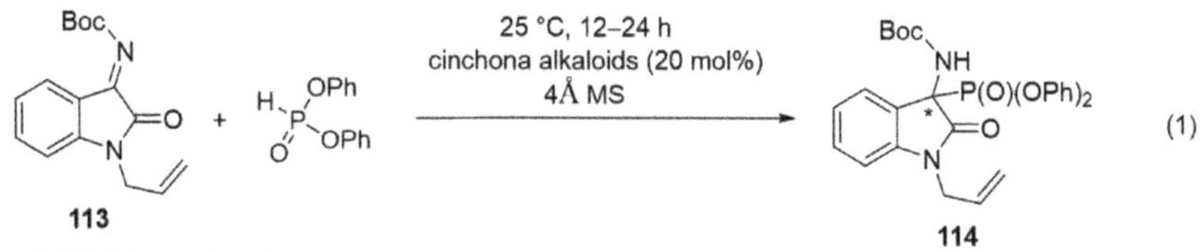


**113**

Boc: tert-butyloxycarbonyl

**114**
48–88%
ee (+): 15–52%
ee (−): 12–94%

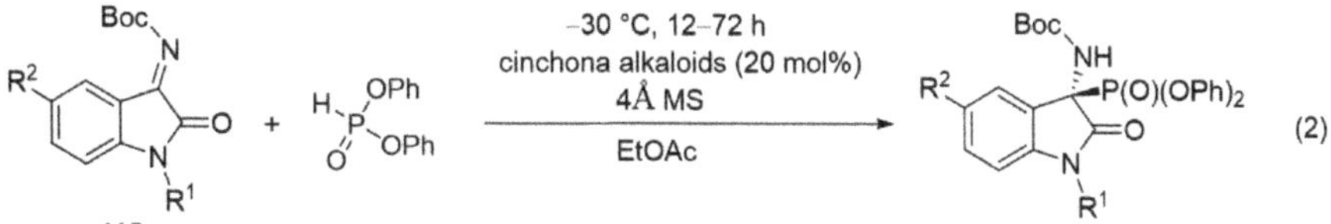


**115**

**116**
71–88%
ee: 71–97%

| | | | | |
|---|---|---|---|---|
| **$R^1$** | $CH_2CHCH_2$ | $CH_2CHCH_2$ | $CH_2CHCH_2$ | $CH_2CHCH_2$ |
| **$R^2$** | H | Cl | Br | I |
| **$R^1$** | $CH_2C(CH_3)CH_2$ | $CH_2CHCHCH_2$ | $CH_2C_6H_5$ | $CH_2C_6H_5$ |
| **$R^2$** | Cl | Cl | H | Cl |
| **$R^1$** | $CH_2C_6H_5$ | $CH_2C_6H_5$ | $CH_2C_6H_5$ | $CH_2C_6H_5$ |
| **$R^2$** | Br | I | MeO | Cl |

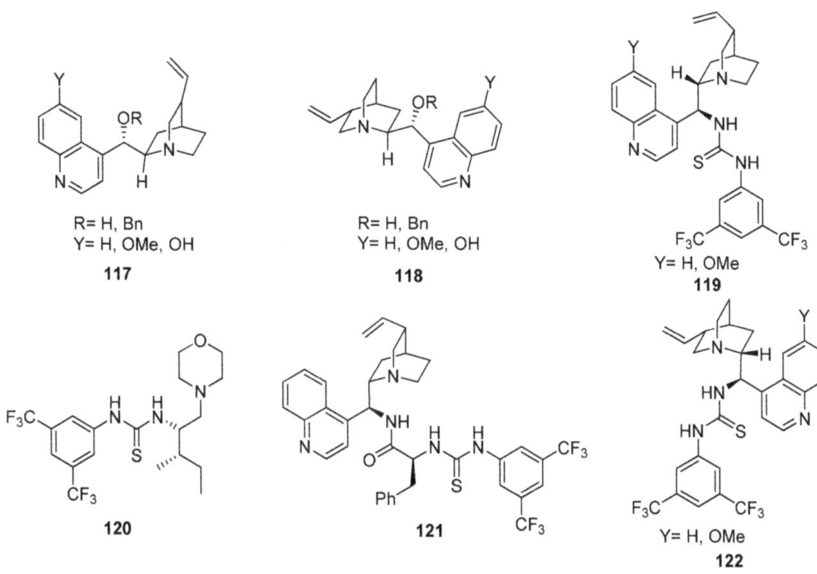


**Scheme 79.** The use of cinchona-derived thiourea catalysts in the aza-Pudovik reaction. MS—molecular sieves.

The aza-Pudovik approach was also useful in the synthesis of (5-nitrofuranoyl)-substituted esters of a phosphonoglycine derivative (**124**). In these cases, $BF_3{\cdot}OEt_2$ was the catalyst (Scheme 80) [116,117].

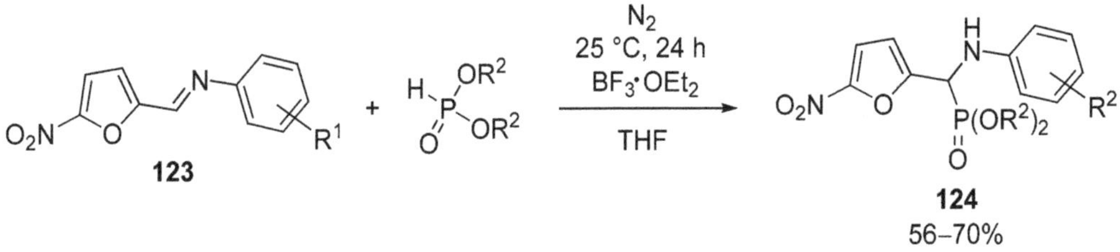


| | | | | | |
|---|---|---|---|---|---|
| **R¹** | 3-Me | 4-Me | 4-MeO | 3-Me | 4-Me |
| **R²** | Me | Me | Me | Et | Et |
| **R¹** | 4-MeO | 2-Me | 3-Me | 4-Me | 4-MeO |
| **R²** | Et | $C_6H_5$ | $C_6H_5$ | $C_6H_5$ | $C_6H_5$ |

**Scheme 80.** Aza-Pudovik reaction applying $BF_3{\cdot}OEt_2$ as the catalyst.

This method was applied to the preparation of the corresponding pyrrole derivatives (**127**). In this case, the imine (**126**) was synthesized in situ (Scheme 81) [118].

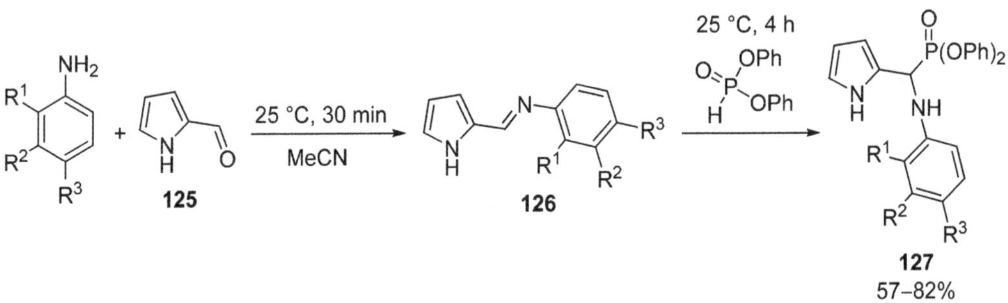


| | | | |
|---|---|---|---|
| **R¹** | H | H | Me |
| **R²** | H | H | H |
| **R³** | H | $NO_2$ | Cl |

**Scheme 81.** Aza-Pudovik reactions starting from the imine of pyrrole carbaldehyde.

In a variation, the imines generated in the reaction of aniline and benzaldehyde derivatives were reacted with diethyl phosphite in boiling ethanol to furnish the corresponding α-aminophosphonates (**129**) in medium yields (Scheme 82) [119].

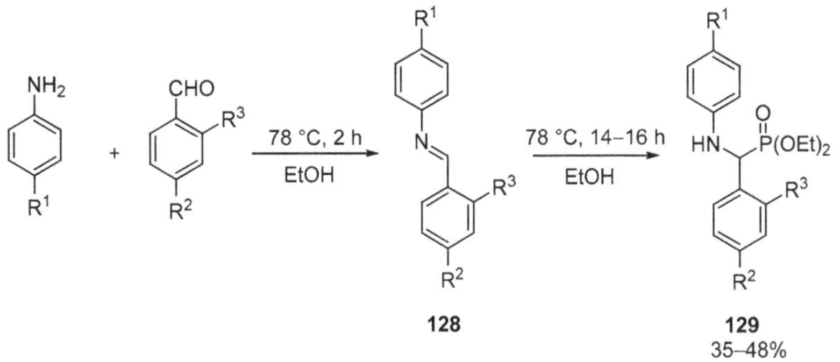

| **R¹** | NO₂ | Cl | Cl | Cl | Cl |
|---|---|---|---|---|---|
| **R²** | Cl | NO₂ | H | MeO | H |
| **R³** | H | H | NO₂ | H | MeO |

**Scheme 82.** Catalyst-free aza-Pudovik reactions.

The imines (**130**) obtained from benzaldehyde were reacted with diethyl phosphite in the presence of $MoO_2Cl_2$ as the catalyst under solvent-free conditions. (Scheme 83) [120].

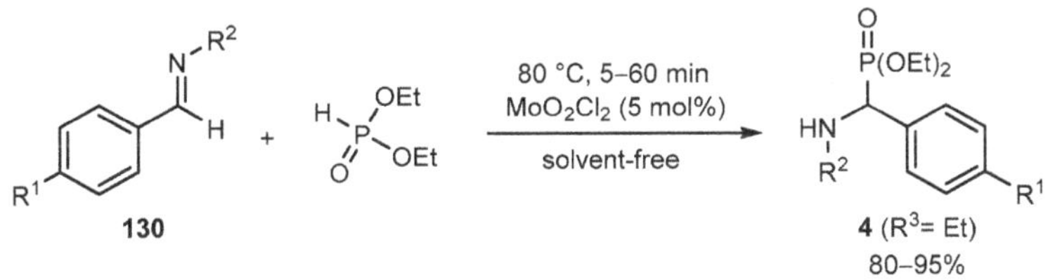

| **R¹** | NC | CF₃ | F | F | H | NO₂ | MeO |
|---|---|---|---|---|---|---|---|
| **R²** | C₆H₅ | C₆H₅ | C₆H₅ | (CH₂)₅CH₃ | C₆H₅ | C₆H₅ | C₆H₅ |

**Scheme 83.** Aza-Pudovik reaction applying $MoO_2Cl_2$ as the catalyst.

α-Aryl-α-aminophosphonates and α-aryl-α-aminophosphine oxides (**132**) were prepared by the MW-assisted Pudovik reaction of benzylideneimines and >P(O)H reagents (Scheme 84) [121].

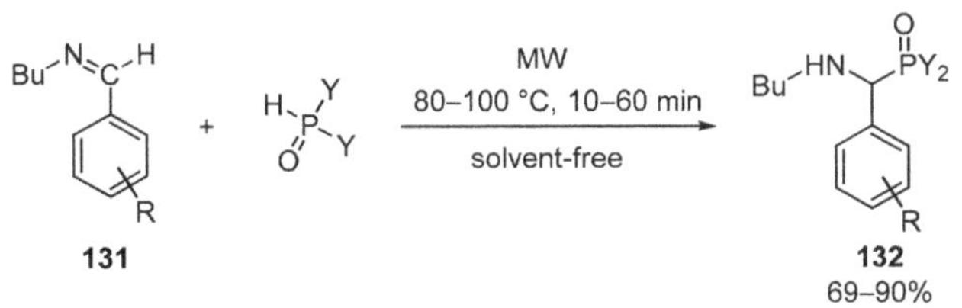

| **R** | H | H | H | H | H | 2-Cl | 2-Cl |
|---|---|---|---|---|---|---|---|
| **Y** | MeO | EtO | BuO | BnO | C₆H₅ | MeO | EtO |
| **R** | 2-Cl | 3-Cl | 3-Cl | 3-Cl | 4-Cl | 4-Cl | 4-Cl |
| **Y** | BuO | MeO | EtO | BuO | MeO | EtO | BuO |

**Scheme 84.** MW-assisted Pudovik reactions.

Poly-(4-vinylbenzaldehyde) (**134**) was prepared by the polymerization of 4-vinylbenzaldehyde (**133**) in DMSO. Postpolymerization modification reactions comprised imine formation (which is not shown here), and the addition of dialkyl phosphite to afford functional polymers. The α-aminophosphonate (**135**) scaffold was a side group (Scheme 85) [122].

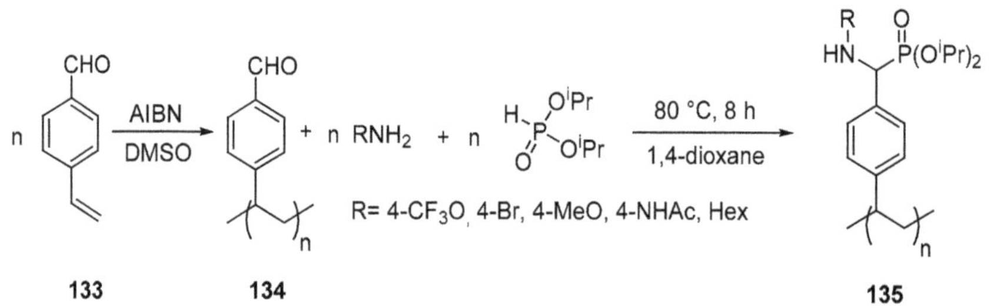


**Scheme 85.** Postpolymerization modification via the Kabachnik–Fields reaction. AIBN—asobisizobutyronitrile.

In another approach, poly(aminophosphonates) were prepared in a one-pot manner including Kabachnik–Fields condensation and polymerization [123]. Functional polymers with bis(phosphonomethyl)amine moieties were also prepared. In this case, phosphorous acid was the P component [124].

Theoretical calculations predicted that the aza-Pudovik reaction under discussion takes place in a single concerted step involving transition state (**136**) formed from the trivalent tautomeric form of dimethyl phosphite and *N*-benzylideneaniline (Scheme 86) [121].

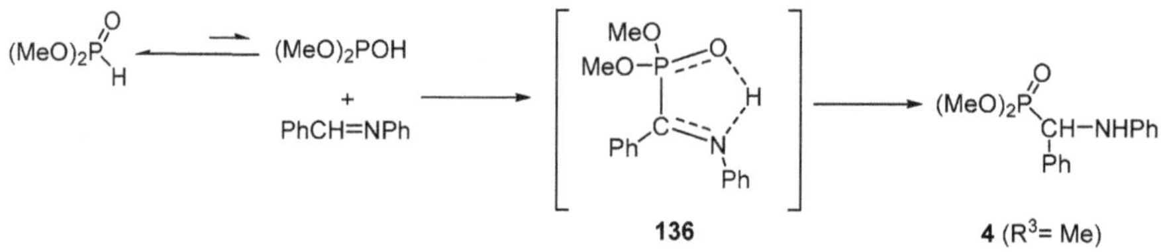


**Scheme 86.** Mechanism for the aza-Pudovik reaction of dimethyl phosphite and *N*-benzylideneaniline.

It was shown that the aza-Pudovik reaction involving the addition of >P(O)H reagents into the unsaturation of imines is a good and atomically efficient route for the preparation of α-aminophosphonic derivatives. As a matter of fact, as was shown in the Introduction, imines are intermediates of the Kabachnik–Fields reactions that may be formed from the oxo component and the amine.

## 5. Conclusions

In conclusion, various methods for the synthesis of α-aminophosphonic derivatives utilizing the Kabachnik–Fields reaction are summarized herein. In this review, different approaches utilizing a wide range of catalysts are summarized, encompassing the results of the last decade. We focused on environmentally friendly points of view. The solvent-free MW-assisted methods are of special importance. The Kabachnik–Fields reaction is also suitable for the synthesis of bis derivatives. Beside >P(O)H reagents, trialkyl phosphites may also be used as the starting materials of the phospha-Mannich condensation. The aza-Pudovik reaction is a special variation for the preparation of α-aminophosphonic derivatives and related compounds.

**Funding:** This project was supported by the National Research, Development and Innovation Office (K119202 and K134318).

**Acknowledgments:** G.K. is grateful to all co-authors appearing in the cited references.

**Conflicts of Interest:** The authors declare no conflict of interest.

## References

1. Keglevich, G.; Bálint, E. The Kabachnik–Fields Reaction: Mechanism and Synthetic Use. *Moecules* **2012**, *17*, 12821–12835. [CrossRef]
2. Kukhar, V.P.; Hudson, H.R. *Aminophosphonic and Aminophosphinic Acids: Chemistry and Biological Activity*; John Wiley & Sons: Chichester, UK, 2000; ISBN 0471891495.
3. Naydenova, E.D.; Todorov, P.T.; Troev, K.D. Recent synthesis of aminophosphonic acids as potential biological importance. *Amino Acids* **2009**, *38*, 23–30. [CrossRef] [PubMed]
4. Abdel-Rahman, R.M.; Ali, T.E.; Abdel-Kariem, S.M. Methods for synthesis of N-heterocyclyl/heteroaryl- α-aminophosphonates and α-(azaheterocyclyl)phosphonates. *Arkivoc* **2016**, *2016*, 183–211. [CrossRef]
5. Review on the Synthesis of α-Aminophosphonate Derivatives. *Chem. Sci. Trans.* **2019**, *8*, 359–367. [CrossRef]
6. Kabachnik, M.I.; Medved, T.Y. New synthesis of aminophosphonic acids. *Dokl. Akad. Nauk SSSR* **1952**, *83*, 689–692.
7. Fields, E.K. The Synthesis of Esters of Substituted Amino Phosphonic Acids1a. *J. Am. Chem. Soc.* **1952**, *74*, 1528–1531. [CrossRef]
8. Mucha, A.; Kafarski, P.; Berlicki, Ł. Remarkable Potential of the α-Aminophosphonate/Phosphinate Structural Motif in Medicinal Chemistry. *J. Med. Chem.* **2011**, *54*, 5955–5980. [CrossRef] [PubMed]
9. Kafarski, P.; Lejczak, B. Biological Activity of Aminophosphonic Acids. *Phosphorus Sulfur Silicon Relat. Elem.* **1991**, *63*, 193–215. [CrossRef]
10. Kafarski, P. Aminophosphonic Acids of Potential Medical Importance. *Curr. Med. Chem. Agents* **2001**, *1*, 301–312. [CrossRef] [PubMed]
11. Berlicki, L.; Kafarski, P. Computer-Aided Analysis and Design of Phosphonic and Phosphinic Enzyme Inhibitors as Potential Drugs and Agrochemicals. *Curr. Org. Chem.* **2005**, *9*, 1829–1850. [CrossRef]
12. Lejczak, B.; Kafarski, P. Biological Activity of Aminophosphonic Acids and Their Short Peptides. In *Topics in Heterocyclic Chemistry—Phosphorous Heterocycles I*; Gupta, R.P., Bansal, R.K., Eds.; Springer: Berlin, Germany, 2009; Volume 20, pp. 31–63.
13. Cherkasov, R.A.; Galkin, V.I. The Kabachnik–Fields reaction: Synthetic potential and the problem of the mechanism. *Russ. Chem. Rev.* **1998**, *67*, 857–882. [CrossRef]
14. Keglevich, G.; Kiss, N.Z.; Menyhárd, D.K.; Fehérvári, A.; Csontos, I. A study on the kabachnik–fields reaction of benzaldehyde, cyclohexylamine, and dialkyl phosphites. *Heteroat. Chem.* **2012**, *23*, 171–178. [CrossRef]
15. Keglevich, G.; Fehérvári, A.; Csontos, I. A study on the Kabachnik-Fields reaction of benzaldehyde, propylamine, and diethyl phosphite by in situ Fourier transform IR spectroscopy. *Heteroat. Chem.* **2011**, *22*, 599–604. [CrossRef]
16. Kafarski, P.; Gorniak, M.G.V.; Andrasiak, I. Kabachnik-Fields Reaction Under Green Conditions—A Critical Overview. *Curr. Green Chem.* **2015**, *2*, 218–222. [CrossRef]
17. Keglevich, G.; Szekrényi, A. Eco-Friendly Accomplishment of the Extended Kabachnik—Fields Reaction; A Solvent- and Catalyst-Free Microwave-Assisted Synthesis of α- Aminophosphonates and α-Aminophosphine Oxides. *Lett. Org. Chem.* **2008**, *5*, 616–622. [CrossRef]
18. Ranu, B.C.; Hajra, A. A simple and green procedure for the synthesis of α-aminophosphonate by a one-pot three-component condensation of carbonyl compound, amine and diethyl phosphite without solvent and catalyst. *Green Chem.* **2002**, *4*, 551–554. [CrossRef]
19. Kabachnik, M.M.; Zobnina, E.V.; Beletskaya, I.P. Catalyst-Free Microwave-Assisted Synthesis of α-Aminophosphonates in a Three-Component System: R1C(O)R2-(EtO)2P(O)H-RNH2. *Synlett* **2005**, *2005*, 1393–1396. [CrossRef]
20. Mu, X.-J.; Lei, M.-Y.; Zou, J.-P.; Zhang, W. Microwave-assisted solvent-free and catalyst-free Kabachnik–Fields reactions for α-amino phosphonates. *Tetrahedron Lett.* **2006**, *47*, 1125–1127. [CrossRef]
21. Zahouily, M.; Elmakssoudi, A.; Mezdar, A.; Rayadh, A.; Sebti, S. Uncatalysed Preparation of α-Amino Phosphonates under Solvent Free Conditions. *J. Chem. Res.* **2005**, *2005*, 324–327. [CrossRef]
22. Prauda, I.; Greiner, I.; Ludányi, K.; Keglevich, G. Efficient Synthesis of Phosphono- and Phosphinoxidomethylated N-Heterocycles under Solvent-Free Microwave Conditions. *Synth. Commun.* **2007**, *37*, 317–322. [CrossRef]
23. Keglevich, G.; Szekrenyi, A.; Sipos, M.; Ludányi, K.; Greiner, I. Synthesis of cyclic aminomethylphosphonates and aminomethyl-arylphosphinic acids by an efficient microwave-mediated phospha-mannich approach. *Heteroat. Chem.* **2008**, *19*, 207–210. [CrossRef]
24. Shuvalov, M.V.; Maklakova, S.Y.; Rudakova, E.V.; Kovaleva, N.V.; Makhaeva, G.F.; Podrugina, T.A. New Possibilities of the Kabachnik–Fields and Pudovik Reactions in the Phthalocyanine-Catalyzed Syntheses of α-Aminophosphonic and α-Aminophosphinic Acid Derivatives. *Russ. J. Gen. Chem.* **2018**, *88*, 1761–1775. [CrossRef]
25. Cabrita, I.R.; Sousa, S.C.; Florindo, P.R.; Fernandes, A.C. Direct Aminophosphonylation of aldehydes catalyzed by cyclopentadienyl ruthenium(II) complexes. *Tetrahedron* **2018**, *74*, 1817–1825. [CrossRef]

26. Awad, M.K.; Abdel-Aal, M.F.; Atlam, F.M.; Hekal, H.A. Design, synthesis, molecular modeling, and biological evaluation of novel α-aminophosphonates based quinazolinone moiety as potential anticancer agents: DFT, NBO and vibrational studies. *J. Mol. Struct.* **2018**, *1173*, 128–141. [CrossRef]
27. Disale, S.T.; Kale, S.R.; Kahandal, S.S.; Srinivasan, T.G.; Jayaram, R.V. Choline chloride·2ZnCl2 ionic liquid: An efficient and reusable catalyst for the solvent free Kabachnik–Fields reaction. *Tetrahedron Lett.* **2012**, *53*, 2277–2279. [CrossRef]
28. Ordóñez, M.; Viveros-Ceballos, J.L.; Estudillo, I.R. Stereoselective Synthesis of α-Aminophosphonic Acids through Pudovik and Kabachnik-Fields Reaction. In *Amino Acid—New Insights and Roles in Plant and Animal*; IntechOpen: Rijeka, Croatia, 2017; pp. 1328–1365.
29. Ohara, M.; Nakamura, S.; Shibata, N. Direct Enantioselective Three-Component Kabachnik-Fields Reaction Catalyzed by Chiral Bis(imidazoline)-Zinc(II) Catalysts. *Adv. Synth. Catal.* **2011**, *353*, 3285–3289. [CrossRef]
30. Essid, I.; Touil, S. Efficient and Green One-Pot Multi-Component Synthesis of α-Aminophosphonates Catalyzed by Zinc Triflate. *Curr. Org. Synth.* **2017**, *14*, 272–278. [CrossRef]
31. Ewies, E.F.; El-Hussieny, M.; El-Sayed, N.F.; Fouad, M.A. Design, synthesis and biological evaluation of novel α-aminophosphonate oxadiazoles via optimized iron triflate catalyzed reaction as apoptotic inducers. *Eur. J. Med. Chem.* **2019**, *180*, 310–320. [CrossRef]
32. Das, S.; Rawal, P.; Bhattacharjee, J.; Devadkar, A.; Pal, K.; Gupta, P.; Panda, T.K. Indium promoted C(sp3)–P bond formation by the Domino A3-coupling method—A combined experimental and computational study. *Inorg. Chem. Front.* **2021**, *8*, 1142–1153. [CrossRef]
33. Teimouri, A.; Chermahini, A.N.; Narimani, M. Three component coupling catalyzed by nickel (II) chloride hexahydrate: Synthesis of α-amino phosphonates. *Chiang Mai J. Sci.* **2015**, *42*, 228–237.
34. Hou, J.-T.; Gao, J.-W.; Zhang, Z.-H. NbCl5: An efficient catalyst for one-pot synthesis of α-aminophosphonates under solvent-free conditions. *Appl. Organomet. Chem.* **2010**, *25*, 47–53. [CrossRef]
35. Che, J.-Y.; Xu, X.-Y.; Tang, Z.-L.; Gu, Y.-C.; Shi, D.-Q. Synthesis and herbicidal activity evaluation of novel α-amino phosphonate derivatives containing a uracil moiety. *Bioorganic Med. Chem. Lett.* **2016**, *26*, 1310–1313. [CrossRef]
36. Jafari, A.A.; Nazarpour, M.; Abdollahi-Alibeik, M. CeCl3·7H2O-catalyzed one-pot Kabachnik-Fields reaction: A green protocol for three-component synthesis of α-aminophosphonates. *Heteroat. Chem.* **2010**, *21*, 397–403. [CrossRef]
37. Agawane, S.M.; Nagarkar, J.M. Nano ceria catalyzed synthesis of α-aminophosphonates under ultrasonication. *Tetrahedron Lett.* **2011**, *52*, 3499–3504. [CrossRef]
38. Sreelakshmi, P.; Santhisudha, S.; Reddy, G.R.; Subbarao, Y.; Peddanna, K.; Apparao, C.; Reddy, C.S. Nano-Cuo–Au-catalyzed solvent-free synthesis of α-aminophosphonates and evaluation of their antioxidant and α-glucosidase enzyme inhibition activities. *Synth. Commun.* **2018**, *48*, 1148–1163. [CrossRef]
39. Reddy, K.M.K.; Santhisudha, S.; Mohan, G.; Peddanna, K.; Rao, C.A.; Reddy, C.S. Nano Gd2O3 catalyzed synthesis and anti-oxidant activity of new α-aminophosphonates. *Phosphorus Sulfur Silicon Relat. Elem.* **2016**, *191*, 933–938. [CrossRef]
40. Saberi, D.; Cheraghi, S.; Mahdudi, S.; Akbari, J.; Heydari, A. Dehydroascorbic acid (DHAA) capped magnetite nanoparticles as an efficient magnetic organocatalyst for the one-pot synthesis of α-aminonitriles and α-aminophosphonates. *Tetrahedron Lett.* **2013**, *54*, 6403–6406. [CrossRef]
41. Shaibuna, M.; Sreekumar, K. Experimental Investigation on the Correlation between the Physicochemical Properties and Catalytic Activity of Six DESs in the Kabachnik-Fields Reaction. *ChemBioChem* **2020**, *5*, 13454–13460. [CrossRef]
42. Rostamnia, S.; Xin, H.; Nouruzi, N. Metal–organic frameworks as a very suitable reaction inductor for selective solvent-free multicomponent reaction: IRMOF-3 as a heterogeneous nanocatalyst for Kabachnik–Fields three-component reaction. *Microporous Mesoporous Mater.* **2013**, *179*, 99–103. [CrossRef]
43. Khatri, C.K.; Satalkar, V.B.; Chaturbhuj, G.U. Sulfated polyborate catalyzed Kabachnik-Fields reaction: An efficient and eco-friendly protocol for synthesis of α-amino phosphonates. *Tetrahedron Lett.* **2017**, *58*, 694–698. [CrossRef]
44. Ordonez, M.; Tibhe, G.; Bedolla-Medrano, M.; Cativiela, C. Phenylboronic Acid as Efficient and Eco-Friendly Catalyst for the One-Pot, Three-Component Synthesis of α-Aminophosphonates under Solvent-Free Conditions. *Synlett* **2012**, *23*, 1931–1936. [CrossRef]
45. Ordóñez, M.; Bedolla-Medrano, M.; Hernández-Fernández, E. Phenylphosphonic Acid as Efficient and Recyclable Catalyst in the Synthesis of α-Aminophosphonates under Solvent-Free Conditions. *Synlett* **2014**, *25*, 1145–1149. [CrossRef]
46. Hellal, A.; Chafaa, S.; Chafai, N.; Touafri, L. Synthesis, antibacterial screening and DFT studies of series of α-amino-phosphonates derivatives from aminophenols. *J. Mol. Struct.* **2017**, *1134*, 217–225. [CrossRef]
47. Rostamnia, S.; Hassankhani, A. Application of biodegradable supramolecular polymer-supported catalyst for multicomponent synthesis of α-aminophosphonates Kabachnik–Fields reaction. *Supramol. Chem.* **2014**, *26*, 736–739. [CrossRef]
48. Cherkasov, R.A.; Garifzyanov, A.R.; Koshkin, S.A. Synthesis of α-Aminophosphine Oxides with Chiral Phosphorus and Carbon Atoms. *Phosphorus Sulfur Silicon Relat. Elem.* **2011**, *186*, 782–784. [CrossRef]
49. Cherkasov, R.A.; Garifzyanov, A.R.; Koshkin, S.A. Synthesis of optically active α-aminophosphine oxides and enantioselective membrane transport of acids with their participation. *Russ. J. Gen. Chem.* **2011**, *81*, 773–774. [CrossRef]
50. Vagapova, L.I.; Burilov, A.R.; Voronina, J.K.; Syakaev, V.V.; Sharafutdinova, D.R.; Amirova, L.R.; Pudovik, M.A.; Garifzyanov, A.R.; Sinyashin, O.G. Phosphorylated Aminoacetal in the Synthesis of New Acyclic, Cyclic, and Heterocyclic Polyphenol Structures. *Heteroat. Chem.* **2014**, *25*, 178–185. [CrossRef]

51. Vagapova, L.I.; Burilov, A.R.; Amirova, L.R.; Voronina, J.K.; Garifzyanov, A.R.; Abdrachmanova, N.F.; Pudovik, M.A. New aminophosphonates (aminophosphine oxides) containing acetal groups in reactions with polyatomic phenols. *Phosphorus Sulfur Silicon Relat. Elem.* **2016**, *191*, 1527–1529. [CrossRef]
52. Gangireddy, C.S.R.; Chinthaparthi, R.R.; Mudumala, V.R.; Mamilla, M.; Arigala, U.R.S. An Efficient Green Synthesis of a New Class of α-Aminophosphonates under Microwave Irradiation Conditions in the Presence of PS/ P TSA. *Heteroat. Chem.* **2014**, *25*, 147–156. [CrossRef]
53. Gundluru, M.; Badavath, V.N.; Shaik, H.Y.; Sudileti, M.; Nemallapudi, B.R.; Gundala, S.; Zyryanov, G.V.; Cirandur, S.R. Design, synthesis, cytotoxic evaluation and molecular docking studies of novel thiazolyl α-aminophosphonates. *Res. Chem. Intermed.* **2021**, *47*, 1139–1160. [CrossRef]
54. Nayab, R.S.; Maddila, S.; Krishna, M.P.; Titinchi, S.J.; Thaslim, B.S.; Chintha, V.; Wudayagiri, R.; Nagam, V.; Tartte, V.; Chinnam, S.; et al. In silico molecular docking and in vitro antioxidant activity studies of novel α-aminophosphonates bearing 6-amino-1,3-dimethyl uracil. *J. Recept. Signal Transduct.* **2020**, *40*, 166–172. [CrossRef] [PubMed]
55. Hellal, A.; Chafaa, S.; Touafri, L. An eco-friendly procedure for the efficient synthesis of diethyl α-aminophosphonates in aqueous media using natural acids as a catalyst. *Korean J. Chem. Eng.* **2016**, *33*, 2366–2373. [CrossRef]
56. Thirumurugan, P.; Nandakumar, A.; Priya, N.S.; Muralidaran, D.; Perumal, P. KHSO4-mediated synthesis of α-amino phosphonates under a neat condition and their 31P NMR chemical shift assignments. *Tetrahedron Lett.* **2010**, *51*, 5708–5712. [CrossRef]
57. Reddy, P.S.; Reddy, P.V.G.; Reddy, S.M. Phosphomolybdic acid promoted Kabachnik–Fields reaction: An efficient one-pot synthesis of α-aminophosphonates from 2-cyclopropylpyrimidine-4-carbaldehyde. *Tetrahedron Lett.* **2014**, *55*, 3336–3339. [CrossRef]
58. Reddy, P.S.; Reddy, M.V.K.; Reddy, P.V.G. Camphor-derived thioureas: Synthesis and application in asymmetric Kabachnik-Fields reaction. *Chin. Chem. Lett.* **2016**, *27*, 943–947. [CrossRef]
59. Tillu, V.; Dumbre, D.; Wakharkar, R.; Choudhary, V. One-pot three-component Kabachnik–Fields synthesis of α-aminophosphonates using H-beta zeolite catalyst. *Tetrahedron Lett.* **2011**, *52*, 863–866. [CrossRef]
60. Taran, J.; Ramazani, A.; Aghahosseini, H.; Gouranlou, F.; Tarasi, R.; Khoobi, M.; Joo, S.W. One-pot three-component syntheses of α-aminophosphonates from a primary amine, quinoline-4-carbaldehyde and a phosphite in the presence of MCM-41@PEI as an efficient nanocatalyst. *Phosphorus Sulfur Silicon Relat. Elem.* **2017**, *192*, 776–781. [CrossRef]
61. Fan, W.; Queneau, Y.; Popowycz, F. The synthesis of HMF-based α-amino phosphonatesviaone-pot Kabachnik–Fields reaction. *RSC Adv.* **2018**, *8*, 31496–31501. [CrossRef]
62. Nadiveedhi, M.R.; Nuthalapati, P.; Gundluru, M.; Yanamula, M.R.; Kallimakula, S.V.; Pasupuleti, V.R.; Avula, V.K.R.; Vallela, S.; Zyryanov, G.V.; Balam, S.K.; et al. Green Synthesis, Antioxidant, and Plant Growth Regulatory Activities of Novel α-Furfuryl-2-alkylaminophosphonates. *ACS Omega* **2021**, *6*, 2934–2948. [CrossRef] [PubMed]
63. Rostamnia, S.; Amini, M. Ultrasonic and Lewis acid ionic liquid catalytic system for Kabachnik-Fields reaction. *Chem. Pap.* **2014**, *68*, 834–837. [CrossRef]
64. Eyckens, D.J.; Henderson, L.C. Synthesis of α-aminophosphonates using solvate ionic liquids. *RSC Adv.* **2017**, *7*, 27900–27904. [CrossRef]
65. Qu, Z.; Chen, X.; Yuan, J.; Bai, Y.; Chen, T.; Qu, L.; Wang, F.; Li, X.; Zhao, Y. New synthetic methodology leading to a series of novel heterocyclic α-aminophosphonates: A very attractive expansion of Kabachnik–Fields reaction. *Tetrahedron* **2012**, *68*, 3156–3159. [CrossRef]
66. Tajti, Á.; Tóth, N.; Rávai, B.; Csontos, I.; Szabó, P.T.; Bálint, E. Study on the Microwave-Assisted Batch and Continuous Flow Synthesis of *N*-Alkyl-Isoindolin-1-One-3-Phosphonates by a Special Kabachnik–Fields Condensation. *Molecules* **2020**, *25*, 3307. [CrossRef]
67. Lewkowski, J.; Moya, M.R. The formation of dimethyl amino(pyrene-1-yl)methylphosphonates in the Kabachnik-Fields reaction with dibenzyl phosphite, pyrene-1-carboxaldehyde and a non-aromatic amine in methanol. *Phosphorus Sulfur Silicon Relat. Elem.* **2017**, *192*, 713–718. [CrossRef]
68. Sampath, C.; Harika, P.; Revaprasadu, N. Design, green synthesis, anti-microbial, and anti-oxidant activities of novel α-aminophosphonates via Kabachnik-Fields reaction. *Phosphorus Sulfur Silicon Relat. Elem.* **2016**, *191*, 1081–1085. [CrossRef]
69. Kumar, M.A.; Lee, K.D. A Simple and Catalyst-Free One-Pot Synthesis of α-Aminophosphonates in Polyethylene Glycol. *Phosphorus Sulfur Silicon Relat. Elem.* **2012**, *187*, 899–905. [CrossRef]
70. Azizi, K.; Karimi, M.; Heydari, A. A catalyst-free synthesis of α-aminophosphonates in glycerol. *Tetrahedron Lett.* **2014**, *55*, 7236–7239. [CrossRef]
71. Bazine, I.; Bendjedid, S.; Boukhari, A. Potential antibacterial and antifungal activities of novel sulfamidophosphonate derivatives bearing the quinoline or quinolone moiety. *Arch. Pharm.* **2021**, *354*, e2000291. [CrossRef] [PubMed]
72. Keglevich, G.; Szekrényi, A.; Kovács, R.; Grün, A. Microwave Irradiation as a Useful Tool in Organophosphorus Syntheses. *Phosphorus Sulfur Silicon Relat. Elem.* **2009**, *184*, 1648–1652. [CrossRef]
73. Bálint, E.; Tóth, R.E.; Keglevich, G. Synthesis of alkyl α-aminomethyl-phenylphosphinates and N,N-bis(alkoxyphenylphosphinylmethyl)amines by the microwave-assisted Kabachnik-Fields reaction. *Heteroat. Chem.* **2016**, *27*, 323–335. [CrossRef]
74. Hudson, H.R.; Tajti, Á.; Bálint, E.; Czugler, M.; Karaghiosoff, K.; Keglevich, G. Microwave-assisted synthesis of α-aminophosphonates with sterically demanding α-aryl substituents. *Synth. Commun.* **2020**, *50*, 1446–1455. [CrossRef]

75. Bálint, E.; Takács, J.; Drahos, L.; Juranovič, A.; Kočevar, M.; Keglevich, G. α-Aminophosphonates and α-Aminophosphine Oxides by the Microwave-Assisted Kabachnik-Fields Reactions of 3-Amino-6-methyl-2H-pyran-2-ones. *Heteroat. Chem.* **2013**, *24*, 221–225. [CrossRef]
76. Tajti, Á.; Szatmári, E.; Perdih, F.; Keglevich, G.; Bálint, E. Microwave-Assisted Kabachnik-Fields Reaction with Amino Alcohols as the Amine Component. *Molecules* **2019**, *24*, 1640. [CrossRef] [PubMed]
77. Balint, E.; Fazekas, E.; Drahos, L.; Keglevich, G. The Synthesis of N,N-Bis(dialkoxyphosphinoylmethyl)- and N,N-Bis(diphenylphosphinoylmethyl)glycine Esters by the Microwave-Assisted Double Kabachnik-Fields Reaction. *Heteroat. Chem.* **2013**, *24*, 510–515. [CrossRef]
78. Bálint, E.; Fazekas, E.; Kóti, J.; Keglevich, G. Synthesis of N,N-Bis(dialkoxyphosphinoylmethyl)- and N,N-Bis(diphenylphosphinoylmethyl)-β- and γ-amino acid Derivatives by the Microwave-Assisted Double Kabachnik-Fields Reaction. *Heteroat. Chem.* **2014**, *26*, 106–115. [CrossRef]
79. Bálint, E.; Tripolszky, A.; Hegedűs, L.; Keglevich, G. Microwave-assisted synthesis of N,N-bis(phosphinoylmethyl)amines and N,N,N-tris(phosphinoylmethyl)amines bearing different substituents on the phosphorus atoms. *Beilstein J. Org. Chem.* **2019**, *15*, 469–473. [CrossRef] [PubMed]
80. Tajti, Á.; Balint, E.; Keglevich, G. Synthesis of Ethyl Octyl α-Aminophosphonate Derivatives. *Curr. Org. Synth.* **2016**, *13*, 638–645. [CrossRef]
81. Bálint, E.; Fazekas, E.; Tripolszky, A.; Kangyal, R.; Milen, M.; Keglevich, G. Synthesis of α-Aminophosphonate Derivatives by Microwave-Assisted Kabachnik–Fields Reaction. *Phosphorus Sulfur Silicon Relat. Elem.* **2015**, *190*, 655–659. [CrossRef]
82. Keglevich, G.; Szekrényi, A.; Szöllősy, Á.; Drahos, L. Synthesis of Bis(phosphonatomethyl)-, Bis(phosphinatomethyl)-, and Bis(phosphinoxidomethyl)amines, as Well as Related Ring Bis(phosphine) Platinum Complexes. *Synth. Commun.* **2011**, *41*, 2265–2272. [CrossRef]
83. Balint, E.; Fazekas, E.; Pinter, G.; Szöllősy, Á.; Holczbauer, T.; Czugler, M.; Drahos, L.; Körtvélyesi, T.; Keglevich, G. P(O)CH2)amine Derivatives Obtained by the Double Kabachnik–Fields Reaction with Cyclohexylamine; Quantum Chemical and X-Ray Study of the Related Bidentate Chelate Platinum Complexes. *Curr. Org. Chem.* **2012**, *16*, 547–554. [CrossRef]
84. Bálint, E.; Fazekas, E.; Pongrácz, P.; Kollár, L.; Drahos, L.; Holczbauer, T.; Czugler, M.; Keglevich, G. N-Benzyl and N-aryl bis(phospha-Mannich adducts): Synthesis and catalytic activity of the related bidentate chelate platinum complexes in hydroformylation. *J. Organomet. Chem.* **2012**, *717*, 75–82. [CrossRef]
85. Bálint, E.; Tajti, Á.; Kalocsai, D.; Mátravölgyi, B.; Karaghiosoff, K.; Czugler, M.; Keglevich, G. Synthesis and utilization of optically active α-aminophosphonate derivatives by Kabachnik-Fields reaction. *Tetrahedron* **2017**, *73*, 5659–5667. [CrossRef]
86. Bálint, E.; Tajti, A.; Tripolszky, A.; Keglevich, G. Synthesis of platinum, palladium and rhodium complexes of α-aminophosphine ligands. *Dalton Trans.* **2018**, *47*, 4755–4778. [CrossRef]
87. Tripolszky, A.; Zoboki, L.; Bálint, E.; Kóti, J.; Keglevich, G. Microwave-assisted synthesis of α-aminophosphine oxides by the Kabachnik-Fields reaction applying amides as the starting materials. *Synth. Commun.* **2019**, *49*, 1047–1054. [CrossRef]
88. Bálint, E.; Tripolszky, A.; Jablonkai, E.; Karaghiosoff, K.; Czugler, M.; Mucsi, Z.; Kollár, L.; Pongrácz, P.; Keglevich, G. Synthesis and use of α-aminophosphine oxides and N,N-bis(phosphinoylmethyl)amines—A study on the related ring platinum complexes. *J. Organomet. Chem.* **2016**, *801*, 111–121. [CrossRef]
89. Keglevich, G.; Rádai, Z. α-Hydroxyphosphonates as intermediates in the Kabachnik–Fields reaction: New proof of their reversible formation. *Tetrahedron Lett.* **2020**, *61*, 151961. [CrossRef]
90. Kiss, N.Z.; Kaszás, A.; Drahos, L.; Mucsi, Z.; Keglevich, G. A neighbouring group effect leading to enhanced nucleophilic substitution of amines at the hindered α-carbon atom of an α-hydroxyphosphonate. *Tetrahedron Lett.* **2012**, *53*, 207–209. [CrossRef]
91. Kiss, N.Z.; Rádai, Z.; Mucsi, Z.; Keglevich, G. Synthesis of α-aminophosphonates from α-hydroxyphosphonates; a theoretical study. *Heteroat. Chem.* **2016**, *27*, 260–268. [CrossRef]
92. Bálint, E.; Tajti, Á.; Dzielak, A.; Hägele, G.; Keglevich, G. Microwave-assisted synthesis of (aminomethylene)bisphosphine oxides and (aminomethylene)bisphosphonates by a three-component condensation. *Beilstein J. Org. Chem.* **2016**, *12*, 1493–1502. [CrossRef] [PubMed]
93. Li, X.-A.; Li, J.-Y.; Yang, B.; Yang, S.-D. Catalyst-free three-component reaction to synthesize chiral α-amino phosphine oxides. *RSC Adv.* **2014**, *4*, 39920–39923. [CrossRef]
94. Tibhe, G.D.; Reyes-Gonzalez, M.A.; Cativiela, C.; Ordonez, M. Microwave-assisted High Diastereoselective Synthesis of α-Aminophosphonates under Solvent and Catalyst Free-conditions. *J. Mex. Chem. Soc.* **2017**, *56*, 94. [CrossRef]
95. Reddy, C.B.; Kumar, K.S.; Kumar, M.A.; Reddy, M.V.N.; Krishna, B.S.; Naveen, M.; Arunasree, M.; Raju, C.N. PEG-SO3H catalyzed synthesis and cytotoxicity of α-aminophosphonates. *Eur. J. Med. Chem.* **2012**, *47*, 553–559. [CrossRef] [PubMed]
96. Xu, D.-Z.; Yu, Y.-Q. A Simple and Green Procedure for the One-Pot Synthesis of α-Aminophosphonates with Quaternary Ammonium Salts as Efficient and Recyclable Reaction Media. *Synth.* **2015**, *47*, 1869–1876. [CrossRef]
97. Milen, M.; Ábrányi-Balogh, P.; Dancsó, A.; Frigyes, D.; Pongó, L.; Keglevich, G. T3P®-promoted Kabachnik–Fields reaction: An efficient synthesis of α-aminophosphonates. *Tetrahedron Lett.* **2013**, *54*, 5430–5433. [CrossRef]
98. Wu, M.; Liu, R.; Wan, D. Convenient One-Pot Synthesis of α-Amino Phosphonates in Water Usingp-Toluenesulfonic Acid as Catalyst for the Kabachnik-Fields Reaction. *Heteroat. Chem.* **2013**, *24*, 110–115. [CrossRef]
99. Ando, K.; Egami, T. Facile synthesis of α-amino phosphonates in water by Kabachnik-Fields reaction using magnesium dodecyl sulfate. *Heteroat. Chem.* **2011**, *22*, 358–362. [CrossRef]

100. Li, X.-C.; Gong, S.-S.; Zeng, D.-Y.; You, Y.-H.; Sun, Q. Highly efficient synthesis of α-aminophosphonates catalyzed by hafnium(IV) chloride. *Tetrahedron Lett.* **2016**, *57*, 1782–1785. [CrossRef]
101. Fang, D.; Jiao, C.; Ni, C. SO3H-functionalized ionic liquids catalyzed the synthesis of α-aminophosphonates in aqueous media. *Heteroat. Chem.* **2010**, *21*, 546–550. [CrossRef]
102. Gao, G.; Chen, M.-N.; Mo, L.-P.; Zhang, Z.-H. Catalyst free one-pot synthesis of α-aminophosphonates in aqueous ethyl lactate. *Phosphorus Sulfur Silicon Relat. Elem.* **2018**, *194*, 528–532. [CrossRef]
103. Dar, B.; Singh, A.; Sahu, A.; Patidar, P.; Chakraborty, A.; Sharma, M.; Singh, B. Catalyst and solvent-free, ultrasound promoted rapid protocol for the one-pot synthesis of α-aminophosphonates at room temperature. *Tetrahedron Lett.* **2012**, *53*, 5497–5502. [CrossRef]
104. Hajinasiri, R.; Hossaini, Z.; Rostami-Charati, F. Efficient synthesis of α-aminophosphonates via one-pot reactions of aldehydes, amines, and phosphates in ionic liquid. *Heteroat. Chem.* **2011**, *22*, 625–629. [CrossRef]
105. Esmaeilpour, M.; Zahmatkesh, S.; Javidi, J.; Rezaei, E. A green one-pot three-component synthesis of α-aminophosphonates under solvent-free conditions and ultrasonic irradiation using $Fe_3O_4$@$SiO_2$-imid-PMAn as magnetic catalyst. *Phosphorus Sulfur Silicon Relat. Elem.* **2017**, *192*, 530–537. [CrossRef]
106. Karimi-Jaberi, Z.; Amiri, M. One-pot synthesis of α-aminophosphonates catalyzed by boric acid at room temperature. *Heteroat. Chem.* **2010**, *21*, 96–98. [CrossRef]
107. Fang, N.; Yang, J.; Ni, C. Dicationic ionic liquids as recyclable catalysts for one-pot solvent-free synthesis of α-aminophosphonates. *Heteroat. Chem.* **2010**, *22*, 5–10. [CrossRef]
108. Borse, A.U.; Patil, N.L.; Patil, M.N.; Mali, R.S. Synthetic utility of Kabachnik–Fields reaction: A convenient one-pot three-component synthesis of N-phenyl isoquinolone-1-phosphonates. *Tetrahedron Lett.* **2012**, *53*, 6940–6942. [CrossRef]
109. Ordóñez, M.; Tibhe, G.; Zamudio-Medina, A.; Viveros-Ceballos, J. An Easy Approach for the Synthesis of N-Substituted Isoindolin-1-ones. *Synth.* **2012**, *2012*, 569–574. [CrossRef]
110. Reyes-González, M.A.; Zamudio-Medina, A.; Ordóñez, M. Practical and high stereoselective synthesis of 3-(arylmethylene)isoindolin-1-ones from 2-formylbenzoic acid. *Tetrahedron Lett.* **2012**, *53*, 5756–5758. [CrossRef]
111. Viveros-Ceballos, J.L.; Cativiela, C.; Ordóñez, M. One-pot three-component highly diastereoselective synthesis of isoindolin-1-one-3-phosphonates under solvent and catalyst free-conditions. *Tetrahedron Asymmetry* **2011**, *22*, 1479–1484. [CrossRef]
112. Milen, M.; Dancsó, A.; Földesi, T.; Slégel, P.; Volk, B. Propylphosphonic anhydride (T3P®) mediated one-pot three-component synthesis of racemic dialkyl (2-substituted-3-oxo-2,3-dihydro-1H-isoindol-1-yl)phosphonates. *Tetrahedron* **2016**, *72*, 5091–5099. [CrossRef]
113. Reddy, S.S.; Rao, V.K.; Krishna, B.S.; Reddy, C.S.; Rao, P.V.; Raju, C.N. Synthesis, Antimicrobial, and Antioxidant Activity of New α-Aminophosphonates. *Phosphorus Sulfur Silicon Relat. Elem.* **2011**, *186*, 1411–1421. [CrossRef]
114. Fu, X.; Loh, W.-T.; Zhang, Y.; Chen, T.; Ma, T.; Liu, H.; Wang, J.; Tan, C.-H. Chiral Guanidinium Salt Catalyzed Enantioselective Phospha-Mannich Reactions. *Angew. Chem.* **2009**, *121*, 7523–7526. [CrossRef]
115. Kumar, A.; Sharma, V.; Kaur, J.; Kumar, V.; Mahajan, S.; Kumar, N.; Chimni, S.S. Cinchona-derived thiourea catalyzed hydrophosphonylation of ketimines—An enantioselective synthesis of α-amino phosphonates. *Tetrahedron* **2014**, *70*, 7044–7049. [CrossRef]
116. Lewkowski, J.; Morawska, M.; Karpowicz, R.; Rychter, P.; Rogacz, D.; Lewicka, K. Novel (5-nitrofurfuryl)-substituted esters of phosphonoglycine—Their synthesis and phyto- and ecotoxicological properties. *Chemosphere* **2017**, *188*, 618–632. [CrossRef]
117. Lewkowski, J.; Morawska, M.; Kowalczyk, A. Antibacterial action of (5-nitrofurfuryl)-derived aminophosphonates and their parent imines. *Chem. Pap.* **2018**, *73*, 365–374. [CrossRef]
118. Lewkowski, J.; Morawska, M.; Kaczmarek, A.; Rogacz, D.; Rychter, P. Novel N-Arylaminophosphonates Bearing a Pyrrole Moiety and Their Ecotoxicological Properties. *Molecules* **2017**, *22*, 1132. [CrossRef]
119. Wang, Q.; Yang, L.; Ding, H.; Chen, X.; Wang, H.; Tang, X. Synthesis, X-ray crystal structure, DNA/protein binding and cytotoxicity studies of five α-aminophosphonate N-derivatives. *Bioorganic Chem.* **2016**, *69*, 132–139. [CrossRef] [PubMed]
120. De Noronha, R.G.; Romão, C.C.; Fernandes, A.C. MoO2Cl2 as a novel catalyst for the synthesis of α-aminophosphonates. *Catal. Commun.* **2011**, *12*, 337–340. [CrossRef]
121. Bálint, E.; Tajti, Á.; Ádám, A.; Csontos, I.; Karaghiosoff, K.; Czugler, M.; Ábrányi-Balogh, P.; Keglevich, G. The synthesis of α-aryl-α-aminophosphonates and α-aryl-α-aminophosphine oxides by the microwave-assisted Pudovik reaction. *Beilstein J. Org. Chem.* **2017**, *13*, 76–86. [CrossRef]
122. Kakuchi, R.; Theato, P. Efficient Multicomponent Postpolymerization Modification Based on Kabachnik-Fields Reaction. *ACS Macro Lett.* **2014**, *3*, 329–332. [CrossRef]
123. Zhang, Y.; Zhao, Y.; Yang, B.; Zhu, C.; Wei, Y.; Tao, L. 'One pot' synthesis of well-defined poly(aminophosphonate)s: Time for the Kabachnik–Fields reaction on the stage of polymer chemistry. *Polym. Chem.* **2013**, *5*, 1857–1862. [CrossRef]
124. Bachler, P.R.; Schulz, M.D.; Sparks, C.A.; Wagener, K.B.; Sumerlin, B.S. Aminobisphosphonate Polymers via RAFT and a Multicomponent Kabachnik-Fields Reaction. *Macromol. Rapid Commun.* **2015**, *36*, 828–833. [CrossRef] [PubMed]

*molecules*

*Article*

# Targeted Synthesis of 3,3′-, 3,4′- and 3,6′-Phenylpropanoid Sucrose Esters

**Wong Pooi Wen Kathy [1,2], Li Lin Ong [1,2], Surabhi Devaraj [1], Duc Thinh Khong [1] and Zaher M. A. Judeh [1,*]**

1 School of Chemical and Biomedical Engineering, Nanyang Technological University, 62 Nanyang Drive, N1.2–B1-14, Singapore 637459, Singapore; pwong003@e.ntu.edu.sg (W.P.W.K.); long008@e.ntu.edu.sg (L.L.O.); surabhi.devaraj@gmail.com (S.D.); thinh@smart.mit.edu (D.T.K.)

2 Institute of Health Technologies, Interdisciplinary Graduate School, Nanyang Technological University, 61 Nanyang Drive, ABN-02b-07, Singapore 637335, Singapore

* Correspondence: zaher@ntu.edu.sg; Tel.: +65-6790-6738; Fax: +65-6794-7553

**Abstract:** In this study, we report on an orthogonal strategy for the precise synthesis of 3,3′-, 3,4′-, and 3,6′-phenylpropanoid sucrose esters (PSEs). The strategy relies on carefully selected protecting groups and deprotecting agents, taking into consideration the reactivity of the four free hydroxyl groups of the key starting material: di-isopropylidene sucrose **2**. The synthetic strategy is general, and potentially applies to the preparation of many natural and unnatural PSEs, especially those substituted at 3-, 3′-, 4′- and 6′-positions of PSEs.

**Keywords:** phenylpropanoid sucrose esters; natural products; orthogonal protection; selective acylation of sugar; antidiabetic compounds

## 1. Introduction

Phenylpropanoid sucrose esters (PSEs, Figure 1) are plant-derived compounds and possess many biological activities, including inhibitory activities against both α-glucosidases and α-amylase [1]. For example, the PSEs Lapathoside D, Lapathoside C, Hydropiperoside, Vanicoside B, and Diboside A showed variable levels of inhibitory activities against α-glucosidase and α-amylase [2–5]. Recently, we proposed PSEs as promising alpha-glucosidase inhibitors (AGIs) that have a better side effect profile than commercial AGIs [6–10]. AGIs possess an excellent efficacy and safety record, and are represented by the commercial drugs acarbose (the gold standard), voglibose, and miglitol. They function by inhibiting the α-glucosidase enzymes responsible for hydrolyzing carbohydrates in the small intestine, thereby restricting its absorption into the bloodstream [11]. However, commercial AGIs cause serious gastrointestinal (GI) side effects such as flatulence, abdominal distension, and diarrhoea [12]. The side effects hamper patient compliance and acceptability, and limit the wide use of these effective drugs [13]. Based on a preliminary structure–activity relationship (SAR) study [6,9,10], we demonstrated that their in vitro inhibition of α-glucosidase and α-amylase depended on the type, number, and position of the phenylpropanoid moieties on the sucrose core and the presence/absence of the di-isopropylidene bridges (Figure 1). The study also identified *O*-3 substituents as favorable for increased level of inhibition of α-glucosidase [6,9,10]. Additionally, the di-isopropylidene bridges favorably reduce the inhibition of α-amylase and minimally affect the inhibition of α-glucosidase [6,9,10]. These results were further corroborated by silico docking and molecular modelling studies. Furthermore, we demonstrated the efficacy of a tetrafeuloyl PSE in a mouse model and found it to be as effective as acarbose in controlling the rise in post-prandial blood glucose levels. The reduction in the inhibition of α-amylase was shown to reduce the side effects of AGIs [14,15]. However, there is a lack of comprehensive and systematic SAR studies identifying the contribution of the type, number, and position of the phenylpropanoid moiety to the inhibition activity. This can be attributed to difficulties in synthesizing PSEs with the precise structures needed for such SAR studies. Previously, we synthesized PSEs through a simple acylation reaction [16,17]. Direct synthesis of substituted PSEs by reacting 2,1′:4,6-di-*O*-diisopropylidene sucrose 2 with substituted cinnamoyl chlorides gave mixtures of differently acylated products depending on the reaction conditions, concentration, and the type of substituted cinnamoyl chloride used, which compromised the yields and complicated the purification process [16,17]. This process cannot be used to synthesize the precisely substituted PSEs required for comprehensive SAR studies.

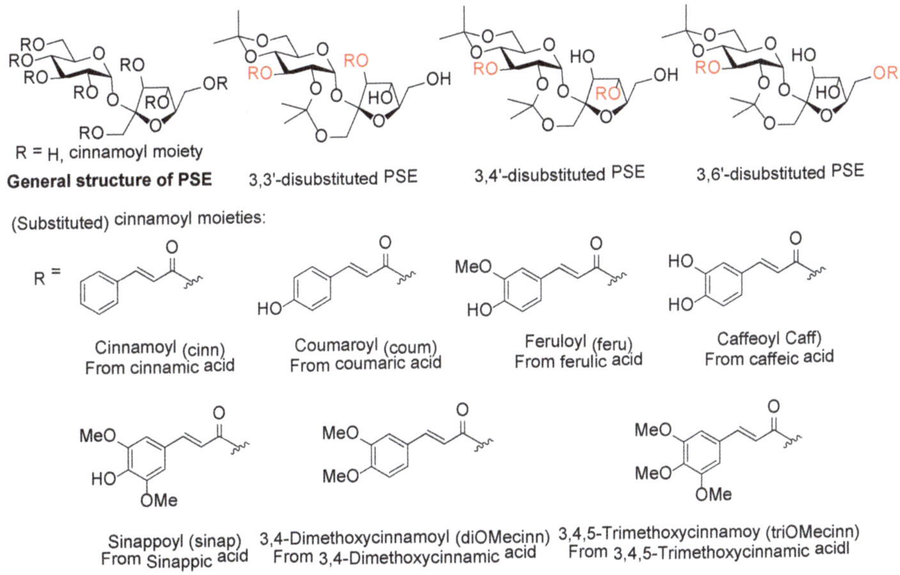


**Figure 1.** General structure of PSE and the targeted 3,3′-, 3,4′-, and 3,6′-di-substituted PSEs.

Herein, we report on the precise synthesis of 3,3′-, 3,4′-, and 3,6′-di-substituted PSEs as potential AGIs. The strategy is designed to also be applicable to other natural and unnatural PSEs.

## 2. Results and Discussion

The inhibition of α-glucosidase and α-amylase varies depending on the type and position of the (substituted) cinnamoyl moieties on the sucrose core (Figure 1) [1–3,15]. Therefore, the targeted 3,3′-, 3,4′-, and 3,6′-di-substituted PSEs are designed with commonly found (substituted) cinnamoyl moieties in natural PSEs, including cinnamoyl, coumaroyl, feruloyl, caffeoyl, sinapoyl, 3,4-dimethoxycinnamoyl, and 3,4,5-trimethoxy cinnamoyl moieties (Figure 1). The di-substituted PSEs are designed with di-isopropylidene bridges since they can have a beneficial effect through the reduction of α-amylase inhibition, which is believed to reduce GI side effects [12].

## 3. Synthesis of 3,3′-di-Substituted PSEs

The synthesis of 3,3′-di-substituted PSEs began with the reaction of sucrose **1** with 2-methoxypropene to give di-isopropylidene sucrose **2** in 65% yield, following the process of Falkenhagen et al. (Scheme 1) with some modifications [16–18]. The dual protection of the 4′-OH and 6′-OH of di-isopropylidene **2** was accomplished using 1,3-dichloro-1,1,3,3-tetraisopropyldisiloxane to give TPDIS-sucrose **3** in 75% yield [19]. Subsequently, Steglich esterification of **3** with cinnamic acid, OTBS-coumaric acid, OTBS-ferulic acid, OTBS-sinapic acid, OTBS-caffeic acid, 3,4-dimethoxycinnamic acid, and 3,4,5-trimethoxycinnamic acid (Figure 1) gave the corresponding 3,3′-di-acylated products **4–10** in 22–48% yield, along with the 3′-mono-acylated counterparts **11–17** [12] in 27–49% yield (Scheme 1). The formation of 3′-mono-acylated compounds **11–17** is attributed to the higher nucleophilicity of 3′-OH in comparison to 3-OH [16,17]. Attempts to increase the yield of 3,3′-di-acylated products **4–10** by using higher equivalents of the acids and increasing the reaction time and temperature were unsuccessful. Finally, removal of the protecting TBS and/or TIPDS groups using $NEt_3.3HF$ gave the corresponding 3,3′-di-substituted PSEs **18–24** in 54–97% yield (Scheme 1).

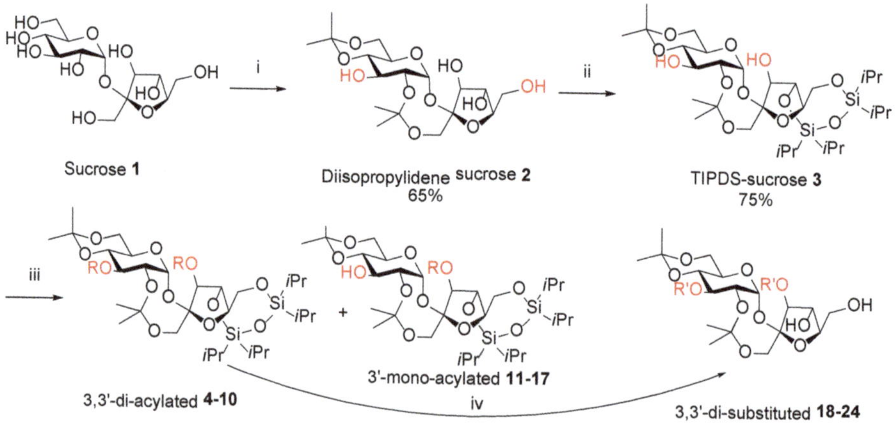


**4**: R=cinn 48%
**5**: R=OTBS-coum 37%
**6**: R=OTBS-feru 30%
**7**: R=OTBS-sinap 22%
**8**: R=OTBS-caff 34%
**9**: R=diOMecinn 29%
**10**: R=triOMecinn 34%

**11**: R=cinn 35%
**12**: R=OTBS-coum 49%
**13**: R=OTBS-feru 35%
**14**: R=OTBS-sinap 27%
**15**: R=OTBS-caff 27%
**16**: R=diOMecinn 55%
**17**: R=triOMecinn 36%

**18**: R'=cinn 67%
**19**: R'=coum 58%
**20**: R'=feru 88%
**21**: R'=sinap 90%
**22**: R'=caff 54%
**23**: R'=diOMecinn 65%
**24**: R'=triOMecinn 97%

Reagents and conditions: i. 2-methoxypropene (4.7 equiv), *p*-TsOH (0.0023 equiv), dry DMF, $N_2$ atmosphere, 1 week; ii. 1,3-dichloro-1,1,3,3-tetraisopropyldisiloxane (1.1 equiv), pyridine, rt, 6 h; iii. acid (4 equiv), EDC.HCl (4 equiv), DMAP (0.1 equiv), $CH_2Cl_2$, rt, 1 week; iv. 1.56 M $NEt_3{\cdot}3HF$ (3 equiv), $NEt_3$ (2 equiv), pyridine, rt, 12 h.

**Scheme 1.** Synthesis of 3,3′-di-substituted PSEs.

## 4. Synthesis of 3,4′-di-Substituted PSEs

The precise synthesis of 3,4′-di-substituted PSEs is shown in Scheme 2. Since the primary 6′-OH of di-isopropylidene sucrose **2** is the most nucleophilic, it was protected first using *tert*-butyldimethylsilyl chloride (TBSCl); the reaction gave 6′-*O*-TBS **25** in 95% yield. Subsequent protection of 3′-OH with benzyl chloroformate (*CbzCl*) gave 3′-*O*-Cbz **26** in 75% yield. 3′-*O*-Cbz **26** was obtained as the major product since 3′-OH is the most reactive among the three OH groups of 6′-*O*-TBS **25** due to fewer steric effects. Next, Steglich reaction between 3′-*O*-Cbz **26** and cinnamic acid, OTBS-coumaric acid, OTBS-ferulic acid, OTBS-sinapic acid, OTBS-caffeic acid, 3,4-dimethoxycinnamic acid, and 3,4,5-trimethoxycinnamic acid gave the corresponding 3,4′-di-acylated products **27–32** in 14–36% yield, along with 4′-mono-acylated products **33–38** [12] in 35–62% yield, respectively (Scheme 2). Again, attempts to increase the yield of 3,4′-di-acylated products **27–32** by increasing the acid equivalents as well as the reaction temperature and time were unsuccessful. In this case, the 4′-OH proved to be more nucleophilic than the 3-OH, as indicated by the formation of 4′-mono-acylated products in high yield. Subsequently, removal of the Cbz protecting groups using $Pd(OAc)_2$ and the TBS protecting groups using $NEt_3.3HF$ gave 3,4′-di-substituted PSEs **39–44** in 22–49% yields over two steps (Scheme 2).

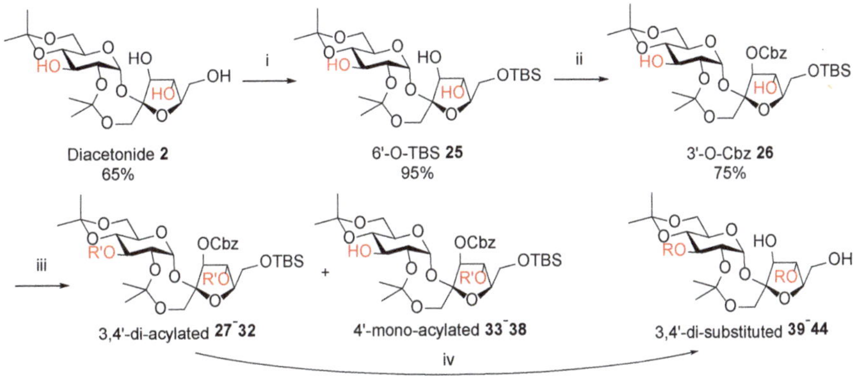


| | | | | | | | |
|---|---|---|---|---|---|---|---|
| **27**: R=R'=OTBS-coum | 36% | **33**: R=OTBS-coum | 62% | **39**: R=coum | 49% |
| **28**: R=R'=OTBS-feru | 25% | **34**: R=OTBS-feru | 35% | **40**: R=feru | 26% |
| **29**: R=R'=OTBS-sinap | 31% | **35**: R=OTBS-sinap | 41% | **41**: R=sinap | 26% |
| **30**: R=R'=OTBS-caff | 14% | **36**: R=OTBS-caff | 37% | **42**: R=caff | 22% |
| **31**: R=R'=diOMecinn | 30% | **37**: R=diOMecinn | 39% | **43**: R=diOMecinn | 30% |
| **32**: R=R'=triOMecinn | 36% | **38**: R=triOMecinn | 35% | **44**: R=triOMecinn | 31% |

Reagents and conditions: i. TBSCl (1.2 equiv), $NEt_3$ (2.4 equiv), DMAP (0.1 equiv), $CH_2Cl_2$' rt, 12 h; ii. CbzCl (1.5 equiv), TMEDA (3 equiv), DMAP (0.1 equiv), $CH_2Cl_2$' rt, 12 h; iii. acid (4 equiv), EDC.HCl (4 equiv), DMAP (0.1 equiv), $CH_2Cl$, rt, 1 week; iv. (a) $Pd(OAc)_2$ (0.1 equiv), $NEt_3$ (0.16 equiv), $Et_3SiH$ (1.6 equiv), $CH_2Cl_2$, rt, 12 h; (b). 1.56M $NEt_3$.3HF (3 equiv), $NEt_3$ (2 equiv), pyridine, rt, 12 h.

**Scheme 2.** Synthesis of 3,4′-di-substituted PSEs.

## 5. Synthesis of 3,6′-di-Substituted PSEs

The synthesis of 3,6′-di-substituted PSEs began with protecting the 4′-OH group of 6′-*O*-TBS **25** with *p*-nitrobenzoyl chloride (PNBCl) to give 4′-OPNB **45** in 70% yield (Scheme 3). Removal of the TBS protecting group of **45** using $NEt_3$.3HF gave compound **46**. Subsequent Steglich reaction between compound **46** and cinnamic acid, acetyl-coumaric acid, acetyl-ferulic acid, acetyl-sinapic acid, OTBS-caffeic acid, 3,4-dimethoxycinnamic acid, and 3,4,5-trimethoxycinnamic acid gave the corresponding 3,6′-di-acylated compounds **47–53** in 66–79% yield, along with traces of other compounds thought to be the mono-acylated counterparts. In this case, the yields were much higher in comparison to 3,3′- and 3,4′-di-acylated compounds due to higher nucleophilicity and less steric hindrance of the primary 6′-OH. We purposely protected coumaric, ferulic, and sinapic acids with acetyl groups rather than the usual TBS since these groups can be removed simultaneously in one step during the removal of the Cbz and PNB groups using $Mg(OMe)_2$. Acetylation of caffeic acid posed problems, so in this case, OTBS-caffeic acid was used. Finally, simultaneous removal of the Cbz, PNB, and acetyl groups of **47–49**, **52** and **53** with $Mg(OMe)_2$ gave 3,6′-di-substituted PSEs **54–56**, **59**, and **60** in 21–90% yield, respectively (Scheme 3). During the reactions, TLC showed two to three spots indicating stepwise deprotection; the reaction was deemed complete when only one spot was observed. However, while $Mg(OMe)_2$ removed the Cbz and PNB groups of 3,6′-diacylated **50**, it failed to remove its acetyl group and gave compound **61** in 53% yield. Piperidine successfully removed the acetyl group of compound **61** to give the required 3,6′-di-substituted PSE **57** in 45% yield. In the case of 3,6′-diacylated **51**, Cbz and PNB groups were removed using $Mg(OMe)_2$ to give compound **62** in 82% yield, which upon removal of its TBS groups using $NEt_3$.3HF gave 3,6′-di-substituted PSE **58** in 94% yield (Scheme 3). Copies of the [1] H NMR, [13] C [1] NMR, and 2D NMR spectra of the synthesized compounds are available online (Supplementary Materials).

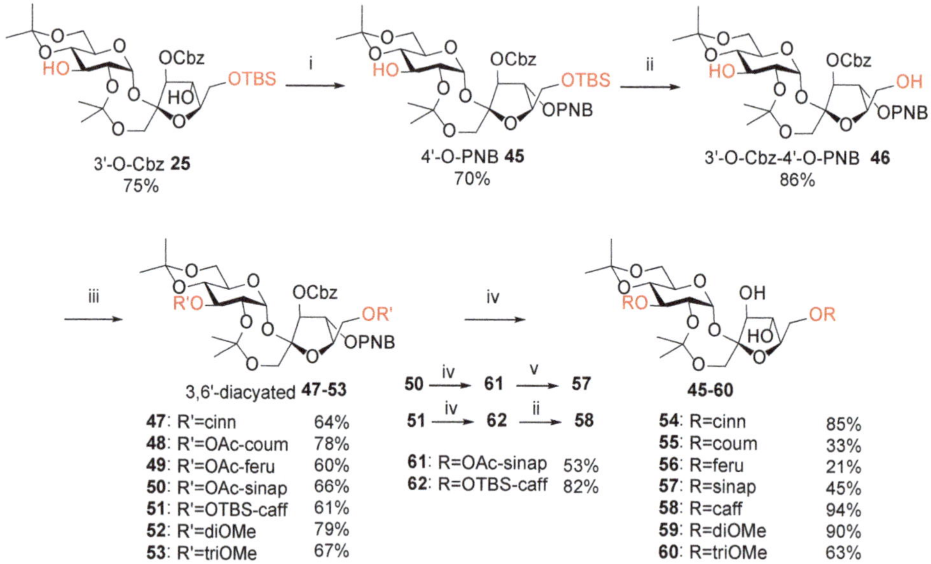

Reagents and conditions: i. PNBCl (1.5 equiv), $NEt_3$ (3 equiv), DMAP (0.1 equiv), $CH_2Cl_2$' 4 °C (ice bath), 12 h; ii. 1.56 M 3HF.$NEt_3$ (3 equiv), $NEt_3$ (2 equiv), pyridine, rt, 12 hours; iii. Acid (4 equiv), EDC.HCl (4 equiv), DMAP (0.1 equiv), $CH_2Cl$, 2 weeks, reflux at 50 °C; vi. $Mg(OMe)_2$ (0.5 equiv), 1:9 THF/MeOH, rt, 12 h; v. Piperidine (4 equiv), 5:1 EtOH/THF, rt, 12 h.

**Scheme 3.** Synthesis of 3,6′-di-substituted PSEs.

The strategy took advantage of the slight differences in reactivates of the four OH groups on the key compound di-isopropylidene sucrose **2**. The above routes gave the required PSEs with the correct substitution patterns at 3,3′-, 3,4′- and 3,6′- positions, as confirmed via 2D NMR experiments (see supporting information).

The synthesized compounds in this work will decipher the role of the O-3 substituents in inhibition through comprehensive SAR studies.

## 6. Conclusions

We successfully developed a precise synthesis of 3,3′-, 3,4′-, and 3,6′-di-substituted PSEs using an orthogonal protection/deprotection strategy. The synthetic strategy has a wider application for the preparation of many natural and unnatural PSEs, especially those substituted at O-3, O-4′, and O-6′ positions such as Helonioside A, Lapathoside C, and Lapathoside D. Future work will investigate the synthesized PSEs as part of a comprehensive SAR study to develop lead antidiabetic AGIs with a better side effect profile.

**Supplementary Materials:** The following supporting information can be downloaded. Copies of the [1] H NMR, [13] C [1] NMR, and 2D NMR spectra of the synthesized compounds are available online.

**Author Contributions:** Conceptualization, W.P.W.K. and Z.M.A.J.; methodology, W.P.W.K., L.L.O., D.T.K. and S.D.; validation, W.P.W.K. and L.L.O.; formal analysis, W.P.W.K.; investigation, W.P.W.K.; data curation, W.P.W.K.; writing—original draft preparation, W.P.W.K.; writing—review and editing, D.T.K., S.D. and Z.M.A.J.; visualization, W.P.W.K.; supervision, Z.M.A.J.; project administration, Z.M.A.J.; funding acquisition, Z.M.A.J. All authors have read and agreed to the published version of the manuscript.

**Funding:** This research was funded by the College of Engineering (Startup Grant), Nanyang Technological University, Singapore.

**Data Availability Statement:** Not applicable.

**Acknowledgments:** We thank Nanyang Technological University, Singapore for financial support (CoE, Startup Grant).

**Conflicts of Interest:** The authors declare no conflict of interest.

**Sample Availability:** Samples of the compounds are not from the authors.

## References

1. Panda, P.; Appalashetti, M.; Judeh, Z.M.A. Phenylpropanoid sucrose esters: Plant-derived natural products as potential leads for new therapeutics. *Curr. Med. Chem.* **2011**, *18*, 3234–3251. [CrossRef] [PubMed]
2. Fan, P.; Terrier, L.; Hay, A.-E.; Marston, A.; Hostettmann, K. Antioxidant and enzyme inhibition activities and chemical profiles of Polygonum sachalinensis F.Schmidt ex Maxim (Polygonaceae). *Fitoterapia* **2010**, *81*, 124–131. [CrossRef] [PubMed]
3. Kawai, Y.; Kumagai, H.; Kurihara, H.; Yamazaki, K.; Sawano, R.; Inoue, N. β-Glucosidase inhibitory activities of phenylpropanoid glycosides, vanicoside A and B from Polygonum sachalinense rhizome. *Fitoterapia* **2006**, *77*, 456–459. [CrossRef] [PubMed]
4. Adisakwattana, S.; Chantarasinlapin, P.; Thammarat, H.; Yibchok-Anun, S. A series of cinnamic acid derivatives and their inhibitory activity on intestinal α-glucosidase. *J. Enzyme Inhib. Med. Chem.* **2009**, *24*, 1194–1200. [CrossRef] [PubMed]
5. Liu, T.; Yip, Y.M.; Song, L.; Feng, S.; Liu, Y.; Lai, F.; Zhang, D.; Huang, D. Inhibiting enzymatic starch digestion by the phenolic compound diboside A: A mechanistic and in silico study. *Food Res. Int.* **2013**, *54*, 595–600. [CrossRef]
6. Surabhi, D.R. Studies on Bioactivity of Phenylpropanoid Sucrose Esters. Ph.D. Thesis, Nanyang Technological University, Singapore, 2017.
7. Lin, O.L. Development of Phenylpropanoid Sucrose Esters as Antidiabetic Lead Compounds. Ph.D. Thesis, Nanyang Technological University, Interdisciplinary Graduate School (NTU Institute for Health Technologies), Singapore, 2018.
8. Wong, P.W.K. Investigation of Phenylpropanoid Sucrose Esters as Antidiabetic Compounds. Ph.D. Thesis, Nanyang Technological University, Interdisciplinary Graduate School (NTU Institute for Health Technologies), Singapore, 2020.
9. Devaraj, S.; Yip, Y.M.; Panda, P.; Ong, L.L.; Wong, P.W.K.; Zhang, D.; Ali, Y.; Judeh, Z. Feruloyl Sucrose Esters: Potent and Selective Inhibitors of α-glucosidase and α-amylase. *Curr. Med. Chem.* **2021**, *68*, 1–16. [CrossRef] [PubMed]
10. Devaraj, S.; Yip, Y.M.; Panda, P.; Ong, L.L.; Wong, P.W.K.; Zhang, D.; Ali, Y.; Judeh, Z. Cinnamoyl Sucrose Esters as Alpha Glucosidase Inhibitors for the Treatment of Diabetes. *Molecules* **2021**, *26*, 469. [CrossRef] [PubMed]
11. Bell, D.S.; O'Keefe, J.H.; Jellinger, P. Postprandial dysmetabolism: The missing link between diabetes and cardiovascular events? *Endocr. Pract.* **2008**, *14*, 112–124. [CrossRef] [PubMed]
12. Aoki, K.; Muraoka, T.; Ito, Y.; Tagashi, Y.; Teraushi, Y. Comparison of adverse gastrointestinal effects of acarbose and miglitol in healthy men: A crossover study. *Intern. Med.* **2010**, *49*, 1085–1087. [CrossRef] [PubMed]
13. Moses, R.G. Combination therapy for patients with type 2 diabetes: Repaglinide in combination with metformin. *Expert Rev. Endocrinol. Metab.* **2010**, *5*, 331–342. [CrossRef] [PubMed]
14. Derosa, G.; Maffioli, P. α-Glucosidase inhibitors and their use in clinical practice. *Arch. Med. Sci.* **2012**, *8*, 899–906. [CrossRef] [PubMed]
15. Kelley, D.E.; Bidot, P.; Freedman, Z.; Haag, B.; Podlecki, D.; Rendell, M.; Schimel, D.; Weiss, S.; Taylor, T.; Krol, A.; et al. Efficacy and safety of acarbose in insulin-treated patients with type 2 diabetes. *Diabetes Care* **1998**, *21*, 2056–2061. [CrossRef] [PubMed]
16. Panda, P.; Appalashetti, M.; Natarajan, M.; Mary, C.-P.; Venkatraman, S.S.; Judeh, Z.M.A. Synthesis and antiproliferative activity of helonioside A, 3′,4′,6′-tri-O-feruloylsucrose, lapathoside C and their analogs. *Eur. J. Med. Chem.* **2012**, *58*, 418–430. [CrossRef] [PubMed]
17. Panda, P.; Appalashetti, M.; Natarajan, M.; Chan-Park, M.B.; Venkatraman, S.S.; Judeh, Z.M.A. Synthesis and antitumor activity of lapathoside D and its analogs. *Eur. J. Med. Chem.* **2012**, *53*, 1–12. [CrossRef] [PubMed]
18. Poschalko, A.; Rohr, T.; Gruber, H.; Bianco, A.; Guichard, G.; Briand, J.-P.; Weber, V.; Falkenhagen, D. SUBPOL: A Novel Sucrose-Based Polymer Support for Solid-Phase Peptide Synthesis and Affinity Chromatography Applications. *J. Am. Chem. Soc.* **2003**, *125*, 13415–13426. [CrossRef] [PubMed]
19. Sato, K.-I.; Sakai, K.; Tsushima, K.; Akai, S. The first total synthesis of telephiose A. *Tetrahedron Lett.* **2007**, *48*, 3745–3748. [CrossRef]

molecules

MDPI

*Article*

# Cinnamoyl Sucrose Esters as Alpha Glucosidase Inhibitors for the Treatment of Diabetes

**Surabhi Devaraj [1], Yew Mun Yip [2], Parthasarathi Panda [1,†], Li Lin Ong [1,3], Pooi Wen Kathy Wong [1,3], Dawei Zhang [2,4] and Zaher Judeh [1,*]**

1 School of Chemical and Biomedical Engineering, Nanyang Technological University, 62 Nanyang Drive, N1.2–B1-14, Singapore 637459, Singapore; surabhi.devaraj@gmail.com (S.D.); panda.ju06@gmail.com (P.P.); long008@e.ntu.edu.sg (L.L.O.); pwong003@e.ntu.edu.sg (P.W.K.W.)

2 School of Physical and Mathematical Sciences, Nanyang Technological University, 21 Nanyang Link, Singapore 637371, Singapore; yipy0010@e.ntu.edu.sg (Y.M.Y.); sunstar53@126.com (D.Z.)

3 Institute of Health Technologies, Interdisciplinary Graduate School, Nanyang Technological University, 61 Nanyang Drive, ABN-02b-07, Singapore 637335, Singapore

4 School of Physics and Engineering, Henan University of Science and Technology, Luoyang 471000, China

* Correspondence: Zaher@ntu.edu.sg; Tel.: +65-6790-6738; Fax: +65-6794-7553

† Current Address: Dr. B.C. Roy College of Pharmacy & Allied Health Sciences, Dr. Meghnad Saha Sarani, Bidhan Nagar, Durgapur, West Bengal 713206, India.

**Abstract:** Cinnamoyl sucrose esters (CSEs) were evaluated as AGIs and their enzyme inhibition activity and potency were compared with gold standard acarbose. The inhibition activity of the CSEs against α-glucosidase and α-amylase depended on their structure including the number of the cinnamoyl moieties, their position, and the presence or absence of the acetyl moieties. The inhibitory values of the CSEs **2–9** generally increases in the order of mono-cinnamoyl moieties < di-cinnamoyl ≤ tri-cinnamoyl < tetra-cinnamoyl. This trend was supported from both in vitro and in silico results. Both tetra-cinnamoyl CSEs **5** and **9** showed the highest α-glucosidase inhibitory activities of 77 ± 5%, 74 ± 9%, respectively, against acarbose at 27 ± 4%, and highest α-amylase inhibitory activities of 98 ± 2%, 99 ± 1%, respectively, against acarbose at 93 ± 2%. CSEs **3**, **4**, **6**, **7**, **8** showed desired higher inhibition of α-glucosidase than α-amylase suggesting potential for further development as AGIs with reduced side effects. Molecular docking studies on CSEs **5** and **9** attributed the high inhibition of these compounds to multiple π-π interactions and favorable projection of the cinnamoyl moieties (especially O-3 cinnamoyl) in the enzyme pockets. This work proposes CSEs as new AGIs with potentially reduced side effects.

**Keywords:** phenylpropanoid sucrose esters; glycosides; natural products; α-glucosidase inhibition; α-amylase inhibition; anti-diabetic

## 1. Introduction

Alpha Glucosidase Inhibitors (AGIs) acarbose, voglibose, and miglitol are effective oral antidiabetic drugs [1]. They function by inhibiting the digestive α-glucosidase and α-amylase enzymes that break down starch and other oligosaccharides. [1] They have a better safety profile compared to other drugs such as insulin, sulphonylureas, biguanides, meglitinides, thiazolidinediones, and SGLT-2 inhibitors [2,3]. However, they are often accompanied by severe gastrointestinal side effects such as flatulence, diarrhea, and bloating, which limit patient acceptance and compliance [4]. The side effects are caused by the fermentation of undigested carbohydrates in the large intestine due to excessive AGIs inhibition of α-amylase [5]. Therefore, it is highly desirable to develop effective AGIs but without these side effects. Such AGIs should have high selectivity causing high inhibition of α-glucosidase and low inhibition of α-amylase.

Phenylpropanoid sucrose esters (PSEs) are naturally occurring compounds isolated from various plant species such as Arecaceae, Liliaceae, Polygonaceae, Rosaceae, Brassicaceae, and Smilaceae [6]. PSEs feature a sucrose core acylated with one or more phenylpropanoid (trans-PhCH=CH-CO-) moieties such as cinnamoyl, coumaroyl, feruloyl, caffeoyl, and/or sinapoyl moieties [7]. Their extracts were used in various traditional and folk medicines for treating various illnesses [8]. They exhibit a wide range of biological activities including anticancer, antibacterial, antiplasmodial, antioxidant, and acetylcholine esterase inhibitory activities [6,7,9–19]. Additionally, PSEs show variable α-glucosidase and α-amylase inhibitory activities depending on the type, number, and position of the phenylpropanoid moieties on the sucrose core. Examples of these biologically active PSEs include lapathoside C [14], lapathoside D [14], hydropiperoside [14], vanicoside B [14], and diboside A [11] (Figure 1). Several other phenylpropanoid glycosides also showed excellent α-glucosidase and α-amylase inhibition activities [20–25].

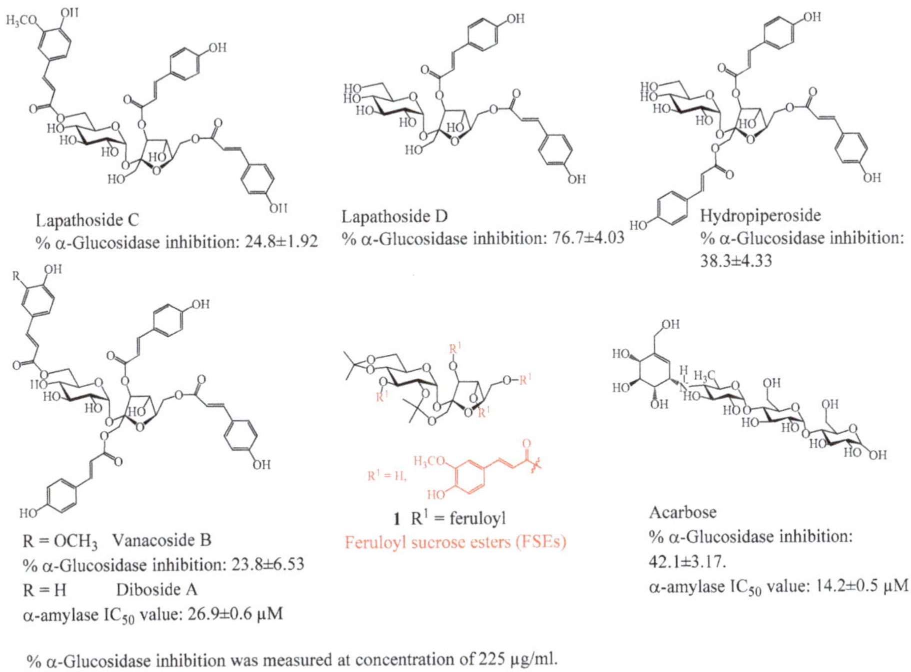


**Figure 1.** Phenylpropanoid sucrose esters (PSEs) with % α-glucosidase and α-amylase inhibitory activities. Also shown is the general structure of feruloyl sucrose ester (FSE) and acarbose.

We have earlier reported that feruloyl sucrose esters (FSEs) (Figure 1) function as selective AGIs and has the potential to eliminate the side effects associated with the commercial AGIs [26]. FSEs desirably showed higher % inhibition of α-glucosidase and lower inhibition of α-amylase in comparison to acarbose as the AGI gold standard [26]. Specifically, FSE **1** (Figure 2) significantly reduced blood glucose excursion in STZ-treated mice compared to control (starch only) mice. The diisopropylidene bridges, position, and the number of the feruloyl substituents on the sucrose core were key determinants of the selectivity and % inhibition of α-glucosidase and α-amylase [26]. Further research is advantageous to assess other phenylpropanoid moieties beside the feruloyl moieties to obtain lead AGIs candidate for further development.

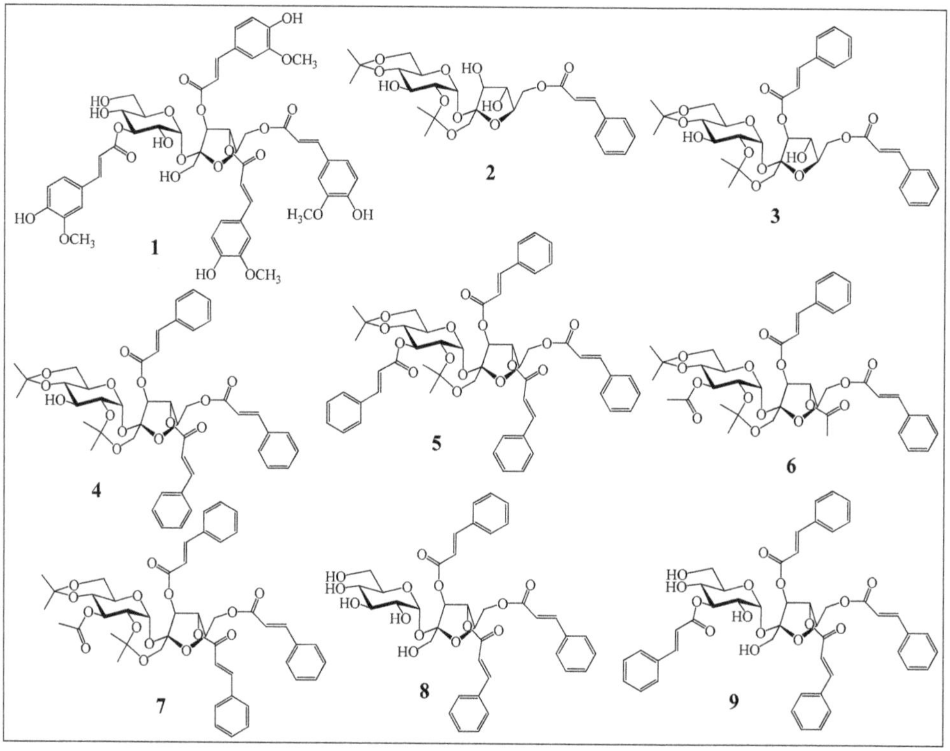

**Figure 2.** Structures of the investigated cinnamoyl sucrose esters (CSEs) **2–9** along with FSE **1**.

Herein, we evaluate cinnamoyl sucrose esters (CSEs) as AGIs and compare their % α-glucosidase and α-amylase inhibition activities with gold standard acarbose. The factors that influence the selectivity and inhibition of the enzymes are also discussed.

## 2. Results and Discussions

### *2.1. Design and Synthesis of Cinnamoyl Sucrose Esters* 2–9

The inhibition activities of α-glucosidase and α-amylase using natural PSEs [26] and FSEs synthesized in our laboratory [26,27] depended on the structural features of these compounds. Therefore, CSEs **2–9** were specifically designed to differ in: (i) the number of cinnamoyl moieties, (ii) the degree of acetylation of the sucrose core, and (iii) the presence or absence of the diisopropylidene bridges on sucrose core (Figure 2). These bridges control the degree of flexibility between the glucose and fructose moieties of the sucrose core. CSEs **2–9** were also designed to complement and compare with our inhibition studies using a small library of FSEs such as **1** (Figure 2). CSEs **2–9** were synthesized by cinnamoylation of 2,1′:4,6-di-*O*-isopropylidene sucrose with cinnamoyl chlorides in dry pyridine according to our previous work (Scheme 1) [19]. Acetylation of the cinnamoylated compounds was then achieved using acetic anhydride to give the acetylated CSEs [19].

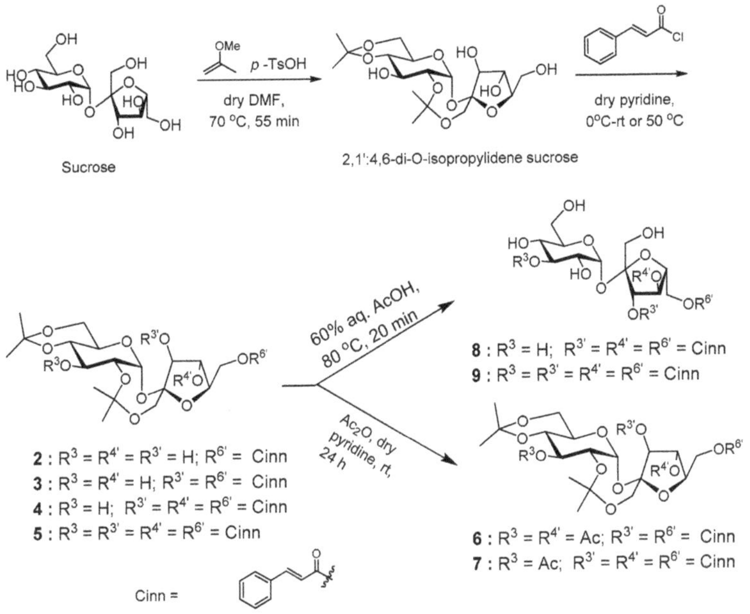

**Scheme 1.** Synthesis of CSEs **2–9**.

### 2.2. *Inhibition of α-Glucosidase and α-Amylase by Cinnamoyl Sucrose Esters* **2–9** *In Vitro*

CSEs **2–9** were screened for α-glucosidase and α-amylase inhibition at their maximum solubility limit of 25 μg/mL (Figure 3). Acarbose, the gold standard AGI drug, was used as a reference standard at the same concentration. Except for CSE **2**, all CSEs investigated showed inhibition of both α-glucosidase and α-amylase, and the inhibition was mainly influenced by the number of the cinnamoyl substituents on the sucrose core and to a lesser extent by the acetyl moieties and the diisopropylidene bridges. CSE **2** with one cinnamoyl moiety did not show significant inhibition activity of both enzymes, in agreement with the inhibition results using FSE with one feruloyl moiety. Both CSEs **3** and **4** with diisopropylidene bridges and free OH groups showed similar α-glucosidase inhibition of 35 ± 5% and 32 ± 3%, respectively, and similar α-amylase inhibition activities of 9 ± 5% and 8 ± 4%, respectively (Figure 3). In both cases, the % α-glucosidase inhibition was >4 times higher than the % α-amylase inhibition. An additional cinnamoyl at O-3 as in CSE **5**, caused a huge increase in the % α-glucosidase inhibition to 77 ± 5 and even a bigger increase in the α-amylase inhibition to 98 ± 2%. Again, these results agree with the inhibition trend observed in the case of FSEs where moieties at O-3 lead to higher enzyme inhibition.[26] Capping of the hydroxyl moieties of CSEs **3** and **4** with acetyl protecting groups to give CSEs **6** and **7** respectively, resulted in a similar increase in both the α-glucosidase inhibition (46 ± 3% and 46 ± 2%, respectively) and α-amylase inhibitions (14 ± 4% and 13 ± 7%, respectively). In both cases, the % α-glucosidase inhibition remained roughly >4 times higher than the % α-amylase inhibition as seen in the case of free OH in CSEs **3** and **4**. The modest increase in selectivity may be attributed to the steric effects that the acetyl groups cause, which favors better docking of CSEs **6** and **7** at the active sites of the enzymes. Though the increase in inhibition was modest, acylation of the OH groups with other larger acetyl groups could be a means to influence the inhibition activities. CSE **8** without the diisopropylidene or acetyl groups exhibited a similar α-glucosidase inhibition value of 34 ± 4% as compared to its counterpart, CSEs **4** with 32 ± 3%. However, it's α-amylase inhibition value of 16 ± 2% is double that of CSEs **4** at 8 ± 4%. These results once again clearly show that the diisopropylidene bridges on the sucrose core have no significant influence on α-glucosidase inhibition: a similar trend observed in the case of FSEs. CSE **9** with four cinnamoyl moieties and no diisopropylidene bridges showed α-glucosidase inhibition of 74 ± 9%, which is similar to its counterpart CSE **5** with an inhibition value of 77 ± 5%. Interestingly, both CSEs **9** and **5** showed similar α-amylase inhibition values at 99 ± 1% and 98 ± 2%, respectively. This result disagrees with the observations from the FSEs where the inhibition activity decreases in the presence of the diisopropylidene bridges [26]. There was no significant increase in the % inhibition of both enzymes with the increase in the number of cinnamoyl moieties from three to four (compare values for CSEs **5** vs. **9**, and **4** vs. **8**). This observation contrasts with the results observed in the case of FSEs [26]. This is attributed to the lack of hydrogen bonding, which is observed in the case of FSEs from docking studies [26]. In the case of FSEs, hydrogen bonding increased the % inhibition of the enzymes due to stronger interactions with the enzyme moieties [26]. However, the inhibition values of CSEs **5** and **9** with four cinnamoyl moieties, were several folds higher than those of the CSEs **3**, **4**, **6**, and **7** with two of three cinnamoyl moieties, indicating that the number of substituents on the sucrose core plays a key role in enzyme inhibition. CSEs **3**, **4**, **6**, **7**, and **8** showed similar α-glucosidase inhibition values as compared to acarbose at 27 ± 4% (Figure 3). However, CSEs **5** and **9** with four cinnamoyl moieties had almost double the inhibitory values compare to acarbose making them more potent inhibitors. Interestingly, except for CSEs **5** and **9**, the rest of the CSEs had much lower % α-amylase inhibition values compared to α-glucosidase inhibition. This selectivity is important for reducing the gastrointestinal side effects.

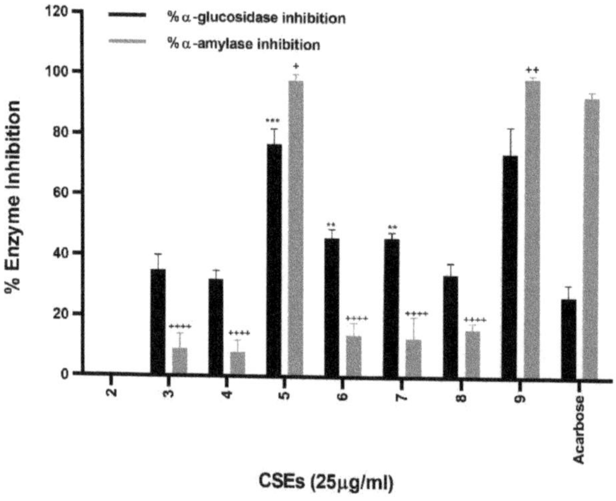


**Figure 3.** Percentage inhibition of α-glucosidase and α-amylase by CSEs **2–9** with acarbose as the reference standard. Inhibition values are expressed as means ± SD; $n = 3$. CSEs showing less than 5% enzyme inhibition are considered to have No Significant Activity (NSA). ** $p \leq 0.01$, *** $p \leq 0.001$, for significant change in α-glucosidase inhibition compared with Acarbose; + $p \leq 0.05$, ++ $p \leq 0.01$, ++++ $p \leq 0.0001$ for significant change in α-amylase inhibition compared with Acarbose.

The general inhibitory values of the CSEs **2–9** increase in the following order, mono-cinnamoyl moieties < di-cinnamoyl ≤ tri-cinnamoyl < tetra-cinnamoyl. The diisopropylidene bridges and acetyl groups have a modest impact on the inhibition values. In many aspects, the investigated CSEs showed similar trends observed in the case of FSEs but also contrasted in some aspects.

The $IC_{50}$ values for CSEs **5** and **9** were calculated for α-glucosidase and α-amylase inhibition. In the case of α-glucosidase, both CSEs **5** and **9** showed similar $IC_{50}$ values of 9 ± 3 µM, which is over 36-fold lower than acarbose at 328 ± 7 µM making them much more potent inhibitors than acarbose (Table 1). In the case of α-amylase, CSEs **5** and **9** showed $IC_{50}$ values of 1 ± 0.2 μM and 0.8 ± 0.1 μM, respectively, which are five-fold less than the value for acarbose 5 ± 0.1 μM (Table 1). Unlike acarbose, which is far more potent inhibitor of α-amylase than α-glucosidase, CSEs **5** and **9** displayed potent inhibition of both the enzymes.

**Table 1.** $IC_{50}$ [a] values for α-glucosidase and α-amylase inhibition by CSEs **5** and **9**.

| Entry | CSE | $IC_{50}$ Value (μM) | $IC_{50}$ Value (μM) |
|---|---|---|---|
| | | α-Glucosidase | α-Amylase |
| 1 | 5 | 9 ± 3 | 1 ± 0.2 |
| 2 | 9 | 9 ± 3 | 0.8 ± 0.1 |
| 3 | Acarbose | 328 ± 7 | 5 ± 0.1 |

[a] $IC_{50}$ values are expressed as means ± SD; $n$ = 3; $IC_{50}$ values were calculated using a dose-response curve in GraphPad PRISM software.

## 2.3. Molecular Docking of CSE 9 with α-Glucosidase

CSE **9** was docked with α-glucosidase to determine its binding modes and interactions. Since the protein structure of yeast α-glucosidase is unavailable, a homology model was built using yeast isomaltase (PDB ID 3A4A). The site of docking, as well as the amino acid residues that interact with the CSE **9**, are presented in the binding modes and the Ligand Interaction Diagrams (LIDs) (Figures 4 and 5). The cinnamoyl moiety at O-3 has three π-π stacking interactions with the amino acid residues, PHE178, ARG442, and TYR72. This corroborates with the increased inhibition observed in the in vitro results with the incorporation of the cinnamoyl moiety at O-3 (Figure 3). The cinnamoyl moieties at O-3′ and O-6′ interact with HIS280 and PHE314, respectively, through π-π stacking interactions. The cinnamoyl moiety at O-6′ also forms a salt bridge with LYS156 (Figure 4). We hypothesize that the high inhibition value of CSE **9** at 74 ± 9% is attributed to multiple π-π interactions, projection of the cinnamoyl moiety at O-3 (depicted in yellow Figure 4) into the active site of the enzyme, and stabilization of its conformation facilitated by the other moieties at O-3′, O-4′ and O-6′. Unlike the cases of FSEs, though the number of hydrogen bonds that CSE **9** forms is limited due to a lack of aromatic OH groups, π-π interaction, and other hydrophobic interactions make up for this to give high inhibition of α-glucosidase [26].

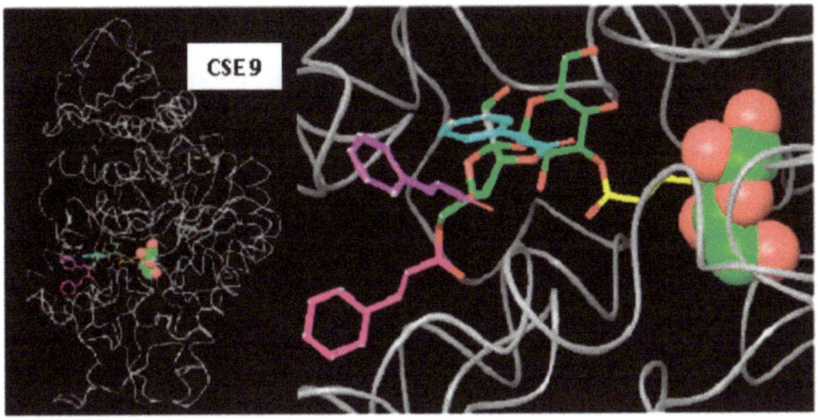


**Figure 4.** Binding mode picture for CSE **9** docked with α-glucosidase.

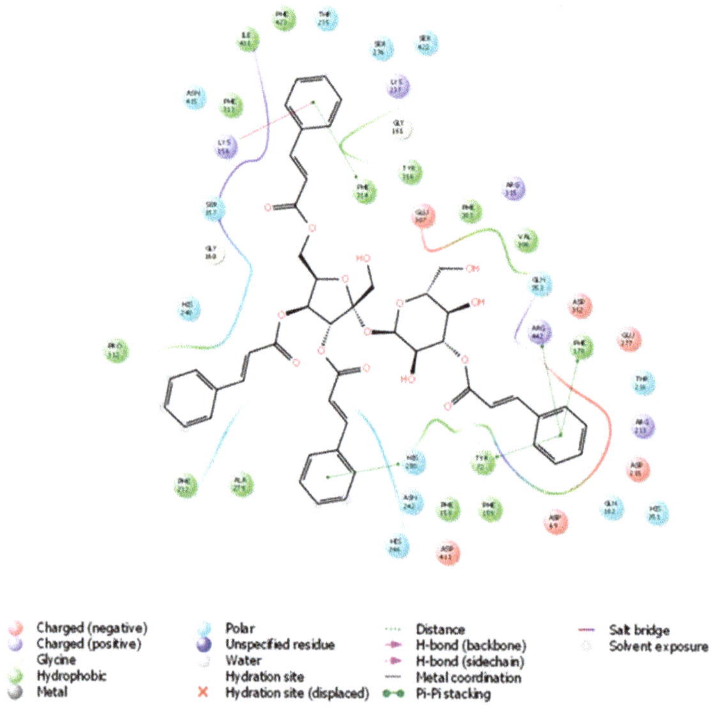

**Figure 5.** Ligand Interaction Diagram for CSE **9** docked with α-glucosidase.

*2.4. Molecular Docking of CSEs* **9** *and* **5** *with α-Amylase*

CSEs **5** and **9** were chosen since CSE **5** has a restricted configuration due to the bridging of the glucose and fructose moieties by the diisopropylidene rings while CSE **9** is more flexible. Binding mode pictures and the Ligand Interaction diagrams of CSEs **5** and **9** are presented in Figures 6 and 7, respectively. Both CSEs **5** and **9** docked in a similar region around amino acid residues 50–63; 145–151; 197–200; 233–240; and 300–306 (depicted in red in Figure 7). From the LID of CSE **5**, the cinnamoyl moiety at O-3 is involved in π-π stacking interactions with HIE 305 and TRP 58. This highlights the importance of the cinnamoyl at O-3 for inhibition of α-amylase. CSE **9**, which has greater conformational flexibility, has greater interactions with the enzyme. Hence, the cinnamoyl moiety at O-3 forms a hydrogen bond with TYR 151, and the cinnamoyl at O-3′ shows π-π stacking with TYR 151. The cinnamoyl moiety at O-6′ shows π-π stacking with HIE 305, and OH-2′ forms a hydrogen bond with GLY 306. The high inhibition of CSEs **5** and **9** could be attributed to multiple π-π interactions and favorable projection of the cinnamoyl moiety at O-3 in the active site of the enzyme. It is noted that these compounds show similar interactions to the FSEs except they lack phenolic OH bonding with the residues.

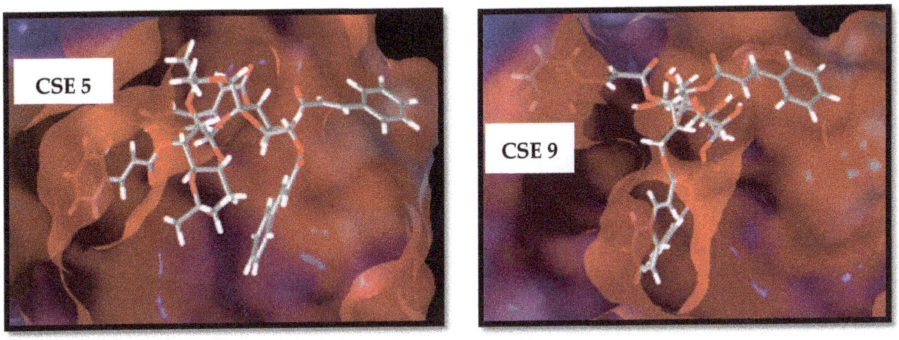


**Figure 6.** Binding mode pictures for CSEs **5** and **9** docked with α-amylase.

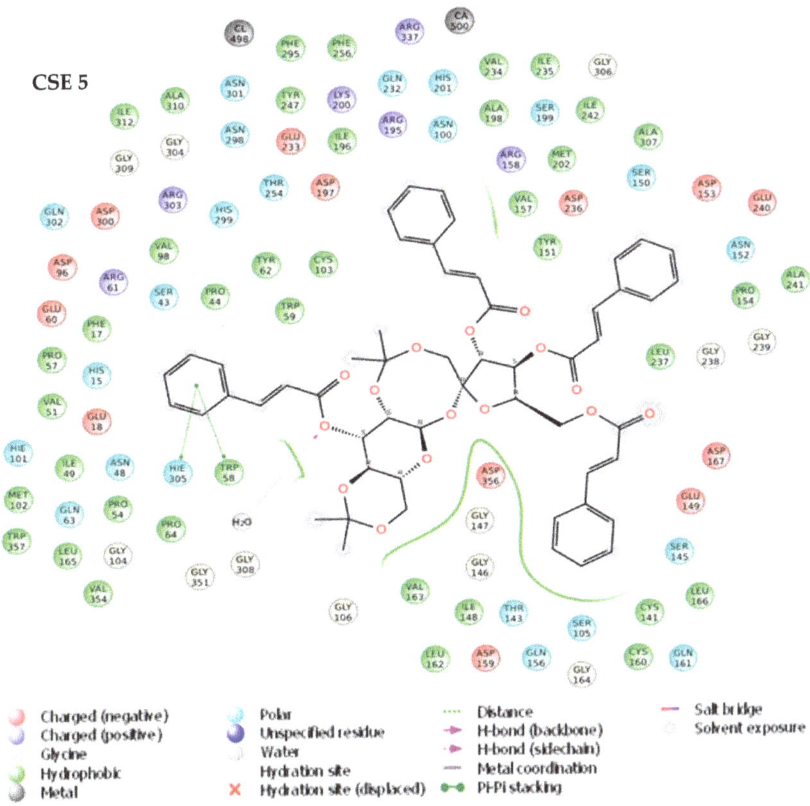


**Figure 7.** *Cont.*

**CSE 9**

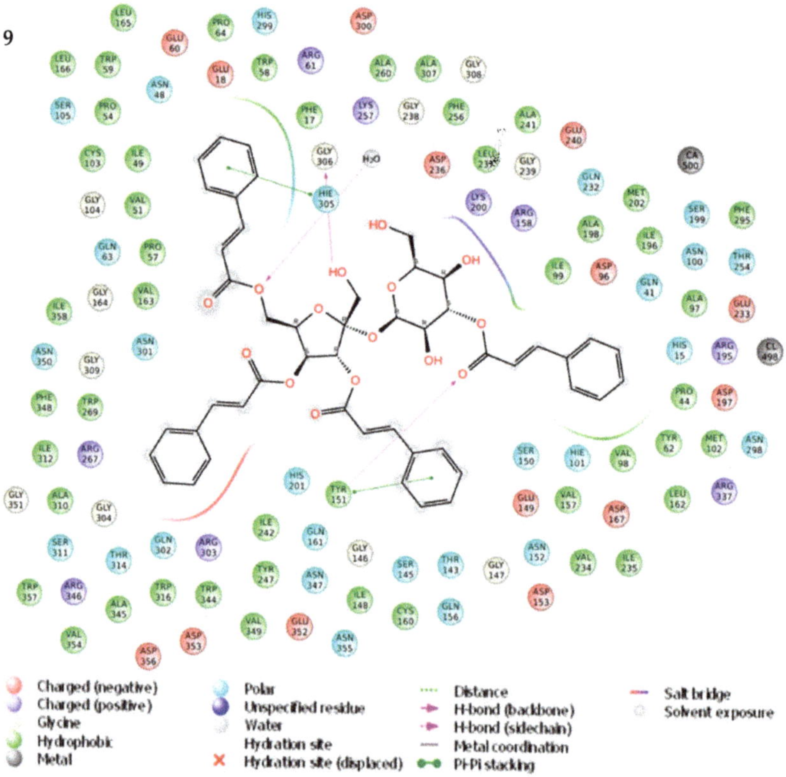


**Figure 7.** Ligand Interaction Diagrams for CSEs **5** and **9** docked with α-amylase.

## 3. Methods

### 3.1. Chemicals

All the chemicals and reagents used in this study were purchased from Sigma Aldrich (α-glucosidase, α-amylase from porcine pancreas, acarbose, 4-nitrophenyl α-D-glucopyranoside (PNPG), Dinitro Salicylic Acid (DNSA), DMSO, $NaHPO_4$, $Na_2HPO_4$).

### 3.2. *In Vitro α-Glucosidase Inhibition Assay*

α-Glucosidase inhibition was tested according to previously reported methods with some modifications [28]. 8 µL of CSEs or control (Acarbose) in DMSO were added to 115 µL of 0.1 M sodium phosphate buffer pH 7.0 in a 96 well microtiter plate (50 µg/mL final concentration). Fifty microliters of yeast α-glucosidase enzyme solution (0.5 U/mL in phosphate buffer) was added to the wells. The plate was incubated at 37 °C for 15 min. Next, 25 µL of 2.5 mM PNPG (4-nitrophenyl α-D-glucopyranoside) substrate solution (in phosphate buffer) was added. The microplate was incubated at 37 °C for another 15 min. The absorbance was then measured using a microplate reader at 405 nm. The percentage inhibition was calculated using the formula:

$$\% \, inhibition = \frac{\Delta Abs_{control} - \Delta Abs_{sample}}{\Delta Abs_{control}} \times 100$$

### 3.3. *In Vitro α-Amylase Inhibition Assay*

α-amylase inhibition was tested using previously reported methods [11] 50 μL of the CSEs or control (Acarbose) in DMSO (final concentration 50 μg/mL) were taken in test tubes to which 100 μL of porcine pancreatic α-amylase (5 U/mL) and 460 μL of 0.05 M sodium phosphate buffer pH 6.8 were added. The tubes were then incubated at 37 °C for 10 min. Next, 450 μL of 0.5% starch solution was added and the tubes were incubated for a further 20 min at 37 °C. Finally, 500 μL of Dinitro Salicylic Acid (DNSA) reagent was added and the tubes were placed in a boiling water bath for 15 min. The absorbance of the tubes was recorded at 540 nm and the % inhibition calculated using the same formula as for α-glucosidase,

$$\%\ inhibition\ = \frac{\Delta Abs_{control} - \Delta Abs_{sample}}{\Delta Abs_{control}} \times 100$$

### 3.4. *Calculation of $IC_{50}$ and Statistical Analysis for Enzyme Inhibition*

All measurements were performed in triplicates and the values. The $IC_{50}$ values for selected CSEs were calculated by plotting a dose-response curve for a range of concentrations of the CSEs (0–25 μg/mL) for the selected CSEs (data not shown) and regression analysis was done using Graphpad Prism software using the in-built function.

### 3.5. *Molecular Docking of the CSE **9** with α-Glucosidase*

A suitable template for building a homology model for α-glucosidase was found using the 'BLAST' algorithm. Yeast isomaltase (PDB ID: 3A4A) *(Saccharomyces cerevisiae)* which shared 72% sequence identity and 85% similarity with yeast α-glucosidase was used as a template to construct the homology model [11]. AutoDock was used for docking simulations and Maestro was used to visualize the binding modes. Receptor preparation was done by first removing water molecules and then adding Gasteiger charges and hydrogen atoms. Maximum number of rotatable bonds was chosen to increase the flexibility of the docked ligand. The site that houses the glucose molecule in the yeast isomaltase was chosen to be the gridded binding site. Lamarckian Genetic algorithm was chosen for the docking and a total of 100 binding modes were chosen.

### 3.6. *Molecular Docking of the CSEs **5** and **9** with α-Amylase*

The molecular interaction of the CSEs with porcine pancreatic α-amylase was studied using Schrödinger's Maestro software. The enzyme porcine pancreatic α-amylase (PDB ID: 1OSE) was imported and the structure processed using the Protein Preparation Wizard module. The receptor grid was generated based on the coordinates of the bound acarbose in the crystal structure, known as the primary binding site [11]. The Glide suite was used to perform the docking of the CSEs with the Extra Precision (XP) option. Water molecules that are 5 Å away from the primary binding site were retained during the docking. Residues that possess bonds containing hydroxyl and thiol groups as well as single bonds not having a specific chirality in the ligands were considered to be flexible.

## 4. Conclusions

Cinnamoyl sucrose esters inhibited α-glucosidase and α-amylase to different extents and the inhibition activity depended on the structure of these compounds. Selective inhibition of α-glucosidase over α-amylase to eliminate the side effects is achievable by tuning the number of cinnamoyl moieties, their positions, diisopropylidene bridges, and the acetyl groups. Among the eight compounds tested, CSEs **5** and **9**, with four cinnamoyl moieties, showed much higher inhibition of α-glucosidase than acarbose and near complete inhibition of α-amylase. Both showed much higher $IC_{50}$ values than acarbose. From the in silico docking studies, the high inhibition of CSEs **5** and **9** is thought to be due to multiple π-π interactions and favorable projection of the cinnamoyl moieties (especially O-3 cinnamoyl) in the enzyme pockets. This work demonstrates the potential of CSEs as AGIs. Further studies on developing phenylpropanoid sucrose esters as AGIs with minimum side effects are underway in our lab.

**Author Contributions:** Synthesis of compounds: P.P.; inhibition studies: S.D.; writing and revising the manuscript: S.D., P.P., P.W.K.W., Y.M.Y., and Z.J.; discussion of results: S.D., P.P., P.W.K.W., L.L.O., Y.M.Y., D.Z. and Z.J.; in silico studies: S.D., Y.M.Y., and D.Z.; supervision: D.Z. and Z.J. All authors have read and agreed to the published version of the manuscript.

**Funding:** We wish to acknowledge financial support from Nanyang Technological University, College of Engineering Start Up Grant.

**Conflicts of Interest:** The authors declare no conflict of interest.

## References

1. Derosa, G.; Maffioli, P. α-Glucosidase Inhibitors and Their Use in Clinical Practice. *Arch. Med. Sci.* **2012**, *8*, 899–906. [CrossRef] [PubMed]
2. Akkati, S.; Sam, K.G.; Tungha, G. Emergence of Promising Therapies in Diabetes Mellitus. *J. Clin. Pharmacol.* **2011**, *51*, 796–804. [CrossRef] [PubMed]
3. Levetan, C. Oral Antidiabetic Agents in Type 2 Diabetes. *Curr. Med. Res. Opin.* **2007**, *23*, 945–952. [CrossRef] [PubMed]
4. Kumar, R.V.; Sinha, V.R. Newer Insights into the Drug Delivery Approaches of α-Glucosidase Inhibitors. *Expert Opin. Drug Deliv.* **2012**, *9*, 403–416. [CrossRef]
5. Kelley, D.E.; Bidot, P.; Freedman, Z.; Haag, B.; Podlecki, D.; Rendell, M.; Schimel, D.; Weiss, S.; Taylor, T.; Krol, A.; et al. Efficacy and Safety of Acarbose in Insulin-Treated Patients with Type 2 Diabetes. *Diabetes Care* **1998**, *21*, 2056–2061. [CrossRef]
6. Panda, P.; Appalashetti, M.; Judeh, Z.M.A. Phenylpropanoid Sucrose Esters: Plant-Derived Natural Products as Potential Leads for New Therapeutics. *Curr. Med. Chem.* **2011**, *18*, 3234–3251. [CrossRef]
7. Panda, P. Synthesis and Anticancer Activity of Phenylpropanoid Sucrose Esters. Ph.D. Thesis, Nanyang Technological University, Singapore, 2016.
8. Kurkin, V.A. Phenylpropanoids from Medicinal Plants: Distribution, Classification, Structural Analysis, and Biological Activity. *Chem. Nat. Compd.* **2003**, *39*, 87–110. [CrossRef]
9. Nhiem, N.X.; Van Kiem, P.; Van Minh, C.; Ban, N.K.; Cuong, N.X.; Tai, B.H.; Kim, Y.H. Phenylpropanoid Glycosides from Heterosmilax Erythrantha and Their Antioxidant Activity. *Arch. Pharm. Res.* **2009**, *32*, 1373–1377. [CrossRef]
10. Gao, X.; Wang, W.; Wei, S.; Li, W. Review of Pharmacological Effects of Glycyrrhiza Radix and Its Bioactive Compounds. *Zhongguo Zhong Yao Za Zhi* **2009**, *21*, 2695–2700.
11. Liu, T.; Yip, Y.M.; Song, L.; Feng, S.; Liu, Y.; Lai, F.; Zhang, D.; Huang, D. Inhibiting Enzymatic Starch Digestion by the Phenolic Compound Diboside A: A Mechanistic and in Silico Study. *Food Res. Int.* **2013**, *54*, 595–600. [CrossRef]
12. Kiem, P.V.; Nhiem, N.X.; Cuong, N.X.; Hoa, T.Q.; Huong, H.T.; Huong, L.M.; Minh, C.V.; Kim, Y.H. New Phenylpropanoid Esters of Sucrose from Polygonum Hydropiper and Their Antioxidant Activity. *Arch. Pharm. Res.* **2008**, *31*, 1477–1482. [CrossRef] [PubMed]
13. Chan, H.-H.; Sun, H.-D.; Reddy, M.V.B.; Wu, T.-S. Potent Alpha-Glucosidase Inhibitors from the Roots of Panax Japonicus C. A. Meyer Var. Major. *Phytochemistry* **2010**, *71*, 1360–1364. [CrossRef] [PubMed]
14. Fan, P.; Terrier, L.; Hay, A.-E.; Marston, A.; Hostettmann, K. Antioxidant and Enzyme Inhibition Activities and Chemical Profiles of Polygonum Sachalinensis F.Schmidt Ex Maxim (Polygonaceae). *Fitoterapia* **2010**, *81*, 124–131. [CrossRef] [PubMed]
15. Wan, C.; Yuan, T.; Cirello, A.L.; Seeram, N.P. Antioxidant and α-Glucosidase Inhibitory Phenolics Isolated from Highbush Blueberry Flowers. *Food Chem.* **2012**, *135*, 1929–1937. [CrossRef] [PubMed]
16. Suo, M.; Ohta, T.; Takano, F.; Jin, S. Bioactive Phenylpropanoid Glycosides from Tabebuia Avellanedae. *Molecules* **2013**, *18*, 7336–7345. [CrossRef]
17. Kumagai, H.; Kawai, Y.; Sawano, R.; Kurihara, H.; Yamazaki, K.; Inoue, N. Antimicrobial Substances from Rhizomes of the Giant Knotweed Polygonum Sachalinense against the Fish Pathogen Photobacterium Damselae Subsp. Piscicida. *Z. Naturforsch. C* **2005**, *60*, 39–44. [CrossRef]
18. Kawai, Y.; Kumagai, H.; Kurihara, H.; Yamazaki, K.; Sawano, R.; Inoue, N. Beta-Glucosidase Inhibitory Activities of Phenylpropanoid Glycosides, Vanicoside A and B from Polygonum Sachalinense Rhizome. *Fitoterapia* **2006**, *77*, 456–459. [CrossRef]
19. Panda, P.; Appalashetti, M.; Natarajan, M.; Chan-Park, M.B.; Venkatraman, S.S.; Judeh, Z.M.A. Synthesis and Antitumor Activity of Lapathoside D and Its Analogs. *Eur. J. Med. Chem.* **2012**, *53*, 1–12. [CrossRef]
20. Meyre-Silva, C.; Cechinel-Filho, V. A Review of the Chemical and Pharmacological Aspects of the Genus Marrubium. *Curr. Pharm. Des.* **2010**, *16*, 3503–3518. [CrossRef]
21. Boudjelal, A.; Henchiri, C.; Siracusa, L.; Sari, M.; Ruberto, G. Compositional Analysis and in Vivo Anti-Diabetic Activity of Wild Algerian *Marrubium vulgare* L. Infusion. *Fitoterapia* **2012**, *83*, 286–292. [CrossRef]
22. Benalla, W.; Bellahcen, S.; Bnouham, M. Antidiabetic Medicinal Plants as a Source of Alpha Glucosidase Inhibitors. *Curr. Diabetes Rev.* **2010**, *6*, 247–254. [CrossRef] [PubMed]

23. Kim, J.-S.; Kwon, Y.-S.; Sa, Y.-J.; Kim, M.-J. Isolation and Identification of Sea Buckthorn (*Hippophae rhamnoides*) Phenolics with Antioxidant Activity and α-Glucosidase Inhibitory Effect. *J. Agric. Food Chem.* **2011**, *59*, 138–144. [CrossRef] [PubMed]
24. Mncwangi, N.; Chen, W.; Vermaak, I.; Viljoen, A.M.; Gericke, N. Devil's Claw-a Review of the Ethnobotany, Phytochemistry and Biological Activity of Harpagophytum Procumbens. *J. Ethnopharmacol.* **2012**, *143*, 755–771. [CrossRef] [PubMed]
25. Andrade Cetto, A.; Wiedenfeld, H.; Revilla, M.C.; Sergio, I.A. Hypoglycemic Effect of Equisetum Myriochaetum Aerial Parts on Streptozotocin Diabetic Rats. *J. Ethnopharmacol.* **2000**, *72*, 129–133. [CrossRef]
26. Devaraj, S. Development of Phenylpropanoid Sucrose Esters as Lead Drug Candidates for Alpha Glucosidase Inhibition. Ph.D. Thesis, Nanyang Technological University, Singapore, 2016.
27. Panda, P.; Appalashetti, M.; Natarajan, M.; Mary, C.-P.; Venkatraman, S.S.; Judeh, Z.M.A. Synthesis and Antiproliferative Activity of Helonioside A, 3′,4′,6′-Tri-O-Feruloylsucrose, Lapathoside C and Their Analogs. *Eur. J. Med. Chem.* **2012**, *58*, 418–430. [CrossRef] [PubMed]
28. Yan, J.; Zhang, G.; Pan, J.; Wang, Y. α-Glucosidase Inhibition by Luteolin: Kinetics, Interaction and Molecular Docking. *Int. J. Biol. Macromol.* **2014**, *64*, 213–223. [CrossRef]

molecules

MDPI

*Communication*

# Practical Synthesis of 2-Iodosobenzoic Acid (IBA) without Contamination by Hazardous 2-Iodoxybenzoic Acid (IBX) under Mild Conditions

**Hideyasu China [1,2,*], Nami Kageyama [2], Hotaka Yatabe [2], Naoko Takenaga [3] and Toshifumi Dohi [2,*]**

[1] Department of Medical Bioscience, Nagahama Institute of Bio-Science and Technology, 1266, Tamuracho Nagahama-shi, Shiga 526-0829, Japan
[2] College of Pharmaceutical Sciences, Ritsumeikan University, 1-1-1 Nojihigashi, Kusatsu, Shiga 525-8577, Japan; ph0093ei@ed.ritsumei.ac.jp (N.K.); ph0090ir@ed.ritsumei.ac.jp (H.Y.)
[3] Faculty of Pharmacy, Meijo University, 150 Yagotoyama, Tempaku-ku, Nagoya 468-8503, Japan; ntakenag@meijo-u.ac.jp
* Correspondence: h_china@nagahama-i-bio.ac.jp (H.C.); td1203@ph.ritsumei.ac.jp (T.D.)

**Abstract:** We report a convenient and practical method for the preparation of nonexplosive cyclic hypervalent iodine(III) oxidants as efficient organocatalysts and reagents for various reactions using Oxone® in aqueous solution under mild conditions at room temperature. The thus obtained 2-iodosobenzoic acids (IBAs) could be used as precursors of other cyclic organoiodine(III) derivatives by the solvolytic derivatization of the hydroxy group under mild conditions of 80 °C or lower temperature. These sequential procedures are highly reliable to selectively afford cyclic hypervalent iodine compounds in excellent yields without contamination by hazardous pentavalent iodine(III) compound.

**Keywords:** cyclic organoiodine(III) compounds; Oxone®; water, solvolytic functionalization, mild condition, metal-free, 2-iodosobenzoic acid

## 1. Introduction

Cyclic hypervalent iodine reagents, such as 2-iodosobenzoic acid (IBA) and 2-iodoxybenzoic acid (IBX) are nonmetallic green oxidants with excellent recyclability [1–3]. IBA and IBX can be regenerated from 2-iodobenzoic acid (2-IB) without requiring an external ligand except for water in this reoxidation step. This is because the carboxy group adjacent to the iodine atom serves as an endogenous ligand. Recently, IBA, a representative trivalent cyclic hypervalent iodine oxidant, has been used as a catalyst and reagent in various reactions, i.e., decarboxylative alkynylation [4,5], decarboxylative acylarylation [6], oxyalkenylation [7], oxyarylation [8], oxidative C–H arylation [9], C–H hydroxylation [10], C-H oxidation [11,12], ring-opening hydrazination [13], and asymmetric intramolecular α-cyclopropanation [14]. IBA derivatives containing OAc [15–28], OMe [29–32], OTs [33–35], OTf [36,37], Cl [38–42], F [43–45], CN [46], $N_3$ [47–54], $CF_3$ [55,56], $OCOCF_3$ [57], alkynyl [58–62] ligands instead of the hydroxy group have also found application in various reactions (Figure 1).

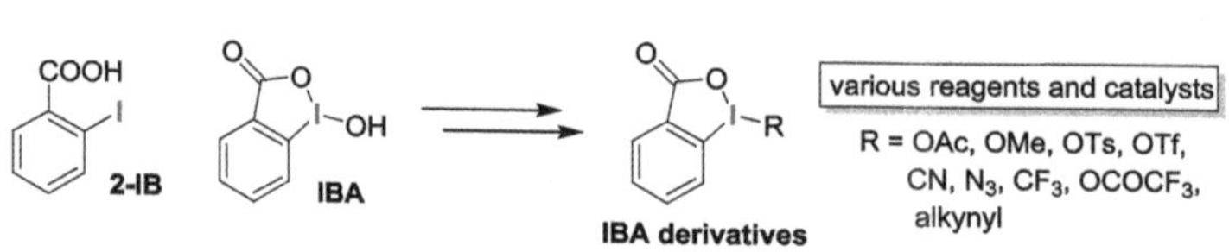


**Figure 1.** 2-Iodosobenzoic acid (IBA) and its precursor 2-iodobenzoic acid (2-IB).

Although IBAs can be prepared from 2-IBs by existing methods (Figure 2) [63–66], the development of a safer and more efficient method for their synthesis is highly desirable.

As shown in Figure 2, IBAs can be further oxidized to pentavalent cyclic hypervalent IBXs [67], which need to be prevented for the preparation of IBAs [68–70], mainly due to the explosive nature of IBXs on heating and impact, while IBXs are useful in some small-scale reactions [71–76]. Thus, contamination by IBX in the IBA products should be avoided for long-term safe storage or large-scale use.

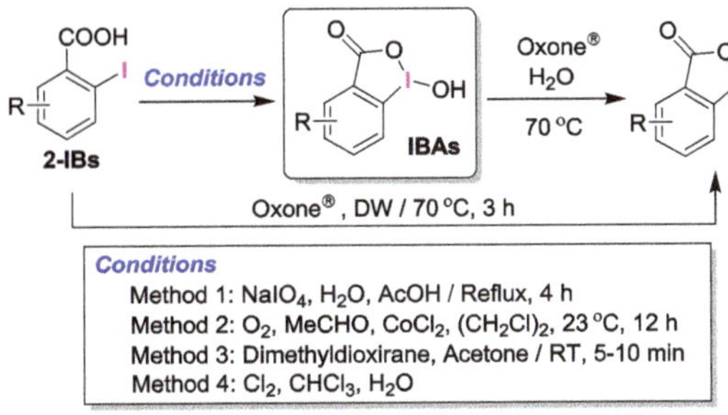


**Figure 2.** Synthesis of 2-iodosobenzoic acids (IBAs) and 2-iodoxybenzoic acids (IBXs) from 2-iodobenzoic acids (2-IBs).

In recent decades, many reactions using Oxone®, which is an inexpensive and commercially available stable triple salt ($2KHSO_5/KHSO_4/K_2SO_4$), have been developed for practical synthetic purposes [77]. In particular, the use of Oxone® as a re-oxidant for pentavalent hypervalent iodine reagents is drawing attention for catalytic oxidation reactions [78–92]. The reaction systems for alcohol oxidations [78–84] involving in situ generated active hypervalent iodine(V) species are optimized on the basis of the preparative conditions of IBX from 2-IB at 70 °C [93]. Meanwhile, oxidative lactonizations from modified 2-IBs using Oxone® occur at room temperature [85–87]. In this context, the generation of nonexplosive trivalent cyclic hypervalent iodines, i.e., IBA and its analogs, using Oxone® can be expected to provide a convenient and safe synthetic procedure; however, to best of our knowledge, the selective preparation of IBAs using Oxone® has not been reported so far.

Recently, we reported that IBAs generated in a reaction system containing 2-IB and Oxone® play a catalytic role in the selective oxidation of alkoxybenzenes to *p*-quinones [94]. This resulted in the development of the practical method herein reported for the selective preparation of IBAs under mild conditions.

## 2. Results and Discussion

### 2.1. *Selective Synthesis of IBA and Its Analogs*

We started our investigation on the selective preparation of IBAs by evaluating the solvent effects on the oxidation of 2-IB **1a** using 1.0 equivalent of Oxone® to obtain IBA **2a** as a representative compound, and the results are summarized in Figure 3. First, the reaction in water led to the successful production of IBA **2a** in 82% yield (Figure 3, entry 2), whereas IBA **2a** was not produced in organic solvent in the absence of water (no reaction because Oxone® was not dissolved) (see entry 1). This result indicates that water plays an essential role in the formation of IBA. Therefore, we assumed that an aqueous system similar to the selective formation of *p*-quinone from alkoxybenzenes catalyzed by 2-IB **1a** with Oxone® [94] could be suitable for the present reaction. We then investigated in detail the effect of a series of organic solvents on the aqueous preparation of IBA **2a** using Oxone®.

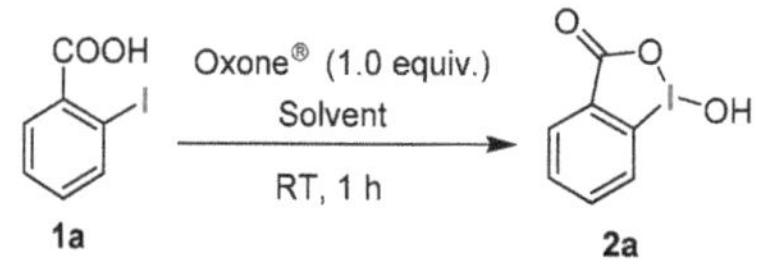


| Entry | Solvent | Yield (%) |
|---|---|---|
| 1 | MeCN | 0 |
| 2 | $H_2O$ | 82 |
| 3 | MeCN / $H_2O$ (1/1) | 80 |
| 4 | THF / $H_2O$ (1/1) | 63 |
| 5 | Dioxane / $H_2O$ (1/1) | 93 |
| 6 | Benzene / $H_2O$ (1/1) | 5 |
| 7 | DMF / $H_2O$ (1/1) | 92 |
| 8 | MeOH / $H_2O$ (1/1) | 91 (1.4)[1)] |
| 9 | EtOH / $H_2O$ (1/1) | 94 (0.8)[2)] |
| 10 | TFE / $H_2O$ (1/1) | 78 (0.4)[3)] |

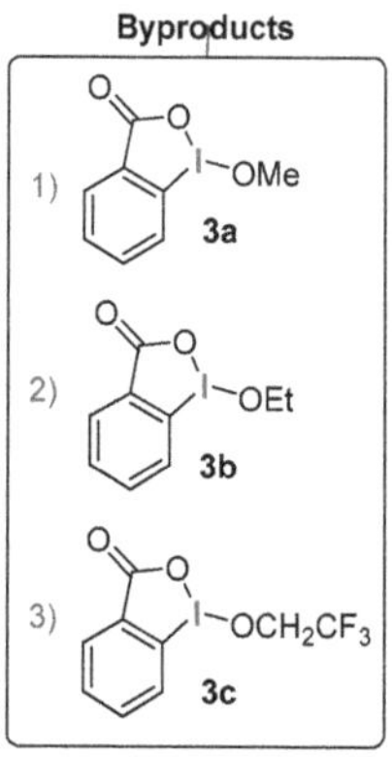


**Figure 3.** Solvent effect on the selective synthesis of IBA **2a** from 2-IB **1a** using Oxone®.

Various water-miscible organic solvents were investigated to dissolve 2-IB **1a** in this reaction. The preparation of IBA **2a** using acetonitrile (MeCN) in aqueous condition (Figure 3, entry 3) was similar to that performed in the absence of organic solvents (Figure 3, entry 2). Tetrahydrofuran (THF), dioxane, benzene and *N,N*-dimethylformamide (DMF) were also examined, finding that the use of highly polar dioxane and DMF led to excellent yields of IBA **2a** (Figure 3, entries 5 and 7), whereas benzene, the least polar solvent among these aprotic solvents, significantly reduced the yield of the desired product (Figure 3, entry 6). The reason for this very low yield IBA formation was interpreted as being due to that benzene forms a two-phase system and interferes with the dissolution of 2-IB into water. Protic solvents such as MeOH, EtOH and 2,2,2-trifuoroethanol (TFE) gave IBA **2a** in high yields; however, they also worked as a ligand for IBA, causing the formation of very small amounts of ligand-exchanged byproducts **3a–c** (Figure 3, entries 8–10). The white solid IBA **2a** obtained after the water and acetone washings did not contain any other byproducts. Although this result indicated that protic organic solvents were not suitable for the selective preparation of IBAs, it also revealed that the IBA hydroxyl group could undergo substitution reactions under mild conditions (vide infra). The yields indicated in Figure 3 are almost equal to the conversion of 2-IB **1a**.

Next, we investigated the substrate scope for the synthesis of IBAs using Oxone® under aqueous conditions with MeCN, and the results are shown in Figure 4. MeCN was used as a component of the solvent to dissolve substrates **1**. By oxidation of 5-substituted 2-IBs, IBAs **2b–d** containing fluoro-, chloro-, and bromo-substituents were smoothly obtained in excellent yields from the corresponding halo-substituted 2-IBs **1b–d**. From 2-IBs **1e–j** with electron-donating groups such as methyl-, methoxy-, and acethoxy-substituents (**1e–g**) and electron-withdrawing groups such as trifluoromethyl-, nitro- and cyano-substituents (**1h–j**), the desired IBAs **2e–j** were also produced in good yields. However, 2-IB bearing a hydroxy-substituent **1k** afforded the desired product **2k** in a moderate yield under the same conditions. In the oxidation of 4-substituted 2-IBs, fluoro-, chloro-, bromo-, trifluoromethyl-, and carboxy-substituted IBAs **2l–p** were obtained in excellent yields from the corresponding 2-IBs **1l–p**. In addition, the oxidized products of 4,5-disubstituted 2-IBs containing difluoro-substituents **2q** and dimethoxy-substituents **2r** were obtained in high yields. Meanwhile, with regard to 3-substituted 2-IBs, the reaction of methyl-substituted **1t** with a slight excess of Oxone® afforded the expected IBA **2t** in a good yield, whereas the yield of bromo-substituted IBA **2s** was lower even at the elevated temperature and in the presence of a large excess of Oxone®. Steric effects are probably important in the formation of the cyclic $\lambda^3$-iodanes. Indeed, the presence of a substituent at the *ortho* position of the iodine atom (3-position) interfered in the synthesis of the corresponding product for 3-bromo-substituted 2-IB **1s**. In the case of 6-substituted 2-IBs, fluoro-substituted IBA **2u** and methyl-substituted **2v** were obtained in good yields. Finally, the reaction of 3-iodonaphthalene-2-carboxylic acid **3** under the present conditions led to the expected tricyclic hypervalent iodine compound **4** in an excellent yield (Scheme 1).

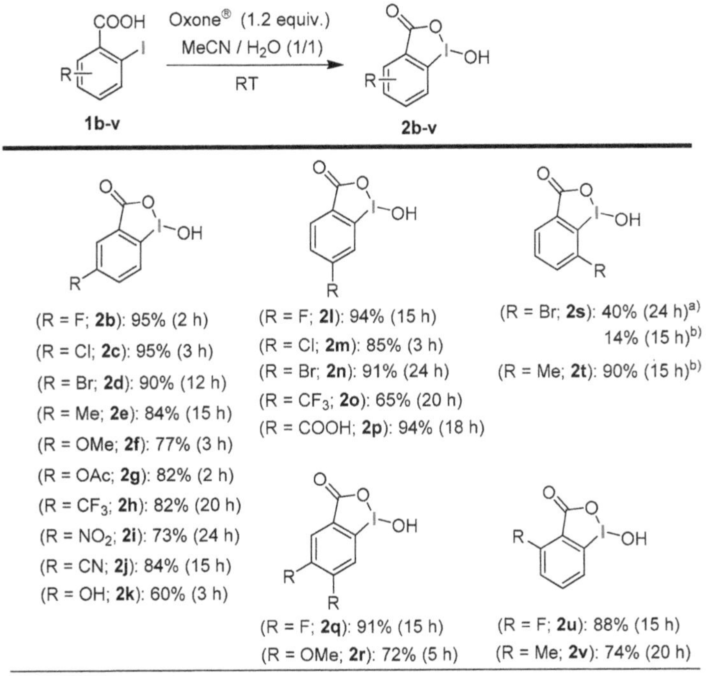


**Figure 4.** Substrate scope of the selective preparation of IBAs **2b–v** using Oxone® under aqueous conditions. (a) This reaction was performed at 30 °C in the presence of 1.2 equivalents of Oxone®. (b) Performed using 5 equivalents of Oxone® at 40 °C.

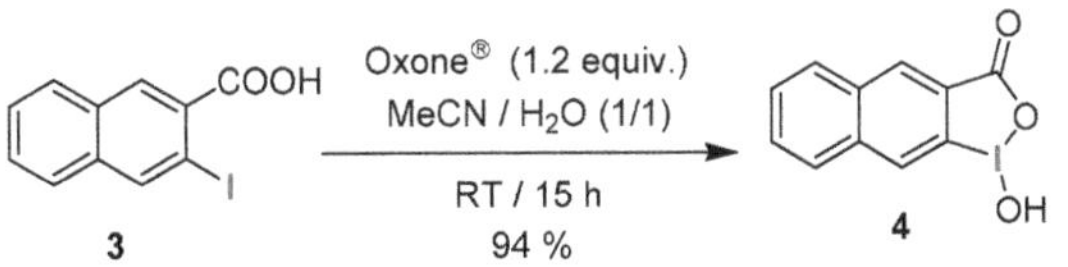


**Scheme 1.** Synthesis of tricyclic hypervalent iodine compound **4**.

*2.2. IBAs Synthesis Using Ferric Effect*

As mentioned in Section 2.1, our present method can selectively afford trivalent cyclic hypervalent iodine IBA at room temperature without contamination by pentavalent iodine byproduct. The mild conditions used contributed favorably to this product selectivity. Interestingly, we further found that iron ion in tap water (TW), which contained iron ion (5.8 μM or less), contribute to the IBA formation, whereas calcium and magnesium ions as main minerals in TW do not affect the selectivity. Indeed, IBA **2a** was selectively produced from 2-IB **1a** by heating even at 100 °C in DW containing 5 mol% $FeCl_3$ (Scheme 2, left).

On the other hand, IBX was instead formed as a main product in the absence of $FeCl_3$ in deionized water (DW) [93]. Other ferric salts such as $Fe(NO_3)$, $Fe(OTf)_3$, and $FeSO_4$ had similar effects. In addition, it was found that pentavalent IBX **5** was converted to IBA **2a** in the presence of a catalytic amount of $FeCl_3$ at 100 °C (Scheme 2, right), while the formation of unidentified high- and low-polar decomposition products were detected in the water and the acetone washing solution, respectively. Here, 2-IB **1a** was not produced. These results would indicate that overoxidation of IBA **2a** to pentavalent IBX **5** was strongly prevented by ferric salts. Thus, the effect of the metal ion in the decomposition of hazardous IBX **5** is also a significant key factor to ensure the safety for our trivalent cyclic hypervalent iodine synthesis under heating conditions.

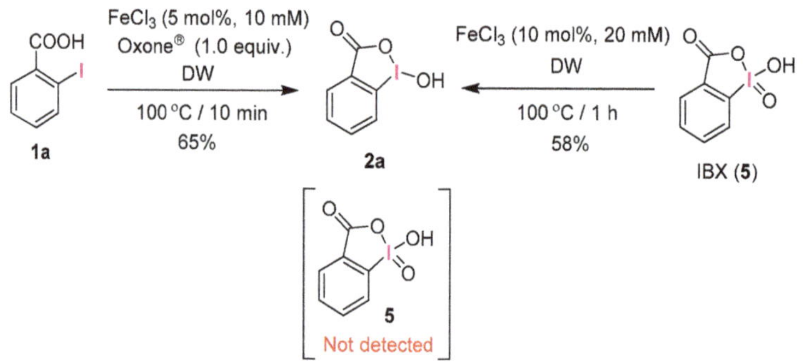


**Scheme 2.** Effect of a ferric salt on the selective synthesis of IBA **2a**.

The reaction time in the synthesis of IBAs was significantly shortened by heating. In the investigation of the heating conditions for the synthesis of IBA **2a** in 0.2 M 2-IB **1a** in the presence of 2.5 mol% $FeCl_3$ for 10 min, the required amount of Oxone® and the reaction temperature were thus optimized to 60 °C (Figure 5a) and 1.0 equivalent (Figure 5b), respectively. The yield of IBA **2a** was very sensitive to the reaction time, which dropped from 83% for 10 min to 70% for 1 h. IBA may be decomposed to small molecules in the presence of excess Oxone®; it has been reported that Oxone® causes oxidative cleavage of the aromatic ring [95]. Without Oxone®, we also confirmed that IBA **2a** was hardly decomposed under the conditions of Scheme 2 in the presence of 1.0 equivalent of $H_2SO_4$ and 10 mol% $FeCl_3$ at 100 °C for 10 min, while only 64% of IBA **2a** was recovered by replacing $H_2SO_4$ in the presence of Oxone® under the same conditions. Thus, the excess uses of Oxone® and performing the reaction at high temperature would decrease the IBA yield as shown in Figure 5a,b.

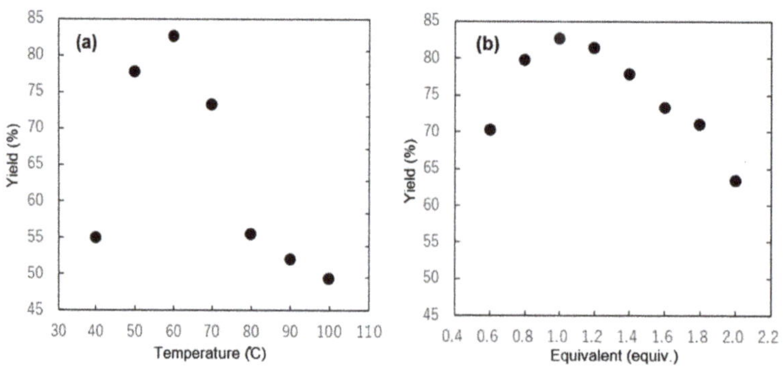


**Figure 5.** Optimization of (**a**) temperature using 1.0 equivalent of Oxone® and (**b**) amount of Oxone® at 60 °C for the synthesis of IBA **2a** from 2-IB **1a** in the presence of 2.5 mol% $FeCl_3$ (MeCN/DW (1/1)).

This optimized heating method could be applied to the synthesis of IBAs **2a–j** (Scheme 3). 2-IB **1a** as well as the substrates **1b–d** and **1g–j** that are tolerable to over-oxidation at this temperature were successfully converted to the desired IBAs **2a–d** and **2g–j** in high yields. However, the transformation of 2-IB having an electron-rich functional group, i.e., methoxy-substituted 2-IB **1f**, resulted in low yield of the corresponding IBA **2f** due to the formation of 2-carboxy-*p*-benzoquinone by the oxidation with Oxone®. Therefore, in order to apply the heating conditions, the stability of the product to oxidation must be considered.

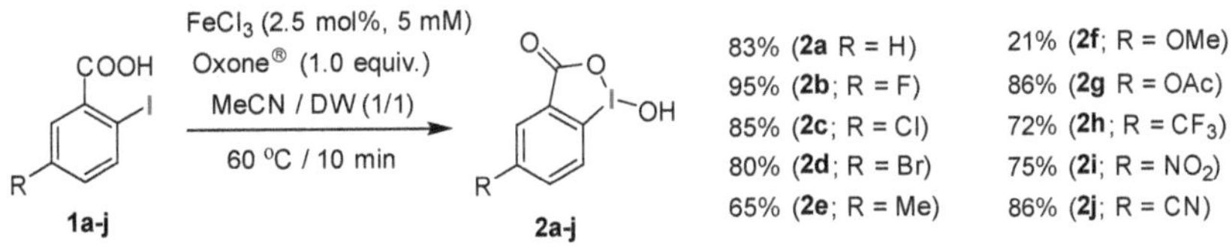


**Scheme 3.** Short-time selective synthesis of IBAs **2a–j** in the presence of ferric salt.

## 2.3. IBA Derivatives

As previously mentioned, when IBA **2a** was synthesized in an aqueous solution with alcohols, alkoxy-substituted derivatives **3a–c** were obtained as byproducts by substitution of the hydroxyl ligand of IBA **2a** (see Figure 3), implying the potential of the solvolytic ligand exchange of IBA **2a** under mild conditions. For the ligand derivatization of IBAs, the water molecule is an obstacle because the ligand exchanges of the IBA hydroxy group are reversible. Thus, molecular sieves with a pore diameter of 3 Å (MS3Å) was used for the solvolytic functionalization of IBA **2a** in dehydrated protic solvent (Figure 6). The quantitative derivatization to benziodoxole methoxide (IB-OMe) **6a** was achieved by heating IBA **2a** at 60 °C in MeOH (Figure 6, entry 1). Upon treatment at 80 °C, benziodoxole ethoxide (IB-OEt) **6b** and benziodoxole 2,2,2-trifluoroethoxide (IB-$OCH_2CF_3$) **6c** were also produced in high yields by the ligand exchange reaction with EtOH and TFE, respectively (Figure 6, entries 2 and 3). Benziodoxole *n*-propoxide (IB-$O^n$Pr) **6d** was obtained in 98% yield using $^n$PrOH at 70 °C (Figure 6, entry 4), and benziodoxole isopropoxide (IB-$O^i$Pr) **6e** was produced in 52% yield at 60 °C in the presence of $^i$PrOH (Figure 6, entry 5). In the cases of IB-$O^n$Pr **6d** and IB-$O^i$Pr **6e**, the temperature control was essential to suppress the formation of a 2-IB-IBA condensate as a byproduct; here, the formation of 2-IB **1a** can be explained in terms of the alcohol oxidation by IBA. It is known that secondary alcohols are readily oxidized by IBA [83]. No unwanted byproduct was found during the transformation to benziodoxole hexafluoroisopropoxide (IB-$OCH(CF_3)_2$) **6f** using hexafluoroisopropanol (HFIP) at 80 °C (Figure 6, entry 6), which is most likely due to the stability of HFIP against oxidation. Indeed, the condensate between 2-IB and IBA appeared during the reaction for benziodoxole *n*-buthoxide (IB-$O^n$Bu) **6g** using an oxidizable primary alcohol, $^n$BuOH, at 80 °C, whereas such byproduct was not observed in the synthesis of benziodoxole *tert*-buthoxide (IB-$O^t$Bu) **6h** using $^t$BuOH as a solvent inert to oxidation. Nevertheless, IB-$O^n$Bu **6g** could be selectively obtained by heat treatment at 60 °C without the formation of the condensate.

Using AcOH as a solvent, the solvolytic method was further applied to the synthesis of benziodoxole acetate (IB-OAc) **7a** and its analogs (R-IB-OAc) **7b–i** from the corresponding IBAs **2a–i** (Scheme 4). IB-OAc **7a** was easily produced in good yield by ligand exchange of IBA **2a** with AcOH at room temperature. Similarly, these transformations successfully afforded R-IB-OAc **7b–d** containing fluoro-, chloro-, and bromo-substituents; **7e–g** with electron-donating methyl-, methoxy-, and acethoxy-groups; and **7h** and **7i** bearing an electron-withdrawing trifluoromethyl- and nitro-substituent, respectively.

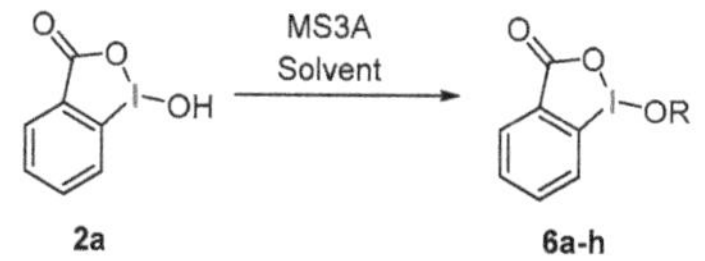


| Entry | Solvent | Time (h) | Temperature (°C) | Product | Yield (%) |
|---|---|---|---|---|---|
| 1 | MeOH | 2 | 60 | R = Me (**6a**) | 100 |
| 2 | EtOH | 1 | 80 | R = Et (**6b**) | 98 |
| 3 | TFE | 1 | 80 | R = $CH_2CF_3$ (**6c**) | 94 |
| 4 | $^n$PrOH | 3 | 70 | R = $^n$Pr (**6d**) | 98 |
| 5 | $^i$PrOH | 15 | 60 | R = $^i$Pr (**6e**) | 52 |
| 6 | HFIP | 1 | 80 | R = $CH(CF_3)_2$ (**6f**) | 83 |
| 7 | $^n$BuOH | 18 | 60 | R = $^n$Bu (**6g**) | 75 |
| 8 | $^t$BuOH | 2 | 80 | R = $^t$Bu (**6h**) | 49 |

**Figure 6.** Benziodoxole alkoxides **6a–h** by solvolytic functionalization of IBA **2a**.

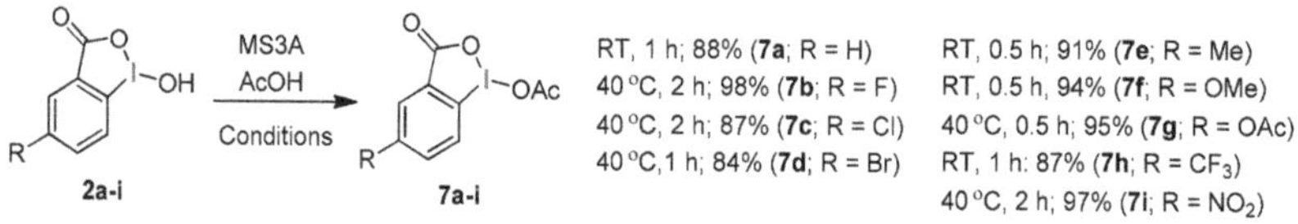


**Scheme 4.** Transformation of IBAs **2a–i** to benziodoxole acetates **7a–i**.

## 3. Materials and Methods

### 3.1. General Information

Substrates **1i** [96], **1k** [97], **1n** [98], **1o** [98], **1p** [99], **1q** [100], **1s** [101], **1t** [98], **1v** [102], and **3** [65] were prepared by Sandmeyer reaction of the corresponding anthranilic acids. Substrate **1g** [84] was synthesized by acetylation of compound **1k**. Substrate **1j** [103] is derived from 5-bromo-anthranilic acid methyl ester. $^1$H, $^{13}$C, and $^{19}$F nuclear magnetic resonance (NMR) spectra were recorded on ECS 400 and ECX 500 NMR spectrometers (JEOL Ltd., Tokyo, Japan) using deuterated dimethyl sulfoxide (DMSO-d6) or chloroform ($CDCl_3$) as a solvent. Chemical shifts (δ) are reported in parts per million (ppm) relative to tetramethylsilane (δ = 0 ppm) as an internal standard for $^1$H and $^{13}$C NMR spectra and hexafluoroacetone (δ = −84.6 ppm) as an internal standard for $^{19}$F NMR spectra. Coupling constants (*J*) are reported in Hertz (Hz), and the multiplicity is reported according to the following convention: singlet (s), doublet (d), double doublet (dd), double double doublet (ddd), double triplet (dt), triplet (t), triple doublet (td), quartet (q), quintet (quin), sextet (sext), septet (sep), and multiplet (m). Data are reported as follows: Chemical shift (number of protons, multiplicity, coupling constants). Infrared (IR) spectra were recorded on a JASCO FT/IR-4200 spectrometer (JASCO Co., Tokyo, Japan) on diffuse reflectance method using KBr powder. Absorptions are expressed in reciprocal centimeter ($cm^{-1}$). High resolution mass spectra (HRMS) obtained by the direct analysis in real time (DART) method were recorded on a Thermo Scientific Exactive Plus Orbitrap (Thermo Fisher Scientific, Inc., Waltham, MA, USA).

### 3.2. Synthesis of IBA Analogues

#### 3.2.1. General Procedure for the Synthesis of IBAs 2a–v and 4

To a solution of 2-IBs (1.0 mmol) in MeCN (5 mL) was added Oxone® (738 mg, 1.2 mmol) and $H_2O$ (TW for Figure 3; Figure 4, Scheme 1 or DW for Scheme 2; Scheme 3, 5 mL). After the mixture was stirred at room temperature for the appropriate time (see Figure 4 and Scheme 1), the product was filtered under reduced pressure. The residue was washed with water and acetone to obtain the corresponding IBAs **2a–v** and **4** (see Supplementary Materials for $^1$H NMR spectroscopic data) as a white powder.

3.2.2. 1-Hydroxy-1λ$^3$-benzo[d][1,2]iodaoxol-3(1H)-one (**2a**)

$^1$H NMR (400 MHz, DMSO-*d6*): δ 7.72 (1H, td, *J* = 7.3, 0.9 Hz, H5), 7.86 (1H, d, *J* = 8.2 Hz, H3), 7.97 (1H, ddd, *J* = 8.7, 7.4, 1.8 Hz, H4), 8.03 (1H, dd, *J* = 7.8, 1.4 Hz, H6), 8.08 (1H, s) ppm. $^{13}$C NMR (100 MHz, DMSO-*d6*): δ 120.3 (C2), 126.2 (C3), 130.3 (C5), 131.0 (C1), 131.4 (C6), 134.4 (C4), 167.7 (COOH) ppm. IR (ATR, KBr): *ν* 2936 (OH), 1616 (C=O), 1566 (C=O) cm$^{-1}$. Mp: 243–244 °C. $^1$H and $^{13}$C NMR data are consistent with those reported in the literature [33].

3.2.3. 5-Fluoro-1-hydroxy-1λ$^3$-benzo[d][1,2]iodaoxol-3(1H)-one (**2b**)

$^1$H NMR (500 MHz, DMSO-*d6*): δ 7.76 (1H, dd, *J* = 8.3, 2.6 Hz), 7.79–7.88 (2H, m), 8.21 (1H, s) ppm. $^{13}$C NMR (125 MHz, DMSO-*d6*): δ 114.2, 117.3 (d, *J* = 22.7 Hz), 121.7 (d, *J* = 23.8 Hz), 128.3 (d, *J* = 8.4 Hz), 134.1 (d, *J* = 7.2 Hz), 163.9 (d, *J* = 246.8 Hz), 166.4 (d, *J* = 2.4 Hz) ppm. $^{19}$F NMR (470 MHz, DMSO-*d6*): δ −116.2 (dt, *J* = 5.7, 8.6 Hz) ppm. IR (ATR, KBr): *ν* 2904 (OH), 1635 (C=O), 1577 (C=O) cm$^{-1}$. Mp: 241–242 °C. $^1$H and $^{13}$C NMR data are consistent with those reported in the literature [104].

3.2.4. 5-Chloro-1-hydroxy-1λ$^3$-benzo[d][1,2]iodaoxol-3(1H)-one (**2c**)

$^1$H NMR (400 MHz, DMSO-*d6*): δ 7.81 (1H, d, *J* = 8.7 Hz), 7.95 (1H, d, *J* = 2.3 Hz), 8.03 (1H, dd, *J* = 8.7, 2.3 Hz), 8.28 (1H, s) ppm. $^{13}$C NMR (100 MHz, DMSO-*d6*): δ 118.6, 128.1, 130.3, 133.5, 134.0, 135.8, 166.3 ppm. IR (ATR, KBr): *ν* 2905 (OH), 1624 (C=O), 1560 (C=O) cm$^{-1}$. Mp: 294–295 °C. $^1$H and $^{13}$C NMR data are consistent with those reported in the literature [105].

3.2.5. 5-Bromo-1-hydroxy-1λ$^3$-benzo[d][1,2]iodaoxol-3(1H)-one (**2d**)

$^1$H NMR (400 MHz, DMSO-*d6*): δ 7.74 (1H, d, *J* = 8.7 Hz), 8.07 (1H, d, *J* = 2.3 Hz), 8.15 (1H, dd, *J* = 8.7, 2.3 Hz), 8.27 (1H, s) ppm. $^{13}$C NMR (100 MHz, DMSO-*d6*): δ 119.5, 124.2, 128.3, 133.3, 133.7, 136.8, 166.2 ppm. IR (ATR, KBr): *ν* 2884 (OH), 1617 (C=O), 1557 (C=O) cm$^{-1}$. Mp: 236–238 °C. $^1$H and $^{13}$C NMR data are consistent with those reported in the literature [106].

3.2.6. 1-Hydroxy-5-methyl-1λ$^3$-benzo[d][1,2]iodaoxol-3(1H)-one (**2e**)

$^1$H NMR (400 MHz, DMSO-*d6*): δ 2.48 (3H, s), 7.70 (1H, d, *J* = 8.2 Hz), 7.79 (1H, dd, *J* = 8.7, 1.8 Hz), 7.85 (1H, s), 8.01 (1H, s) ppm. $^{13}$C NMR (100 MHz, DMSO-*d6*): δ 20.1, 116.7, 125.9, 131.3, 131.4, 135.2, 140.4, 167.7 ppm. IR (ATR, KBr): *ν* 3054 (OH), 1622 (C=O), 1569 (C=O) cm$^{-1}$. Mp: 212–214 °C. $^1$H and $^{13}$C NMR data are consistent with those reported in the literature [105].

3.2.7. 1-Hydroxy-5-methoxy-1λ$^3$-benzo[d][1,2]iodaoxol-3(1H)-one (**2f**)

$^1$H NMR (400 MHz, DMSO-*d6*): δ 3.89 (3H, s), 7.52 (1H, d, *J* = 2.7 Hz), 7.55 (1H, dd, *J* = 8.7, 2.8 Hz), 7.67 (1H, d, *J* = 9.2 Hz), 8.04 (1H, s) ppm. $^{13}$C NMR (100 MHz, DMSO-*d6*): δ 55.8, 108.9, 114.8, 121.5, 127.0, 132.9, 161.4, 167.4 ppm. IR (ATR, KBr): *ν* 2953 (OH), 1620 (C=O), 1577 (C=O) cm$^{-1}$. Mp: 217–218 °C. $^1$H and $^{13}$C NMR data are consistent with those reported in the literature [105].

3.2.8. 1-Hydroxy-3-oxo-1,3-dihydro-1λ$^3$-benzo[d][1,2]iodaoxol-5-yl acetate (**2g**)

$^1$H NMR (500 MHz, DMSO-*d6*): δ 2.33 (3H, s), 7.74 (1H, dd, *J* = 8.6, 2.3 Hz), 7.77 (1H, d, *J* = 2.3 Hz), 7.84 (1H, d, *J* = 8.6 Hz), 8.16 (1H, s) ppm. $^{13}$C NMR (125 MHz, DMSO-*d6*): δ 20.8, 116.1, 124.2, 127.4, 127.9, 133.0, 152.5, 166.8, 169.0 ppm. IR (ATR, KBr): *ν* 2891 (OH), 1759 (C=O), 1604 (C=O), 1559 (C=O) cm$^{-1}$. Mp: 207–208 °C. HRMS (DART, m/z) calcd for $C_9H_8IO_5$ $[M + H]^+$: 322.9411; found: 322.9413.

3.2.9. 1-Hydroxy-5-(trifluoromethyl)-1λ$^3$-benzo[d][1,2]iodaoxol-3(1H)-one (**2h**)

$^1$H NMR (500 MHz, DMSO-*d6*): δ 8.08 (1H, d, *J* = 8.0 Hz), 8.21 (1H, s), 8.33 (1H, d, *J* = 8.1 Hz), 8.38 (1H, s) ppm. $^{13}$C NMR (125 MHz, DMSO-*d6*): δ 123.4 (q, *J* = 271.0 Hz), 125.5, 127.1 (d, *J* = 3.6 Hz), 127.9, 130.6 (d, *J* = 2.4 Hz), 131.6 (q, *J* = 32.6 Hz), 132.9, 166.3 ppm. $^{19}$F NMR (470 MHz, DMSO-*d6*): δ −64.5 ppm. IR (ATR, KBr): *ν* 2854 (OH), 1597 (C=O), 1559 (C=O) cm$^{-1}$. Mp: 233–235 °C. HRMS (DART, m/z) calcd for $C_8H_5F_3IO_3$ [M + H]$^+$: 332.9230; found: 332.9227.

3.2.10. 1-Hydroxy-5-nitro-1λ$^3$-benzo[d][1,2]iodaoxol-3(1H)-one (**2i**)

$^1$H NMR (400 MHz, DMSO-*d6*): δ 8.10 (1H, d, *J* = 8.7 Hz), 8.54 (1H, s), 8.57 (1H, d, *J* = 2.3 Hz), 8.73 (1H, dd, *J* = 8.7, 2.8 Hz) ppm. $^{13}$C NMR (100 MHz, DMSO-*d6*): δ 124.8, 127.7, 128.1, 128.2, 133.4, 149.7, 165.9 ppm. IR (ATR, KBr): *ν* 2834 (OH), 1617 (C=O), 1572 (C=O), 1541 (C=O) cm$^{-1}$. Mp: 214–216 °C. $^1$H and $^{13}$C NMR data are consistent with those reported in the literature [107].

3.2.11. 1-Hydroxy-3-oxo-1,3-dihydro-1λ$^3$-benzo[d][1,2]iodaoxole-5-carbonitrile (**2j**)

$^1$H NMR (500 MHz, DMSO-*d6*): δ 8.01 (1H, d, *J* = 8.6 Hz), 8.32–8.41 (3H, m) ppm. $^{13}$C NMR (125 MHz, DMSO-*d6*): δ 113.5, 117.3, 126.4, 127.7, 132.9, 134.2, 137.0, 166.0 ppm. IR (ATR, KBr): *ν* 2903 (OH), 1625 (C=O), 1582 (C=O), 1561 (C=O) cm$^{-1}$. Mp: 234–236 °C. HRMS (DART, m/z) calcd for $C_8H_5INO_3$ [M + H]$^+$: 289.9309; found: 289.9310.

3.2.12. 1,5-Dihydroxy-1λ$^3$-benzo[d][1,2]iodaoxol-3(1H)-one (**2k**)

$^1$H NMR (400 MHz, DMSO-*d6*): δ 7.36 (1H, dd, *J* = 8.7, 2.7 Hz), 7.40 (1H, d, *J* = 2.3 Hz), 7.57 (1H, d, *J* = 9.2 Hz), 7.94 (1H, s) ppm. $^{13}$C NMR (100 MHz, DMSO-*d6*): δ 106.6, 117.1, 122.0, 127.0, 132.8, 159.7, 167.6 ppm. IR (ATR, KBr): *ν* 3447 (OH), 3234 (OH), 1576 (C=O) cm$^{-1}$. Mp: 230–232 °C. HRMS (DART, m/z) calcd for $C_7H_6IO_4$ [M + H]$^+$: 280.9305; found: 280.9304.

3.2.13. 6-Fluoro-1-hydroxy-1λ$^3$-benzo[d][1,2]iodaoxol-3(1H)-one (**2l**)

$^1$H NMR (500 MHz, DMSO-*d6*): δ 7.53–7.60 (2H, m), 8.01 (1H, dd, *J* = 8.0, 5.2 Hz), 8.21 (1H, s) ppm. $^{13}$C NMR (125 MHz, DMSO-*d6*): δ 113.5 (d, *J* = 27.4 Hz), 118.0 (d, *J* = 22.7 Hz), 122.8 (d, *J* = 8.4 Hz), 128.3, 132.9 (d, *J* = 8.4 Hz), 166.0 (d, *J* = 254.0 Hz), 166.7 ppm. $^{19}$F NMR (470 MHz, DMSO-*d6*): δ −109.0 (dt, *J* = 5.8, 8.6 Hz) ppm. IR (ATR, KBr): *ν* 3091 (OH), 1636 (C=O), 1586 (C=O) cm$^{-1}$. Mp: 206–208 °C. $^1$H and $^{13}$C NMR data are consistent with those reported in the literature [105].

3.2.14. 6-Chloro-1-hydroxy-1λ$^3$-benzo[d][1,2]iodaoxol-3(1H)-one (**2m**)

$^1$H NMR (400 MHz, DMSO-*d6*): δ 7.75 (1H, d, *J* = 1.8 Hz), 7.78 (1H, dd, *J* = 7.8, 1.8 Hz), 7.96 (1H, d, *J* = 8.2, 2.3 Hz), 8.27 (1H, s) ppm. $^{13}$C NMR (100 MHz, DMSO-*d6*): δ 122.1, 125.7, 130.6, 130.7, 132.2, 139.3, 166.7 ppm. IR (ATR, KBr): *ν* 2854 (OH), 1607 (C=O), 1557 (C=O) cm$^{-1}$. Mp: 212–214 °C. $^1$H NMR data is consistent with those reported in the literature [94].

3.2.15. 6-Bromo-1-hydroxy-1λ$^3$-benzo[d][1,2]iodaoxol-3(1H)-one (**2n**)

$^1$H NMR (500 MHz, DMSO-*d6*): δ 7.80–7.98 (3H, m), 8.23 (1H, s) ppm. $^{13}$C NMR (125 MHz, DMSO-*d6*): δ 122.1, 127.9, 128.5, 131.0, 132.5, 133.5, 166.8 ppm. IR (ATR, KBr): *ν* 2844 (OH), 1602 (C=O), 1556 (C=O) cm$^{-1}$. Mp: 222–224 °C. HRMS (DART, m/z) calcd for $C_7H_5BrIO_3$ [M + H]$^+$: 342.8461; found: 342.8460.

3.2.16. 1-Hydroxy-6-(trifluoromethyl)-1λ$^3$-benzo[d][1,2]iodaoxol-3(1H)-one (**2o**)

$^1$H NMR (400 MHz, DMSO-*d6*): δ 8.06 (1H, s), 8.10 (1H, d, *J* = 8.1 Hz), 8.20 (1H, d, *J* = 8.0 Hz), 8.38 (1H, s) ppm. $^{13}$C NMR (100 MHz, DMSO-*d6*): δ 121.7, 123.1 (d, *J* = 3.6 Hz), 123.4 (d, *J* = 270.7 Hz), 127.6 (d, *J* = 3.6 Hz), 131.9, 133.9 (q, *J* = 32.2 Hz), 135.4, 166.4 ppm.

$^{19}$F NMR (370 MHz, DMSO-*d6*): δ −64.6 ppm. IR (ATR, KBr): ν 2871 (OH), 1616 (C=O), 1560 (C=O) cm$^{-1}$. Mp: 216–217 °C. $^{1}$H and $^{13}$C NMR data are consistent with those reported in the literature [12].

3.2.17. 1-Hydroxy-3-oxo-1,3-dihydro-1λ$^{3}$-benzo[d][1,2]iodaoxole-6-carboxylic acid (**2p**)

$^{1}$H NMR (500 MHz, DMSO-*d6*): δ ppm. $^{13}$C NMR (125 MHz, DMSO-*d6*): δ ppm. IR (ATR, KBr): ν 2832 (OH), 1704 (C=O), 1616 (C=O), 1558 (C=O) cm$^{-1}$. Mp: 291–293 °C. HRMS (DART, m/z) calcd for $C_8H_6IO_5$ [M + H]$^+$: 308.9254; found: 308.9252.

3.2.18. 5,6-Difluoro-1-hydroxy-1λ$^{3}$-benzo[d][1,2]iodaoxol-3(1H)-one (**2q**)

$^{1}$H NMR (500 MHz, DMSO-*d6*): δ 7.73 (1H, dd, *J* = 9.2, 6.9 Hz), 7.97 (1H, dd, *J* = 9.7, 7.4 Hz), 8.37 (1H, s) ppm. $^{13}$C NMR (125 MHz, DMSO-*d6*): δ 115.5 (d, *J* = 22.7 Hz), 119.2 (d, *J* = 19.1 Hz), 129.16 (d, *J* = 2.4 Hz), 129.20 (d, *J* = 3.6 Hz), 151.3 (dd, *J* = 263.5, 13.1 Hz), 153.7 (dd, *J* = 256.4, 14.3 Hz), 165.9 ppm. $^{19}$F NMR (470 MHz, DMSO-*d6*): δ −138.7–138.5 (m), −132.6–132.4 (m) ppm. IR (ATR, KBr): ν 2895 (OH), 1624 (C=O), 1591 (C=O) cm$^{-1}$. Mp: 201–203 °C. HRMS (DART, m/z) calcd for $C_7H_4F_2IO_3$ [M + H]$^+$: 300.9168; found: 300.9170.

3.2.19. 1-Hydroxy-5,6-dimethoxy-1λ$^{3}$-benzo[d][1,2]iodaoxol-3(1H)-one (**2r**)

$^{1}$H NMR (500 MHz, DMSO-*d6*): δ 3.89 (6H, s), 7.24 (1H, s), 7.46 (1H, s), 7.95 ppm. $^{13}$C NMR (125 MHz, DMSO-*d6*): δ 55.9, 56.0, 107.4, 110.7, 112.4, 123.9, 150.6, 154.1, 167.8 ppm. IR (ATR, KBr): ν 3016 (OH), 1592 (C=O), 1559 (C=O) cm$^{-1}$. Mp: 201–203 °C. $^{1}$H and $^{13}$C NMR data are consistent with those reported in the literature [46].

3.2.20. 7-Bromo-1-hydroxy-1λ$^{3}$-benzo[d][1,2]iodaoxol-3(1H)-one (**2s**)

$^{1}$H NMR (500 MHz, DMSO-*d6*): δ 7.60 (1H, t, *J* = 7.7 Hz), 7.97 (1H, dd, *J* = 7.7, 1.5 Hz), 8.02 (1H, dd, *J* = 7.5, 1.2 Hz) ppm. $^{13}$C NMR (125 MHz, DMSO-*d6*): δ 119.6, 130.0, 133.1, 135.4, 140.5, 146.1, 167.0 ppm. IR (ATR, KBr): ν 3273 (OH), 1647 (C=O) cm$^{-1}$. Mp: 154–155 °C. HRMS (DART, m/z) calcd for $C_7H_5BrIO_3$ [M + H]$^+$: 342.8461; found: 342.8462.

3.2.21. 1-Hydroxy-7-methyl-1λ$^{3}$-benzo[d][1,2]iodaoxol-3(1H)-one (**2t**)

$^{1}$H NMR (400 MHz, DMSO-*d6*): δ 2.79 (3H, s), 7.57–7.73 (2H, m), 7.90 (1H, d, *J* = 6.9 Hz) ppm. $^{13}$C NMR (100 MHz, DMSO-*d6*): δ 19.6, 128.7, 132.0, 132.6, 137.9, 139.1, 147.4, 167.9 ppm. IR (ATR, KBr): ν 1672 (C=O) cm$^{-1}$. Mp: 164–166 °C. $^{1}$H NMR data are consistent with those reported in the literature [106].

3.2.22. 4-Fluoro-1-hydroxy-1λ$^{3}$-benzo[d][1,2]iodaoxol-3(1H)-one (**2u**)

$^{1}$H NMR (400 MHz, DMSO-*d6*): δ 7.51 (1H, dd, *J* = 10.1, 8.2 Hz), 7.71 (1H, d, *J* = 7.7 Hz), 7.90 (1H, td, *J* = 8.2, 4.6 Hz), 8.24 (1H, s) ppm. $^{13}$C NMR (100 MHz, DMSO-*d6*): δ 118.6 (d, *J* = 22.0 Hz), 119.2 (d, *J* = 11.5 Hz), 122.5 (d, *J* = 3.8 Hz), 123.2, 134.3 (d, *J* = 8.6 Hz), 163.8 (d, *J* = 4.8 Hz), 163.8 (d, *J* = 264.4 Hz) ppm. $^{19}$F NMR (375 MHz, DMSO-*d6*): δ −114.7 (dd, *J* = 15.2, 4.9 Hz) ppm. IR (ATR, KBr): ν 3091 (OH), 1636 (C=O), 1586 (C=O) cm$^{-1}$. Mp: 213–214 °C. $^{1}$H and $^{13}$C NMR data are consistent with those reported in the literature [106,108].

3.2.23. 1-Hydroxy-4-methyl-1λ$^{3}$-benzo[d][1,2]iodaoxol-3(1H)-one (**2v**)

$^{1}$H NMR (400 MHz, DMSO-*d6*): δ 2.70 (3H, s), 7.48–7.55 (1H, m), 7.72–7.80 (2H, m), 7.94 (1H, s) ppm. $^{13}$C NMR (100 MHz, DMSO-*d6*): δ 20.4, 122.2, 124.2, 128.2, 133.3, 133.4, 144.3, 168.0 ppm. IR (ATR, KBr): ν 2926 (OH), 1625 (C=O), 1584 (C=O) cm$^{-1}$. Mp: 212–213 °C. $^{1}$H and $^{13}$C NMR data are consistent with those reported in the literature [106].

3.2.24. 1-Hydroxy-1λ$^3$-naphtho[2,3-d][1,2]iodaoxol-3(1H)-one (**4**)

$^1$H NMR (400 MHz, DMSO-*d6*): δ 7.76 (2H, m), 8.14–8.33 (2H, m), 8.29 (1H, d, *J* = 8.2 Hz), 8.39 (1H, s), 8.69 (1H, s) ppm. $^{13}$C NMR (100 MHz, DMSO-*d6*): δ 115.9, 126.3, 127.8, 127.9, 128.1, 128.9, 129.3, 131.7, 132.8, 135.8, 167.7 ppm. IR (ATR, KBr): ν 3053 (OH), 1698 (C=O), 1607 (C=O), 1559 (C=O) cm$^{-1}$. Mp: 164–165 °C. $^1$H and $^{13}$C NMR data are consistent with those reported in the literature [107].

### 3.3. *Synthesis of Benziodoxole Alkoxides*

3.3.1. General Procedure for the Synthesis of Benziodoxole Alkoxides (**6**)

To a suspension of IBA **2a** (264 mg, 1.0 mmol) in an appropriate alcohol (10 mL) was added MS3Å (1 g). After the mixture was stirred under the appropriate conditions (see Figure 6), MS3Å was filtered using $CH_2Cl_2$, and the solvents were then removed by evaporation. The residue was washed with hexane and filtered to remove the corresponding alcohol completely. The residue was dissolved with $CH_2Cl_2$ and the extract was then filtered through filter paper to remove unreacted substrate. Removal of the solvent by evaporation gave the corresponding benziodoxole alkoxides **6a–h** as a white powder.

3.3.2. 1-Methoxy-1λ$^3$-benzo[d][1,2]iodaoxol-3(1H)-one (**6a**)

$^1$H NMR (500 MHz, $CDCl_3$): δ 4.29 (3H, s), 7.70 (1H, t, *J* = 7.7 Hz), 7.78 (1H, d, *J* = 8.1 Hz), 7.91 (1H, ddd, *J* = 8.6, 6.9, 1.2 Hz), 8.28 (1H, dd, *J* = 7.5, 1.2 Hz) ppm. $^{13}$C NMR (125 MHz, $CDCl_3$): δ 62.3, 118.6, 126.0, 130.6, 131.0, 132.9, 135.1, 168.0 ppm. IR (ATR, KBr): ν 1653 (C=O) cm$^{-1}$. Mp: 161–163 °C. $^1$H and $^{13}$C NMR data are consistent with those reported in the literature [28,109].

3.3.3. 1-Ethoxy-1λ$^3$-benzo[d][1,2]iodaoxol-3(1H)-one (**6b**)

$^1$H NMR (500 MHz, $CDCl_3$): δ 1.35 (3H, t, *J* = 6.9 Hz), 4.30 (2H, q, *J* = 6.9 Hz), 7.70 (1H, t, *J* = 7.4 Hz), 7.79 (1H, d, *J* = 8.9 Hz), 7.89 (1H, td, *J* = 8.6, 1.8 Hz), 8.28 (1H, dd, *J* = 7.2, 2.0 Hz) ppm. $^{13}$C NMR (125 MHz, $CDCl_3$): δ 19.0, 69.9, 118.8, 125.9, 130.7, 131.0, 132.9, 135.0, 168.0 ppm. IR (ATR, KBr): ν 1655 (C=O) cm$^{-1}$. Mp: 123–125 °C. $^1$H and $^{13}$C NMR data are consistent with those reported in the literature [109].

3.3.4. 1-(2,2,2-trifluoroethoxy)-1λ$^3$-benzo[d][1,2]iodaoxol-3(1H)-one (**6c**)

$^1$H NMR (500 MHz, $CDCl_3$): δ 4.52 (2H, q, *J* = 8.6 Hz), 7.74 (1H, t, *J* = 7.5 Hz), 7.86 (1H, d, *J* = 8.0 Hz), 7.97 (1H, ddd, *J* = 8.0, 6.9, 1.2 Hz), 8.27 (1H, dd, *J* = 7.5, 1.2 Hz) ppm. $^{13}$C NMR (125 MHz, $CDCl_3$): δ 69.7 (q, *J* = 34.2 Hz), 119.0, 123.5 (q, *J* = 278.2 Hz), 126.5, 129.5, 131.4, 133.2, 135.9, 167.9 ppm. $^{19}$F NMR (470 MHz, $CDCl_3$): δ −77.2 (q, *J* = 9.1 Hz) ppm. IR (ATR, KBr): ν 1646 (C=O) cm$^{-1}$. Mp: 139–141 °C. HRMS (DART, m/z) calcd for $C_9H_7F_3IO_3$ $[M + H]^+$: 346.9386; found: 346.9384.

3.3.5. 1-Propoxy-1λ$^3$-benzo[d][1,2]iodaoxol-3(1H)-one (**6d**)

$^1$H NMR (500 MHz, $CDCl_3$): δ 1.02 (3H, t, *J* = 7.5 Hz), 1.72 (2H, sext, *J* = 7.1 Hz), 4.20 (2H, t, *J* = 6.6 Hz), 7.70 (1H, t, *J* = 7.2 Hz), 7.79 (1H, d, *J* = 8.6 Hz), 7.89 (1H, t, *J* = 7.2 Hz), 8.28 (1H, d, *J* = 7.5 Hz) ppm. $^{13}$C NMR (125 MHz, $CDCl_3$): δ 10.1, 26.5, 76.0, 118.9, 125.9, 130.7, 130.9, 132.8, 135.0, 167.9 ppm. IR (ATR, KBr): ν 1651 (C=O) cm$^{-1}$. Mp: 146–148 °C. HRMS (DART, m/z) calcd for $C_{10}H_{12}IO_3$ $[M + H]^+$: 306.9826; found: 306.9823.

3.3.6. 1-Isopropoxy-1λ$^3$-benzo[d][1,2]iodaoxol-3(1H)-one (**6e**)

$^1$H NMR (500 MHz, $CDCl_3$): δ 1.36 (6H, d, *J* = 6.3 Hz), 4.33 (1H, sep, *J* = 6.1 Hz), 7.69 (1H, t, *J* = 7.4 Hz), 7.82 (1H, d, *J* = 7.5 Hz), 7.88 (1H, td, *J* = 7.8, 1.5 Hz), 8.28 (1H, dd, *J* = 7.5, 1.7 Hz) ppm. $^{13}$C NMR (125 MHz, $CDCl_3$): δ 25.2, 75.6, 119.1, 126.0, 130.8, 130.9, 132.7, 134.8, 168.0 ppm. IR (ATR, KBr): ν 1653 (C=O) cm$^{-1}$. Mp: 253–254 °C. $^1$H and $^{13}$C NMR data are consistent with those reported in the literature [109].

3.3.7. 1-((1,1,1,3,3,3-hexafluoropropan-2-yl)oxy)-1λ$^3$-benzo[d][1,2]iodaoxol-3(1H)-one **(6f)**

$^1$H NMR (500 MHz, $CDCl_3$): δ 4.80 (1H, sep, $J$ = 5.8 Hz), 7.74 (1H, ddd, $J$ = 8.0, 7.5, 1.4 Hz), 7.97–8.04 (2H, m), 8.24 (1H, dd, $J$ = 7.4, 1.2 Hz) ppm. $^{13}$C NMR (125 MHz, $CDCl_3$): δ 76.1 (quin, $J$ = 32.5 Hz), 119.4, 122.2 (q, $J$ = 283.8 Hz), 127.3, 128.5, 131.6, 133.3, 136.4, 168.1 ppm. $^{19}$F NMR (470 MHz, $CDCl_3$): δ −76.0 (d, $J$ = 5.7 Hz) ppm. IR (ATR, KBr): ν 1661 (C=O) cm$^{-1}$. Mp: 148–149 °C. HRMS (DART, m/z) calcd for $C_{10}H_6F_6IO_3$ [M + H]$^+$: 414.9260; found: 414.9258.

3.3.8. 1-Butoxy-1λ$^3$-benzo[d][1,2]iodaoxol-3(1H)-one **(6g)**

$^1$H NMR (500 MHz, $CDCl_3$): δ 0.98 (3H, t, $J$ = 7.5 Hz), 1.46 (2H, sext, $J$ = 7.4 Hz), 1.68 (2H, quin, $J$ = 7.2 Hz), 4.24 (2H, t, $J$ = 6.6 Hz), 7.70 (1H, t, $J$ = 7.5 Hz), 7.78 (1H, d, $J$ = 8.0 Hz), 7.89 (1H, t, $J$ = 7.5 Hz), 8.28 (1H, d, $J$ = 7.5 Hz) ppm. $^{13}$C NMR (125 MHz, $CDCl_3$): δ 13.9, 19.0, 35.4, 74.2, 118.9, 125.9, 130.7, 131.0, 132.9, 135.0, 167.9 ppm. IR (ATR, KBr): ν 1650 (C=O) cm$^{-1}$. Mp: 143–144 °C. $^1$H and $^{13}$C NMR data are consistent with those reported in the literature [110].

3.3.9. 1-(tert-Butoxy)-1λ$^3$-benzo[d][1,2]iodaoxol-3(1H)-one **(6h)**

$^1$H NMR (500 MHz, $CDCl_3$): δ 1.41 (9H, s), 7.67 (1H, ddd, $J$ = 8.1, 7.5, 1.8 Hz), 7.83–7.91 (2H,m), 8.26 (1H, dd, $J$ = 8.1, 1.8 Hz) ppm. $^{13}$C NMR (125 MHz, $CDCl_3$): δ 30.4, 78.6, 119.6, 126.2, 130.8, 131.0, 132.4, 134.7, 168.0 ppm. IR (ATR, KBr): ν 1659 (C=O) cm$^{-1}$. Decomp: 265 °C. HRMS (DART, m/z) calcd for $C_{11}H_{13}IO_3$ [M + H]$^+$: 320.9982; found: 320.9980.

*3.4. Synthesis of Benziodoxole Acetates*

3.4.1. General Procedure for the Synthesis of Benziodoxole Acetates (7)

MS3Å (0.5 g) was added to a suspension of IBAs **2a–i** (0.50 mmol) in AcOH (5 mL), and the mixture was stirred under the appropriate conditions (see Scheme 4). Then, MS3Å was filtered using $CH_2Cl_2$, and the solvents were removed by evaporation. The residue was washed with ether and filtered to remove AcOH completely. The resulting residue was dissolved with $CH_2Cl_2$, and the extract was then filtered through filter paper to remove unreacted substrate. After solvent removal by evaporation, the corresponding benziodoxole acetates **7a–i** were obtained as a white powder.

3.4.2. 3-Oxo-1λ$^3$-benzo[d][1,2]iodaoxol-1(3H)-yl acetate **(7a)**

$^1$H NMR (500 MHz, $CDCl_3$): δ 2.27 (3H, s), 7.72 (1H, td, $J$ = 7.5, 1.2 Hz), 7.94 (1H, ddd, $J$ = 8.6, 6.9, 1.2 Hz), 8.01 (1H, d, $J$ = 8.6 Hz), 8.25 (1H, dd, $J$ = 7.5, 1.2 Hz) ppm. $^{13}$C NMR (125 MHz, $CDCl_3$): δ 20.2, 118.3, 128.9, 129.2, 131.2, 133.1, 136.1, 168.1, 176.3 ppm. IR (ATR, KBr): ν 1684 (C=O) cm$^{-1}$. Mp: 220–222 °C. $^1$H and $^{13}$C NMR data are consistent with those reported in the literature [109].

3.4.3. 5-Fluoro-3-oxo-1λ$^3$-benzo[d][1,2]iodaoxol-1(3H)-yl acetate **(7b)**

$^1$H NMR (500 MHz, $CDCl_3$): δ 2.26 (3H, s), 7.64 (1H, ddd, $J$ = 8.6, 7.7, 2.9 Hz), 7.94–8.00 (2H, m) ppm. $^{13}$C NMR (125 MHz, $CDCl_3$): δ 20.2, 111.3, 120.0 (d, $J$ = 23.8 Hz), 123.7 (d, $J$ = 22.7 Hz), 131.0 (d, $J$ = 8.3 Hz), 131.8 (d, $J$ = 7.2 Hz), 165.0 (d, $J$ = 252.8 Hz), 166.8, 176.4 ppm. $^{19}$F NMR (470 MHz, $CDCl_3$): δ −110.8 (td, $J$ = 7.2, 4.3 Hz) ppm. IR (ATR, KBr): ν 1696 (C=O) cm$^{-1}$. Mp: 225–226 °C. $^1$H and $^{13}$C NMR data are consistent with those reported in the literature [111].

3.4.4. 5-Chloro-3-oxo-1λ$^3$-benzo[d][1,2]iodaoxol-1(3H)-yl acetate **(7c)**

$^1$H NMR (500 MHz, $CDCl_3$): δ 2.27 (3H, s), 7.87 (1H, dd, $J$ = 8.6, 2.3 Hz), 7.93 (1H, d, $J$ = 9.2 Hz), 8.22 (1H, d, $J$ = 1.7 Hz) ppm. $^{13}$C NMR (125 MHz, $CDCl_3$): δ 20.2, 115.5, 130.4, 130.9, 133.0, 136.0, 138.8, 166.7, 176.4 ppm. IR (ATR, KBr): ν 1698 (C=O)

$cm^{-1}$. Mp: 244–245 °C. $^{1}H$ and $^{13}C$ NMR data are consistent with those reported in the literature [105].

3.4.5. 5-Bromo-3-oxo-1λ$^{3}$-benzo[d][1,2]iodaoxol-1(3H)-yl acetate (**7d**)

$^{1}H$ NMR (500 MHz, $CDCl_3$): δ 2.27 (3H, s), 7.85 (1H, d, $J$ = 9.2 Hz), 8.01 (1H, dd, $J$ = 8.6, 2.3 Hz), 8.37 (1H, d, $J$ = 1.8 Hz) ppm. $^{13}C$ NMR (125 MHz, $CDCl_3$): δ 20.2, 116.5, 126.6, 130.7, 131.0, 136.1, 138.9, 166.6, 176.4 ppm. IR (ATR, KBr): $\nu$ 1680 (C=O) $cm^{-1}$. Mp: 226–228 °C. $^{1}H$ and $^{13}C$ NMR data are consistent with those reported in the literature [112].

3.4.6. 5-Methyl-3-oxo-1λ$^{3}$-benzo[d][1,2]iodaoxol-1(3H)-yl acetate (**7e**)

$^{1}H$ NMR (500 MHz, $CDCl_3$): δ 2.25 (3H, s), 2.56 (3H, s), 7.73 (1H, dd, $J$ = 8.6, 1.7 Hz), 7.84 (1H, d, $J$ = 8.6 Hz), 8.07 (1H, d, $J$ = 1.8 Hz) ppm. $^{13}C$ NMR (125 MHz, $CDCl_3$): δ 20.3, 20.8, 114.6, 128.9, 133.6, 137.1, 142.3, 168.3, 176.4 ppm. IR (ATR, KBr): $\nu$ 1682 (C=O), 1659 (C=O) $cm^{-1}$. Mp: 215–217 °C. $^{1}H$ and $^{13}C$ NMR data are consistent with those reported in the literature [105].

3.4.7. 5-Methoxy-3-oxo-1λ$^{3}$-benzo[d][1,2]iodaoxol-1(3H)-yl acetate (**7f**)

$^{1}H$ NMR (500 MHz, $CDCl_3$): δ 2.25 (3H, s), 3.94 (3H, s), 7.46 (1H, dd, $J$ = 9.2, 2.9 Hz), 7.74 (1H, d, $J$ = 2.9 Hz), 7.81 (1H, d, $J$ = 8.6 Hz) ppm. $^{13}C$ NMR (125 MHz, $CDCl_3$): δ 20.3, 56.2, 106.8, 115.9, 124.5, 129.7, 130.6, 162.7, 168.1, 176.4 ppm. IR (ATR, KBr): $\nu$ 1697 (C=O), 1681 (C=O), 1656 (C=O) $cm^{-1}$. Mp: 207–209 °C. $^{1}H$ and $^{13}C$ NMR data are consistent with those reported in the literature [105].

3.4.8. 3-Oxo-1λ$^{3}$-benzo[d][1,2]iodaoxole-1,5(3H)-diyl diacetate (**7g**)

$^{1}H$ NMR (500 MHz, $CDCl_3$): δ 2.26 (3H, s), 2.37 (3H, s), 7.68 (1H, dd, $J$ = 8.9, 2.6 Hz), 7.96–8.02 (2H, m) ppm. $^{13}C$ NMR (125 MHz, $CDCl_3$): δ 20.3, 21.1, 113.6, 126.2, 129.8, 130.3, 130.9, 153.6, 167.2, 168.7, 176.5 ppm. IR (ATR, KBr): $\nu$ 1690 (C=O) $cm^{-1}$. Mp: 153–154 °C. HRMS (DART, m/z) calcd for $C_{11}H_{10}IO_6$ $[M + H]^+$: 364.9517; found: 364.9518.

3.4.9. 3-Oxo-5-(trifluoromethyl)-1λ$^{3}$-benzo[d][1,2]iodaoxol-1(3H)-yl acetate (**7h**)

$^{1}H$ NMR (500 MHz, $CDCl_3$): δ 2.29 (3H, s), 8.14 (1H, dd, $J$ = 8.6, 1.7 Hz), 8.20 (1H, d, $J$ = 8.6 Hz), 8.52 (1H, d, $J$ = 1.7 Hz) ppm. $^{13}C$ NMR (125 MHz, $CDCl_3$): δ 20.2, 121.9, 122.8 (q, $J$ = 271.4 Hz), 130.1 (d, $J$ = 3.6 Hz), 130.4 (d, $J$ = 9.5 Hz), 132.4 (d, $J$ = 2.4 Hz), 134.5 (q, $J$ = 33.8 Hz), 166.7, 176.5 ppm. $^{19}F$ NMR (470 MHz, $CDCl_3$): δ −64.9 ppm. IR (ATR, KBr): $\nu$ 1692 (C=O), 1647 (C=O) $cm^{-1}$. Mp: 212–213 °C. HRMS (DART, m/z) calcd for $C_{10}H_7F_3IO_4$ $[M + H]^+$: 374.9336; found: 374.9334.

3.4.10. 5-Nitro-3-oxo-1λ$^{3}$-benzo[d][1,2]iodaoxol-1(3H)-yl acetate (**7i**)

$^{1}H$ NMR (500 MHz, $CDCl_3$): δ 2.30 (3H, s), 8.27 (1H, d, $J$ = 9.2 Hz), 8.71 (1H, dd, $J$ = 9.0, 2.5 Hz), 9.04 (1H, d, $J$ = 2.3 Hz) ppm. $^{13}C$ NMR (125 MHz, $CDCl_3$): δ 20.2, 124.1, 127.6, 129.8, 131.0, 131.5,150.8, 165.7, 176.6 ppm. IR (ATR, KBr): $\nu$ 1705 (C=O), 1665 (C=O) $cm^{-1}$. Mp: 209–210 °C. $^{1}H$ and $^{13}C$ NMR data are consistent with those reported in the literature [107].

## 4. Conclusions

We have presented a practical synthetic method for IBA from 2-IB without contamination by hazardous pentavalent IBX using cost-effective Oxone® in aqueous solution. This highly safe, convenient method operates under mild conditions such as room temperature, which contrasts with traditional method using reflux conditions and expensive $NaIO_4$ in AcOH solution. The use of mild conditions circumvents the problem of the formation of byproducts such as potentially explosive pentavalent cyclic hypervalent iodine compound, i.e., IBX; the contamination of IBX into IBA is generally not desired for safety reasons. The reaction time can be shortened by heating; in this case, addition of a ferric salt in our reaction system can effectively suppress the formation of IBX as byproducts. In addition, a convenient derivatization of the hydroxy group of IBAs by solvolytic treatment is presented. These derivatizations were generally achieved under mild conditions below 80 °C. Our methods, which do not require any chromatography technique, can be performed safely and would be suitable for large-scale synthesis.

**Supplementary Materials:** Supplementary materials are available online, $^1$H NMR spectroscopic data for the compounds **2a–v** and **4**.

**Author Contributions:** H.C. found the selective reaction to obtain IBAs using Oxone® and the solvolytic functionalization for IBA and drafted the manuscript; N.K., H.Y., and N.T. also contributed to the experiments; T.D. directed this study as a project and finalized the manuscript with critical discussion. All authors have read and agreed to the published version of the manuscript.

**Funding:** This work was financially supported by a Grant-in-Aid for Scientific Research (C) (JSPS KAKENHI Grant Number JP19K05466) from JSPS and the Ritsumeikan Global Innovation Research Organization (R-GIRO) project. H.C. also acknowledges support from a Grant-in-Aid for Early-Career Scientists (JSPS KAKENHI Grant Number 20K15103) from JSPS.

**Institutional Review Board Statement:** Not applicable.

**Informed Consent Statement:** Not applicable.

**Data Availability Statement:** The data presented in this study are available in the communication.

**Conflicts of Interest:** The authors declare no conflict of interest.

**Sample Availability:** Samples of the compounds are not available from the authors.

## References

1. Zhdankin, V.V. Organoiodine(V) reagents in organic synthesis. *J. Org. Chem.* **2011**, *76*, 1185–1197. [CrossRef]
2. Singh, F.V.; Wirth, T. Hypervalent iodine-catalyzed oxidative functionalizations including stereoselective reactions. *Chem. Asian J.* **2014**, *9*, 950–971. [CrossRef] [PubMed]
3. Yoshimura, A.; Zhdankin, V.V. Advances in synthetic applications of hypervalent iodine compounds. *Chem. Rev.* **2016**, *116*, 3328–3435. [CrossRef] [PubMed]
4. Tan, H.; Ji, W.; Wang, L. Sunlight-driven decarboxylative alkynylation of α-keto acids with bromoacetylenes by hypervalent iodine reagent catalysis: A facile approach to ynones. *Angew. Chem. Int. Ed.* **2015**, *54*, 8374–8377. [CrossRef] [PubMed]
5. Wang, D.; Zhang, L.; Luo, S. Enantioselective decarboxylative α-alkynylation of β-ketocarbonyls via a catalytic α-imino radical Intermediate. *Org. Lett.* **2017**, *19*, 4924–4927. [CrossRef]
6. Yang, S.; Tan, H.; Ji, W.; Zhang, X.; Li, P. Visible light-induced decarboxylative acylarylation of phenyl propiolates with α-oxocarboxylic acids to coumarins catalyzed by hypervalent iodine reagents under transition metal-free conditions. *Adv. Synth. Catal.* **2017**, *359*, 443–453. [CrossRef]
7. Sun, X.; Liu, T.; Yang, Y.-T.; Gu, Y.-J.; Liu, Y.W.; Ji, Y.G.; Luo, K.; Zhu, J.; Wu, L. Visible-light-promoted regio- and stereoselective oxyalkenylation of phosphinyl allenes. *Adv. Synth. Catal.* **2020**, *362*, 2701–2708. [CrossRef]
8. Ball, L.T.; Lloyd-Jones, G.C.; Russell, C.A. Gold-catalysed oxyarylation of styrenes and mono- and *gem*-disubstituted olefins facilitated by an iodine(III) oxidant. *Chem. Eur. J.* **2012**, *18*, 2931–2937. [CrossRef] [PubMed]
9. Hata, K.; Segawa, Y.; Itami, K. Pyridylidene ligand facilitates gold-catalyzed oxidative C–H arylation of heterocycles. *Beilstein. J. Org. Chem.* **2015**, *11*, 2737–2746. [CrossRef] [PubMed]
10. Hu, J.; Lan, T.; Sun, Y.; Chen, H.; Yao, J.; Rao, Y. Unactivated C(sp$^3$)–H hydroxylation through palladium catalysis with $H_2O$ as the oxygen source. *Chem. Commun.* **2015**, *51*, 14929–14932. [CrossRef] [PubMed]
11. Bindu, V.H.; Parvathaneni, S.P.; Rao, V.J. Iodosobenzoic acid (IBA) catalysed benzylic and aromatic C–H oxidations. *Catal. Lett.* **2017**, *147*, 1434–1440. [CrossRef]
12. Li, G.-X.; Morales-Rivera, C.A.; Gao, F.; Wang, Y.; He, G.; Liu, P.; Chen, G. A unified photoredox-catalysis strategy for C(sp$^3$)–H hydroxylation and amidation using hypervalent iodine. *Chem. Sci.* **2017**, *8*, 7180–7185. [CrossRef]
13. Wang, D.; Ren, R.; Zhu, C. Manganese-promoted ring-opening hydrazination of cyclobutanols: Synthesis of alkyl hydrazines. *J. Org. Chem.* **2016**, *81*, 8043–8049. [CrossRef]
14. Ye, L.; Gu, Q.-S.; Tian, Y.; Meng, X.; Chen, G.-C.; Liu, X.-Y. Radical asymmetric intramolecular α-cyclopropanation of aldehydes towards bicyclo[3.1.0]hexanes containing vicinal all-carbon quaternary stereocenters. *Nat. Commun.* **2018**, *9*, 1–13. [CrossRef]
15. Amos, S.G.E.; Nicolai, S.; Waser, J. Photocatalytic umpolung of *N*- and *O*-substituted alkenes for the synthesis of 1,2-amino alcohols and diols. *Chem. Sci.* **2020**, *11*, 11274–11279. [CrossRef]
16. He, X.-K.; Lu, J.; Zhang, A.-J.; Zhang, Q.-Q.; Xu, G.-Y.; Xuan, J. Bi-OAc-accelerated C3-H alkylation of quinoxaline-2(1*H*)-ones under visible-light irradiation. *Org. Lett.* **2020**, *22*, 5984–5989. [CrossRef]

17. Li, J.; Liu, Z.; Wu, S.; Chen, Y. Acyl radical smiles rearrangement to construct hydroxybenzophenones by photoredox catalysis. *Org. Lett.* **2019**, *21*, 2077–2080. [CrossRef] [PubMed]
18. Fang, Z.; Wang, Y.; Wang, Y. Synthesis of 4-iodoisoquinolin-1(2*H*)-ones by a dirhodium (II)-catalyzed 1,4-bisfunctionalization of isoquinolinium iodide salts. *Org. Lett.* **2019**, *21*, 434–438. [CrossRef] [PubMed]
19. Wu, L.; Hao, Y.; Lin, Y.; Wang, Q. Visible-light-induced intramolecular $sp^3$-C-H oxidation of 2-alkyl-substituted benzamides for the synthesis of functionalized iminoisobenzofurans. *Chem. Commun.* **2019**, *55*, 13908–13911. [CrossRef] [PubMed]
20. Wang, N.; Gu, Q.-S.; Li, Z.-L.; Li, Z.; Guo, Y.-L.; Guo, Z.; Liu, X.-Y. Direct photocatalytic synthesis of medium-sized lactams by C−C bond cleavage. *Angew. Chem. Int. Ed.* **2018**, *57*, 14225–14229. [CrossRef] [PubMed]
21. Pawar, G.G.; Robert, F.; Grau, E.; Cramail, H.; Landais, Y. Visible-light photocatalyzed oxidative decarboxylation of oxamic acids: A green route to urethanes and ureas. *Chem. Commun.* **2018**, *54*, 9337–9340. [CrossRef] [PubMed]
22. Jia, K.; Zhang, F.; Huang, H.; Chen, Y. Visible-light-induced alkoxyl radical generation enables selective $C(sp^3)$–$C(sp^3)$ bond cleavage and functionalizations. *J. Am. Chem. Soc.* **2016**, *138*, 1514–1517. [CrossRef]
23. Li, G.-X.; Morales-Rivera, C.A.; Wang, Y.; Gao, F.; He, G.; Liu, P.; Chen, G. Photoredox-mediated Minisci C–H alkylation of *N*-heteroarenes using boronic acids and hypervalent iodine. *Chem. Sci.* **2016**, *7*, 6407–6412. [CrossRef]
24. Ji, W.; Tan, H.; Wang, M.; Li, P.; Wang, L. Photocatalyst-free hypervalent iodine reagent catalyzed decarboxylative acylarylation of acrylamides with α-oxocarboxylic acids driven by visible-light irradiation. *Chem. Commun.* **2016**, *52*, 1462–1465. [CrossRef] [PubMed]
25. Dai, J.-J.; Zhang, W.-M.; Shu, Y.-J.; Sun, Y.-Y.; Xu, J.; Feng, Y.-S.; Xu, H.-J. Deboronative cyanation of potassium alkyltrifluoroborates *via* photoredox catalysis. *Chem. Commun.* **2016**, *52*, 6793–6796. [CrossRef] [PubMed]
26. Huang, H.; Zhang, G.; Chen, Y. Dual hypervalent iodine (III) reagents and photoredox catalysis enable decarboxylative ynonylation under mild conditions. *Angew. Chem. Int. Ed.* **2015**, *54*, 7872–7876. [CrossRef] [PubMed]
27. Zhang, D.; Gao, F.; Nian, Y.; Zhou, Y.; Jiang, H.; Liu, H. Palladium-catalyzed picolinamide-directed coupling of $C(sp^2)$–H and $C(sp^2)$–H: A straightforward approach to quinolinone and pyridone scaffolds. *Chem. Commun.* **2015**, *51*, 7509–7511. [CrossRef]
28. Shan, G.; Yang, X.; Zong, Y.; Rao, Y. An efficient palladium-catalyzed C-H alkoxylation of unactivated methylene and methyl groups with cyclic hypervalent iodine ($I^{3+}$) oxidants. *Angew. Chem. Int. Ed.* **2013**, *52*, 13606–13610. [CrossRef]
29. Zong, Y.; Rao, Y. Developing Pd (II) catalyzed double $sp^3$ C–H alkoxylation for synthesis of symmetric and unsymmetric acetals. *Org. Lett.* **2014**, *16*, 5278–5281. [CrossRef] [PubMed]
30. Sun, X.; Yao, X.; Zhang, C.; Rao, Y. Pd (II) catalyzed *ortho* C–H iodination of phenylcarbamates at room temperature using cyclic hypervalent iodine reagents. *Chem. Commun.* **2015**, *51*, 10014–10017. [CrossRef]
31. Yu, Q.-Y.; Zhong, H.-M.; Sun, W.-W.; Zhang, S.-J.; Cao, P.; Dong, X.-P.; Qin, H.-B.; Liu, J.-K.; Wu, B. Palladium-catalyzed $C(sp^3)-H$ functionalization at the C3 position of L-pipecolinic acid derivatives. *Asian J. Org. Chem.* **2016**, *5*, 608–612. [CrossRef]
32. Yang, B.; Xu, X.-H.; Qing, F.-L. Synthesis of difluoroalkylated arenes by hydroaryldifluoromethylation of alkenes with α,α-difluoroarylacetic acids under photoredox catalysis. *Org. Lett.* **2016**, *18*, 5956–5959. [CrossRef]
33. Nappi, M.; He, C.; Whitehurst, W.G.; Chappell, B.G.N.; Gaunt, M.J. Selective reductive elimination at alkyl palladium(IV) by dissociative ligand ionization: Catalytic $C(sp^3)-H$ amination to azetidines. *Angew. Chem. Int. Ed.* **2018**, *57*, 3178–3182. [CrossRef] [PubMed]
34. Muraki, T.; Togo, H.; Yokoyama, M. Synthetic use of 1-(*p*-toluenesulfonyloxy)-1,2-benziodoxol-3(1*H*)-one: Iodination of aromatic rings. *Synlett* **1998**, *3*, 286–288. [CrossRef]
35. Muraki, T.; Togo, H.; Yokoyama, M. Reactivity and synthetic utility of 1-(arenesulfonyloxy)benziodoxolones. *J. Org. Chem.* **1999**, *64*, 2883–2889. [CrossRef]
36. Harper, M.J.; Emmett, E.J.; Bower, J.F.; Russell, C.A. Oxidative 1,2-difunctionalization of ethylene via gold-catalyzed oxyarylation. *J. Am. Chem. Soc.* **2017**, *139*, 12386–12389. [CrossRef]
37. Yoshimura, A.; Nguyen, K.C.; Klasen, S.C.; Postnikov, P.S.; Yusubov, M.S.; Saito, A.; Nemykin, V.N.; Zhdankin, V.V. Hypervalent iodine-catalyzed synthesis of 1,2,4-oxadiazoles from aldoximes and nitriles. *Asian J. Org. Chem.* **2016**, *5*, 1128–1133. [CrossRef]
38. Vinayak, B.; Ravindrakumar, P.V.; Ramana, D.V.; Chandrasekharam, M. Revisiting 1-chloro-1,2-benziodoxol-3-one: Efficient *ortho*-chlorination of aryls under aqueous conditions. *New J. Chem.* **2018**, *42*, 8953–8959. [CrossRef]
39. Parvathaneni, S.P.; Perumgani, P.C. Regioselective chlorination of aryl C−H bonds with hypervalent iodine(III) reagent 1-chloro-1,2-benziodoxol-3-one. *Asian J. Org. Chem.* **2018**, *7*, 324–327. [CrossRef]
40. Jia, Y.; Chen, L.; Zhang, H.; Zheng, Y.; Jiang, Z.-X.; Yang, Z. Electrophilic chloro(ω-alkoxy)lation of alkenes employing 1-chloro-1,2-benziodoxol-3-one: Facile synthesis of β-chloroethers. *Org. Biomol. Chem.* **2018**, *16*, 7203–7213. [CrossRef]
41. Wang, M.; Zhang, Y.; Wang, T.; Wang, C.; Xue, D.; Xiao, J. Story of an age-old reagent: An electrophilic chlorination of arenes and heterocycles by 1-chloro-1,2-benziodoxol-3-one. *Org. Lett.* **2016**, *18*, 1976–1979. [CrossRef] [PubMed]
42. Egami, H.; Yoneda, T.; Uku, M.; Ide, T.; Kawato, Y.; Hamashima, Y. Difunctionalization of alkenes using 1-chloro-1,2-benziodoxol-3-(1*H*)-one. *J. Org. Chem.* **2016**, *81*, 4020–4030. [CrossRef] [PubMed]
43. Xing, B.; Ni, C.; Hu, J. Hypervalent iodine(III)-catalyzed Balz–Schiemann fluorination under mild conditions. *Angew. Chem. Int. Ed.* **2018**, *57*, 9896–9900. [CrossRef]
44. Jiang, X.; Zheng, C.; Lei, L.; Lin, K.; Yu, C. Synthesis of 2-oxindoles from substituted indoles by hypervalent-iodine oxidation. *Eur. J. Org. Chem.* **2018**, *2018*, 1437–1442. [CrossRef]

45. Jiang, X.; Li, G.; Yu, C. A Diels-Alder reaction/oxa-Michael addition/acyloin rearrangement cascade on tropolonic substrates. *Tetrahedron Lett.* **2018**, *59*, 1506–1510. [CrossRef]
46. Vaillant, F.L.; Wodrich, M.D.; Waser, J. Room temperature decarboxylative cyanation of carboxylic acids using photoredox catalysis and cyanobenziodoxolones: A divergent mechanism compared to alkynylation. *Chem. Sci.* **2017**, *8*, 1790–1800. [CrossRef] [PubMed]
47. Li, X.; Qi, X.; Hou, C.; Chen, P.; Liu, G. Palladium(II)-catalyzed enantioselective azidation of unactivated alkenes. *Angew. Chem. Int. Ed.* **2020**, *59*, 17239–17244. [CrossRef]
48. Wang, Y.; Wang, N.; Zhao, J.; Sun, M.; You, H.; Fang, F.; Li, Z.-Q. Visible-light-promoted site-specific and diverse functionalization of a C($sp^3$)-C($sp^3$) bond adjacent to an arene. *ACS Catal.* **2020**, *10*, 6603–6612. [CrossRef]
49. Wang, Y.; Hu, X.; Morales-Rivera, C.A.; Li, G.-X.; Huang, X.; He, G.; Liu, P.; Chen, G. Epimerization of tertiary carbon centers via reversible radical cleavage of unactivated C($sp^3$)-H bonds. *J. Am. Chem. Soc.* **2018**, *140*, 9678–9684. [CrossRef]
50. Shen, K.; Wang, Q. Copper-catalyzed alkene aminoazidation as a rapid entry to 1,2-diamines and installation of an azide reporter onto azaheterocycles. *J. Am. Chem. Soc.* **2017**, *139*, 13110–13116. [CrossRef] [PubMed]
51. Li, L.; Li, Z.-L.; Wang, F.-L.; Guo, Z.; Cheng, Y.-F.; Wang, N.; Dong, X.-W.; Fang, C.; Liu, J.; Hou, C.; et al. Radical aryl migration enables diversity-oriented synthesis of structurally diverse medium/macro- or bridged-rings. *Nat. Commun.* **2016**, *7*, 13852. [CrossRef]
52. Wang, Y.; Li, G.-X.; Yang, G.; He, G.; Chen, G. A visible-light-promoted radical reaction system for azidation and halogenation of tertiary aliphatic C–H bonds. *Chem. Sci.* **2016**, *7*, 2679–2683. [CrossRef] [PubMed]
53. Sharma, A.; Hartwig, J.F. Metal-catalyzed azidation of tertiary C-H bonds suitable for late-stage functionalization. *Nature* **2015**, 600–604. [CrossRef]
54. Fumagalli, G.; Rabet, P.T.G.; Boyd, S.; Greaney, M.F. Three-component azidation of styrene-type double bonds: Light-switchable behavior of a copper photoredox catalyst. *Angew. Chem. Int. Ed.* **2015**, *54*, 11481–11484. [CrossRef] [PubMed]
55. Liu, T.; Zhu, J.; Sun, X.; Cheng, L.; Wu, L. $I_2$/TBHP mediated divergent C($sp^3$)-P cleavage of allenylphosphine oxides: Substituent-controlled regioselectivity. *Adv. Synth. Catal.* **2019**, *361*, 3532–3537. [CrossRef]
56. Jiang, H.; He, Y.; Cheng, Y.; Yu, S. Radical alkynyltrifluoromethylation of alkenes initiated by an electron donor–acceptor complex. *Org. Lett.* **2017**, *19*, 1240–1243. [CrossRef]
57. Mangaonkar, S.R.; Kole, P.B.; Singh, F.V. Oxidation of organosulfides to organosulfones with trifluoromethyl 3-oxo-1$\lambda^3$,2-benziodoxole-1(3*H*)-carboxylate as an oxidant. *Synlett* **2018**, *29*, 199–202. [CrossRef]
58. Shen, K.; Wang, Q. Copper-catalyzed aminoalkynylation of alkenes with hypervalent iodine reagents. *Chem. Sci.* **2017**, *8*, 8265–8270. [CrossRef]
59. Mukherjee, S.; Garza-Sauchez, R.A.; Tlahuext-Aca, A.; Glorius, F. Alkynylation of $C_{sp}{}^2$(O)-H bonds enabled by photoredox-mediated hydrogen-atom transfer. *Angew. Chem. Int. Ed.* **2017**, *56*, 14723–14726. [CrossRef]
60. Nicolai, S.; Waser, J. Pd(0)-catalyzed oxy- and aminoalkynylation of olefins for the synthesis of tetrahydrofurans and pyrrolidines. *Org. Lett.* **2011**, *13*, 6324–6327. [CrossRef]
61. Brand, J.P.; Waser, J. Direct alkynylation of thiophenes: Cooperative activation of TIPS–EBX with gold and Brønsted acids. *Angew. Chem. Int. Ed.* **2010**, *49*, 7304–7307. [CrossRef] [PubMed]
62. González, D.F.; Brand, J.P.; Waser, J. Asymmetric synthesis of 4-amino-4*H*-chromenes by organocatalytic oxa-Michael/aza-Baylis–Hillman tandem reactions. *Chem. Eur. J.* **2010**, *16*, 9457–9461.
63. Baker, G.P.; Mann, G.; Sheppard, N.; Tetlow, A.J. The structure of *o*-iodosobenzoic acid and of certain derivatives. *J. Chem. Soc.* **1965**, 3721–3728. [CrossRef]
64. Kraszkiewicz, L.; Skulski, L. Optimized syntheses of iodylarenes from iodoarenes, with sodium periodate as the oxidant. *Part II. Arkivoc* **2003**, *6*, 120–125. [CrossRef]
65. Bosset, C.; Coffinier, R.; Peioto, P.A.; Assal, M.E.; Miqueu, K.; Sotiropoulos, M.; Pouységu, L.; Quideau, S. Asymmetric hydroxylative phenol dearomatization promoted by chiral binaphthylic and biphenylic iodanes. *Angew. Chem. Int. Ed.* **2014**, *53*, 9860–9864. [CrossRef] [PubMed]
66. Maity, A.; Hyun, S.-M.; Powers, D.C. Oxidase catalysis via aerobically generated hypervalent iodine intermediates. *Nat. Chem.* **2018**, *10*, 200–204. [CrossRef]
67. Chandrasekar, S.; Sekar, G. An efficient synthesis of iminoquinones by a chemoselective domino *ortho*-hydroxylation/oxidation/imidation sequence of 2-aminoarylketones. *Org. Biomol. Chem.* **2016**, *14*, 3053–3060. [CrossRef]
68. Wirth, T. IBX—New reactions with an old reagent. *Angew. Chem. Int. Ed.* **2001**, *40*, 2812–2814. [CrossRef]
69. Ladziata, U.; Zhdankin, V.V. Hypervalent iodine(V) reagents in organic synthesis. *Arkivoc* **2006**, *9*, 26–58. [CrossRef]
70. Sharma, P.; Kaur, N.; Pareek, A.; Kishore, D. An insight in to general features of IBX (2-iodoxybenzoic acid). *Sci. Revs. Chem. Commun.* **2013**, *3*, 16–42.
71. Plumb, J.B.; Harper, D.J. IBX is reported to be a shock-sensitive explosive. *Chem. Eng. News* **1990**, *68*, 3.
72. Dess, D.B.; Martin, J.C.J. A useful 12-I-5 triacetoxyperiodinane (the Dess-Martin periodinane) for the selective oxidation of primary or secondary alcohols and a variety of related 12-I-5 species. *J. Am. Chem. Soc.* **1991**, *113*, 7277–7287. [CrossRef]
73. Boeckmann, R.K.; Shao, P.; Mullins, J.J. The Dess-Martin periodinane: 1,1,1-triacetoxy-1,1-dihydro-1,2-benziodoxolo-3(1H)-one. *Org. Synth.* **2000**, *77*, 141–152.

74. More, J.D.; Finney, N.S. A simple and advantageous protocol for the oxidation of alcohols with *o*-iodoxybenzoic acid (IBX). *Org. Lett.* **2002**, *4*, 3001–3003. [CrossRef]
75. Tiffner, M.; Stockhammer, L.; Schörgenhumer, J.; Röser, K.; Waser, M. Towards an asymmetric organocatalytic α-azidation of β-ketoesters. *Molecules* **2018**, *23*, 1142. [CrossRef]
76. Bernini, R.; Barontini, M.; Spatafora, C. New lipophilic piceatannol derivatives exhibiting antioxidant activity prepared by aromatic hydroxylation with 2-iodoxybenzoic acid (IBX). *Molecules* **2009**, *14*, 4669–4681. [CrossRef]
77. Hussain, H.; Green, I.R.; Ahmed, I. Journey describing applications of oxone in synthetic chemistry. *Chem. Rev.* **2013**, *113*, 3329–3371. [CrossRef]
78. Thottumkara, A.P.; Bowsher, M.S.; Vinod, T.K. In situ generation of *o*-iodoxybenzoic acid (IBX) and the catalytic use of it in oxidation reactions in the presence of oxone as a co-oxidant. *Org. Lett.* **2005**, *7*, 2933–2936. [CrossRef] [PubMed]
79. Uyanik, M.; Akakura, M.; Ishihara, K. 2-Iodoxybenzenesulfonic acid as an extremely active catalyst for the selective oxidation of alcohols to aldehydes, ketones, carboxylic acids, and enones with oxone. *J. Am. Chem. Soc.* **2009**, *131*, 251–262. [CrossRef]
80. Miura, T.; Nakashima, K.; Tada, N.; Itoh, A. An effective and catalytic oxidation using recyclable fluorous IBX. *Chem. Commun.* **2011**, *47*, 1875–1877. [CrossRef]
81. Moorthy, J.N.; Senapati, K.; Parida, K.N.; Jhulki, S.; Sooraj, K.; Nair, N.N. *Twist* does a *twist* to the reactivity: Stoichiometric and catalytic oxidations with *twisted* tetramethyl-IBX. *J. Org. Chem.* **2011**, *76*, 9593–9601. [CrossRef] [PubMed]
82. Ishihara, K.; Uyanik, M.; Crockett, R. 2-Iodoxy-5-methylbenzenesulfonic acid-catalyzed selective oxidation of 4-bromobenzyl alcohol to 4-bromobenzaldehyde or 4-bromobenzoic acid with oxone. *Org. Synth.* **2012**, *89*, 105–114.
83. Bikshapathi, R.; Prathima, P.S.; Rao, V.J. Hypervalent iodine catalysis for selective oxidation of Baylis–Hillman adducts *via* in situ generation of *o*-iodoxybenzoic acid (IBX) from 2-iodosobenzoic acid (IBA) in the presence of oxone. *New J. Chem.* **2016**, *40*, 10300–10304. [CrossRef]
84. Yakura, T.; Fujiwara, T.; Yamada, A.; Nambu, H. 2-Iodo-*N*-isopropyl-5-methoxybenzamide as a highly reactive and environmentally benign catalyst for alcohol oxidation. *Beilstein J. Org. Chem.* **2018**, *14*, 971–978. [CrossRef] [PubMed]
85. Mishra, A.K.; Moorthy, J.N. Mechanochemical catalytic oxidations in the solid state with *in situ*-generated modified IBX from 3,5-di-*tert*-butyl-2-iodobenzoic acid (DTB-IA)/Oxone. *Org. Chem. Front.* **2017**, *4*, 343–349. [CrossRef]
86. Jhulki, S.; Seth, S.; Mondal, M.; Moorthy, J.N. Facile organocatalytic domino oxidation of diols to lactones by in situ-generated TetMe-IBX. *Tetrahedron* **2014**, *70*, 2286–2293. [CrossRef]
87. Yakura, T.; Horiuchi, Y.; Nishimura, Y.; Yamada, A.; Nambu, H.; Fujiwara, T. Efficient oxidative cleavage of tetrahydrofuran-2-methanols to γ-lactones by a 2-iodobenzamide catalyst in combination with Oxone®. *Adv. Synth. Catal.* **2016**, *358*, 869–873. [CrossRef]
88. Yakura, T.; Yamauchi, Y.; Tian, Y.; Omoto, M. Catalytic hypervalent iodine oxidation of *p*-dialkoxybenzenes to *p*-quinones using 4-iodophenoxyacetic acid and Oxone®. *Chem. Pharm. Bull.* **2008**, *56*, 1632–1634. [CrossRef] [PubMed]
89. Yakura, T.; Tian, Y.; Yamauchi, Y.; Omoto, M.; Konishi, T. Catalytic hypervalent iodine oxidation using 4-iodophenoxyacetic acid and Oxone®: Oxidation of *p*-alkoxyphenols to *p*-benzoquinones. *Chem. Pharm. Bull.* **2009**, *57*, 252–256. [CrossRef]
90. Zagulyaeva, A.A.; Banek, C.T.; Yusubov, M.S.; Zhdankin, V.V. Hofmann rearrangement of carboxamides mediated by hypervalent iodine species generated in situ from iodobenzene and oxone: Reaction scope and limitations. *Org. Lett.* **2010**, *12*, 4644–4647. [CrossRef] [PubMed]
91. Yakura, T.; Omoto, M.; Yamauchi, Y.; Tian, Y.; Ozono, A. Hypervalent iodine oxidation of phenol derivatives using a catalytic amount of 4-iodophenoxyacetic acid and Oxone® as a co-oxidant. *Tetrahedron* **2010**, *66*, 5833–5840. [CrossRef]
92. Ren, J.; Lu, L.; Xu, J.; Yu, T.; Zeng, B.-B. Selective oxidation of 1-tetralones to 1,2-naphthoquinones with IBX and to 1,4-naphthoquinones with Oxone® and 2-iodobenzoic acid. *Synthesis* **2015**, *47*, 2270–2280. [CrossRef]
93. Frigerio, M.; Santagostino, M.; Sputore, S. A user-friendly entry to 2-iodoxybenzoic acid (IBX). *J. Org. Chem.* **1999**, *64*, 4537–4538. [CrossRef]
94. China, H.; Tanihara, K.; Sasa, H.; Kikushima, K.; Dohi, T. Regiodivergent oxidation of alkoxyarenes by hypervalent iodine/oxone® system. *Catal. Today* **2020**, *348*, 2–8. [CrossRef]
95. Parida, K.N.; Moorthy, J.N. Synthesis of *o*-carboxyarylacrylic acids by room temperature oxidative cleavage of hydroxynaphthalenes and higher aromatics with Oxone. *J. Org. Chem.* **2015**, *80*, 8354–8360. [CrossRef]
96. Costello, J.P.; Ferreira, E.M. Regioselectivity influences in platinum-catalyzed intramolecular alkyne O-H and N-H additions. *Org. Lett.* **2019**, *21*, 9934–9939. [CrossRef]
97. Koguchi, S.; Mihoya, A.; Mimura, M. Alcohol oxidation via recyclable hydrophobic ionic liquid-supported IBX. *Tetrahedron* **2016**, *72*, 7633–7637. [CrossRef]
98. Boelke, A.; Kuczmera, T.J.; Caspers, L.D.; Lork, E.; Nachtsheim, B.J. Iodolopyrazolium salts: Synthesis, derivatizations, and applications. *Org. Lett.* **2020**, *22*, 7261–7266. [CrossRef]
99. Kalaj, M.; Mimeni, M.R.; Bentz, K.C.; Barcus, K.S.; Palomba, J.M.; Paesani, F.; Cohen, S.M. Halogen bonding in UiO-66 frameworks promotes superior chemical warfare agent simulant degradation. *Chem. Commun.* **2019**, *55*, 3481–3484. [CrossRef]
100. Sun, W.; Cama, L.D. Preparation of 6H-benzo[c]chromenes as estrogen receptor modulators. *PCT Int. Appl.* **2004**, *WO 2004073612*, A2.
101. Caspers, L.D.; Spils, J.; Damrath, M.; Lork, E.; Nachtsheim, B.J. One-pot synthesis and conformational analysis of six-membered cyclic iodonium salts. *J. Org. Chem.* **2020**, *85*, 9161–9178. [CrossRef] [PubMed]

102. Miles, K.C.; Le, C.C.; Stambuli, J.P. Direct carbocyclizations of benzoic acids: Catalyst-controlled synthesis of cyclic ketones and the development of tandem aHH (acyl Heck-Heck) reactions. *Chem. Eur. J.* **2014**, *20*, 11336–11339. [CrossRef]
103. Hamley, P.; Pimm, A.; Tinker, A. Preparation of spiro[pyridoisoindolequinazoline] derivatives and analogs as nitric oxide synthase inhibitors. *PCT Int. Appl.* **1999**, *WO 9901455*, A1.
104. Declas, N.; Vaillant, F.L.; Waser, J. Revisiting the Urech synthesis of hydantoins: Direct access to enantiopure 1,5-substituted hydantoins using cyanobenziodoxolone. *Org. Lett.* **2019**, *21*, 524–528. [CrossRef] [PubMed]
105. Bertho, S.; Rey-Rodriguez, R.; Colas, C.; Retailleau, P.; Gillaizeau, I. Regio- and stereoselective iron-catalyzed oxyazidation of enamides using a hypervalent iodine reagent. *Chem. Eur. J.* **2017**, *23*, 17674–17677. [CrossRef] [PubMed]
106. Lu, B.; Wu, J.; Yoshikai, N. Palladium-catalyzed condensation of *N*-aryl imines and alkynylbenziodoxolones to form multisubstituted furans. *J. Am. Chem. Soc.* **2014**, *136*, 11598–11601. [CrossRef]
107. Chen, M.; Huang, Z.-T.; Zheng, Q.-Y. Organic base-promoted enantioselective electrophilic cyanation of β-keto esters by using chiral phase-transfer catalysts. *Org. Biomol. Chem.* **2015**, *13*, 8812–8816. [CrossRef]
108. Hari, D.P.; Waser, J. Enantioselective copper-catalyzed oxy-alkynylation of diazo compounds. *J. Am. Chem. Soc.* **2017**, *139*, 8420–8423. [CrossRef]
109. Mocci, F.; Uccheddu, G.; Frongia, A.; Cerioni, G. Solution structure of some $\lambda^3$ iodanes: An $^{17}$O NMR and DFT study. *J. Org. Chem.* **2007**, *72*, 4163–4168. [CrossRef]
110. Ito, E.; Fukushima, T.; Kawakami, T.; Murakami, K.; Itami, K. Catalytic dehydrogenative C–H imidation of arenes enabled by photo-generated hole donation to sulfonimide. *Chem* **2017**, *2*, 383–392. [CrossRef]
111. Jia, K.; Pan, Y.; Chen, Y. Selective carbonyl-C ($sp^3$) bond cleavage to construct ynamides, ynoates, and ynones by photoredox catalysis. *Angew. Chem. Int. Ed.* **2017**, *56*, 2478–2481. [CrossRef]
112. Iinuma, M.; Moriyama, K.; Togo, H. Oxidation of alcohols to aldehydes or ketones with 1-acetoxy-1,2-benziodoxole-3(1*H*)-one derivatives. *Eur. J. Org. Chem.* **2014**, *2014*, 772–780. [CrossRef]

*molecules*

MDPI

*Review*

# Kitamura Electrophilic Fluorination Using HF as a Source of Fluorine

**Jianlin Han [1,*], Greg Butler [2], Hiroki Moriwaki [3], Hiroyuki Konno [4], Vadim A. Soloshonok [5,6,*] and Tsugio Kitamura [7]**

1. Jiangsu Co-Innovation Center of Efficient Processing and Utilization of Forest Resources, College of Chemical Engineering, Nanjing Forestry University, Nanjing 210037, Jiangsu, China
2. Oakwood Chemical, Inc. 730 Columbia Hwy. N, Estill, SC 29918, USA; gbutler@oakwoodchemical.com
3. Hamari Chemical Ltd., 1-4-29 Kunijima, Higashi-Yodogawa-ku, Osaka 533-0024, Japan; hiroki-moriwaki@hamari.co.jp
4. Department of Biological Engineering, Graduate School of Science and Engineering, Yamagata University, Yonezawa, Yamagata 992-8510, Japan; konno@yz.yamagata-u.ac.jp
5. Department of Organic Chemistry I, Faculty of Chemistry, University of the Basque Country UPV/EHU, Paseo Manuel Lardizábal 3, 20018 San Sebastián, Spain
6. IKERBASQUE, Basque Foundation for Science, Plaza Bizkaia, 48011 Bilbao, Spain
7. Department of Chemistry and Applied Chemistry, Saga University, 1 Honjo-machi, Saga 840-8502, Japan; kitamura@cc.saga-u.ac.jp

* Correspondence: hanjl@njfu.edu.cn (J.H.); vadym.soloshonok@ehu.es (V.A.S.)

Academic Editor: Maged Henary
Received: 4 April 2020; Accepted: 27 April 2020; Published: 30 April 2020

**Abstract:** This review article focused on the innovative procedure for electrophilic fluorination using HF and in situ generation of the required electrophilic species derived from hypervalent iodine compounds. The areas of synthetic application of this approach include fluorination of 1,3-dicarbonyl compounds, aryl-alkyl ketones, styrene derivatives, α,β-unsaturated ketones and alcohols, homoallyl amine and homoallyl alcohol derivatives, 3-butenoic acids and alkynes.

**Keywords:** electrophilic fluorination; hydrogen fluoride; hypervalent iodine; fluorination reagents; bioactive compounds

## 1. Introduction

Over the last two decades, the chemistry of fluorine-containing compounds has emerged as one of the exciting areas of multidisciplinary research. The most notable impact of fluorine can be seen in materials [1–10], agriculture [11–13] and health-related industries [14–22]. To sustain the continuous advancement and pace of the innovations enabled by fluorine, many research groups are focusing on new methodological inventions allowing for more selective and economical syntheses of structurally diverse fluoro-organic compounds [23–28]. For instance, the recent progress in asymmetric synthesis of fluorine-containing tailor-made amino acids [29–48] was stimulated by growth in their applications to drug design [49] magnetic resonance imaging [50,51], positron emission tomography [52,53], and peptide/protein engineering [54–60]. Nevertheless, while some complex polyfunctional fluorine-containing molecules possessing useful properties represent the ultimate target of synthetic chemistry, more fundamental research still focuses on the formation of the C–F bond. In this regard, electrophilic fluorination is one of the most pioneering and rapidly developing areas of study [61–67]. Conceptually, this approach requires a carbon-centered nucleophile and an electrophilic source of fluorine. While the former is a well-established chemical unit, the "electrophilic fluorine" is still a rather exotic and mechanistically controversial entity [68–71]. The major thrust of research activity in this field was centered on the development of the corresponding reagents capable of releasing the required "electrophilic fluorine". The most successful results have been achieved utilizing compounds with N–F bonds. For example, as presented in Figure 1, 1-chloromethyl-4-fluoro-1,4-diazoniabicyclo[2.2.2]octane bis(tetrafluoroborate) (**1**), introduced by Professor E. Banks [72], also known as Selectfluor, is one of the best reagents used as a source of "electrophilic fluorine". Other reagents, developed by Professor N. Shibata [73–76], are *N*-fluoro-*N*-(methylsulfonyl)methanesulfonamide (Me-NFSI) (**2**), 3,5-di-*tert*-butyl-*N*-((3,5-di-*tert*-butyl-4-methoxyphenyl)sulfonyl)-*N*-fluoro-4-methoxybenzenesulfonamide (NFBSI) (**3**) and axially chiral NFSIs (**4**), which can be used for enantioselective fluorination [77]. All these reagents are shelf-stable, easy to handle and operationally convenient to use for various synthetic applications [78–81]. However, the preparation of N-F reagents usually requires molecular fluorine [72,82], rendering them rather expensive and not practical for large-scale syntheses.

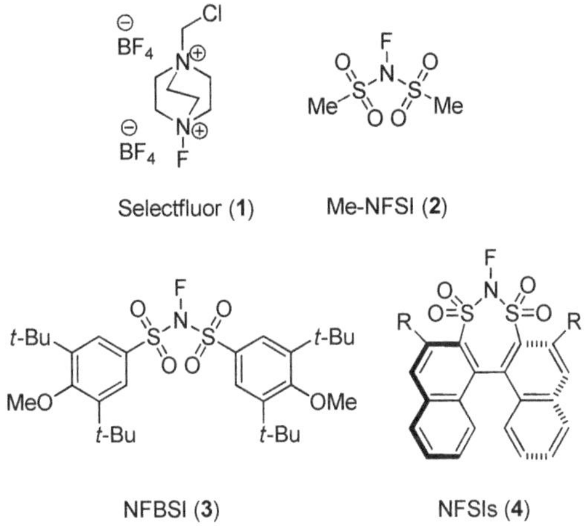


**Figure 1.** Some commercially available N–F electrophilic fluorination reagents.

From the standpoint of practicality, the application of HF, as a source of fluorine, with the in situ formation of the electrophilic species, would offer an attractive alternative as a general methodology for "electrophilic" formation of a C–F bond. In this review article, we discuss the use of hypervalent iodine compounds, as electrophilic centers, and HF as a source of fluorine, creatively assembled in a one-pot sequence, allowing one to perform "electrophilic fluorination" of various types of organic compounds. The synthetic generality and practicality of these methods is critically discussed.

## 2. Fluorination of 1,3-Dicarbonyl Compounds

### 2.1. Iodosylbenzene-Mediated Fluorination

In 2011, Professor T. Kitamura's group has reported that mixing ethyl 3-oxo-3-phenylpropionate (**5**) with 1.2 equivalents of a hypervalent iodine compound and excess (10-fold) of 55% aqueous HF resulted in formation of the corresponding ethyl 2-fluoro-3-oxo-3-phenylpropionate (**6**) in up to 98% chemical yield (Scheme 1) [83].

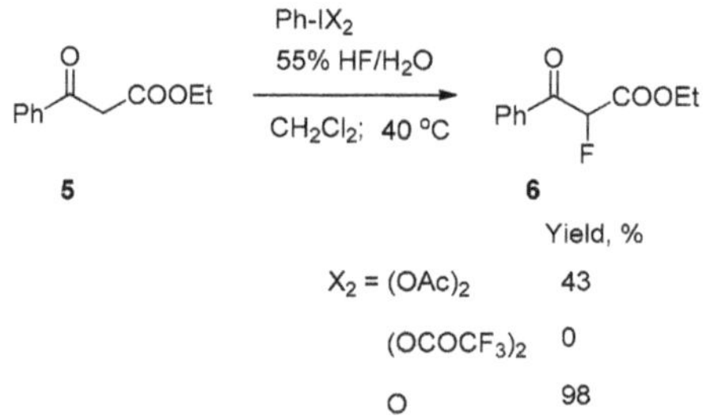


**Scheme 1.** Fluorination of 3-oxo-3-phenylpropionate **5** using HF as a source of fluorine.

It was found that the nature of a hypervalent iodine compound played a key role in the reaction, affording an excellent yield of 98% of product **6** with the application of iodosylbenzene (PhIO). The outcome of this reaction, the substitution of acidic hydrogen in **5** by fluorine, is classified as "electrophilic" fluorination and was previously reported using $F_2$ [84], $XeF_2$ [85–87] fluoroxy compounds [88–94], N–F compounds [95–102] of type 1–4 (Figure 1) and (difluoroiodo)toluene [103,104]; all of them are typical electrophilic fluorination reagents.

The mechanistic rationale for the reaction is presented in Scheme 2. It postulates the in situ formation of (difluoroiodo)benzene **7** from iodosylbenzene and two equivalents of hydrogen fluoride. The reaction of **7** with the enol **8** gives rise to intermediate **9**, followed by the nucleophilic substitution of the iodine species to afford fluorinated compound **6** along with iodobenzene **10** as the final reaction products.

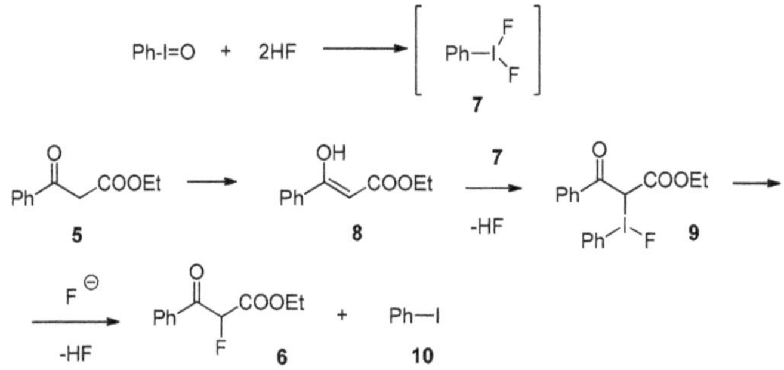


**Scheme 2.** Mechanistic rationale of the "electrophilic" fluorination of 3-oxo-3-phenylpropionate **5** to 2-fluoro-3-oxo-3-phenylpropionate **6**.

Some support for the proposed mechanistic pathway can be derived from the reactions of iodonium ylides with HF and HCl [105]. As shown in Scheme 3, iodonium ylide **11** can be prepared in quantitative yield by the reaction of keto ester **5** with (diacetoxyiodo)benzene in the presence of KOH in MeCN [106].

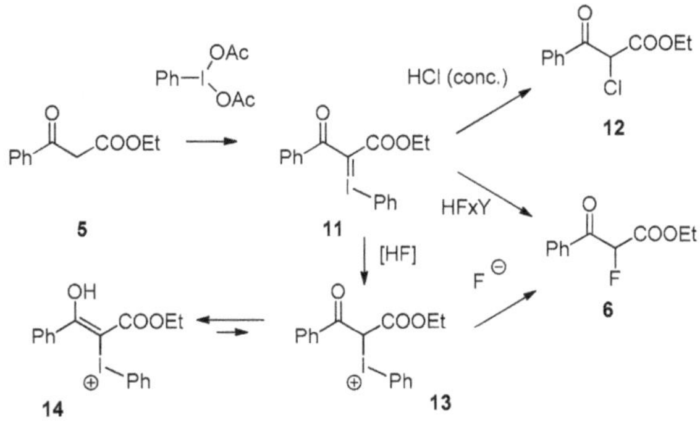

**Scheme 3.** Synthesis of iodonium ylide **11** and its reactions with HF and HCl.

The reaction of iodonium ylide **11** with concentrated aqueous HCl, conducted in dichloromethane at ambient temperature, gave chlorinated product **12** in 55% yield [105]. Similar yields of fluorination product **6** were also obtained under the same conditions in the reactions of **11** with various HF reagents, such as 55% aqueous HF and TEA·3HF [105]. The noticeably lower chemical yields of **6** obtained in the reactions of iodonium ylide **11** with HF reagents (vs 98%), as compared with the reactions of **5** with HF in the presence of PhIO (Schemes 1 and 2) can be explained by enolization of intermediate **13** to vinyliodonium salt **14**, further reactions of which give complex mixtures of products.

Meticulous investigations of HF/PhIO reactivity revealed that this new approach has a general synthetic application for fluorination of various compounds bearing the acidic $CH_2$ moiety, such as 3-keto-esters, 1,3-diketones and malonic acid derivatives, summarized in Scheme 4.

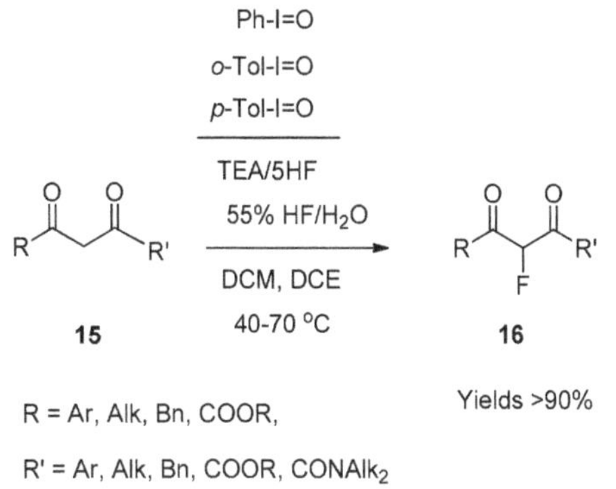

**Scheme 4.** General synthetic applications of HF/PhIO for "electrophilic" fluorination of 1,3-dicarbonyl compounds.

Optimization of the reaction conditions and reagents revealed that besides the original iodosylbenzene, its derivatives, such as *p*- and *o*-iodosyltoluene, can also be used successfully, and in some cases, even give better chemical yields as compared with unsubstituted iodosylbenzene [107,108]. For example, fluorination of amide derivatives of 3-keto-esters **15** (R′ = $CONAlk_2$) with HF/PhIO affords the corresponding products **16** with relatively low (<50%) yield, while the application of *o*-iodosyltoluene allows for improved yields of the target products **16** (up to 93%). The source of the HF has also been examined in detail showing that other HF reagents such as complexes with triethylamine and pyridine can be successfully used in place of aqueous HF. Of particular importance is the wide synthetic generality of this approach. Thus, 3-keto esters **15** bearing an aromatic ring with electron-withdrawing or donating substituents can be successfully used as substrates. In the case of derivatives **15** featuring alkyl groups (R and/or R′ = Alk) the chemical yields of the corresponding fluorinated products **16** are a bit lower (~50–70%), likely due to possible enolization.

### 2.2. Catalytic Iodoarene-Mediated Fluorination

Considering the postulated reaction mechanism (Scheme 2) involving eventual transformation (reduction) of iodosylbenzene to iodobenzene **10**, the final reaction product, the authors posited that providing in situ efficient oxidation of the latter to iodosylbenzene, would allow for a catalytic version of this process. Indeed, a significant breakthrough was made with the application of *m*-CPBA as a terminal oxidant [109]. As presented in Scheme 5, the Ar-I, used in catalytic amounts, undergoes a three-step transformation: oxidation to Ar-IO, reaction with HF to produce Ar-$IF_2$ and reaction with the enolate form of **15** giving rise to the target product **16**.

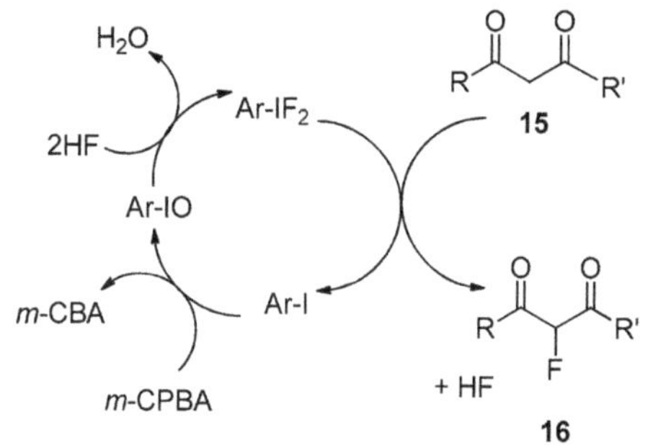


**Scheme 5.** Proposed catalytic cycle of the iodoarene-mediated "electrophilic" fluorination.

The optimized conditions for this catalytic "electrophilic" fluorination method are presented in Scheme 6 and included the following: as low as 20 mol% ArI, 55% aq. HF as a source of fluorine, *m*-CPBA as the oxidizing reagent and 1,2-dichloroethane as a solvent. The reactions are conducted at 49 °C and can be easily scaled up. The overall synthetic generality of this catalytic process is rather similar to the stoichiometric version.

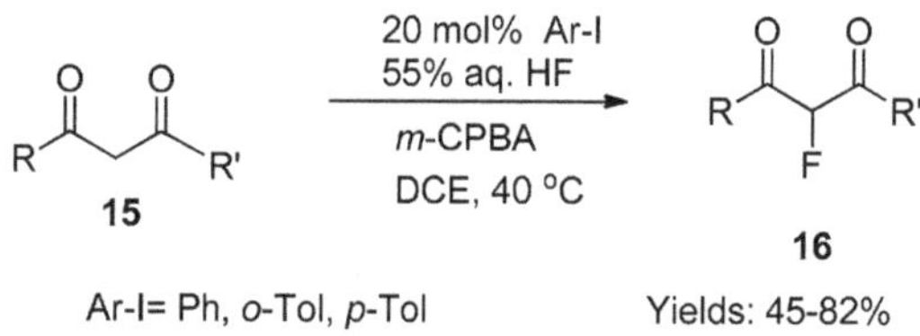


**Scheme 6.** "Electrophilic" fluorination using a catalytic amount of Ar-I.

The catalytic version can be used for fluorination of 3-keto-esters and 1,3-diketones bearing substituted aromatic, aliphatic, ester as well as amide groups. It should be notated, however, that the yields of target products **16** are a bit lower as compared with the results obtained in the reactions using a stoichiometric amount of the corresponding iodoarene. Furthermore, in most of the cases, application of *o*-Tol-I gave the best conversion of the starting 1,3-dicarbonyl compounds **15** and highest yields of fluorinated products **16**.

## 3. Fluorination of Aryl-Alkyl Ketones

Synthesis of fluorinated derivatives of monocarbonyl compounds, such as ketones and aldehydes, are of high importance in fluoro-organic chemistry [110–121]. These types of fluorinated derivatives are of proven synthetic value as building blocks for the preparation of a variety of polyfunctional fluorine-containing compounds of biological interest [30,122–128]. In particular, these derivatives can be easily transformed to the corresponding fluorinated amines and amino acids via biomimetic transamination [129–131]. General approaches for the preparation of α-fluoro-ketones include the following: two-step sequence of halogenation followed by nucleophilic substitution using fluoride [132–136] or a two-step process, involving the generation of the corresponding enolates, followed by fluorination using typical electrophilic fluorination reagents [137–139].

It was found that the direct application of Kitamura's approach, using PhIO/hydrofluoric acid, for fluorination of acetophenone (Scheme 7) gives very low yields of the target product **17**.

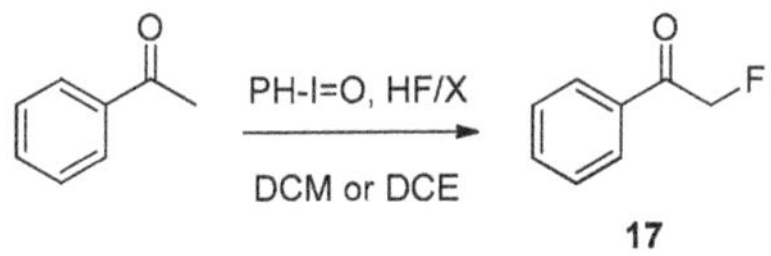


| HF/X | Yield |
|---|---|
| 55% HF | 7 |
| HF/TEA | 79 |

**Scheme 7.** Fluorination of acetophenone.

However, careful examination of various reaction conditions and reagents allowed for the discovery that the presence of water is detrimental for the fluorination process. The most likely reason is a reduction of fluoride's nucleophilicity by coordination with water molecules. Consequently, it was found that the application of a triethylamine/5HF complex as a fluorine source provides for a smooth fluorination process affording α-fluoro-acetophenone **17** in a good yield [140]. Further research revealed that this reaction can be generally applied for various aryl-alkyl ketones (Scheme 8). Among possible sources of hypervalent iodine, *p*-iodosyltoluene (4-$MeC_6H_4IO$), *p*-chloloiodosylbenzene (4-$ClC_6H_4IO$), and *p*-iodosyl(trifluoromethyl)benzene (4-$CF_3C_6H_4IO$) gave generally good results. Optimized reaction conditions included TEA/5HF in DCE (1,2-dichloroethane) at 60 °C for 24 h. Under these conditions, chemical yields of aryl-fluoromethyl ketones **19** varied between 70–85%. Of particular interest is the application of this reaction for α-fluorination of substrates derived from aryl-benzyl ketone **20**, higher alkyl derivatives such as **21** and **22**, haloalkyl **23** and cyclic compounds **24**.

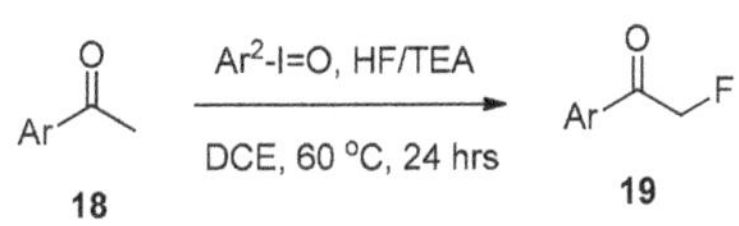


$Ar^2$ = Ph, *p*-Me-Ph, *o*-Me-Ph, *p*-$CF_3$-Ph, *p*-Cl-Ph

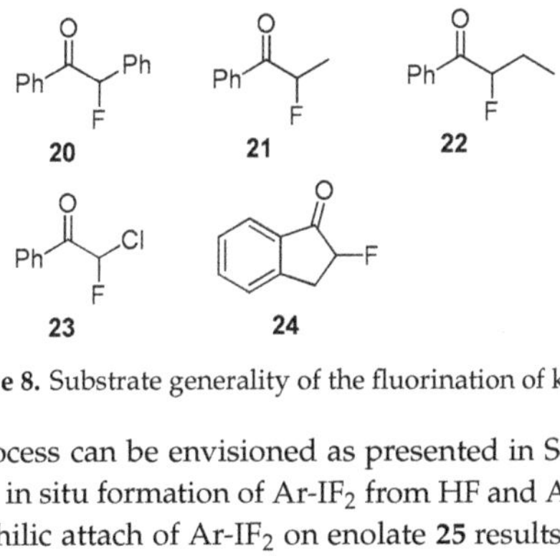


**Scheme 8.** Substrate generality of the fluorination of ketones.

Mechanistically, the process can be envisioned as presented in Scheme 9. There are two first independent steps including in situ formation of Ar-$IF_2$ from HF and Ar-I=O, and enolization of the starting ketone **24**. Electrophilic attach of Ar-$IF_2$ on enolate **25** results in intermediate **26**, which is subjected to nucleophilic substitution with a fluoride ion giving rise to the final product **27**. The net result of this reaction sequence is the "electrophilic fluorination" of **24** to **27**.

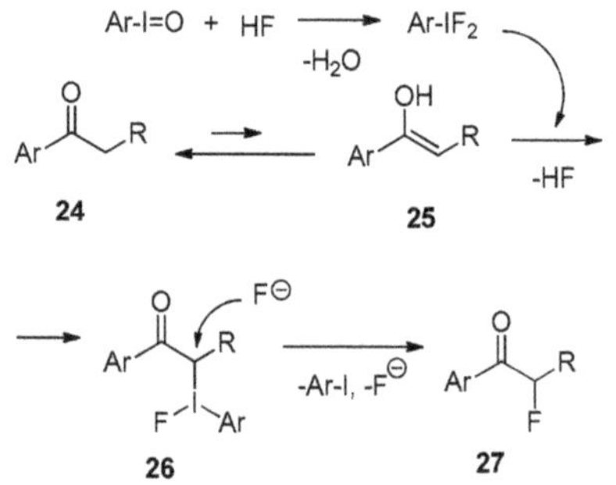

**Scheme 9.** Proposed mechanism for electrophilic fluorination.

## 4. Fluorination of Styrene Derivatives

In sharp contrast to a trifluoromethyl group, the $CHF_2$ group is still rather scarcely represented among marketed pharmaceuticals [14–22]. Known biological properties of difluoromethyl-containing compounds [141], clearly suggest that the application of this fluorinated motif might be as successful as that already established for the trifluoromethylated compounds. The major reason for the current significantly lesser application of a $CHF_2$ group in drug design is, most definitely, a lack of synthetic methods allowing for convenient installation of this functionality. Thus, most generally used methods include reaction of organozinc reagents with potassium bromodifluoroacetate [142], fluorination of gem-bistriflates and gem-dihalides [143–146], fluorodecarboxylation of dicarboxylic acids [147,148] and chlorodifluoromethylation followed by the elimination of HCl and migration of the double bond [149].

### *4.1. Hypervalent Iodine-Mediated Fluorination*

#### 4.1.1. Stoichiometric Hypervalent Iodine Reagents

The synthesis of difluoromethyl-containing compounds via reaction of styrene derivatives with fluorinated hypervalent iodine reagents or iodine in the presence $XeF_2$ [150–156] is also a known method. However, the necessity of preparing hypervalent iodine compounds or the use of $XeF_2$ limits its synthetic applications. With this in mind, Kitamura's approach was examined for the fluorination of styrene substrates [157]. As presented in Scheme 10, a series of hypervalent reagents were screened and the trifluoroacetoxy derivatives were identified as the best.

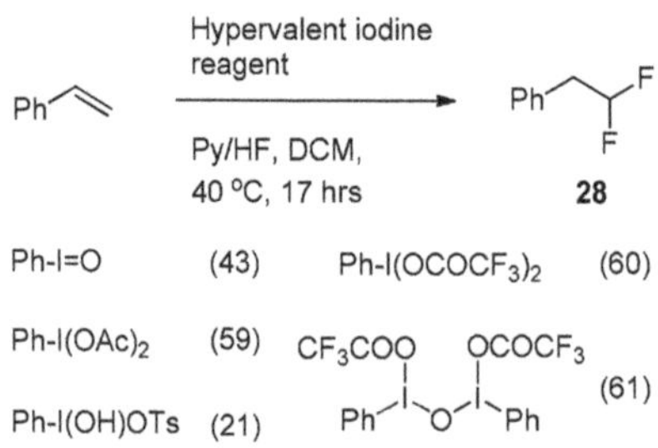

**Scheme 10.** Fluorination of styrene.

It should also be noted that a separate optimization study showed that a complex of HF with pyridine was found to serve as a superior source of nucleophilic fluoride. Thus, under these optimized conditions, the target fluorinated product **28** was prepared in greater than 60% yield [157].

Application of these reaction conditions for fluorination of various substituted styrenes gave rather good results. This approach was applied to substrates **29** (Scheme 11) bearing alkyl, halo and OAc-type substituents in the *o*-, *m*- or *p*-position on the phenyl ring. The chemical yields of difluorinated products **30** ranged from 50% to 93%.

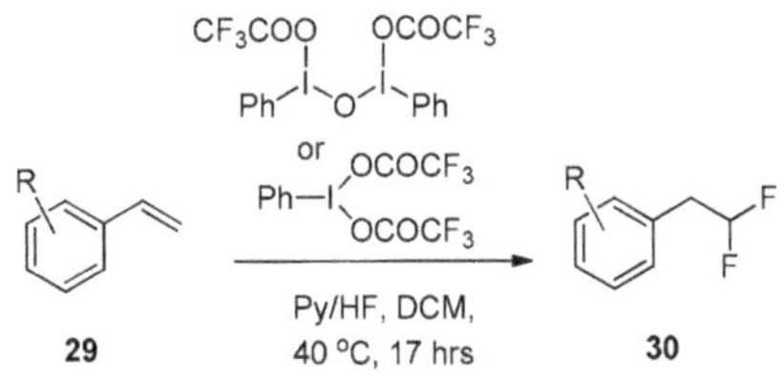


**Scheme 11.** Generality of styrene fluorination using hypervalent iodine and HF complex with pyridine.

Some structural limitations of this method may arise from a mechanism involving the migration of an aryl group. As presented in Scheme 12, in situ generated electrophilic hyper-iodide reagent **30**, reacts with starting styrene **29** to form three-ring intermediate **31** which is opened with fluoride to afford mono-fluorinated compound **32**. The latter proceeds to a second spirocyclic three-ring intermediate **33** with the elimination of Ar-I. The final step of the process is the nucleophilic opening of **33** with fluoride to give the difluorinated product **30**. One can assume that the stability of intermediate **33** will be strongly influenced by the electronic properties of the substituents on the aromatic ring. Nevertheless, as mentioned above, moderately electron-donating/withdrawing substituents, such as alkyl groups and halogens, can be tolerated giving product **30** with synthetically attractive chemical yields.

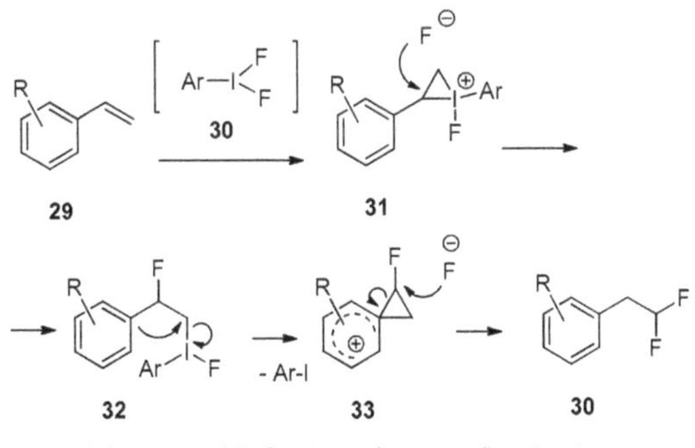


**Scheme 12.** Mechanism of styrene fluorination.

4.1.2. Catalytic Hypervalent Iodine Reactions

The catalytic version (Scheme 13) of this process was realized with application of 4-iodotoluene, HF/Py complex and *m*-CPBA, as the oxidizing reagent [157].

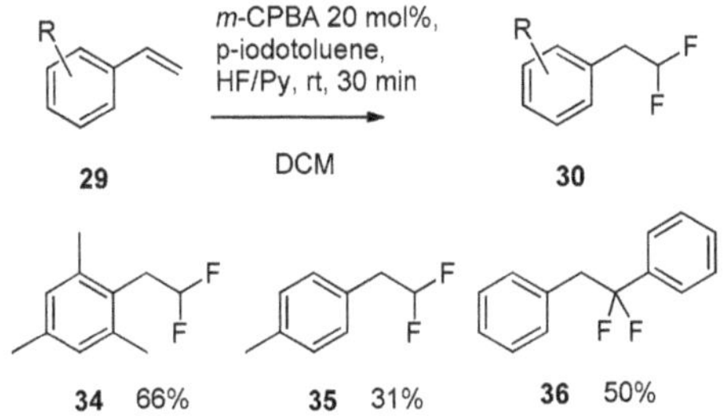


**Scheme 13.** Catalytic version of styrene fluorination.

However, the outcome of the catalytic reactions was not entirely successful as difluoro products **30** were generally isolated in relatively low yields of about 50%. The highest yield (66%) in the series was obtained for the electron-rich trimethyl derivative **34**. In sharp contrast, mono-methyl substituted compound **35** was prepared in only 31% yield. It is interesting to note that fluorination of 1,1-diphenylethene resulted in rearranged difluoro compound **36** isolated in 50% yield.

## 5. Fluorination of α,β-Unsaturated Ketones and Alcohols

One may assume that a chemically similar process can also be realized for fluorination of other types of unsaturated compounds [158]. For example, as presented in Scheme 14, it was found that α,β-unsaturated ketones of general structure **37** can be converted to ketones **38** featuring α-aryl and difluoromethyl groups [159].

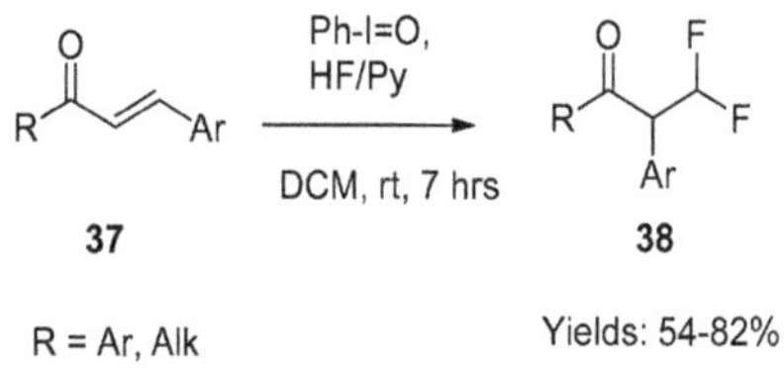


**Scheme 14.** Fluorination of α,β-unsaturated ketones.

Substrate generality in this reaction is rather broad as the substituent R in starting **37** can be a methyl, long-chain alkyl, *tert*-butyl, aromatic or heteroaromatic group. Furthermore, the aromatic ring on the carbonyl carbon can bear electron-withdrawing or -donating groups, including $NO_2$, halogens, Alk-O and Ac-NH. The aromatic group on the unsaturated C=C fragment is migrating during the reaction to the α-position, relatively to the carbonyl, and therefore is a bit more sensitive to the nature of substitution. Nevertheless, alkyl and halogen groups on the para position of the Ar moiety seem to be perfectly tolerated [159].

A catalytic version of this process was successfully realized using *m*-CPBA for the in situ oxidation of *p*-Tol-I to *p*-Tol-I=O. Optimized conditions included *p*-Tol-I (0.2 mol%), HF/Py (40 mol%) and (1.3 mol%). Substrate generality under the catalytic conditions was not compromised, however, the chemical yields were about 5–10% lower when compared with those obtained for the reactions conducted with stoichiometric amounts of the *p*-Tol-I=O [159].

Of particular interest are the results reported for the fluorination of cinnamyl alcohol derivatives [160]. As presented in Scheme 15, starting compounds **39** were treated with Ph-I=O and HF/Py in dichloromethane to furnish fluorinated products **40**.

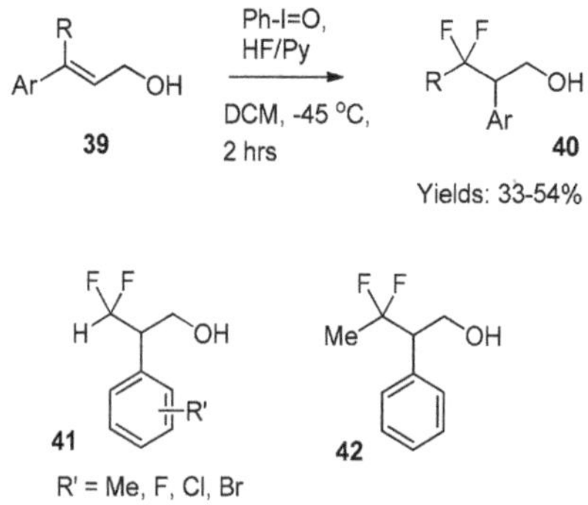


**Scheme 15.** Fluorination of cinnamyl alcohol derivatives.

It should be noted that this type of fluorination required low reaction temperature due to the sensitive nature of the cinnamyl alcohol functionality. Similar to the previously discussed fluorination of compounds with conjugated C=C bonds, the reactions occurred with migration of the Ar group. Substrate generality study of these reactions was limited to two types of products, featuring difluoromethyl **41** and difluoroethyl groups **42**.

## 6. Cyclization–Fluorination Cascade

### 6.1. Homoallyl Amine Derivatives

Compounds containing the 3-fluoropyrrolidine moiety possessing a wide spectrum of biological properties. Some of them have been developed as dipeptidyl peptidase inhibitors [160–163], glucokinase activators [164] prolyl oligopeptidase inhibitors [165] and purine nucleoside phosphorylase inhibitors [166]. The most commonly used synthetic approach for preparation of 3-fluoropyrrolidines is based on fluorine substitution for hydroxy group in 3-hydroxylpyrrolidines [167–171]. Another approach, based on aminofluorination of alkenes [172–176], is more practical allowing both ring construction and introduction of a fluorine atom in one convenient synthetic sequence. It was found that the aminofluorination version of this approach can be successfully realized using the Kitamura fluorination protocol. As presented in Scheme 16, treatment of homoallyl amines **43** with a hypervalent iodine reagent and HF/Py afforded 3-fluoropyrrolidines **44** with respectable yields ranging from 50% to 87% [177].

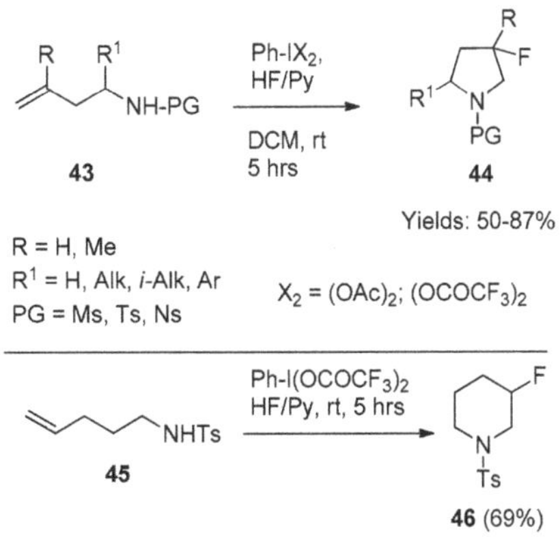


**Scheme 16.** Intramolecular aminofluorination of homoallyl amine via cyclization-fluorination cascade.

Optimization of the reaction conditions in terms of hypervalent iodine reagent and source of HF found that a combination of HF/Py and $PhI(OCOCF_3)_2$ or $PhI(OAc)_2$ was superior to other compounds such as $PhI(OAc)_2$ and aqueous 55% HF and PhI(OH)OTs and HF/TEA complex [177]. As for the starting homoallyl amines, protection of the amino group with strong electron-withdrawing groups such as Ts, Ms or Ns, was found to be essential for the successful transformation. From the standpoint of generality, the process was shown to be applicable for a reasonably wide range of compounds with the substituent R bearing hydrogen or alkyl groups and with the $R^1$ representing hydrogen, alkyl, bulky iso-alkyl and aryl groups. Quite remarkably, the reaction can be used for preparation of six-membered rings, as represented by the transformation of *N*-tosyl-4-pentenylamine **45** to *N*-tosyl-3-fluoropiperidine **46**, in 69% yield [177].

To obtain information about the reaction mechanism for this intramolecular aminofluorination, the authors conducted a competitive reaction between homoallyl amines **47** and **48** (Scheme 17).

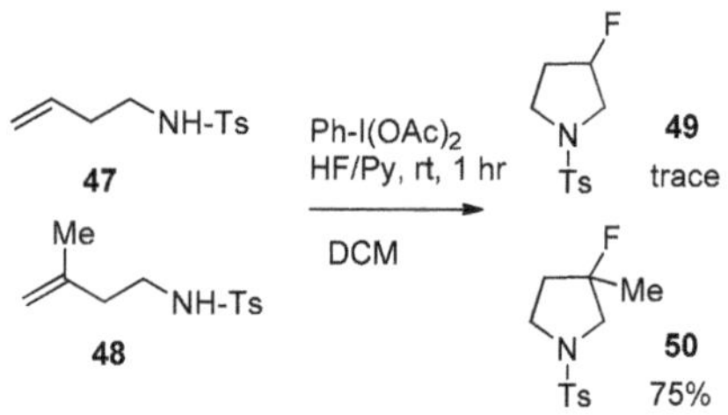


**Scheme 17.** Competitive intramolecular aminofluorination.

To this end, an equimolar mixture of **47** and **48** was subjected to the aminofluorination reaction using Ph-I(OAc)$_2$ and HF/Py. It was found that, almost exclusively, homoallyl amine **48** was transformed to 3-fluoro-3-methylpyrrolidine **50**, while product **49**, derived from homoallyl amine **47**, was detected in the reaction mixture only in trace amounts. This result strongly suggested that the hypervalent iodine reagent preferentially reacts with the more electron-rich olefinic moiety. Based on the outcome of this competitive reaction, the authors proposed the following reaction mechanism, presented in Scheme 18.

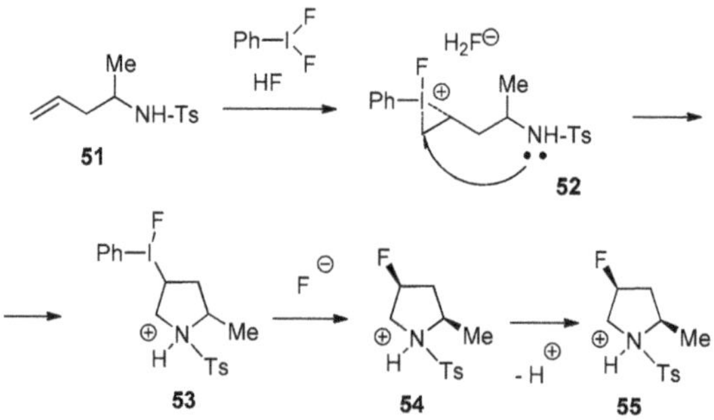

**Scheme 18.** Mechanism of the intramolecular aminofluorination.

According to the proposed mechanism, the formed in situ (difluoroiodo)benzene is activated by HF and interacts with the nucleophilic double bond of homoallyl amine **51** resulting in formation of the cyclic iodonium salt **52**. The three-membered ring is opened next by the nitrogen, attacking the terminal carbon by the bridged iodonium salts **52** to afford pyrrolidine **53**. The formation of intermediate **53** is followed by $S_N2$ substitution by a fluoride ion. The final step is the deprotonation of **54** giving rise to the final 3-fluoropyrrolidine product **55**.

*6.2. Homoallyl Alcohol and 3-butenoic Acid Derivatives*

An interesting extension of this reaction cascade was demonstrated for other types of polyfunctional olefins, such as homoallyl alcohols and 3-butenoic acid derivatives [178]. The fluorination-cyclization cascade of homoallyl alcohols **56** (Scheme 19) was performed using the reagent system of PhI(OPiv)$_2$ and HF/Py in dichloromethane. The target fluorinated tetrahydrofuran derivatives **57** were isolated with reasonably good 54–65% yields as a mixture of cis- and trans-isomers.

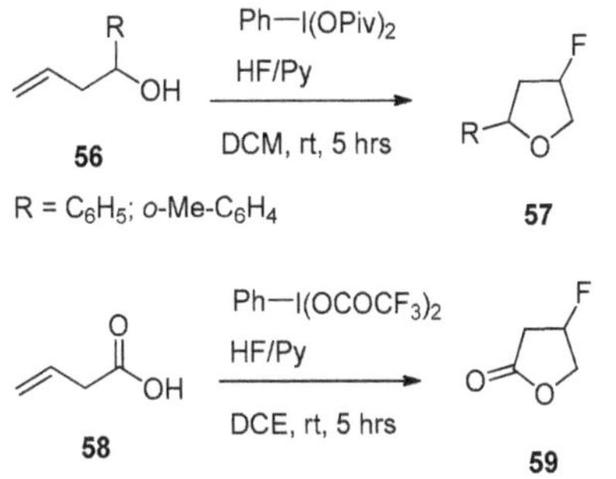

**Scheme 19.** Fluorination of homoallyl alcohols and 3-butenoic acid derivatives.

Under similar conditions, except using Ph-I($OCOCF_3$)$_2$ as the hypervalent iodine reagent and dichloroethane as a solvent, butenoic acid **58** was transformed to fluorinated butyrolactone **59** in 45% yield. The structure of products **57** and **59** is consistent with the above-discussed mechanism (Scheme 18) for the fluorination-cyclization cascade. Thus, in the cases of homoallyl alcohols **56** and 3-butenoic acid **58** the oxygen of the hydroxy group acts as the nucleophilic element attacking the terminal carbon of the corresponding intermediate bridged iodonium salts of type **52**, to complete the cyclization step.

## 7. Reactions with Alkynes

One of the most recent developments in this chemistry is the synthesis of β-fluorovinyliodonium salts via the reaction of alkynes with hypervalent iodine reagents in the presence of HF (Scheme 20) [179].

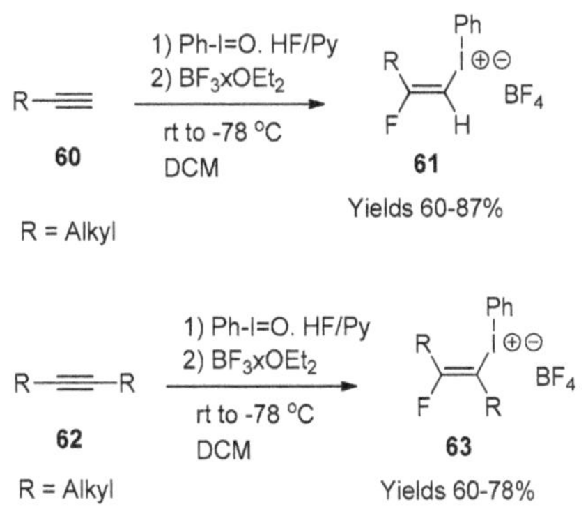

**Scheme 20.** Synthesis of β-fluorovinyliodonium salts by the reaction of alkynes with hypervalent iodine/HF reagent.

It should be noted that direct application of the conditions developed for the reactions of various C=C unsaturated compounds was found to be ineffective for alkynes. In a series of preliminary experiments, it was determined that Ph-$IF_2$ needed some additional activation by a Lewis acid, such as $BF_3{\cdot}OEt_2$. Indeed, treatment of mono-alkyl substituted alkynes **60** with Ph-I=O and HF/Py, followed by the addition of $BF_3{\cdot}OEt_2$, resulted in the formation of β-fluorovinyliodonium salts **61** with a respectable chemical yield. Compound **61** is quite stable to be isolated and fully characterized. In terms of generality one can mention that the alkyl group could bear in its terminal position some functionalities, such as aromatic or heterocyclic rings, a protected alcohol or ester group. The reactions are highly regio- and stereospecific as the fluorine being added to the most substituted carbon on **60** and products **61** are obtained as trans-isomers only. This set of conditions can also be successfully applied to symmetrically disubstitute alkynes **62**. The corresponding β-fluorovinyliodonium salts **63** were obtained exclusively as trans-isomers with 60–78% yields. The proposed mechanism for the reactions of Ph-I=O and HF/Py reagents with alkynes is presented in Scheme 21.

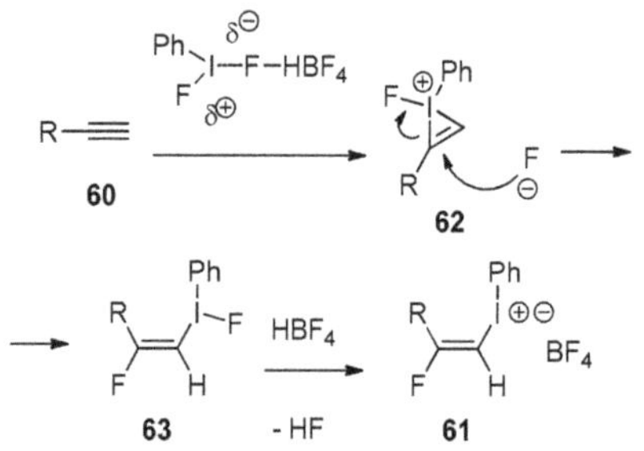


**Scheme 21.** Proposed mechanism for the reactions of alkynes with Ph-I=O and HF/Py in the presence of $BF_3{\cdot}OEt_2$.

According to the proposed mechanism, the in situ generated $PhIF_2$ is activated by $HBF_4$ and undertakes the electrophilic addition to alkyne **60** affording bridged three-membered iodonium species **62**. Intermediate **62** is subjected to the nucleophilic attack of fluoride ions leading to the formation of (*E*)-β-vinyliodonium fluorides **63**. The final step in this sequence is the ligand exchange with $HBF_4$ yielding final product **61**. It should be emphasized that the geometric configuration of **63** is controlled by the ring-opening of iodonium species **62** with fluoride ion.

## 8. Conclusions

The chemistry discussed in this review article is based on the original idea of the application of HF as a source of fluorine for subsequent "electrophilic" formation of a C–F bond. The target transformation is achieved via in situ generation of the proper electrophilic species derived from hypervalent iodine compounds. The data reported so far clearly show the great synthetic value of this approach for fluorination of various 1,3-dicarbonyl compounds, aryl-alkyl ketones, styrene derivatives, α,β-unsaturated ketones and alcohols, homoallyl amine and homoallyl alcohol derivatives, 3-butenoic acids and alkynes. The major advantage of this chemistry over alternative approaches is its practicality and very attractive cost-structure, boding well for its application in large-scale synthesis of important drug intermediates or other industrial fluoro-organics. However, there are still some issues that need to be solved, to further increase the synthetic value of this methodology. One critical area of improvement would be the application of more safe and still cheaper sources of HF. Thus, most of the research has been performed using aqueous HF, and its complexes with TEA and Py. One would also suggest HF in complex with THF as an alternative source, which was reported by Professor W. R. Dolbier [179,180]. Finally, further optimization of the reaction conditions, alongside with applications of new sources of HF, leading to increased chemical yield would clearly be in the focus for future research in this exciting area of fundamental fluoro-organic methodology. As a word of caution, we would like to remind the readers that hydrogen fluoride, aqueous or in complexes with pyridine, triethylamine or in any other form, is quite toxic, highly corrosive and can easily penetrate skin and muscles destroying cell membranes and nerves. The reactions should be conducted in a well-ventilated hood using Teflon-lined reactors of tubes.

**Author Contributions:** Conceptualization, J.H. and V.A.S.; validation, V.A.S., G.B. and H.M.; writing—original draft preparation, G.B., H.K. and T.K.; writing—review and editing, V.A.S. and J.H.; supervision, V.A.S. All authors have read and agreed to the published version of the manuscript.

**Funding:** This research was funded by the National Natural Science Foundation of China (No. 21761132021), and IKERBASQUE, Basque Foundation for Science.

**Conflicts of Interest:** The authors declare no conflict of interest.

## References


1. Aspern, N.; Röser, S.; Rad, B.R.; Murmann, P.; Streipert, B.; Mönnighoff, X.; Tillmann, S.D.; Shevchuk, M.; Stubbmann-Kazakova, O.; Röschenthaler, G.V.; et al. Phosphorus additives for improving high voltage stability and safety of lithium ion batteries. *J. Fluorine Chem.* **2017**, *198*, 24–33. [CrossRef]
2. Gschwind, F.; Rodriguez-Garcia, G.; Sandbeck, D.J.S.; Gross, A.; Weil, M.; Fichtner, M.; Hörmann, N. Fluoride ion batteries: Theoretical performance, safety, toxicity, and a combinatorial screening of new electrodes. *J. Fluorine Chem.* **2016**, *182*, 76–90. [CrossRef]
3. Jeong, E.; Lee, B.H.; Doh, S.J.; Park, I.J.; Lee, Y.S. Multifunctional surface modification of an aramid fabric via direct fluorination. *J. Fluorine Chem.* **2012**, *141*, 69–75. [CrossRef]
4. Simone, C.D.; Vaccaro, E.; Scola, D.A. The synthesis and characterization of highly fluorinated aromatic polyimides. *J. Fluorine Chem.* **2019**, *224*, 100–112. [CrossRef]
5. Miyajima, H.; Kasuya, M.C.Z.; Hatanaka, K. New fluorous gelators for perfluorodecalin. *J. Fluorine Chem.* **2019**. [CrossRef]
6. Fersing, C.; Bouhlel, A.; Cantelli, C.; Garrigue, P.; Lisowski, V.; Guillet, B. A Comprehensive Review of Non-Covalent Radiofluorination Approaches Using Aluminum [$^{18}$F] fluoride: Will [$^{18}$F] AlF Replace $^{68}$Ga for Metal Chelate Labeling? *Molecules* **2019**, *24*, 2866. [CrossRef]
7. Norton, R.S.; Leung, E.W.W.; Chandrashekaran, I.R.; MacRaild, C.A. Applications of $^{19}$F-NMR in fragment-based drug discovery. *Molecules* **2016**, *21*, 860. [CrossRef]
8. Bernard-Gauthier, V.; Bailey, J.J.; Berke, S.; Schirrmacher, R. Recent advances in the development and application of radiolabeled kinase inhibitors for PET imaging. *Molecules* **2015**, *20*, 22000–22027. [CrossRef]
9. Pretze, M.; Pietzsch, D.; Mamat, C. Recent trends in bioorthogonal click-radiolabeling reactions using fluorine-18. *Molecules* **2013**, *18*, 8618–8665. [CrossRef]
10. De la Torre, D.G.; Albericio, F. The pharmaceutical industry in 2018. An analysis of FDA drug approvals from the perspective of molecules. *Molecules* **2019**, *24*, 809. [CrossRef]
11. Fujiwara, T.; O'Hagan, D. Successful fluorine-containing herbicide agrochemicals. *J. Fluorine Chem.* **2014**, *167*, 16–29. [CrossRef]
12. Jeschke, P. The unique role of halogen substituents in the design of modern agrochemicals. *Pest Manag. Sci.* **2010**, *66*, 10–27. [CrossRef] [PubMed]
13. Theodoridis, G. Chapter 4: Fluorine-Containing Agrochemicals: An Overview of Recent Developments. In *Advance in Fluorine Science*; Tressaud, A., Ed.; Elsevier: Amsterdam, The Netherlands; Volume 2, pp. 121–175. Available online: https://www.sciencedirect.com/science/article/pii/S1872035806020045 (accessed on 30 April 2020).
14. Isanbor, C.; O'Hagan, D. Fluorine in medicinal chemistry: A review of anticancer agents. *J. Fluorine Chem.* **2006**, *127*, 303–319. [CrossRef]
15. O'Hagan, D. Fluorine in health care: Organofluorine containing blockbuster drugs. *J. Fluorine Chem.* **2010**, *131*, 1071–1081. [CrossRef]
16. Zhu, W.; Wang, J.; Wang, S.; Gu, Z.; Aceña, J.L.; Izawa, K.; Liu, H.; Soloshonok, V.A. Recent advances in the trifluoromethylation methodology and new $CF_3$-containing drugs. *J. Fluorine Chem.* **2014**, *167*, 37–54. [CrossRef]
17. Wang, J.; Sánchez-Roselló, M.; Aceña, J.L.; del Pozo, C.; Sorochinsky, A.E.; Fustero, S.; Soloshonok, V.A.; Liu, H. Fluorine in Pharmaceutical Industry: Fluorine-Containing Drugs Introduced to the Market in the Last Decade (2001–2011). *Chem. Rev.* **2014**, *114*, 2432–2506. [CrossRef]
18. Zhou, Y.; Wang, J.; Gu, Z.; Wang, S.; Zhu, W.; Aceña, J.L.; Soloshonok, V.A.; Izawa, K.; Liu, H. Next Generation of Fluorine-Containing Pharmaceuticals, Compounds Currently in Phase II–III Clinical Trials of Major Pharmaceutical Companies: New Structural Trends and Therapeutic Areas. *Chem. Rev.* **2016**, *116*, 422–518. [CrossRef]
19. Zhu, Y.; Han, J.; Wang, J.; Shibata, N.; Sodeoka, M.; Soloshonok, V.A.; Coelho, J.A.S.; Toste, F.D. Modern Approaches for Asymmetric Construction of Carbon-Fluorine Quaternary Stereogenic Centers: Synthetic Challenges and Pharmaceutical Needs. *Chem. Rev.* **2018**, *118*, 3887–3964. [CrossRef]
20. Mei, H.; Han, J.; Fustero, S.; Medio-Simon, M.; Sedgwick, D.M.; Santi, C.; Ruzziconi, R.; Soloshonok, V.A. Fluorine-Containing Drugs Approved by the FDA in 2018. *Chem. Eur. J.* **2019**, *25*, 11797–11819. [CrossRef]

21. Mei, H.; Remete, A.M.; Zou, Y.; Moriwaki, H.; Fustero, S.; Kiss, L.; Soloshonok, V.A.; Han, J.L. Fluorine-containing drugs approved by the FDA in 2019. *Chin. Chem. Lett.* **2020**. [CrossRef]
22. Liu, J.; Li, Z.; Mei, H.; Soloshonok, V.A.; Han, J.L. Detrifluoroacetylative in Situ Generated Cyclic Fluorinated Enolates for the Preparation of Compounds Featuring a C–F Stereogenic Center. *ACS Omega* **2019**, *4*, 19505–19512. [CrossRef] [PubMed]
23. Liang, T.; Neumann, C.N.; Ritter, T. Introduction of Fluorine and Fluorine-Containing Functional Groups. *Angew. Chem. Int. Ed.* **2013**, *52*, 8214–8264. [CrossRef] [PubMed]
24. Noel, M.; Suryanarayanan, V.; Chellammal, S. A review of recent developments in the selective electrochemical fluorination of organic compounds. *J. Fluorine Chem.* **1997**, *83*, 31–40. [CrossRef]
25. Wu, J. Review of recent advances in nucleophilic C–F bond-forming reactions at sp3 centers. *Tetrahedron Lett.* **2014**, *55*, 4289–4294. [CrossRef]
26. Kuehnel, M.F.; Lentz, D.; Braun, T. Synthesis of Fluorinated Building Blocks by Transition-Metal-Mediated Hydrodefluorination Reactions. *Angew. Chem. Int. Ed.* **2013**, *52*, 3328–3348. [CrossRef]
27. Lectard, S.; Hamashima, Y.; Sodeoka, M. Recent Advances in Catalytic Enantioselective Fluorination Reactions. *Adv. Synth. Catal.* **2010**, *352*, 2708–2732. [CrossRef]
28. Yerien, D.E.; Bonesi, S.; Postigo, A. Fluorination methods in drug discovery. *Org. Biomol. Chem.* **2016**, *14*, 8398–8427. [CrossRef]
29. Soloshonok, V.A.; Cai, C.; Hruby, V.J.; Meervelt, L.V. Asymmetric Synthesis of Novel Highly Sterically Constrained (2*S*,3*S*)-3-Methyl-3-Trifluoromethyl- and (2*S*,3*S*,4*R*)-3-Trifluoromethyl-4-Methylpyroglutamic Acids. *Tetrahedron* **1999**, *55*, 12045–12058. [CrossRef]
30. Han, J.; Sorochinsky, A.E.; Ono, T.; Soloshonok, V.A. Biomimetic Transamination—A Metal-Free Alternative to the Reductive Amination. Application for Generalized Preparation of Fluorine-Containing Amines and Amino Acids. *Curr. Org. Synth.* **2011**, *8*, 281–294.
31. Aceña, J.L.; Sorochinsky, A.E.; Soloshonok, V.A. Asymmetric synthesis of α-amino acids via homologation of Ni(II) complexes of glycine Schiff bases. Part 3: Michael addition reactions and miscellaneous transformations. *Amino Acids* **2014**, *46*, 2047–2073. [CrossRef]
32. Soloshonok, V.A.; Sorochinsky, A.E. Practical Methods for the Synthesis of Symmetrically α,α-Disubstituted-α-Amino Acids. *Synthesis* **2010**, 2319–2344. [CrossRef]
33. Mikami, K.; Fustero, S.; Sánchez-Roselló, M.; Aceña, J.L.; Soloshonok, V.A.; Sorochinsky, A.E. Synthesis of Fluorine Containing β-Amino Acids. *Synthesis* **2011**, 3045–3079.
34. Aceña, J.L.; Sorochinsky, A.E.; Moriwaki, H.; Sato, T.; Soloshonok, V.A. Synthesis of fluorine-containing α-amino acids in enantiomerically pure form via homologation of Ni(II) complexes of glycine and alanine Schiff bases. *J. Fluorine Chem.* **2013**, *155*, 21–38. [CrossRef]
35. Turcheniuk, K.V.; Kukhar, V.P.; Roeschenthaler, G.V.; Acena, J.L.; Soloshonok, V.A.; Sorochinsky, A.E. Recent advances in the synthesis of fluorinated aminophosphonates and aminophosphonic acids. *RSC Adv.* **2013**, *3*, 6693–6716. [CrossRef]
36. Kukhar, V.P. Fluorine-containing amino acids. *J. Fluorine Chem.* **1994**, *69*, 199–205. [CrossRef]
37. Furin, G.G. Some new aspects in the application of perfluoroalkyl halides in the synthesis of fluorine-containing organic compounds. *Russ. Chem. Rev.* **2000**, *69*, 491–522. [CrossRef]
38. Kiss, L.; Fülöp, F. Selective Synthesis of Fluorine-Containing Cyclic β-Amino Acid Scaffolds. *Chem. Rec.* **2018**, *18*, 266–281. [CrossRef]
39. Turcheniuk, K.V.; Poliashko, K.O.; Kukhar, V.P.; Rozhenko, A.B.; Soloshonok, V.A.; Sorochinsky, A.E. Efficient asymmetric synthesis of trifluoromethylated β-aminophosphonates and their incorporation into dipeptides. *Chem. Commun.* **2012**, *48*, 11519–11521. [CrossRef]
40. Röschenthaler, G.V.; Kukhar, V.P.; Kulik, I.B.; Belik, M.Y.; Sorochinsky, A.E.; Rusanov, E.B.; Soloshonok, V.A. Asymmetric synthesis of phosphonotrifluoroalanine and its derivatives using *N-tert*-butanesulfinyl imine derived from fluoral. *Tetrahedron Lett.* **2012**, *53*, 539–542. [CrossRef]
41. Yin, Z.; Moriwaki, H.; Abe, H.; Miwa, T.; Han, J.; Soloshonok, V.A. Large-Scale Asymmetric Synthesis of Fmoc-(S)-2-Amino-6,6,6-Trifluorohexanoic Acid. *ChemistryOpen* **2019**, *8*, 701–704. [CrossRef]
42. Mei, H.; Yin, Z.; Miwa, T.; Moriwaki, H.; Abe, H.; Han, J.; Soloshonok, V.A. Convenient Asymmetric Synthesis of Fmoc-(S)-6,6,6-trifluoro-Norleucine. *Symmetry* **2019**, *11*, 578. [CrossRef]
43. Osipov, S.N.; Kolomiets, A.F.; Bruneau, C.; Picquet, M.; Dixneuf, P.H. Synthesis of fluorine-containing cyclic amino acid derivatives via ring closing olefin metathesis. *Chem. Commun.* **1998**, 2053–2054. [CrossRef]

44. Osipov, S.N.; Artyushin, O.I.; Kolomiets, A.F.; Bruneau, C.; Picquet, M.; Dixneuf, P.H. Synthesis of Fluorine-Containing Cyclic α-Amino Acid and α-Amino Phosphonate Derivatives by Alkene Metathesis. *Eur. J. Org. Chem.* **2001**, 3891–3897. [CrossRef]
45. Tsushima, T.; Kawada, K.; Tsuji, T.; Tawara, K. Fluorine-Containing Amino Acids and Their Derivatives. 4.1 Synthesis and Antibacterial Activity of Threo and Erythro1-Fluorodehydroxylated Chloramphenicol Analogues. *J. Med. Chem.* **1985**, *28*, 253–256. [CrossRef] [PubMed]
46. Osipov, S.N.; Sewald, N.; Kolomiets, A.F.; Fokin, A.V.; Burger, K. Synthesis of α-trifluoromethyl substituted α-amino acid derivatives from methyl 3,3,3-trifluoro-2-diazopropionate. *Tetrahedron Lett.* **1996**, *37*, 615–618. [CrossRef]
47. Konno, T.; Kanda, M.; Ishihara, T.; Yamanaka, H. A novel synthesis of fluorine-containing quaternary amino acid derivatives via palladium-catalyzed allylation reaction. *J. Fluorine Chem.* **2005**, *126*, 1517–1523. [CrossRef]
48. Ayoup, M.S.; Cordes, D.B.; Slawin, A.M.Z.; O'Hagan, D. Fluorine containing amino acids: Synthesis and peptide coupling of amino acids containing the all-cis tetrafluorocyclohexyl motif. *Org. Biomol. Chem.* **2015**, *13*, 5621–5624. [CrossRef]
49. Mei, H.; Han, J.; Klika, K.D.; Izawa, K.; Sato, T.; Meanwell, N.A.; Soloshonok, V.A. Applications of Fluorine-Containing Amino Acids for Drug Design. *Eur. J. Med. Chem.* **2020**, *186*, 111826. [CrossRef]
50. Chen, H.; Viel, S.; Ziarelli, F.; Peng, L. $^{19}$F NMR: A valuable tool for studying biological events. *Chem. Soc. Rev.* **2013**, *42*, 7971–7982. [CrossRef]
51. Marsh, E.N.G.; Suzuki, Y. Using $^{19}$F NMR to probe biological interactions of proteins and peptides. *ACS Chem. Biol.* **2014**, *9*, 1242–1250. [CrossRef]
52. Cai, L.; Lu, S.; Pike, V.W. Chemistry with [$^{18}$F]fluoride ion. *Eur. J. Org. Chem.* **2008**, *2008*, 2853–2873. [CrossRef]
53. Brooks, A.F.; Topczewski, J.J.; Ichiishi, N.; Sanford, M.S.; Scott, P.J.H. Late-Stage [$^{18}$F]Fluorination: New Solutions to Old Problems. *Chem. Sci.* **2014**, *5*, 4545–4553. [CrossRef] [PubMed]
54. Jaeckel, C.; Seufert, W.; Thust, S.; Koksch, B. Evaluation of the molecular interactions of fluorinated amino acids with native polypeptides. *ChemBioChem* **2004**, *5*, 717–720. [CrossRef] [PubMed]
55. Salwiczek, M.; Koksch, B. Effects of fluorination on the folding kinetics of a heterodimeric coiled coil. *ChemBioChem* **2009**, *10*, 2867–2870. [CrossRef] [PubMed]
56. Vagt, T.; Nyakatura, E.; Salwiczek, M.; Jaeckel, C.; Koksch, B. Towards identifying preferred interaction partners of fluorinated amino acids within the hydrophobic environment of a dimeric coiled coil peptide. *Org. Biomol. Chem.* **2010**, *8*, 1382–1386. [CrossRef] [PubMed]
57. Nyakatura, E.K.; Reimann, O.; Vagt, T.; Salwiczek, M.; Koksch, B. Accommodating fluorinated amino acids in a helical peptide environment. *RSC Adv.* **2013**, *3*, 6319–6322. [CrossRef]
58. Buer, B.C.; Chugh, J.; Al-Hashimi, H.M.; Marsh, E.N.G. Using fluorine nuclear magnetic resonance to probe the interaction of membrane-active peptides with the lipid bilayer. *Biochemistry* **2010**, *49*, 5760–5765. [CrossRef]
59. De Kort, D.W.; Rombouts, W.H.; Hoeben, F.J.M.; Janssen, H.M.; As, H.V.; van Duynhoven, J.P.M. Scaling behavior of dendritic nanoparticle mobility in semidilute polymer solutions. *Macromolecules* **2015**, *48*, 7585–7591. [CrossRef]
60. Kubyshkin, V.; Afonin, S.; Kara, S.; Budisa, N.; Mykhailiuk, P.K.; Ulrich, A.S. (*S*)-Trifluoromethyl proline: Evaluation as a structural substitute of proline for solid state 19F-NMR peptide studies. *Org. Biomol. Chem.* **2015**, *13*, 3171–3181. [CrossRef]
61. Taylor, S.D.; Kotoris, C.C.; Hum, G. Recent advances in electrophilic fluorination. *Tetrahedron* **1999**, *55*, 12431–12477. [CrossRef]
62. Szpera, R.; Moseley, D.F.J.; Smith, L.B.; Sterling, A.J.; Gouverneur, V. The Fluorination of C−H Bonds: Developments and Perspectives. *Angew. Chem. Int. Ed.* **2019**, *58*, 14824–14848. [CrossRef] [PubMed]
63. Chen, C.; Fu, L.; Chen, P.; Liu, G. Recent Advances and Perspectives of Transition Metal-Catalyzed Asymmetric Fluorination Reactions. *Chin. J. Chem.* **2017**, *35*, 1781–1788. [CrossRef]
64. Kohlhepp, S.V.; Gulder, T. Hypervalent iodine(III) fluorinations of alkenes and diazo compounds: New opportunities in fluorination chemistry. *Chem. Soc. Rev.* **2016**, *45*, 6270–6288. [CrossRef] [PubMed]
65. Yang, L.; Dong, T.; Revankar, H.M.; Zhang, C.P. Recent progress on fluorination in aqueous media. *Green Chem.* **2017**, *19*, 3951–3992. [CrossRef]

66. Prakash, G.K.S.; Beier, P. Construction of Asymmetric Fluorinated Carbon Centers. *Angew. Chem. Int. Ed.* **2006**, *45*, 2172–2174. [CrossRef]
67. Tredwell, M.; Gouverneur, V. Electrophilic fluorination of organosilanes. *Org. Biomol. Chem.* **2006**, *4*, 26–32. [CrossRef]
68. Davis, F.A.; Han, W.; Murphy, C.K. Selective, electrophilic fluorinations using N-fluoro-o-benzenedisulfonimide. *J. Org. Chem.* **1995**, *60*, 4730–4737. [CrossRef]
69. Differding, E.; Rüegg, G.M. Nucleophilic substitution versus electron transfer: 1. On the mechanism of electrophilic fluorinations. *Tetrahedron Lett.* **1991**, *32*, 3815–3818. [CrossRef]
70. Rozatian, N.; Ashworth, I.W.; Sandford, G.; Hodgson, D.R.W. A quantitative reactivity scale for electrophilic fluorinating reagents. *Chem. Sci.* **2018**, *9*, 8692–8702. [CrossRef]
71. Piana, S.; Devillers, I.; Togni, A.; Rothlisberger, U. The mechanism of catalytic enantioselective fluorination: Computational and experimental studies. *Angew. Chem. Int. Ed.* **2002**, *41*, 979–982. [CrossRef]
72. Banks, R.E.; Mohialdin-Khaffaf, S.N.; Lal, G.S.; Sharif, I.; Syvret, R.G. 1-Alkyl-4-fluoro-1,4-diazoniabicyclo[2.2.2]octane salts: A novel family of electrophilic fluorinating agents. *J. Chem. Soc. Chem. Commun.* **1992**, 595–596. [CrossRef]
73. Shibata, N. Development of shelf-stable reagents for fluoro-functionalization reactions. *Bull. Chem. Soc. Jpn.* **2016**, *89*, 1307–1320. [CrossRef]
74. Yasui, H.; Yamamoto, T.; Ishimaru, T.; Fukuzumi, T.; Tokunaga, E.; Akikazu, K.; Shiro, M.; Shibata, N. *N*-Fluoro-(3,5-di-tert-butyl-4-methoxy)benzenesulfonimide (NFBSI): A sterically demanding electrophilic fluorinating reagent for enantioselective fluorination. *J. Fluorine Chem.* **2011**, *132*, 222–225. [CrossRef]
75. Fukushi, K.; Suzuki, S.; Kamo, T.; Tokunaga, E.; Sumii, Y.; Kagawa, T.; Kawada, K.; Shibata, N. Methyl NFSI: Atom-economical alternative to NFSI shows higher fluorination reactivity under Lewis acid-catalysis and non-catalysis. *Green Chem.* **2016**, *18*, 1864–1868. [CrossRef]
76. Fukushi, K.; Tokunaga, E.; Sumii, Y.; Kagawa, T.; Nagasaki, N.; Shibata, N. Lewis Acid-Catalyzed Selective Mono-fluorination of Malonates Using Me-NFSI. *Fluorine Notes* **2016**, *105*, 3–4.
77. Zhu, C.L.; Maeno, M.; Zhang, F.G.; Shigehiro, T.; Kagawa, T.; Kawada, K.; Shibata, N.; Ma, J.A.; Cahard, D. Chiral N-Fluorodibenzenesulfonimide Analogues for Enantioselective Electrophilic Fluorination and Oxidative Fluorination. *Eur. J. Org. Chem.* **2013**, *29*, 6501–6505. [CrossRef]
78. Shibata, N.; Ishimaru, T.; Nakamura, S.; Toru, T. New approaches to enantioselective fluorination: Cinchona alkaloids combinations and chiral ligands/metal complexes. *J. Fluorine Chem.* **2007**, *128*, 469–483. [CrossRef]
79. Mohar, B.; Baudoux, J.; Plaquevent, J.C.; Cahard, D. Electrophilic Fluorination Mediated by Cinchona Alkaloids: Highly Enantioselective Synthesis of α-Fluoro-α-phenylglycine Derivatives. *Angew. Chem. Int. Ed.* **2001**, *40*, 4214–4216. [CrossRef]
80. Cahard, D.; Audouard, C.; Plaquevent, J.C.; Roques, N. Design, Synthesis, and Evaluation of a Novel Class of Enantioselective Electrophilic Fluorinating Agents: N-Fluoro Ammonium Salts of Cinchona Alkaloids (F-CA-$BF_4$). *Org. Lett.* **2000**, *2*, 3699–3701. [CrossRef]
81. Shibata, N.; Suzuki, E.; Takeuchi, Y. A Fundamentally New Approach to Enantioselective Fluorination Based on Cinchona Alkaloid Derivatives/Selectfluor Combination. *J. Am. Chem. Soc.* **2000**, *122*, 10728–10729. [CrossRef]
82. Umemoto, T.; Nagayoshi, M. N,N′-Difluoro-1,4-diazoniabicyclo[2.2.2]octane Salts, Highly Reactive and Easy-to-Handle Electrophilic Fluorinating Agents. *Bull. Chem. Soc. Jpn.* **1996**, *69*, 2287–2295. [CrossRef]
83. Kitamura, T.; Kuriki, S.; Morshed, M.H.; Hori, Y. A Practical and Convenient Fluorination of 1,3-Dicarbonyl Compounds Using Aqueous HF in the Presence of Iodosylbenzene. *Org. Lett.* **2011**, *13*, 2392–2394. [CrossRef] [PubMed]
84. Chambers, R.D.; Greenhall, M.P.; Hutchinson, J. Direct fluorination of 1, 3-dicarbonyl compounds. *Tetrahedron* **1996**, *52*, 1–8. [CrossRef]
85. Zajc, B.; Zupan, M. Room temperature fluorination of 1, 3-diketones and enol acetates with xenon difluoride. *J. Chem. Soc. Chem. Commun.* **1980**, 759–760. [CrossRef]
86. Yemul, S.S.; Kagan, H.B.; Setton, R. Selective fluorination by $C_{19}XeF_6$. *Tetrahedron Lett.* **1980**, *21*, 277–280. [CrossRef]
87. Zajc, B.; Zupan, M. Fluorination with xenon difluoride. 27. The effect of catalyst on fluorination of 1,3-diketones and enol acetates. *J. Org. Chem.* **1982**, *47*, 573–575. [CrossRef]

88. Inman, C.E.; Oesterling, R.E.; Tyczkowski, E.A. Reactions of Perchloryl Fluoride with Organic Compounds. II. Fluorination of Certain Active Methylene Compounds1. *J. Am. Chem. Soc.* **1958**, *80*, 6533–6535. [CrossRef]
89. Machleidt, H.; Hartmann, V.I. Organische Fluorverbindungen, VI. Reaktionen cyclischer Fluor-carbonyl-Verbindungen. *Liebigs Ann. Chem.* **1964**, *679*, 9–19. [CrossRef]
90. Lerman, O.; Rozen, S. Acetyl hypofluorite, a new moderating carrier of elemental fluorine and its use in fluorination of 1,3-dicarbonyl derivatives. *J. Org. Chem.* **1983**, *48*, 724–727. [CrossRef]
91. Rozen, S.; Brand, M. Direct fluorination of lithium enolates with acetyl hypofluorite. *Synthesis* **1985**, 665–667. [CrossRef]
92. Rozen, S.; Hebel, D. Acyl hypofluorites. A new class of organic compounds. *J. Org. Chem.* **1990**, *55*, 2621–2623. [CrossRef]
93. Rozen, S.; Menahem, Y. A novel fluorinating method for the synthesis of α-fluoroketones. *Tetrahedron Lett.* **1979**, *20*, 725–728. [CrossRef]
94. Stavber, S.; Zupan, M. Room-temperature fluorination of alkenes with caesium fluoroxysulphate. *J. Chem. Soc. Chem. Commun.* **1981**, 795–796. [CrossRef]
95. Banks, R.E.; Murtagh, V.; Tsiliopoulos, E. N-halogeno compounds. Part 12 [1]. Site-specific fluorination of carbanions with perfluoro-N-fluoropiperidine [2]. *J. Fluorine Chem.* **1991**, *52*, 389–401. [CrossRef]
96. Xu, Z.Q.; DesMarteau, D.D.; Gotoh, Y. N-Fluorobis [(perfluoroalkyl) sulfonyl] imides. Efficient reagents for the fluorination of 1, 3-dicarbonyl derivatives. *J. Fluorine Chem.* **1992**, *58*, 71–79. [CrossRef]
97. Banks, R.E.; Lawrence, N.J.; Popplewell, A.L. Efficient electrophilic fluorination of β-dicarbonyl compounds with the selectfluor reagent F-TEDA-$BF_4${1-chloromethyl-4-fluoro-1,4-diazoniabicyclo[2.2.2]octane bis(tetrafluoroborate)}. *J. Chem. Soc. Chem. Commun.* **1994**, 343–344. [CrossRef]
98. Cabrera, I.; Appel, W.K. New fluorinating reagents from acesulfam sweeteners. *Tetrahedron* **1995**, *51*, 10205–10208. [CrossRef]
99. Umemoto, T.; Nagayoshi, M.; Adachi, K.; Tomizawa, G. Synthesis, Properties, and Reactivity of N,N′-Difluorobipyridinium and Related Salts and Their Applications as Reactive and Easy-To-Handle Electrophilic Fluorinating Agents with High Effective Fluorine Content. *J. Org. Chem.* **1998**, *63*, 3379–3385. [CrossRef]
100. Frantz, R.; Hintermann, L.; Perseghini, M.; Broggini, D.; Togni, A. Titanium-catalyzed stereoselective geminal heterodihalogenation of β-ketoesters. *Org. Lett.* **2003**, *5*, 1709–1712. [CrossRef]
101. Gupta, O.D.; Shreeve, J.M. Reactions of trifluoroamine oxide: A new method for selective fluorination of 1, 3-diketones and β-ketoesters. *Tetrahedron Lett.* **2003**, *44*, 2799–2801. [CrossRef]
102. Stavber, G.; Zupan, M.; Stavber, S. Solvent-free fluorination of organic compounds using N–F reagents. *Tetrahedron Lett.* **2007**, *48*, 2671–2673. [CrossRef]
103. Hara, S.; Sekiguchi, M.; Ohmori, A.; Fukuhara, T.; Yoneda, N. Selective fluorination of β-ketoesters using iodotoluene difluoride and a HF–amine complex. *Chem. Commun.* **1996**, 1899–1900. [CrossRef]
104. Yoshida, M.; Fujikawa, K.; Sato, S.; Hara, S. α-Fluorination of β-dicarbonyl compounds using p-iodotoluene difluoride under neutral conditions. *ARKIVOC* **2003**, *6*, 36–42.
105. Gondo, K.; Kitamura, T. Reaction of iodonium ylides of 1, 3-dicarbonyl compounds with HF reagents. *Molecules* **2012**, *17*, 6625–6632. [CrossRef]
106. Goudreau, S.R.; Marcoux, D.; Charette, A.B. General method for the synthesis of phenyliodonium ylides from malonate esters: Easy access to 1,1-cyclopropane diesters. *J. Org. Chem.* **2009**, *74*, 470–473. [CrossRef]
107. Kitamura, T.; Kuriki, S.; Muta, K.; Morshed, M.H.; Muta, K. Facile Synthesis of 2-Fluoro-1, 3-dicarbonyl Compounds with Aqueous Hydrofluoric Acid Mediated by Iodosylarenes. *Synthesis* **2013**, *45*, 3125–3130. [CrossRef]
108. Kitamura, T.; Muta, K.; Oyamada, J. A Convenient Synthesis of 2-Fluoro-and 2-Chloromalonic Esters Mediated by Hypervalent Iodine. *Synthesis* **2015**, *47*, 3241–3245. [CrossRef]
109. Kitamura, T.; Muta, K.; Kuriki, S. Catalytic fluorination of 1, 3-dicarbonyl compounds using iodoarene catalysts. *Tetrahedron Lett.* **2013**, *54*, 6118–6120. [CrossRef]
110. Leroy, J. 1, 2-Difluoroethylenes: Synthesis via fluoro ketones. *J. Org. Chem.* **1981**, *46*, 206–209. [CrossRef]
111. Moughamir, K.; Atmani, A.; Mestdagh, H.; Rolando, C.; Francesch, C. Activation of tetrabutylammonium hydrogen difluoride with pyridine: A mild and efficient procedure for nucleophilic fluorination. *Tetrahedron Lett.* **1998**, *39*, 7305–7306. [CrossRef]

112. Makosza, M.; Bujok, R. Cocatalysis in phase-transfer catalyzed fluorination of alkyl halides and sulfonates. *J. Fluorine Chem.* **2005**, *126*, 209–216. [CrossRef]
113. Fuglseth, E.; Thvedt, T.H.K.; Møll, M.F.; Hoff, B.H. Electrophilic and nucleophilic side chain fluorination of para-substituted acetophenones. *Tetrahedron* **2008**, *64*, 7318–7323. [CrossRef]
114. Chen, Z.; Zhu, W.; Zhen, Z.; Zou, X. One-pot α-nucleophilic fluorination of acetophenones in a deep eutectic solvent. *J. Fluorine Chem.* **2010**, *131*, 340–344. [CrossRef]
115. Li, Y.; Li, X.; Shang, H.; Chen, X.; Ren, X. Diastereoselective Mannich Reactions Using Fluorinated Ketones: Synthesis of Stereogenic Carbon–Fluorine Units. *J. Org. Chem.* **2016**, *81*, 9858–9866. [CrossRef]
116. Xu, Y.S.; Tang, Y.; Feng, H.J.; Liu, J.T.; Hsung, R.P. A Highly Regio-and Stereoselective Synthesis of α-Fluorinated Imides via Fluorination of Chiral Enamides. *Org. Lett.* **2015**, *17*, 572–575. [CrossRef]
117. Saidalimu, I.; Fang, X.; Lv, W.; Yang, X.; He, X.; Zhang, J.; Wu, F. Organocatalytic Asymmetric Michael Addition/Carbon-Carbon Bond Cleavage of Trifluoromethyl α-Fluorinated gem-Diols to Nitroolefins. *Adv. Synth. Catal.* **2013**, *355*, 857–863. [CrossRef]
118. Kitahara, K.; Mizutani, H.; Iwasa, S.; Shibatomi, K. Asymmetric Synthesis of α-Chloro-α-halo Ketones by Decarboxylative Chlorination of α-Halo-β-ketocarboxylic Acids. *Synthesis* **2019**, *51*, 4385–4392. [CrossRef]
119. Katada, M.; Kitahara, K.; Iwasa, S.; Shibatomi, K. Catalyst-free decarboxylative fluorination of tertiary β-keto carboxylic acids. *Synlett* **2018**, *29*, 2408–2411.
120. Krespan, C.G.; Smart, B.E. Fluorocarbanion chemistry. A versatile synthesis of functionalized fluoro ketones. *J. Org. Chem.* **1986**, *51*, 320–326. [CrossRef]
121. Soloshonok, V.A.; Mikami, K.; Yamazaki, T.; Welch, J.T.; Honek, J. (Eds.) *Current Fluoroorganic Chemistry. New Synthetic Directions, Technologies, Materials and Biological Applications*; ACS Symposium Series 949; Oxford University Press: Oxford, UK, 2007.
122. Xiao, X.; Xie, Y.; Su, C.; Liu, M.; Shi, Y. Organocatalytic Asymmetric Biomimetic Transamination: From α-Keto Esters to Optically Active α-Amino Acid Derivatives. *J. Am. Chem. Soc.* **2011**, *133*, 12914–12917. [CrossRef]
123. Liu, M.; Li, J.; Xie, Y.; Shi, Y. An efficient synthesis of optically active trifluoromethyl aldimines via asymmetric biomimetic transamination. *Chem. Commun.* **2013**, *49*, 1404–1406. [CrossRef] [PubMed]
124. Soloshonok, V.A.; Kukhar, V.P. Biomimetic transamination of α-keto perfluorocarboxylic esters. An efficient preparative synthesis of β,β,β-trifluoroalanine. *Tetrahedron* **1997**, *53*, 8307–8314. [CrossRef]
125. Soloshonok, V.A.; Ohkura, H.; Yasumoto, M. Operationally convenient asymmetric synthesis of (*S*)- and (*R*)-3-amino-4,4,4-trifluorobutanoic acid: Part I: Enantioselective biomimetic transamination of isopropyl 4,4,4-trifluoro-3-oxo-butanoate. *J. Fluorine Chem.* **2006**, *127*, 924–929. [CrossRef]
126. Guo, C.; Song, J.; Gong, L.Z. Biomimetic Asymmetric 1,3-Dioplar Cycloaddition: Amino Acid Precursors in Biosynthesis Serve as Latent Azomethine Ylides. *Org. Lett.* **2013**, *15*, 2676–2679. [CrossRef] [PubMed]
127. Soloshonok, V.A.; Soloshonok, I.V.; Kukhar, V.P.; Svedas, V.K. Biomimetic Transamination of α-Alkyl β-Keto Carboxylic Esters. Chemoenzymatic Approach to the Stereochemically Defined α-Alkyl β-Fluoroalkyl β-Amino Acids. *J. Org. Chem.* **1998**, *63*, 1878–1884. [CrossRef]
128. Xiao, X.; Liu, M.; Rong, C.; Xue, F.; Li, S.; Xie, Y.; Shi, Y. An Efficient Asymmetric Biomimetic Transamination of α-Keto Esters to Chiral α-Amino Esters. *Org. Lett.* **2012**, *14*, 5270–5273. [CrossRef]
129. Soloshonok, V.A.; Ono, T.; Soloshonok, I.V. Enantioselective Biomimetic Transamination of β-Keto Carboxylic Acid Derivatives. An Efficient Asymmetric Synthesis of β-Fluoroalkyl-β-Amino Acids. *J. Org. Chem.* **1997**, *62*, 7538–7539.
130. Soloshonok, V.A.; Ono, T. The Effect of Substituents on the Feasibility of Azomethine-Azomethine Isomerization: New Synthetic Opportunities for Biomimetic Transamination. *Tetrahedron* **1996**, *52*, 14701–14712. [CrossRef]
131. Soloshonok, V.A.; Ohkura, H.; Yasumoto, M. Operationally Convenient Asymmetric Synthesis of (*S*)- and (*R*)-3-Amino-4,4,4-trifluorobutanoic Acid. Part II: Enantioselective Biomimetic Transamination of 4,4,4-Trifluoro-3-oxo-*N*-[(*R*)-1-phenylethyl)butanamide. *J. Fluorine Chem.* **2006**, *127*, 930–935. [CrossRef]
132. Barnette, W.E. N-Fluoro-N-alkylsulfonamides: Useful reagents for the fluorination of carbanions. *J. Am. Chem. Soc.* **1984**, *106*, 452–454. [CrossRef]
133. Differding, E.; Lang, R.W. New fluorinating reagents-I. The first enantioselective fluorination reaction. *Tetrahedron Lett.* **1988**, *29*, 6087–6090. [CrossRef]

134. Resnati, G.; DesMarteau, D.D. N-fluorobis [(trifluoromethyl) sulfonyl] imide: An efficient reagent for the. alpha.-fluorination of functionalized carbonyl compounds. *J. Org. Chem.* **1991**, *56*, 4925–4929. [CrossRef]
135. Davis, F.A.; Han, W. N-Fluoro-o-benzenedisulfonimide: A useful new fluorinating reagent. *Tetrahedron Lett.* **1991**, *32*, 1631–1634. [CrossRef]
136. Davis, F.A.; Zhou, P.; Murphy, C.K. Asymmetric fluorination of enolates with N-fluoro 2, 10-(3, 3-dichlorocamphorsultam). *Tetrahedron Lett.* **1993**, *34*, 3971–3974. [CrossRef]
137. Middleton, W.J.; Bingham, E.M. alpha-Fluorination of carbonyl compounds with trifluoromethyl hypofluorite. *J. Am. Chem. Soc.* **1980**, *102*, 4845–4846. [CrossRef]
138. Purrington, S.T.; Lazaridis, N.V.; Bumgardner, C.L. Preparation of α-fluoroaldehydes and α-fluoroketones using dilute fluorine. *Tetrahedron Lett.* **1986**, *27*, 2715–2716. [CrossRef]
139. Umemoto, T.; Kawada, K.; Tomita, K. N-fluoropyridinium triflate and its derivatives: Useful fluorinating agents. *Tetrahedron Lett.* **1986**, *27*. [CrossRef]
140. Kitamura, T.; Muta, K.; Muta, K. Hypervalent Iodine-Promoted α-Fluorination of Acetophenone Derivatives with a Triethylamine· HF Complex. *J. Org. Chem.* **2014**, *79*, 5842–5846. [CrossRef]
141. Rueeger, H.; Lueoend, R.; Rogel, O.; Rondeau, J.M.; Möbitz, H.; Machauer, R.; Jacobson, L.; Staufenbiel, M.; Desrayaud, S.; Neumann, U. Discovery of Cyclic Sulfone Hydroxyethylamines as Potent and Selective β-Site APP-Cleaving Enzyme 1 (BACE1) Inhibitors: Structure-Based Design and in Vivo Reduction of Amyloid β-Peptides. *J. Med. Chem.* **2012**, *55*, 3364–3386. [CrossRef]
142. Levin, V.V.; Zemtsov, A.A.; Struchkova, M.I.; Dilman, A.D. Reactions of organozinc reagents with potassium bromodifluoroacetate. *J. Fluorine Chem.* **2015**, *171*, 97–101. [CrossRef]
143. Dolbier, W.R., Jr.; Okamoto, M. Preparation of 1, 1-difluoroalkanes from aldehydes via 1, 1-bistriflates: Advantageous use of HF–Lewis base reagents. *J. Fluorine Chem.* **2014**, *167*, 96–100. [CrossRef]
144. Bujok, R.; Mlkosza, M. Synthesis of 1, 1-Difluoroalkanes via Phase Transfer Catalysed Reaction of 1, 1-bis-Triflates with KF in the Presence of Cocatalyst-Ph3SnF. *Synlett* **2002**, 1285–1286.
145. Martinez, A.G.; Barcina, J.O.; Rys, A.Z.; Subramanian, L.R. A facile conversion of aliphatic aldehydes to 1, 1-difluoroalkanes. *Tetrahedron Lett.* **1992**, *33*, 7787–7788. [CrossRef]
146. Bloodworth, A.J.; Bowyer, K.J.; Mitchell, J.C. A mild, convenient, halogen-exchange route to gem-difluorides and trifluorides. *Tetrahedron Lett.* **1987**, *28*, 5347–5350. [CrossRef]
147. Patrick, T.B.; Johri, K.K.; White, D.H. Fluoro-decarboxylation with xenon difluoride. *J. Org. Chem.* **1983**, *48*, 4158–4159. [CrossRef]
148. Patrick, T.B.; Johri, K.K.; White, D.H.; Bertrand, W.S.; Mokhtar, R.; Kilbourn, M.R.; Welch, M.J. Replacement of the carboxylic acid function with fluorine. *Can. J. Chem.* **1986**, *64*, 138–141. [CrossRef]
149. Salomon, P.; Zard, S.Z. A Practical Source of Chlorodifluoromethyl Radicals. Convergent Routes to gem-Difluoroalkenes and -dienes and (2,2-Difluoroethyl)-indoles, -azaindoles, and –naphthols. *Org. Lett.* **2014**, *16*, 2926–2929. [CrossRef]
150. Zupan, M.; Pollak, A. Preparation of a polymer-supported aryliodine(III) difluoride and its use to fluorinate olefins to difluorides. *J. Chem. Soc. Chem. Commun.* **1975**, 715–716. [CrossRef]
151. Carpenter, W.R. Aryliodosodifluorides. *J. Org. Chem.* **1966**, *31*, 2688–2689. [CrossRef]
152. Lermontov, S.A.; Rakov, I.M.; Zefirov, N.S.; Stang, P.J. Hexafluoropropene oxide–a fluorinating reagent for the formation of element–fluorine bonds. *J. Fluorine Chem.* **1999**, *93*, 103–106. [CrossRef]
153. Patrick, T.B.; Qian, S. Rearrangement of Phenylethenes on Reaction with Iodine–Xenon Difluoride. *Org. Lett.* **2000**, *2*, 3359–3360. [CrossRef]
154. Hara, S.; Nakahigashi, J.; Ishi-i, K.; Fukuhara, T.; Yoneda, N. Fluorinative ring-contraction of cyclic alkenes with p-iodotoluene difluoride. *Tetrahedron Lett.* **1998**, *39*, 2589–2592. [CrossRef]
155. Sawaguchi, M.; Hara, S.; Yoneda, N. Fluorination of alkenes by iodoarene difluorides. *J. Fluorine Chem.* **2000**, *105*, 313–317. [CrossRef]
156. Zupan, M.; Pollak, A. Fluorination with xenon difluoride. Preparation of aryliodine/III/difluoride. *J. Fluorine. Chem.* **1976**, *7*, 445–447. [CrossRef]
157. Kitamura, T.; Muta, K.; Oyamada, J. Hypervalent Iodine-Mediated Fluorination of Styrene Derivatives: Stoichiometric and Catalytic Transformation to 2,2-Difluoroethylarenes. *J. Org. Chem.* **2015**, *80*, 10431–10436. [CrossRef]
158. Ilchenko, N.O.; Tasch, B.O.A.; Szabo, K.J. Mild Silver-Mediated Geminal Difluorination of Styrenes Using an Air- and Moisture-Stable Fluoroiodane Reagent. *Angew. Chem. Int. Ed.* **2014**, *53*, 12897–12901. [CrossRef]

159. Kitamura, T.; Yoshida, K.; Mizuno, S.; Miyake, A.; Oyamada, J. Difluorination of functionalized aromatic olefins using hypervalent iodine/HF reagents. *J. Org. Chem.* **2018**, *83*, 14853–14860. [CrossRef]
160. Xu, J.; Wei, L.; Mathvink, R.; He, J.; Park, Y.J.; He, H.; Leiting, B.; Lyons, K.A.; Marsilio, F.; Patel, R.A.; et al. Discovery of potent and selective phenylalanine based dipeptidyl peptidase IV inhibitors. *Bioorg. Med. Chem. Lett.* **2005**, *15*, 2533–2536. [CrossRef]
161. Augustyns, K.J.L.; Lambeir, A.M.; Borloo, M.; De Meester, I.; Vedernikova, I.; Vanhoof, G.; Hendriks, D.; Scharpe, S.; Haemers, A. Pyrrolidides: Synthesis and structure-activity relationship as inhibitors of dipeptidyl peptidase IV. *Eur. J. Med. Chem.* **1997**, *32*, 301–309. [CrossRef]
162. Caldwell, C.G.; Chen, P.; He, J.; Parmee, E.R.; Leiting, B.; Marsilio, F.; Patel, R.A.; Wu, J.K.; Eiermann, G.J.; Petrov, A.; et al. Fluoropyrrolidine amides as dipeptidyl peptidase IV inhibitors. *Bioorg. Med. Chem. Lett.* **2004**, *14*, 1265–1268. [CrossRef]
163. Fukushima, H.; Hiratate, A.; Takahashi, M.; Mikami, A.; Saito-Hori, M.; Munetomo, E.; Kitano, K.; Chonan, S.; Saito, H.; Suzuki, A.; et al. Synthesis and structure–activity relationships of potent 4-fluoro-2-cyanopyrrolidine dipeptidyl peptidase IV inhibitors. *Bioorg. Med. Chem.* **2008**, *16*, 4093–4106. [CrossRef]
164. Mao, W.; Ning, M.; Liu, Z.; Zhu, Q.; Leng, Y.; Zhang, A. Design, synthesis, and pharmacological evaluation of benzamide derivatives as glucokinase activators. *Bioorg. Med. Chem.* **2012**, *20*, 2982–2991. [CrossRef] [PubMed]
165. Goossens, F.; Vanhoof, G.; Meester, I.; Augustyns, K.; Borloo, M.; Tourwe, D.; Haemers, A.; Scharpe, S. Development and Evaluation of Peptide-Based Prolyl Oligopeptidase Inhibitors- Introduction of N-Benzyloxycarbonyl-Prolyl-3-Fluoropyrrolidine as a Lead in Inhibitor Design. *Eur. J. Biochem.* **1997**, *250*, 177–183. [CrossRef] [PubMed]
166. Mason, J.M.; Murkin, A.S.; Li, L.; Schramm, V.L.; Gainsford, G.J.; Skelton, B.W. A β-Fluoroamine Inhibitor of Purine Nucleoside Phosphorylase. *J. Med. Chem.* **2008**, *51*, 5880–5884. [CrossRef] [PubMed]
167. Giardina, G.; Dondio, G.; Grugni, M. Facile and Efficient Syntheses of Novel (S)- and (R)-3-Fluoropyrrolidines and 3,3-Difluoropyrrolidine. *Synlett* **1995**, *1995*, 55–57. [CrossRef]
168. Demange, L.; Cluzeau, J.; Ménez, A.; Dugave, C. Synthesis of optically pure N-Boc-protected (2R,3R)- and (2R,3S)-3-fluoroprolines. *Tetrahedron Lett.* **2001**, *42*, 651–653. [CrossRef]
169. Doi, M.; Nishi, Y.; Kiritoshi, N.; Iwata, T.; Nago, M.; Nakano, H.; Uchiyama, S.; Nakazawa, T.; Wakamiya, T.; Kobayashi, Y. Simple and efficient syntheses of Boc- and Fmoc-protected 4(R)- and 4(S)-fluoroproline solely from 4(R)-hydroxyproline. *Tetrahedron* **2002**, *58*, 8453–8459. [CrossRef]
170. Verniest, G.; Piron, K.; Van Hende, E.; Thuring, J.W.; Macdonald, G.; Deroose, F.; De Kimpe, N. Synthesis of aminomethylated 4-fluoropiperidines and 3-fluoropyrrolidines. *Org. Biomol. Chem.* **2010**, *8*, 2509–2512. [CrossRef]
171. Fjelbye, K.; Marigo, M.; Clausen, R.P.; Juhl, K. Diastereodivergent Access to Syn and Anti 3,4-Substituted β-Fluoropyrrolidines: Enhancing or Reversing Substrate Preference. *Org. Lett.* **2016**, *18*, 1170–1173. [CrossRef]
172. Kong, W.; Merino, E.; Nevado, C. Divergent Reaction Mechanisms in the Aminofluorination of Alkenes. *Chimia* **2014**, *68*, 430–435. [CrossRef]
173. Chen, P.; Liu, G. Advancements in Aminofluorination of Alkenes and Alkynes: Convenient Access to β-Fluoroamines. *Eur. J. Org. Chem.* **2015**, *2015*, 4295–4309. [CrossRef]
174. Combettes, L.E.; Lozano, O.; Gouverneur, V. Metal free fluoroamination of allylsilanes: A route to 3-fluoropyrrolidines. *J. Fluorine Chem.* **2012**, *143*, 167–176. [CrossRef]
175. Xu, T.; Qiu, S.; Liu, G. Palladium-Catalyzed Intramolecular Aminofluorination of Styrenes. *Chin. J. Chem.* **2011**, *29*, 2785–2790. [CrossRef]
176. Cui, J.; Jia, Q.; Feng, R.Z.; Liu, S.S.; He, T.; Zhang, C. Boron Trifluoride Etherate Functioning as a Fluorine Source in an Iodosobenzene-Mediated Intramolecular Aminofluorination of Homoallylic Amines. *Org. Lett.* **2014**, *16*, 1442–1445. [CrossRef]
177. Kitamura, T.; Miyake, A.; Muta, K.; Oyamada, J. Hypervalent Iodine/HF Reagents for the Synthesis of 3-Fluoropyrrolidines. *J. Org. Chem.* **2017**, *82*, 11721–11726. [CrossRef]
178. Kitamura, T.; Mizuno, S.; Muta, K.; Oyamada, J. Synthesis of β-Fluorovinyliodonium Salts by the Reaction of Alkynes with Hypervalent Iodine/HF Reagents. *J. Org. Chem.* **2018**, *83*, 2773–2778. [CrossRef]

179. Dolbier, W.R., Jr.; Celewicz, L.; Ohnishi, K. Fluorination reactions with HF/THF medium solvolysis of N-tosyl-O-phenylhydroxylamine. *Tetrahedron Lett.* **1989**, *30*, 4929–4930. [CrossRef]
180. Dolbier, W.R., Jr.; Gray, T.A.; Onnishi, K. Hydrogen Fluoride/Tetrahydrofuran as a Fluorinating Medium. A General Synthesis of 1,1,1,2-Tetrafluoro-2-alkenes. *Synthesis* **1987**, 956–958. [CrossRef]

*molecules*

MDPI

*Article*

# Catalyst-Solvent System for PASE Approach to Hydroxyquinolinone-Substituted Chromeno[2,3-*b*]pyridines Its Quantum Chemical Study and Investigation of Reaction Mechanism

**Fedor V. Ryzhkov [1], Yuliya E. Ryzhkova [1], Michail N. Elinson [1,*], Stepan V. Vorobyev [2], Artem N. Fakhrutdinov [1], Anatoly N. Vereshchagin [1] and Mikhail P. Egorov [1]**

1 N. D. Zelinsky Institute of Organic Chemistry Russian Academy of Sciences, Leninsky pr. 47, 119991 Moscow, Russia; ryzhkov.fe@ya.ru (F.V.R.); julia4912@mail.ru (Y.E.R.); fak.part@gmail.com (A.N.F.); anatoly103@yandex.ru (A.N.V.); mpe@ioc.ac.ru (M.P.E.)

2 Department of Organic Chemistry and Petroleum Chemistry, Gubkin Russian State University of Oil and Gas, 65 Leninsky Prospect, 119991 Moscow, Russia; vorstepan@yandex.ru

* Correspondence: elinson@ioc.ac.ru

Academic Editor: Maged Henary

Received: 4 May 2020; Accepted: 29 May 2020; Published: 31 May 2020

**Abstract:** The Pot, Atom, and Step Economy (PASE) approach is based on the Pot economy principle and unites it with the Atom and Step Economy strategies; it ensures high efficiency, simplicity and low waste formation. The PASE approach is widely used in multicomponent chemistry. This approach was adopted for the synthesis of previously unknown hydroxyquinolinone substituted chromeno[2,3-*b*]pyridines via reaction of salicylaldehydes, malononitrile dimer and hydroxyquinolinone. It was shown that an ethanol-pyridine combination is more beneficial than other inorganic or organic catalysts. Quantum chemical studies showed that chromeno[2,3-*b*]pyridines has potential for corrosion inhibition. Real time $^1$H NMR monitoring was used for the investigation of reaction mechanism and 2-((2*H*-chromen-3-yl)methylene)malononitrile was defined as a key intermediate in the reaction.

**Keywords:** salicylaldehyde; malononitrile dimer; hydroxyquinolinone; chromeno[2,3-*b*]pyridines; multicomponent reactions; PASE approach; corrosion inhibitor; NMR monitoring

## 1. Introduction

Multicomponent reactions (MCRs) employ three or more reactants to obtain heterocycles containing structures of all starting materials in a one-pot process under fixed reaction conditions [1–4]. It provides powerful productivity to satisfy modern green chemistry requirements, but new synthetic strategies with robust efficiency are still demanded. In this connection, the PASE approach has recently emerged [5,6], it is based on the Pot economy principle and unites it with the Atom and Step Economy strategies (PASE), thereby ensuring high efficiency, simplicity and low waste formation [7–10]. Nowadays, it is emerging as a fast-paced research front of organic chemistry [11–16].

Corrosion is a gradual destruction of refined metal by means of reactions with environment. Today it causes heavy losses to the economy [17–19]. Due to electronic configuration of heterocyclic compounds, they are capable of corrosion inhibition or coating metals. The development of PASE approaches to anti-corrosion heterocycles is beneficial for protection of metals.

Chromeno [2,3-*b*]pyridines are heterocycles with special and useful electronic configuration. Thus, they showed gastric antisecretory activity [20], inhibit mitogen-activated protein kinase 2 and suppress expression of tumor necrosis factor alpha (TNFα) in U937 cells [21].

Similar compounds were earlier synthesized via microwave irradiation of aldehydes, malononitrile dimer and kojic acid in EtOH [22]. The synthesis was carried out under reflux conditions in the presence of $Et_3N$ as a catalyst (73–90% yields). Bis-chromeno[2,3-*b*]pyridine derivatives were obtained via reaction of bis-aldehydes, malononitrile dimer and dimedone under reflux conditions. The reaction was carried out for 5 h in EtOH with a large amount of piperidine [23]. Phenyl substituted derivatives were obtained by reaction of benzaldehydes, malononitrile dimer and naphthols (12%–62% yields). The reaction was carried out under reflux conditions in $H_2O$-EtOH with an equivalent amount of $Et_2NH$ [24] and in solvent-free conditions with guanidine hydrochloride catalysis (100 °C, 2 h) [25]. Solvent-free conditions were also used for the transformation of benzaldehydes, malononitrile dimer and coumarin [26]. Carbazole and indole derivatives were synthesized (67–85%) under reflux conditions and microwave irradiation: by reaction of aldehydes, malononitrile dimer and hydroxycarbazole or hydroxyindole in anhydrous EtOH with EtONa [27].

We have already described multicomponent syntheses of chromeno[2,3-*b*]pyridines [28–34]. However, there are no reports on a PASE synthesis of hydroxyquinolinone substituted chromeno[2,3-*b*]pyridines. Therefore, our attention was devoted toward reactions of salicylaldehydes, malononitrile dimer and hydroxyquinolinone. We were interested in developing the PASE method, clarifying reaction mechanism and defining the actual intermediates of the reaction. We were also prompted to carry out quantum chemical studies and estimate chromeno[2,3-*b*]pyridine potential for corrosion inhibition.

## 2. Results and Discussion

### 2.1. PASE Approach

Initially, to examine the reaction of salicylaldehyde **1a**, malononitrile dimer **2** and hydroxyquinolinone **3**, we have carried out multicomponent synthesis of chromeno[2,3-*b*]pyridine **4a** under solvent-free conditions (Scheme 1, Table 1). Previously, AcONa and KF have successfully catalyzed similar processes under solvent-free conditions [32]. AcONa showed better results (Entry 3) than KF (Entry 2) and provided twice the yield as the reaction without catalyst (Entry 1). 'On-water' [33–35] reactions showed almost the same results as solvent-free experiments (Entries 4,5).

Further, we have examined the multicomponent reaction in alcohol media. The reaction in EtOH without catalyst resulted in assembling of chromeno[2,3-*b*]pyridine **4a** in 19% yield (Entry 6), in the presence of AcONa it was formed in 35% yield (Entry 7) whereas organocatalysis by $Et_3N$ and morpholine resulted in 63% and 57% yields (Entries 8 and 9).

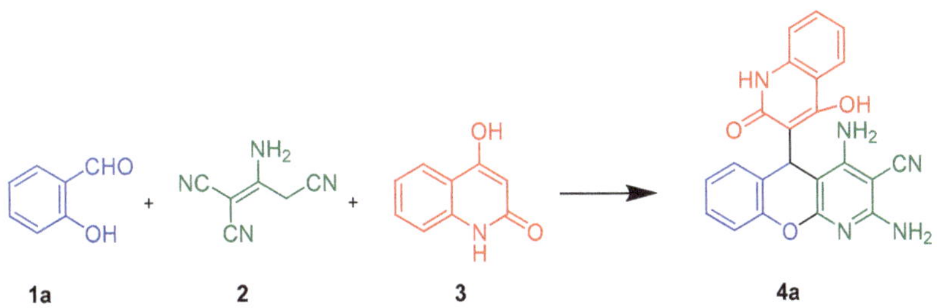


**Scheme 1.** Reaction of salicylaldehyde, malononitrile dimer and hydroxyquinolinone.

**Table 1.** Optimization of reaction conditions [1].

| Entry | Solvent | Catalyst | Time (h) | Temp (°C) | Yield (%) |
|---|---|---|---|---|---|
| 1 | Solvent-free | - | 2 | 80 | 17 |
| 2 | Solvent-free | KF | 2 | 80 | 25 |
| 3 | Solvent-free | AcONa | 2 | 80 | 37 |
| 4 | $H_2O$ | - | 2 | 80 | 16 |
| 5 | $H_2O$ | AcONa | 2 | 80 | 31 |
| 6 | EtOH | - | 2 | 78 | 19 [2] |
| 7 | EtOH | AcONa | 2 | 78 | 35 [2] |
| 8 | EtOH | $Et_3N$ | 2 | 78 | 63 [2] |
| 9 | EtOH | Morph | 2 | 78 | 57 [2] |
| 10 | Py | - | 2 | 116 | 61 [2] |
| 11 | EtOH-Py (4:1) | - | 2 | 78 | 87 [2] |
| 12 | EtOH-Py (3:1) | - | 2 | 78 | 95 [2] |
| 13 | EtOH-Py (2:1) | - | 2 | 78 | 92 [2] |
| 14 | EtOH-Py (3:1) | - | 1 | 78 | 89 [2] |

[1] Reaction conditions **1a** (1 mmol), **2** (1 mmol), **3** (1 mmol) were heated in 4 mL of solvent or without solvent; with 10 mol% of catalyst or without catalyst. [2] Isolated yield, in other cases NMR data.

Pyridine (Py) has been already employed as a solvent and catalyst for similar processes [36]. Refluxing of salicylaldehyde **1a**, malononitrile dimer **2** and hydroxyquinone **3** in Py for 2 h resulted in 61% yield (Entry 10). Py is a good solvent for structures of this type, however, a small amount of chromeno[2,3-*b*]pyridine **4a** always remains dissolved in Py.

Then, reaction in a mixture of EtOH and Py was carried out. In the volumetric range of EtOH:Py (2-4:1), the best yield was in EtOH-Py (3:1) and chromeno[2,3-*b*]pyridine **4a** was isolated in excellent 95% yield (Entry 12).

Figure 1 shows that this organic catalyst is more effective than inorganic KF or AcONa catalysts and the 'EtOH-Py' system is more beneficial than 'solvent-free' and 'on-water' approaches to chromeno[2,3-*b*]pyridine **4a**. Py in EtOH keeps the intermediates dissolved and ensures optimal basicity [37] supporting the reaction.

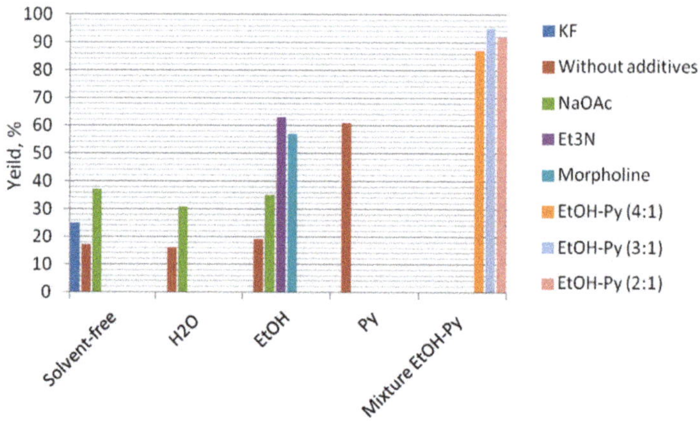


**Figure 1.** Comparison diagram of approaches to chromeno[2,3-*b*]pyridine **4a**. The mixture of EtOH-Py (3:1) provides the best result.

When the reaction in EtOH:Py mixture was finished, the final compound was directly crystallized in pure form after cooling. Under the optimal conditions (Entry12: refluxing for 2 h in 4 mL of EtOH-Py (3:1) mixture) multicomponent reactions of salicylaldehydes **1a–i**, malononitrile dimer **2** and hydroxyquinolinone **3** were carried out. Chromeno[2,3-*b*]pyridines **4a–i** were obtained in 59–98%

yields (Table 2). In general, substitution reduced yields of chromeno[2,3-*b*]pyridines **4b–i**. Presumably, electronic effects were taking place: electron-donating methyl, methoxy and ethoxy groups tended to support higher yields than bromo and nitro groups. The yield of chlorine substituted compound was bigger than in the case of bromo substituted compound due to a mesomeric effect.

**Table 2.** PASE reaction of salicylaldehydes **1a–i**, malononitrile dimer **2** and hydroxyquinolinone **3** [1].

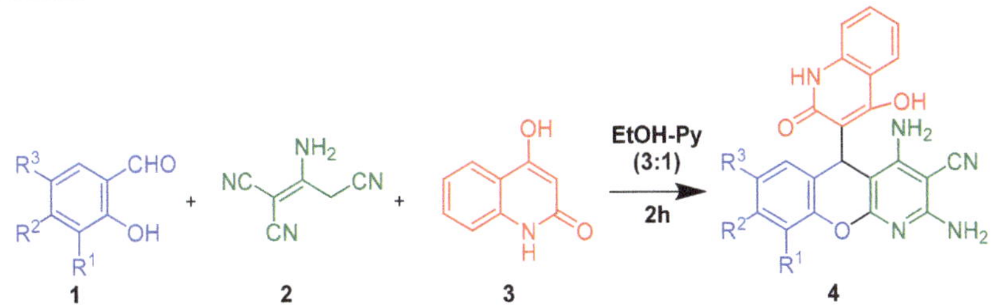


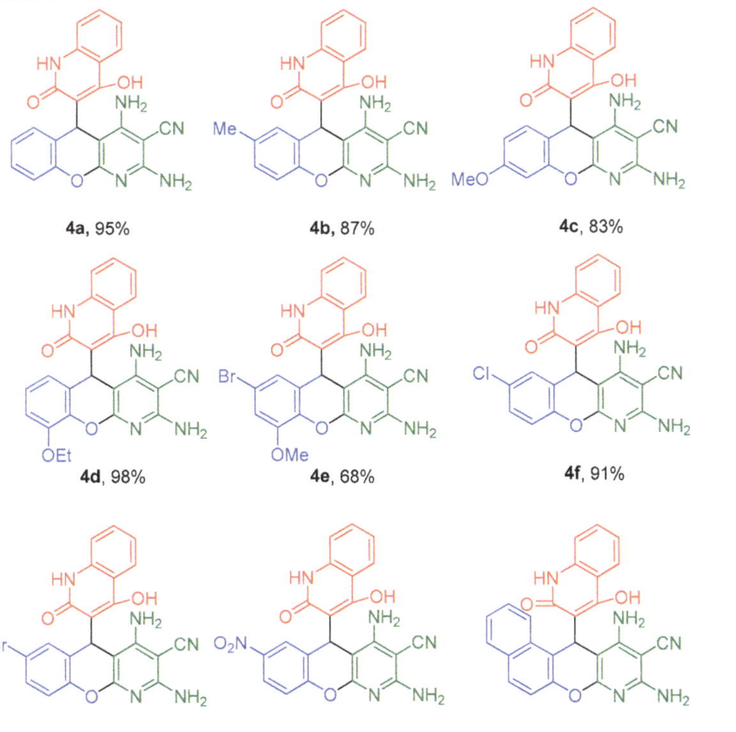


[1] Reaction conditions: **1a–i** (1 mmol), **2** (1 mmol), **3** (1 mmol) were refluxed in 4 mL of EtOH-Py mixture (3:1). Isolated yields.

Considering the mechanism of this multicomponent reaction, several path-ways for the reaction were possible. Salicylaldehyde **1** may have undergone condensation either with malononitrile dimer **2** or hydroxyquinolinone **3** (Scheme 2). Hence, four main pathways of the reaction could be discussed. Path 1 started from Knoevenagel condensation of salicylaldehyde **1** and malononitrile dimer **2**, then cyclization into intermediate **5** proceeded. The cyclization was followed by Michael addition of hydroxyquinolinone **3** and another cyclization. Path 2 [38,39] started from Knoevenagel condensation of salicylaldehyde **1** and malononitrile dimer **2**. Further Michael addition of hydroxyquinolinone **3** to intermediate **7** took place, and subsequent double cyclization of the malononitrile fragment formed chromeno[2,3-*b*]pyridine **4**. Path 3 began with Knoevenagel condensation of salicylaldehyde **1** and hydroxyquinolinone **3**. Formation of chromeno[2,3-*b*]pyridine **4** proceeded via intermediate **8**. In Path 4, salicylaldehyde **1** undergoes condensation with malononitrile dimer **2**, and then double cyclization took place to form intermediate **10**. Further, addition of hydroxyquinolinone **3** formed chromeno[2,3-*b*]pyridine **4**.

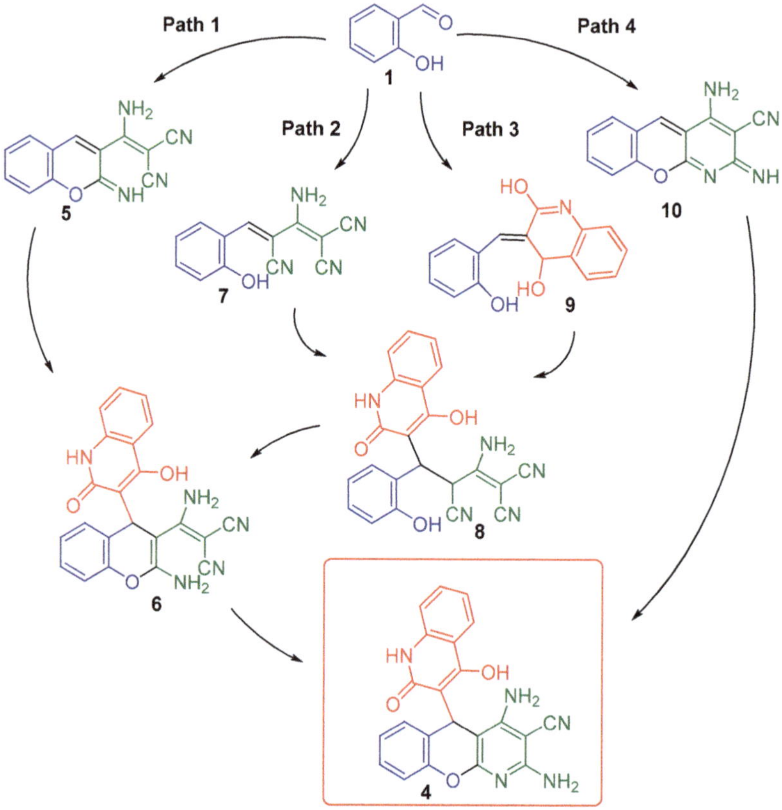


**Scheme 2.** The key intermediates for the possible pathways to chromeno[2,3-*b*]pyridine formation.

In order to gain insight into the reaction mechanism, we have performed $^1$H NMR monitoring, to obtain constituent data on the reaction. To reduce the influence of sample preparation, the transformation of starting materials into chromeno[2,3-*b*]pyridine **4a** was carried out and monitored directly into a spectrometer without catalyst to slow down the reaction.

During the NMR study, six major components were recorded: salicylaldehyde **1a**, malononitrile dimer **2** and hydroxyquinolinone **3**, intermediate **5**, intermediate **7** and chromeno[2,3-*b*]pyridine **4a**. A representative $^1$H NMR spectrum with assignment of peaks showed on Figure 2.

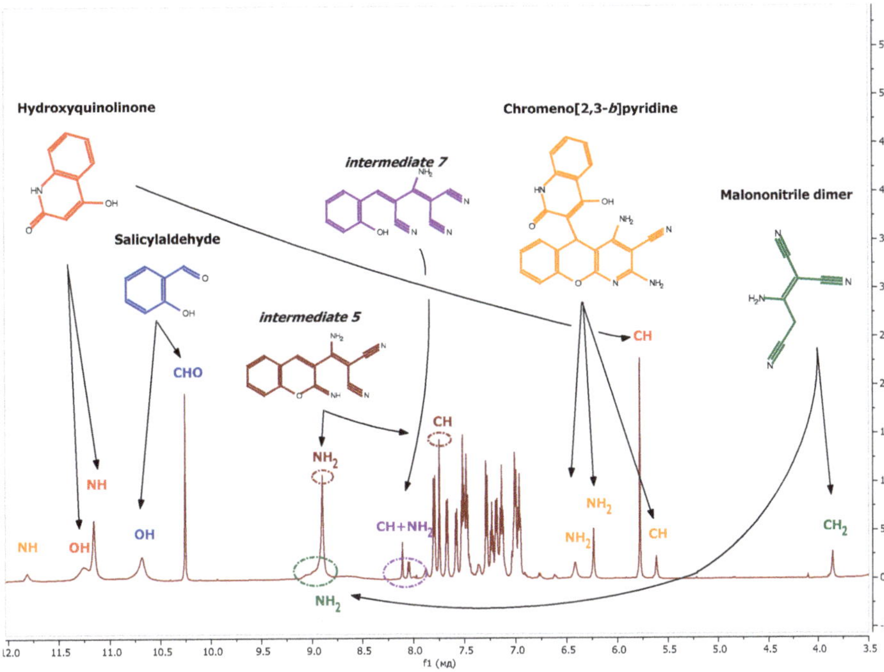


**Figure 2.** Representative $^1$H NMR spectrum of multicomponent reaction in DMSO-$d_6$ at 313 K recorded 2 h after dissolution.

The starting materials are well known (we estimated the presence of salicylaldehyde **1a** by the singlet at 10.25 ppm, malononitrile dimer **2** by the singlet at 3.85 ppm and hydroxyquinolinone by the singlet at 5.78 ppm); compound **4a** is described in this manuscript and was estimated by the signal at 5.61 ppm; intermediate **5** was described previously (7.75 ppm) [40]; intermediate **7** was estimated by the signals at 8.04–8.11 ppm [41].

Figure 3 presents a series of $^1$H NMR spectra for a conversion of starting materials into the final compound **4a** in DMSO-$d_6$. It shows the disappearance of malononitrile dimer **2** (in 20 min to 2 h from the beginning of experiment) and the simultaneous formation of intermediate **7** and intermediate **5**. Intermediate **7** formed by Knoevenagel condensation and it was followed by cyclization into intermediate **5** (Scheme 2). Thus, intermediate **7** was forming and rapidly converting into intermediate **5** (1–3 h of experiment). Eventually the signals of intermediate **7** disappeared.

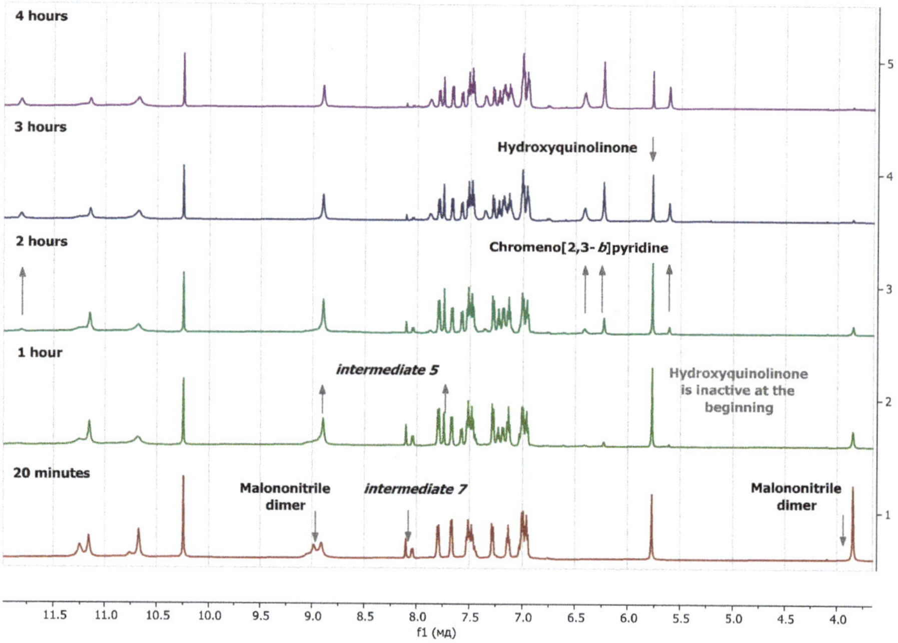


**Figure 3.** Real-time monitoring of chemical reaction by $^1$H NMR spectroscopy in DMSO-$d_6$ at 313 K. The NMR spectra of all the synthesized compounds, as well as the NMR spectra of the real-time monitoring are presented in Supplementary Materials (Figures S1–S42).

As shown in Figure 3, when intermediate **7** disappeared (Figure 3), hydroxyquinolinone **3** signals disappeared and chromeno[2,3-*b*]pyridine **4a** signals appeared. Thus, hydroxyquinolinone **3** took part in Michael addition to the electron-deficient intermediate **5** to form final compound **4a**.

Based on these data and taking into consideration earlier published results [42,43], we suggest that the first stage was a rapid formation of intermediate **7** with expulsion of a hydroxide anion [37]. This hydroxide anion instantly catalyzed a rapid cyclization of intermediate **7** into intermediate **5**. Then, subsequent Michael addition and cyclization formed the chromeno[2,3-*b*]pyridine **4a**.

To prove this conclusion, the intermediate **5** was isolated in a one-step reaction. Further addition of hydroxyquinolinone **3** to the obtained intermediate **5** in a distinct reactor afforded chromeno[2,3-*b*]pyridine **4a**. The reaction conditions were the same as developed for multicomponent process and the yield of chromeno[2,3-*b*]pyridine **4a** was 95% again. More than that, the two-component reaction of salicylaldehyde **1a** and hydroxyquinolinone **3** in a separate reactor did not form intermediate **9**. This experimental data and $^1$NMR monitoring data were consistent with each other. Thus, the results from both intermediate synthesis and $^1$NMR monitoring turned out to be consistent with each other.

Moreover, both $^1$NMR monitoring and experimental data (Tables 1 and 2) revealed no signals of intermediate **9 [44]**: 7.11–7.16 (m, 1H), 7.36 (s, 1H), 7.54–7.58 (m, 1H), 7.67–7.70 (d, 1H, *J* = 8.4 Hz), 7.93–7.99 (m, 4H), 8.45–8.48 (d, 1H, *J* = 8.4 Hz), 10.22 (s, 1H), 11.19 (s, 1H) ppm.

To sum up, we postulated Path 1 for the assembling of chromeno[2,3-*b*]pyridine **4a** in this multicomponent process. The proposed mechanism for the developed reaction is outlined in Scheme 3.

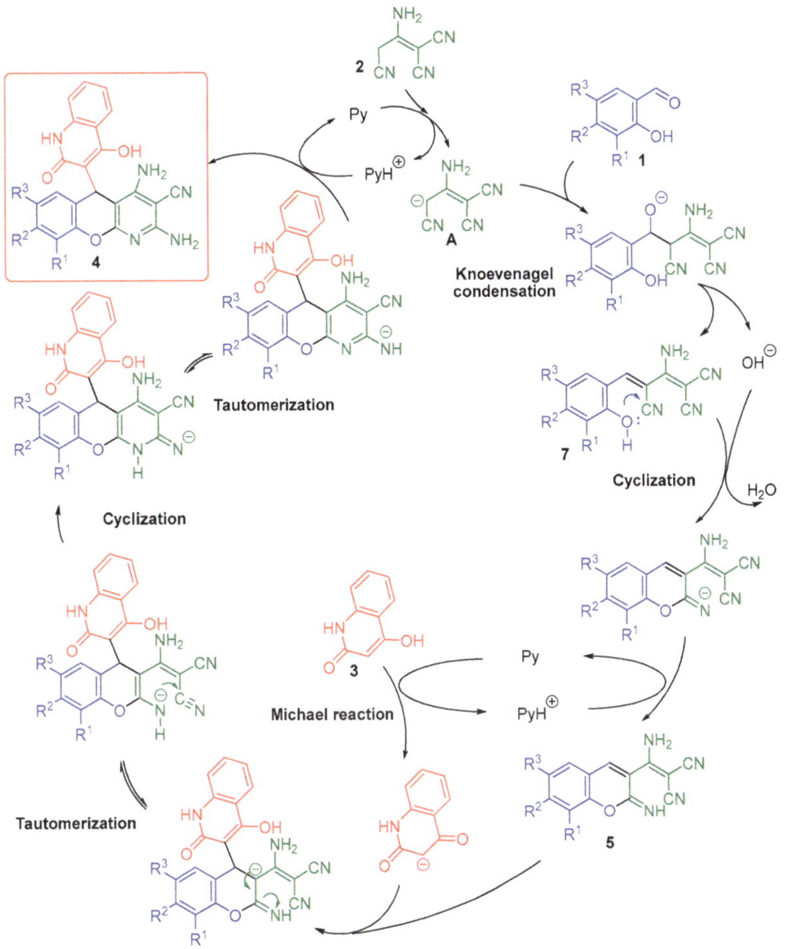


**Scheme 3.** Mechanism of salicylaldehydes **1**, malononitrile dimer **2** and hydroxyquinolinone **3** transformation into chromeno[2,3-*b*]pyridine **4**. Catalytic cycles are simplified.

## 2.2. *Quantum Chemical Investigation*

### 2.2.1. Quantum Chemistry Approach

One of the most well-known corrosion inhibitors are heterocycles, such as azoles [45,46], pyridines [47], several bioorganic compounds [48] and chromenes [49]. The mechanism of their action is the adsorption on the metal's surface (whatever metal is used–copper, steel, brass, etc.). Generally, the greater the number of electron-donating groups in molecule, the higher the probability of adsorption and inhibition activity. As it was shown previously, the inhibitory activity of organic compounds can be predicted properly by quantum-chemical methods [50–52]. This reduces the time of the study and hazardous reactant wasting by selecting the hit-compounds. They must have appropriate electronic properties, which can be estimated by quantum chemistry calculations, to interact with metal's surface.

To estimate electronic properties, the next method can be used [53]: according to Koopman's theorem, the energy of the highest occupied orbital ($E_{HOMO}$) is equal to the ionization potential

**Table 4.** Frontier orbitals of several studied compounds.

| Compound | HOMO | LUMO |
|---|---|---|
| | **In Gas Phase** | |
| 4a | 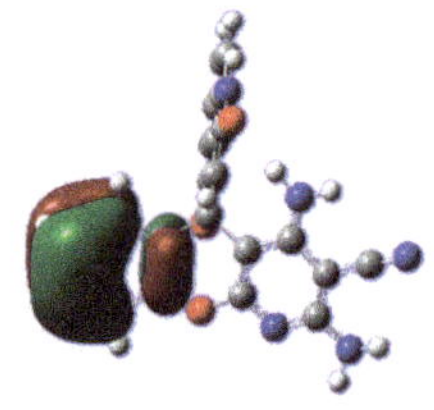 | 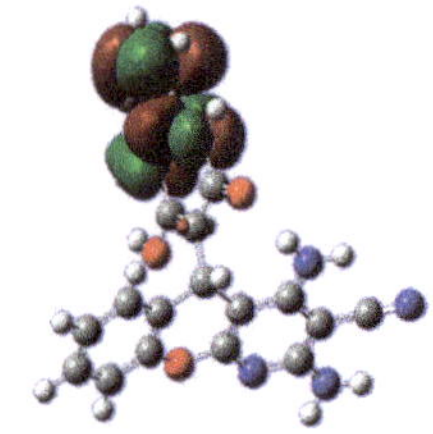 |
| 4e | 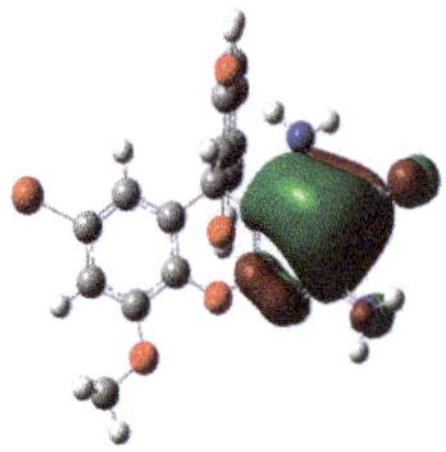 | 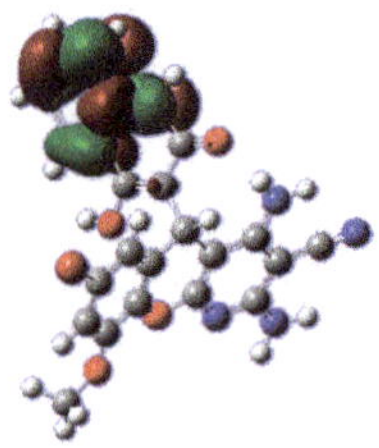 |
| 4h | 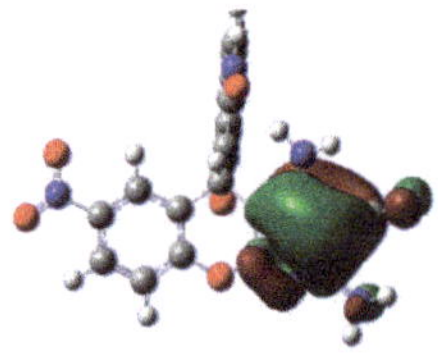 | 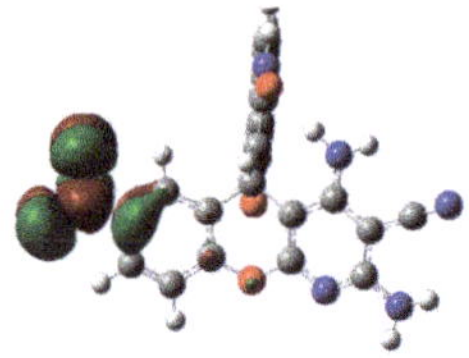 |
| | **Solvated Molecules** | |
| 4c | 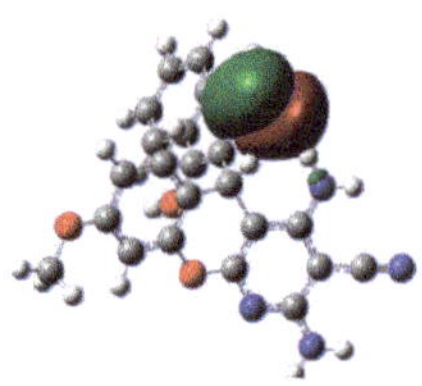 | 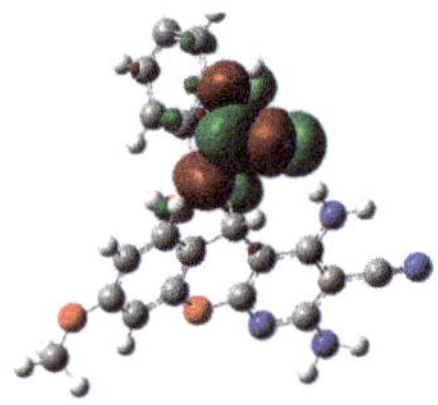 |
| | **Protonated Molecules** | |
| 4a | 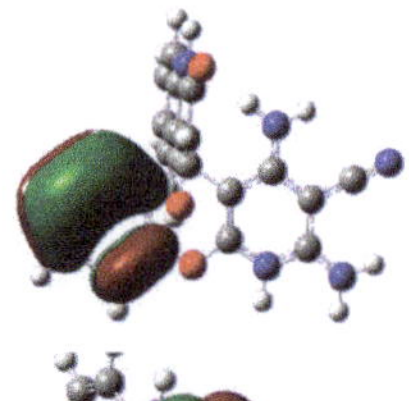 | 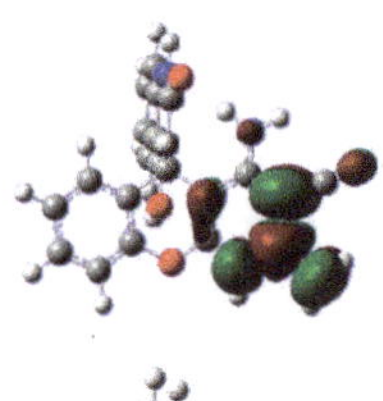 |
| 4h | 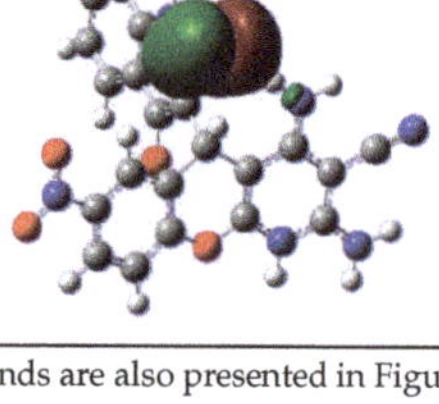 | 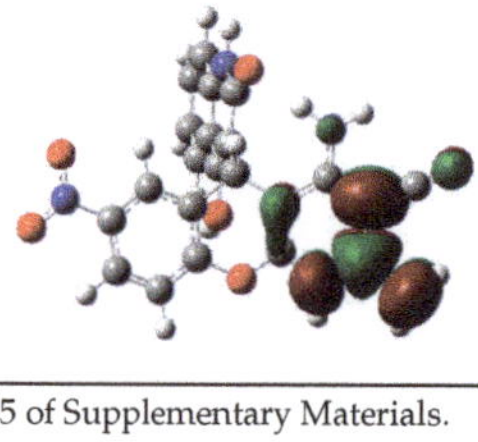 |

Frontier orbitals of these compounds are also presented in Figures S43–S55 of Supplementary Materials.

### 2.2.2. Gas Phase Calculations

During quantum chemical calculations, the structures of the studied compounds were optimized as shown in Figure 4 for **4a**. The chromeno[2,3-*b*]pyridine fragment was not planar and hydroxyquinolinone ring was localized nearly perpendicular to chromeno[2,3-*b*]pyridine ring. Calculated key parameters of the studied compounds **4a–i** are shown in Table 3.

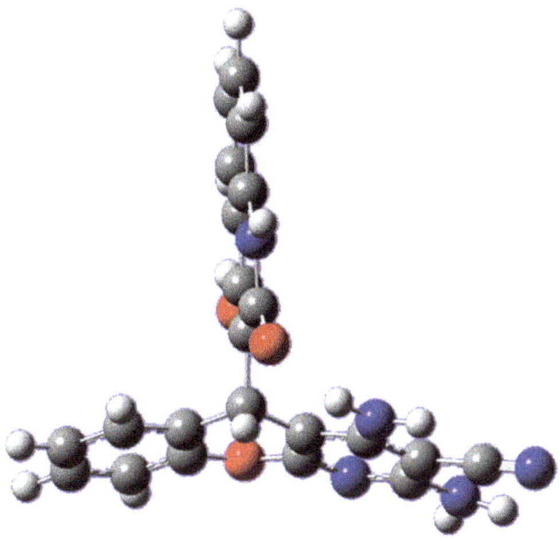

**Figure 4.** Optimized structure for compound **4a** (gas phase).

As mentioned above, corrosion inhibition depends on the energies and distributions of frontier orbitals. For most cases in considered compounds, the HOMOs are localized on the benzene ring atoms of chromeno[2,3-*b*]pyridines, making them sites for interaction with metal cations that formed by dissolving the metal in acid. The LUMOs are localized in the hydroxyquinolinone ring of the substituent. Such a type of distribution of the frontier orbitals is represented in compounds **4a, 4b, 4d** and **4i**. The frontier orbitals of several compounds are shown in Table 4.

Introducing of a strong electron-withdrawing substituent, such as a nitro-group, tended to change the orbital distribution. The HOMO became localized on the atoms of the pyridine ring, and the LUMO on the nitro-group of the substituent (**4h**, Table 4). A similar distribution was observed for the compounds **4e**, **4f** and **4g**: the HOMOs were localized in the pyridine ring, while the LUMOs were in the hydroxyquinolinone ring (Table 4). This was caused by the withdrawing effect of the halogen atom. It is noteworthy that compound **4c** had the same distribution of the orbitals, which was probably related to poor overlapping of oxygen orbital of methoxy-group with ones of benzene ring.

The energy difference is another important parameter. The lower the energy difference of the molecule, the higher the reaction ability (due to easier electron release). For the studied compounds these values were comparable, but **4b**, **4e** and **4i** had the lowest ones. The global electronegativity $\chi$ values for **4b**, **4e** and **4i** were almost twice as low as values calculated for similar tricyclic cationic inhibitors (<7.2 is accepted, [53]). The global electrophilicity index $\omega$ was low as well. It was almost five times lower than the values calculated for the studied inhibitors (<19.3 is accepted, [53]).

### 2.2.3. Solvated Form Calculations

Several parameters changed by taking into consideration the solvation processes. Thus, the frontier orbitals in compounds **4a, 4b, 4d, 4f** and **4i** were located in the same manner as in non-solvated ones, but for **4c**, **4e**, **4g** and **4h** shifting of the HOMOs to the carbonyl atoms of hydroxyquinolinone ring is observed, while the LUMOs remained in the same place (Table 4).

The analysis of the basic parameters (Table 3) shows that assuming solvation led to changing of some values mostly for compound **4h**; we can expect the highest anticorrosive effect from **4b**, **4c** and **4d** due to their low values of general electrophilicity $\omega$, which can be predicted because of electron-donating substituents. The values of electronegativity $\chi$ for **4b**, **4c** and **4d** remained low, almost the same as was calculated for the gas phase. It is noteworthy that the value of the global softness $\sigma$ for these compounds tended to decrease while taking to consideration the solvation effects.

2.2.4. Protonated form Calculations

In the case of a corrosion inhibition study in high acidic media, we must take in consideration the possibility of protonation of our compounds because of the basicity of some functional groups.

As it was shown previously [63], the main center of basicity in aminopyridines is the nitrogen atom in heterocyclic ring. We decided to confirm this statement by calculating the protonation energy for the compound **4a** (Scheme 4).

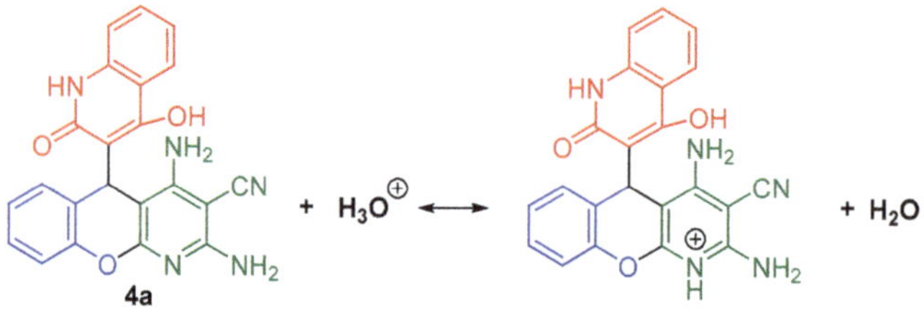

**Scheme 4.** Protonation of chromeno[2,3-*b*]pyridine **4a**.

Proton affinity (PA) is Equation:

$$PA = E_{PyH} + E_{H_2O} - E_{Py} - E_{H_3O^+} \tag{1}$$

where $E_i$–the total energy of the corresponding compound

We found that for the compound **4a** protonation took place on the pyridine ring nitrogen atom, while it was preferable by 15.1 kcal/mol in comparison to the $\alpha$-amino-group protonation and by 14.2 kcal/mol to the $\gamma$-amino-group.

The calculation results confirmed that the protonation took place first on the pyridine ring, so we have not carried out such calculations for the other compounds in order to reduce computation time, and optimized their geometry assuming protonation of the first pyridine position.

The calculation for the protonated molecules shows the great changing of electron density distribution in them. As the nitrogen atom in chromeno[2,3-*b*]pyridine cycle became positively charged and revealed high electron-withdrawing effect, the electron density in the pyridine ring decreased. This process was also strengthened by the influence of the cyano-group in this ring. In all nine compounds the LUMOs were localized on the atoms of pyridine ring, while the HOMOs were localized either on the benzene ring atoms (compounds **4a**, **4b**, **4d**, **4i**, Table 4) or on the carbonyl group of the hydroxyquinolinone ring (compounds **4c**, **4e**, **4f**, **4g**, **4h**, Table 4).

The key parameters remained low for compounds **4a–i** even in the protonated state. Global electrophilicity $\omega$ was extremely low (<60 is acceptable, [53]), the softness $\sigma$ and electronegativity $\chi$ were almost twice as low as the values for known cationic dies (<1 and <10 are acceptable, respectively [53]).

The analysis of the key parameters for the protonated molecules of **4a–i** shows that the highest anticorrosion effect was possessed by the compounds **4b**, **4c** and **4d**, the lowest by **4f** and **4h**. However, despite of the presence of an electron-withdrawing substituent and the high value of global electrophilicity $\omega$, compound **4h** had the highest value of chemical softness $\sigma$, which indicates that this compound can readily react with forming $Fe^{2+}$ ions (soft acid with soft base).

## 3. Materials and Methods

### 3.1. Synthesis

#### 3.1.1. General Information

All melting points were measured with a Gallenkamp melting point apparatus (London, UK). $^{1}$H and $^{13}$C NMR spectra were recorded with Bruker AM–300 spectrometer (Billerica, MA, USA) at ambient temperature. Chemical shifts values were relative to $Me_4Si$. IR spectra were registered with a Bruker ALPHA-T FT-IR spectrometer (Billerica, MA, USA) in KBr pellets. Mass spectra (EI, 70 eV) were obtained directly with a Finnigan MAT INCOS 50 spectrometer (Bremen, Germany). High-resolution mass spectra (HRMS) were measured on a Bruker micrOTOF II instrument (Billerica, MA, USA) using electrospray ionization (ESI).

#### 3.1.2. Synthesis of **4a–i**

Salicylaldehyde **1a–i** (1 mmol), 2-aminoprop-1-ene-1,1,3-tricarbonitrile **2** (0.13 g, 1 mmol) and 4-hydroxyquinolin-2(1*H*)-one **3** (0.16 g, 1 mmol) were refluxed in 4 mL of ethanol–pyridine (3:1) mixture for 2 h. After the reaction was completed, the solid was filtered, washed with well-chilled methanol (3 × 2 mL) and dried to isolate pure substituted 2,4-diamino-5-(4-hydroxy-2-oxo-1,2-dihydroquinolin-3-yl)-5*H*-chromeno[2,3-*b*]pyridine-3-carbonitriles **4a–i**.

2,4-Diamino-5-(4-hydroxy-2-oxo-1,2-dihydroquinolin-3-yl)-5*H*-chromeno[2,3-*b*]pyri-dine-3-carbonitrile **4a**, (white solid, 0.377g, 95%), mp > 350 °C (from Py-EtOH), FTIR (KBr) $cm^{-1}$: 3391, 3184, 2993, 2846, 2201, 1642, 1606, 1399, 1237, 751. $^{1}$H-NMR (400 MHz, DMSO-*d6*) δ 5.58 (s, 1H, CH), 6.31 (s, 2H, $NH_2$), 6.44 (s, 2H, $NH_2$), 6.90–7.05 (m, 3H, Ar), 7.06–7.22 (m, 2H, Ar), 7.28–7.41 (m, 2H, Ar), 7.86 (d, *J* = 7.8 Hz, 1H, Ar), 10.77 (br s, 1H, OH), 11.86 (s, 1H, NH) ppm. $^{13}$C-NMR (100 MHz, DMSO-d6) δ 28.68, 70.32, 88.97, 115.24, 115.41 (2C), 115.61, 116.54, 121.60, 122.16, 123.39, 127.42 (2C), 128.68, 130.76, 137.49, 151.27, 156.72, 159.19, 159.35, 160.19, 164.18. MS (EI, 70 eV) *m/z* (%): 397 ($M^+$, 17), 376 (11), 304 (7), 252 (6), 237 (100), 171 (12), 161 (26), 119 (12), 79 (86), 52 (55). HRMS-ESI: $[M + H]^+$, calcd for $C_{22}H_{16}N_5O_3$ 398.1253, found 398.1252.

2,4-Diamino-5-(4-hydroxy-2-oxo-1,2-dihydroquinolin-3-yl)-7-methyl-5*H*-chromeno[2,3-*b*]pyridine-3-carbonitrile **4b**, (white solid, 0.358g, 87%), mp > 350 °C (from Py-EtOH), FTIR (KBr) $cm^{-1}$: 3419, 3361, 2881, 2845, 2203, 1634, 1580, 1402, 1220, 752. $^{1}$H-NMR (400 MHz, DMSO-*d6*) δ 2.14 (s, 3H, $CH_3$), 5.53 (s, 1H, CH), 6.28 (s, 2H, $NH_2$), 6.41 (s, 2H, $NH_2$), 6.78 (s, 1H, Ar), 6.93 (dd, $^{3}J$ = 16.6 Hz, $^{4}J$ = 8.0 Hz, 2H, Ar), 7.11 (t, *J* = 7.4Hz, 1H, Ar), 7.33 (d, *J* = 7.8 Hz, 1H, Ar), 7.48 (t, *J* = 7.3 Hz, 1H, Ar), 7.86 (d, *J* = 7,8 Hz, 1H, Ar), 10.74 (s, 1H, OH), 11.84 (s, 1H, NH) ppm. $^{13}$C-NMR (100 MHz, DMSO-d6) δ 20.11, 28.64, 70.20, 89.00, 115.18 (2C), 115.61, 116.58, 121.48, 122.14, 123.15, 127.97 (2C), 128.34, 130.73, 132.22, 137.46, 149.20, 156.68, 159.15,159.49 160.09, 164.18. MS (EI, 70 eV) *m/z* (%): 411 ($M^+$, 26), 390 (7), 251 (100), 223 (14), 185 (28), 161 (61), 119 (43), 92 (30), 77 (35), 42 (15). HRMS-ESI: $[M + H]^+$, calcd for $C_{23}H_{18}N_5O_3$ 412.1410, found 412.1402.

2,4-Diamino-5-(4-hydroxy-2-oxo-1,2-dihydroquinolin-3-yl)-8-methoxy-5*H*-chromeno[2,3-*b*]pyridine-3-carbonitrile **4c**, (white solid, 0.355g, 83%), mp > 350°C (from Py-EtOH), FTIR (KBr) $cm^{-1}$: 3428, 3381, 2887, 2836, 2199, 1632, 1607, 1569, 1402, 1201, 761. $^{1}$H-NMR (400 MHz, DMSO-*d6*) δ 3.72 (s, 3H, OMe), 5.50 (s, 1H, CH), 6.29 (s, 2H, $NH_2$), 6.43 (s, 2H, $NH_2$), 6.51–6.65 (m, 2H, Ar), 6.88 (d, *J* = 7.9 Hz, 1H, Ar), 7.11 (t, *J* = 7.2 Hz, 1H, Ar), 7.33 (d, *J* = 7.9 Hz, 1H, Ar), 7.48 (t, *J* = 7.2 Hz, 1H, Ar), 7.86 (d, *J* = 7.3 Hz, 1H, Ar), 10.71 (br s, 1H, OH), 11.83 (s, 1H, NH) ppm. $^{13}$C-NMR (100 MHz, DMSO-d6) δ 28.08, 30.63, 55.21, 70.29, 89.12, 100.60 (2C), 109.69, 115.27, 115.55 (2C), 116.50, 121.43, 122.11, 128.75, 130.64, 137.40, 151.93, 156.68, 158.53, 159.10, 159.97, 164.13. MS (EI, 70 eV) *m/z* (%): 407 (18), 267 (100), 252 (11), 237 (9), 224 (17), 201 (4), 161 (60), 119 (43), 92 (33), 15 (63). HRMS-ESI: $[M + H]^+$, calcd for $C_{23}H_{18}N_5O_4$ 428.1359, found 428.1351.

2,4-Diamino-9-ethoxy-5-(4-hydroxy-2-oxo-1,2-dihydroquinolin-3-yl)-5*H*-chromeno[2,3-*b*]pyridine-3-carbonitrile **4d**, (white solid, 0.433 g, 98%), mp > 350 °C (from Py-EtOH), FTIR (KBr) $cm^{-1}$: 3409, 3372, 2979, 2881, 2202, 1631, 1568, 1483, 1222, 751. $^1$H-NMR (400 MHz, DMSO-*d6*) δ 1.39 (t, *J* = 6.8 Hz, 3H, OEt), 4.04 (m, 2H, OEt), 5.56 (s, 1H, CH), 6.35 (s, 2H, $NH_2$), 6.41 (s, 2H, $NH_2$), 6.52 (d, *J* = 6.4 Hz, 1H, Ar), 6.78–6.90 (m, 2H, Ar), 7.10 (t, *J* = 7.6 Hz, 1H, Ar), 7.33 (d, *J* = 8.1 Hz, 1H, Ar), 7.48 (t, *J* = 7.6 Hz, 1H, Ar), 7.88 (d, *J* = 8.1 Hz, 1H, Ar), 10.80 (s, 1H, OH), 11.83 (s, 1H, NH) ppm. $^{13}$C-NMR (100 MHz, DMSO-d6) δ 14.81, 28.75, 63.62, 70.22, 88.77, 110.79, 115.22, 115.57, 116.55, 119.49 (2C), 121.47, 122.10, 122.90, 124.00, 130.71, 137.43, 140.78, 145.90, 156.64, 159.18 (2C), 160.21, 164.12. MS (EI, 70 eV) *m*/*z* (%): 441 ($M^+$, 19), 412 (18), 392 (26), 281 (74), 253 (77), 187 (14), 161 (100), 119 (57), 92 (42), 29 (95). HRMS-ESI: $[M + H]^+$, calcd for $C_{24}H_{19}N_5O_4$ 442.1510, found 442.1503.

2,4-Diamino-7-bromo-5-(4-hydroxy-2-oxo-1,2-dihydroquinolin-3-yl)-9-methoxy-5*H*-chromeno[2,3-*b*] pyridine-3-carbonitrile **4e**, (white solid, 0.344 g, 68%), mp > 350 °C (from Py-EtOH), FTIR (KBr) $cm^{-1}$: 3445, 3387, 2204, 1639, 1600, 1567, 1398, 1224, 1013, 768. $^1$H-NMR (400 MHz, DMSO-*d6*) δ 3.84 (s, 3H, OMe), 5.53 (s, 1H, CH), 6.33 (s, 2H, $NH_2$), 6.42 (br s, 2H, $NH_2$), 6.64 (s, 1H, Ar), 7.04 (s, 1H, Ar), 7.12 (t, *J* = 7.3 Hz, 1H, Ar), 7.34 (d, *J* = 8.1 Hz, 1H, Ar), 7.50 (t, *J* = 7.3 Hz, 1H, Ar), 7.88 (d, *J* = 7.2 Hz, 1H, Ar), 10.90 (s, 1H, OH), 11.86 (s, 1H, NH) ppm. $^{13}$C-NMR (100 MHz, DMSO-d6) δ 28.64, 56.06, 70.39, 88.34, 113.03, 113.23, 114.08, 115.07, 115.62, 116.37, 121.62, 122.20, 123.27, 125.73, 130.88, 131.78, 137.51, 137.71, 147.67, 156.58, 156.74, 159.13, 163.94. MS (EI, 70 eV) *m*/*z* (%): 507 ($M^+$, 3), 346 (51), 331 (8), 305 (51), 252 (14), 204 (45), 161 (100), 119 (59), 92 (39), 15 (28). HRMS-ESI: $[M + H]^+$, calcd for $C_{23}H_{17}BrN_5O_4$ 506.0464 [$^{79}$Br], 508.0443 [$^{81}$Br], found 506.0458 [$^{79}$Br], 508.0434 [$^{81}$Br].

2,4-Diamino-7-chloro-5-(4-hydroxy-2-oxo-1,2-dihydroquinolin-3-yl)-5*H*-chrome-no[2,3-*b*]pyridine-3-carbonitrile **4f**, (white solid, 0.393 g, 91%), mp > 350°C (from Py-EtOH), FTIR (KBr) $cm^{-1}$: 3393, 3217, 2975, 2894, 2203, 1633, 1607, 1404, 1259, 757. $^1$H-NMR (400 MHz, DMSO-*d6*) δ 5.56 (s, 1H, CH), 6.35 (s, 2H, $NH_2$), 6.47 (br s, 2H, $NH_2$), 6.96 (s, 1H, Ar), 7.06 (d, *J* = 8.7 Hz, 1H, Ar), 7.13 (t, *J* = 7.6 Hz, 1H, Ar), 7.22 (d, *J* = 8.6 Hz, 1H, Ar), 7.34 (d, *J* = 7.9 Hz, 1H, Ar), 7.50 (t, *J* = 7.6 Hz, 1H, Ar), 7.88 (d, *J* = 6.0 Hz, 1H, Ar), 10.89 (br s, 1H, OH), 11.88 (s, 1H, NH) ppm. $^{13}$C-NMR (100 MHz, DMSO-d6) δ 28.73, 70.43, 88.31, 115.15, 115.37, 115.66, 116.39, 117.27 (2C), 121.51, 122.27, 125.62, 126.68, 127.36, 127.48, 130.90, 137.60, 150.23, 156.65, 156.80, 159.20, 163.98. MS (EI, 70 eV) *m*/*z* (%): 431 ($M^+$, 17), 409 (9), 271 (100), 243 (10), 205 (21), 161 (79), 119 (73), 92 (92), 77 (54), 28 (52). HRMS-ESI: $[M + H]^+$, calcd for $C_{22}H_{15}ClN_5O_3$ 432.0863 [$^{35}$Cl], 434.0834 [$^{37}$Cl], found 432.0856 [$^{35}$Cl], 434.0824 [$^{37}$Cl].

2,4-Diamino-7-bromo-5-(4-hydroxy-2-oxo-1,2-dihydroquinolin-3-yl)-5H-chrome-no[2,3-b]pyridine-3-carbonitrile **4g**, (white solid, 0.324 g, 68%), mp > 231–233 °C (from Py-EtOH), FTIR (KBr) $cm^{-1}$: 3343, 3184, 2993, 2846, 2201, 1642, 1609, 1398, 1258, 775. $^1$H-NMR (400 MHz, DMSO-*d6*) δ 5.56 (s, 1H, CH), 6.35 (s, 2H, $NH_2$), 6.46 (br s, 2H, $NH_2$), 7.01 (d, *J* = 8.5 Hz, 1H, Ar), 7.08 (s, 1H, Ar), 7.13 (t, *J* = 7.5 Hz, 1H, Ar), 7.35 (d, *J* = 7.9 Hz, 2H Ar), 7.50 (t, *J* = 7.5 Hz, 1H, Ar), 7.88 (d, *J* = 6.0 Hz, 1H Ar), 10.89 (s, 1H, OH), 11.87 (s, 1H, NH) ppm. $^{13}$C-NMR (100 MHz, DMSO-d6) δ 28.61, 70.43, 88.34, 114.47, 115.07, 115.65 (2C), 116.36, 117.72, 121.52, 122.27, 126.09, 130.23, 130.34, 130.90, 137.56, 150.67, 156.67, 158.92, 159.20, 160.32, 163.90. MS (EI, 70 eV) *m*/*z* (%): 316 ($[M-C_9H_6NO_2]^+$, $^{81}$Br, 2), 314 ($[M-C_9H_6NO_2]^+$, $^{79}$Br, 2), 236 (2), 202 (1), 171 (1), 161 (13), 119 (9), 92 (5), 78 (73), 63 (100), 15 (31). HRMS-ESI: $[M + H]^+$, calcd for $C_{22}H_{14}BrN5O_3$ 476.0353 [$^{79}$Br], 478.0333 [$^{81}$Br], found 476.0324 [$^{79}$Br], 478.0323 [$^{81}$Br].

2,4-Diamino-5-(4-hydroxy-2-oxo-1,2-dihydroquinolin-3-yl)-7-nitro-5*H*-chrome-no[2,3-*b*]pyridine-3-carbonitrile **4h**, (yellow solid, 0.261 g, 59%), mp > 350 °C (from Py-EtOH), FTIR (KBr) $cm^{-1}$: 3357, 3184, 2199, 1661, 1627, 1336, 1242, 1026, 828, 752. $^1$H-NMR (400 MHz, DMSO-*d6*) δ 5.24 (s, 1H, CH), 6.53 (br s, 2H, $NH_2$), 6.56 (s, 2H, $NH_2$), 7.28 (t, *J* = 7.6 Hz, 1H, Ar), 7.34 (d, *J* = 8.3 Hz, 1H Ar), 7.42 (d, *J* = 8.3 Hz, 1H Ar), 7.54 (t, *J* = 7.6 Hz, 1H, Ar), 7.87–7.94 (m, 1H, Ar), 8.02 (d, *J* = 8.3 Hz, 1H Ar), 8.08 (dd, $^3J$ = 7.0 Hz, $^4J$ = 2.6 Hz, 1H, Ar), 9.57 (s, 1H, OH), 11.62 (s, 1H, NH) ppm. $^{13}$C-NMR (100 MHz, DMSO-d6) δ 28.45, 98.42, 107.18, 112.75, 115.20 (2C), 116.43, 116.77, 121.76 (2C), 123.02, 124.14, 126.22, 130.52, 137.22, 143.17, 152.75, 153.74, 154.75, 155.08, 159.76, 161.57. MS (EI, 70 eV) *m*/*z* (%): 294 (11), 247 (10),

236 (3), 190 (3), 161 (20), 150 (100), 122 (65), 78 (16), 63 (31), 18 (32). HRMS-ESI: $[M + H]^+$, calcd for $C_{22}H_{15}N_6O_5$ 443.1104, found 443.1098.

9,11-Diamino-12-(4-hydroxy-2-oxo-1,2-dihydroquinolin-3-yl)-12*H*-benzo[5,6]chromeno[2,3-*b*]pyridine-10-carbonitrile **4i**, (white solid, 0.389 g, 87%), mp > 350 °C (from Py-EtOH), FTIR (KBr) $cm^{-1}$: 3454, 3400, 2875, 2835, 2203, 1634, 1607, 1409, 1239, 755. $^1$H-NMR (400 MHz, DMSO-*d6*) δ 6.06 (s, 1H, CH), 6.35 (s, 2H, $NH_2$), 6.69 (s, 2H, $NH_2$), 7.07 (t, *J* = 7.6 Hz, 1H, Ar), 7.25–7.51 (m, 5H, Ar), 7.76–7.93 (m, 3H, Ar), 8.02 (d, *J* = 8.4 Hz, 1H Ar), 10.82 (s, 1H, OH), 11.95 (s, 1H, NH) ppm. $^{13}$C-NMR (100 MHz, DMSO-d6) δ 26.76, 70.47, 89.08, 114.46, 115.21, 115.58, 116.51, 117.06 (2C), 121.56, 122.13, 122.68, 124.08, 126.83, 128.30, 128.44 (2C), 130.18, 130.78, 131.32, 137.26, 149.24, 156.86, 159.17, 160.96, 163.90. MS (EI, 70 eV) *m*/*z* (%): 429 ($[M-H_2O]^+$, 5), 410 (14), 364 (19), 287 (100), 258 (6), 221 (13), 161 (35), 144 (38), 92 (12), 63 (13). HRMS-ESI: $[M + H]^+$, calcd for $C_{26}H_{18}N_5O_3$ 448.1410, found 448.1401.

### 3.1.3. Isolation of the Intermediate 5

Salicylaldehyde **1a** (0.12 g, 1 mmol) and 2-aminoprop-1-ene-1,1,3-tricarbonitrile **2** (0.13 g, 1 mmol) were stirred at room temperature in 4 mL of ethanol–pyridine (3:1) mixture for 2 h. After the reaction was completed, the solid was filtered, washed with well-chilled methanol (3 × 2 mL) and dried to isolate pure 2-(amino-(2-imino-2*H*-chromen-3-yl)methylene)malononitrile **5**.

2-(Amino-(2-imino-2*H*-chromen-3-yl)methylene)malononitrile **5**, (Yellow solid, 0.208 g, yield 88%), m.p. 272–273 °C (decomp.) (lit [40] m.p. 271–272 °C (decomp.)). $^1$H-NMR (300 MHz, DMSO-d6) δ 7.11–7.31 (m, 2H, 2CH Ar), 7.45–7.63 (m, 2H, 2CH Ar), 7.75 (s, 1H, CH), 8.65 (s, 1H, NH), 8.93 (br.s, 1H, N*H*H), 8.95 (br.s, 1H, NH*H*) ppm.

### 3.1.4. Synthesis of Chromeno[2,3-*b*]pyridine 4a from 2-(amino-(2-imino-2*H*-chromen-3-yl)methylene)malononitrile 5 and 4-hydroxyquinolin-2(1*H*)-one 3

2-(Amino-(2-imino-2*H*-chromen-3-yl)methylene)malononitrile **5** (0.24 g, 1 mmol) and 4-hydroxyquinolin-2(1*H*)-one (0.16 g, 1 mmol) **3** were refluxed in 4 mL of ethanol–pyridine (3:1) mixture for 2 h. After the reaction was completed, the solid was filtered, washed with well-chilled methanol (3 × 2 mL) and dried to isolate pure chromeno[2,3-*b*]pyridine **4a**.

2,4-Diamino-5-(4-hydroxy-2-oxo-1,2-dihydroquinolin-3-yl)-5*H*-chromeno[2,3-*b*]pyridine-3-carbonitrile **3a**, (White solid, 0.377g, 95%), mp > 350°C (from Py-EtOH), $^1$H-NMR (400 MHz, DMSO-*d6*) δ 5.58 (s, 1H, CH), 6.31 (s, 2H, $NH_2$), 6.44 (s, 2H, $NH_2$), 6.90–7.05 (m, 3H, Ar), 7.06–7.22 (m, 2H, Ar), 7.28–7.41 (m, 2H, Ar), 7.86 (d, *J* = 7.8 Hz, 1H, Ar), 10.77 (br s, 1H, OH), 11.86 (s, 1H, NH) ppm.

## 4. Conclusions

In summary, the PASE transformation of salicylaldehydes, malononitrile dimer and hydroxyquinolinone into previously unknown hydroxyquinolinone substituted chromeno[2,3-*b*] pyridines has been found. The proposed EtOH-Py catalyst-solvent system provides an efficient rout to hydroxyquinolinone substituted chromeno[2,3-*b*]pyridines.

The developed approach is facile, it is easy to isolate final compounds directly from reaction mixture and the yields of final compounds are 59%–98%.

During investigation of reaction mechanism using a real-time $^1$H NMR monitoring, 2-((2*H*-chromen-3-yl)methylene)malononitrile was determined and proven as the key intermediate in assembling of chromeno[2,3-*b*]pyridines.

Quantum chemistry calculations showed that hydroxyquinolinone-substituted chromeno[2,3-*b*]pyridines bearing electron-donating groups and hydroxynaphthaldehyde derivatives are prospective compounds for corrosion inhibition. In particular, methyl, methoxy, ethoxy substituted 5-(1,2-dihydroquinolin-3-yl)-5*H*-chromeno[2,3-*b*]pyridines are the most effective among those examined according to calculation.

**Supplementary Materials:** $^1$H and $^{13}$C Spectra of synthesized compounds **4a–i** and intermediate **5** (Figure S1–S22), NMR monitoring spectra (Figure S23–S42), results of quantum chemical calculations with extended decimal point (Table S1) and figures of frontier orbitals (Figure S44–S55) are available online.

**Author Contributions:** Conceptualization: F.V.R. and Y.E.R.; Methodology: F.V.R., Y.E.R. and M.N.E.; writing—original draft preparation: F.V.R., Y.E.R., and S.V.V.; supervision: M.N.E. and M.P.E.; funding acquisition: M.N.E. and M.P.E.; performed the synthesis: Y.E.R.; quantum chemistry simulation: S.V.V.; performed the NMR monitoring: A.N.F.; supervised, wrote and edited the manuscript: F.V.R. and M.N.E; visualization: F.V.R. and A.N.V.; Resources: A.N.V. All authors contributed to writing the manuscript, editing, and reviewing of the manuscript. All authors have read and agreed to the published version of the manuscript.

**Funding:** The authors gratefully acknowledge the financial support of the Russian Foundation for Basic Research (Project 18-03-00212).

**Conflicts of Interest:** There are no conflicts to declare.

## References

1. Dömling, A. Recent developments in isocyanide based multicomponent reactions in applied chemistry. *Chem. Rev.* **2006**, *106*, 17–89. [CrossRef] [PubMed]
2. Dömling, A.; Ugi, I. Multicomponent reactions with isocyanides. *Angew. Chemie Int. Ed.* **2000**, *39*, 3168–3210. [CrossRef]
3. Nair, V.; Rajesh, C.; Vinod, A.U.; Bindu, S.; Sreekanth, A.R.; Mathen, J.S.; Balagopal, L. Strategies for heterocyclic construction via novel multicomponent reactions based on isocyanides and nucleophilic carbenes. *Acc. Chem. Res.* **2003**, *36*, 899–907. [CrossRef] [PubMed]
4. Wan, J.-P.; Liu, Y. Multicomponent reactions promoted by organosilicon reagents. *Curr. Org. Chem.* **2011**, *15*, 2758–2773. [CrossRef]
5. Trost, B.M. The atom economy—A search for synthetic efficiency. *Science* **1991**, *254*, 1471–1477. [CrossRef] [PubMed]
6. Trost, B.M. Atom economy—A challenge for organic synthesis: Homogeneous catalysis leads the way. *Angew. Chemie Int. Ed. English* **1995**, *34*, 259–281. [CrossRef]
7. Clarke, P.A.; Santos, S.; Martin, W.H.C. Combining pot, atom and step economy (PASE) in organic synthesis. Synthesis of tetrahydropyran-4-ones. *Green Chem.* **2007**, *9*, 438–440. [CrossRef]
8. Newhouse, T.; Baran, P.S.; Hoffmann, R.W. The economies of synthesis. *Chem. Soc. Rev.* **2009**, *38*, 3010–3021. [CrossRef]
9. Hayashi, Y. Pot economy and one-pot synthesis. *Chem. Sci.* **2016**, *7*, 866–880. [CrossRef]
10. Khasanov, A.F.; Kopchuk, D.S.; Kim, G.A.; Slepukhin, P.A.; Kovalev, I.S.; Santra, S.; Zyryanov, G.V.; Majee, A.; Chupakhin, O.N.; Charushin, V.N. Pot, Atom, Step Economic (PASE) approach towards (Aza)-2, 2′-Bipyridines: Synthesis and photophysical studies. *ChemistrySelect* **2018**, *3*, 340–347. [CrossRef]
11. Zhang, W.; Yi, W.B. *Pot, Atom, and Step Economy (PASE) Synthesis*; Springer Briefs in Molecular Science; Springer International Publishing: Cham, Switzerland, 2019; ISBN 9783030225964.
12. Zhi, S.; Ma, X.; Zhang, W. Consecutive multicomponent reactions for the synthesis of complex molecules. *Org. Biomol. Chem.* **2019**, *17*, 7632–7650. [CrossRef] [PubMed]
13. Moseev, T.D.; Varaksin, M.V.; Gorlov, D.A.; Nikiforov, E.A.; Kopchuk, D.S.; Starnovskaya, E.S.; Khasanov, A.F.; Zyryanov, G.V.; Charushin, V.N.; Chupakhin, O.N. Direct CH/CLi coupling of 1,2,4-triazines with C6F5Li followed by aza-Diels-Alder reaction as a pot, atom, and step economy (PASE) approach towards novel fluorinated 2,2′-bipyridine fluorophores. *J. Fluor. Chem.* **2019**, *224*, 89–99. [CrossRef]
14. Chen, X.-B.; Xiong, S.-L.; Xie, Z.-X.; Wang, Y.-C.; Liu, W. Three-Component One-Pot Synthesis of Highly Functionalized Bis-Indole Derivatives. *ACS omega* **2019**, *4*, 11832–11837. [CrossRef] [PubMed]
15. Vereshchagin, A.N.; Elinson, M.N.; Anisina, Y.E.; Ryzhkov, F.V.; Novikov, R.A.; Egorov, M.P. PASE Pseudo-Four-Component Synthesis and Docking Studies of New 5-C-Substituted 2,4-Diamino-5*H*-Chromeno[2,3-*b*]pyridine-3-Carbonitriles. *ChemistrySelect* **2017**, *2*, 4593–4597. [CrossRef]
16. Elinson, M.N.; Ryzhkov, F.V.; Nasybullin, R.F.; Vereshchagin, A.N.; Egorov, M.P. Fast Efficient and General PASE Approach to Medicinally Relevant 4*H*,5*H*-Pyrano-[4,3-*b*]pyran-5-one and 4,6-Dihydro-5*H*-pyrano-[3,2-*c*]pyridine-5-one Scaffolds. *Helv. Chim. Acta* **2016**, *99*, 724–731. [CrossRef]

17. Cabeza, L.F.; Illa, J.; Roca, J.; Badia, F.; Mehling, H.; Hiebler, S.; Ziegler, F. Immersion corrosion tests on metal-salt hydrate pairs used for latent heat storage in the 32 to 36 °C temperature range. *Mater. Corros.* **2001**, *52*, 140–146. [CrossRef]
18. NACE—Economic Impact, Assessment of the Global Cost of Corrosion. Available online: http://impact.nace.org/economic-impact.aspx (accessed on 18 January 2020).
19. U.S. Report on Corrosion Costs and Preventive Strategies in the United States. Available online: http://www.corrosioncost.com (accessed on 18 January 2020).
20. Bristol, J.A.; Gold, E.H.; Gross, I.; Lovey, R.G.; Long, J.F. Gastric antisecretory agents. 2. Antisecretory activity of 9-[(aminoalkyl)thio]-9*H*-xanthenes and 5-[(aminoalkyl)thio]-5*H*-[1]benzopyrano-[2,3-*b*]pyridines. *J. Med. Chem.* **1981**, *24*, 1010–1013. [CrossRef]
21. Anderson, D.R.; Hegde, S.; Reinhard, E.; Gomez, L.; Vernier, W.F.; Lee, L.; Liu, S.; Sambandam, A.; Snider, P.A.; Masih, L. Aminocyanopyridine inhibitors of mitogen activated protein kinase-activated protein kinase 2 (MK-2). *Bioorg. Med. Chem. Lett.* **2005**, *15*, 1587–1590. [CrossRef]
22. Tu, X.-J.; Fan, W.; Hao, W.-J.; Jiang, B.; Tu, S.-J. Three-component bicyclization providing an expedient access to Pyrano[2′,3′:5,6]pyrano[2,3-*b*]Pyridines and its derivatives. *ACS Comb. Sci.* **2014**, *16*, 647–651. [CrossRef]
23. Abdelmoniem, A.M.; Ghozlan, S.A.S.; Abdelmoniem, D.M.; Elwahy, A.H.M.; Abdelhamid, I.A. Facile one-pot, three-component synthesis of novel Bis-Heterocycles incorporating 5*H*-chromeno[2,3-*b*]pyridine-3-carbonitrile Derivatives. *J. Heterocycl. Chem.* **2017**, *54*, 2844–2849. [CrossRef]
24. Bardasov, I.N.; Alekseeva, A.U.; Mihailov, D.L.; Ershov, O.V.; Grishanov, D.A. Double heteroannulation reactions of 1-naphthol with alkyl-and arylmethylidene derivatives of malononitrile dimer. *Tetrahedron Lett.* **2015**, *56*, 1830–1832. [CrossRef]
25. Olyaei, A.; Shahsavari, M.S.; Sadeghpour, M. Organocatalytic approach toward the green one-pot synthesis of novel benzo[*f*]chromenes and 12*H*-benzo[5,6]chromeno[2,3-*b*]pyridines. *Res. Chem. Intermed.* **2018**, *44*, 943–956. [CrossRef]
26. Olyaei, A.; Shafie, Z.; Sadeghpour, M. An efficient and one-pot green synthesis of novel 6-oxo-7-aryl-6,7-dihydrochromeno pyrano[2,3-*b*]pyridine derivatives. *Tetrahedron Lett.* **2018**, *59*, 3567–3570. [CrossRef]
27. Zhang, W.; Wang, J.; Mao, J.; Hu, L.; Wu, X.; Guo, C. Three-component domino cyclization of novel carbazole and indole fused pyrano[2,3-*c*]pyridine derivatives. *Tetrahedron Lett.* **2016**, *57*, 1985–1989. [CrossRef]
28. Elinson, M.N.; Vereshchagin, A.N.; Anisina, Y.E.; Egorov, M.P. Efficient Multicomponent Approach to the Medicinally Relevant 5-aryl-chromeno[2,3-*b*]pyridine Scaffold. *Polycycl. Aromat. Compd.* **2020**, *40*, 108–115. [CrossRef]
29. Elinson, M.N.; Vereshchagin, A.N.; Anisina, Y.E.; Krymov, S.K.; Fakhrutdinov, A.N.; Egorov, M.P. Selective multicomponent 'one-pot' approach to the new 5-(4-hydroxy-6-methyl-2-oxo-2*H*-pyran-3-yl)chromeno[2,3-*b*]pyridine scaffold in pyridine-ethanol catalyst/solvent system. *Monatshefte für Chemie Chem. Mon.* **2019**, *150*, 1073–1078. [CrossRef]
30. Elinson, M.; Vereshchagin, A.; Anisina, Y.; Krymov, S.; Fakhrutdinov, A.; Egorov, M. Potassium fluoride catalysed multicomponent approach to medicinally privileged 5-[3-hydroxy-6-(hydroxymethyl)-4*H*-pyran-2-yl] substituted chromeno[2,3-*b*]pyridine scaffold. *Arkivoc* **2019**, *part ii*, 38–49. [CrossRef]
31. Vereshchagin, A.N.; Elinson, M.N.; Anisina, Y.E.; Ryzhkov, F.V.; Goloveshkin, A.S.; Novikov, R.A.; Egorov, M.P. Synthesis, structural, spectroscopic and docking studies of new 5C-substituted 2,4-diamino-5*H*-chromeno[2,3-*b*]pyridine-3-carbonitriles. *J. Mol. Struct.* **2017**, *1146*, 766–772. [CrossRef]
32. Elinson, M.N.; Ryzhkov, F.V.; Korolev, V.A.; Egorov, M.P. Pot, atom and step-economic (PASE) synthesis of medicinally relevant spiro [oxindole-3, 4′-pyrano [4, 3-*b*] pyran] scaffold. *Heterocycl. Commun.* **2016**, *22*, 11–15. [CrossRef]
33. Elinson, M.N.; Nasybullin, R.F.; Ryzhkov, F.V.; Egorov, M.P. Solvent-free and 'on-water' multicomponent assembling of salicylaldehydes, malononitrile and 3-methyl-2-pyrazolin-5-one: A fast and efficient route to the 2-amino-4-(1*H*-pyrazol-4-yl)-4*H*-chromene scaffold. *Comptes Rendus Chim.* **2014**, *17*, 437–442. [CrossRef]

34. Elinson, M.N.; Nasybullin, R.F.; Ryzhkov, F.V.; Zaimovskaya, T.A.; Nikishin, G.I. Solvent-free and 'on-water' multicomponent assembling of aldehydes, 3-methyl-2-pyrazoline-5-one, and malononitrile: Fast and efficient approach to medicinally relevant pyrano[2,3-*c*]pyrazole scaffold. *Monatshefte für Chemie Chem. Mon.* **2015**, *146*, 631–635. [CrossRef]
35. Chanda, A.; Fokin, V. V Organic synthesis "On Water". *Chem. Rev.* **2009**, *109*, 725–748. [CrossRef] [PubMed]
36. Vereshchagin, A.N.; Elinson, M.N.; Anisina, Y.E.; Ryzhkov, F.V.; Goloveshkin, A.S.; Bushmarinov, I.S.; Zlotin, S.G.; Egorov, M.P. Pot, atom and step economic (PASE) synthesis of 5-isoxazolyl-5*H*-chromeno[2,3-*b*]pyridine scaffold. *Mendeleev Commun.* **2015**, *25*, 424–426. [CrossRef]
37. Patai, S.; Israeli, Y. 411. The kinetics and mechanisms of carbonyl–methylene condensations. Part VII. The reaction of malononitrile with aromatic aldehydes in ethanol. *J. Chem. Soc.* **1960**, 2025–2030. [CrossRef]
38. Elinson, M.N.; Vereshchagin, A.N.; Anisina, Y.E.; Goloveshkin, A.S.; Ushakov, I.E.; Egorov, M.P. PASE facile and efficient multicomponent approach to the new type of 5-C-substituted 2,4-diamino-5*H*-chromeno[2,3-*b*]pyridine scaffold. *Mendeleev Commun.* **2018**, *28*, 372–374. [CrossRef]
39. Elinson, M.N.; Gorbunov, S.V.; Vereshchagin, A.N.; Nasybullin, R.F.; Goloveshkin, A.S.; Bushmarinov, I.S.; Egorov, M.P. Chemical and electrocatalytic cascade cyclization of salicylaldehyde with three molecules of malononitrile: 'one-pot' simple and efficient way to the chromeno[2,3-*b*]pyridine scaffold. *Tetrahedron* **2014**, *70*, 8559–8563. [CrossRef]
40. Elinson, M.N.; Vereshchagin, A.N.; Anisina, Y.E.; Fakhrutdinov, A.N.; Goloveshkin, A.S.; Egorov, M.P. Pot-, Atom- and Step-Economic (PASE) Multicomponent approach to the 5-(Dialkylphosphonate)-Substituted 2,4-Diamino-5*H*-chromeno[2,3-*b*]pyridine scaffold. *Eur. J. Org. Chem.* **2019**, *2019*, 4171–4178. [CrossRef]
41. Amer, A.A. Synthesis of Some New Polyfunctionalized Pyridines. *J. Heterocycl. Chem.* **2018**, *55*, 297–301. [CrossRef]
42. Abou Elmaaty, T.; el taweel, M.; Elmougi, S.; Elagamey, A. The condensation of active methylene reagents with salicylaldehyde: Novel synthesis of chromene, azaanthracene, pyrano[3,4-*c*]chromene and chromeno[3,4-*c*]pyridine derivatives. *J. Heterocycl. Chem.* **2004**, *41*, 655–658. [CrossRef]
43. Sakurai, A.; Midorikawa, H.; Hashimoto, Y. The cyclization of ethyl cyanoacetate and salicylaldehyde or 3-methoxysalicylaldehyde with ketones by means of ammonium acetate. *Bull. Chem. Soc. Jpn.* **1970**, *43*, 2925–2933. [CrossRef]
44. Soleiman, H.A.; Koraiem, A.I.M.; Mahmoud, N.Y. Synthesis of new fused hetecrocyclic compounds of benzpyrid-4-one derivatives and their some biological activity. *J. Chin. Chem. Soc.* **2004**, *51*, 553–560. [CrossRef]
45. Finšgar, M.; Milošev, I. Inhibition of copper corrosion by 1,2,3-benzotriazole: A review. *Corros. Sci.* **2010**, *52*, 2737–2749. [CrossRef]
46. Al-Mayouf, A.M.; Al-Ameery, A.K.; Al-Suhybani, A.A. Inhibition of type 304 stainless steel corrosion in 2 M sulfuric acid by some benzoazoles—Time and temperature effects. *Corrosion* **2001**, *57*, 614–620. [CrossRef]
47. Lashgari, M.; Arshadi, M. DFT studies of pyridine corrosion inhibitors in electrical double layer: Solvent, substrate, and electric field effects. *Chem. Phys.* **2004**, *299*, 131–137. [CrossRef]
48. Levin, M.; Wiklund, P.; Leygraf, C. Bioorganic compounds as copper corrosion inhibitors in hydrocarbon media. *Corros. Sci.* **2012**, *58*, 104–114. [CrossRef]
49. Paul, P.K.; Saraswat, V.; Yadav, M. Chromenes as efficient corrosion inhibitor for mild steel in HCl solution. *J. Adhes. Sci. Technol.* **2019**, *33*, 1275–1293. [CrossRef]
50. Khaled, K.; Al-Mobarak, N.A. A predictive model for corrosion inhibition of mild steel by thiophene and its derivatives using artificial neural network. *Int. J. Electrochem. Sci.* **2012**, *7*, 1045–1059.
51. Taylor, C.D. Design and prediction of corrosion inhibitors from quantum chemistry. *J. Electrochem. Soc.* **2015**, *162*, 340–346. [CrossRef]
52. Taylor, C.D.; Chandra, A.; Vera, J.; Sridhar, N. Design and prediction of corrosion inhibitors from quantum chemistry II. A general framework for prediction of effective oil/water partition coefficients and speciation from quantum chemistry. *J. Electrochem. Soc.* **2015**, *162*, 347–353. [CrossRef]
53. Ebenso, E.E.; Kabanda, M.M.; Murulana, L.C.; Singh, A.K.; Shukla, S.K. Electrochemical and quantum chemical investigation of some azine and thiazine dyes as potential corrosion inhibitors for mild steel in hydrochloric acid solution. *Ind. Eng. Chem. Res.* **2012**, *51*, 12940–12958. [CrossRef]
54. Amin, M.A.; Khaled, K.F.; Mohsen, Q.; Arida, H.A. A study of the inhibition of iron corrosion in HCl solutions by some amino acids. *Corros. Sci.* **2010**, *52*, 1684–1695. [CrossRef]

55. Khaled, K.; Fadl-allah, S.; Hammouti, B. Some benzotriazole derivatives as corrosion inhibitors for copper in acidic medium: Experimental and quantum chemical molecular dynamics approach. *Mater. Chem. Phys.* **2009**, *117*, 148–155. [CrossRef]
56. Parr, R.G.; Pearson, R.G. Absolute hardness: Companion parameter to absolute electronegativity. *J. Am. Chem. Soc.* **1983**, *105*, 7512–7516. [CrossRef]
57. Zhang, J.; Liu, J.; Yu, W.; Yan, Y.; You, L.; Liu, L. Molecular modeling of the inhibition mechanism of 1-(2-aminoethyl)-2-alkyl-imidazoline. *Corros. Sci.* **2010**, *52*, 2059–2065. [CrossRef]
58. Sulaiman, K.O.; Onawole, A.T. Quantum chemical evaluation of the corrosion inhibition of novel aromatic hydrazide derivatives on mild steel in hydrochloric acid. *Comput. Theor. Chem.* **2016**, *1093*, 73–80. [CrossRef]
59. Dega-Szafran, Z.; Kania, A.; Nowak-Wydra, B.; Szafran, M. UV, 1H and 13C NMR spectra, and AM1 studies of protonation of aminopyridines. *J. Mol. Struct.* **1994**, *322*, 223–232. [CrossRef]
60. Frisch, M.J.; Trucks, G.W.; Schlegel, H.B.; Scuseria., G.E.; Robb, M.A.; Cheeseman, J.R.; Scalmani, G.; Barone, V.; Mennucci, B.; Petersson, G.A.; et al. *Gaussian 09*; Revision C.01; Gaussian, Inc.: Wallingford, CT, USA, 2009.
61. Becke, A.D. Becke's three parameter hybrid method using the LYP correlation functional. *J. Chem. Phys.* **1993**, *98*, 5648–5652. [CrossRef]
62. Metri, N.; Sallenave, X.; Plesse, C.; Beouch, L.; Aubert, P.-H.; Goubard, F.; Chevrot, C.; Sini, G. Processable star-shaped molecules with triphenylamine core as hole-transporting materials: Experimental and theoretical approach. *J. Phys. Chem. C* **2012**, *116*, 3765–3772. [CrossRef]
63. Cances, E.; Mennucci, B.; Tomasi, J. A new integral equation formalism for the polarizable continuum model: Theoretical background and applications to isotropic and anisotropic dielectrics. *J. Chem. Phys.* **1997**, *107*, 3032–3041. [CrossRef]


**Sample Availability:** Samples of the compounds **4a–i** are available from the authors.

molecules

MDPI

Article

# Mono- and Diamination of 4,6-Dichloropyrimidine, 2,6-Dichloropyrazine and 1,3-Dichloroisoquinoline with Adamantane-Containing Amines †

Alisa D. Kharlamova [1], Anton S. Abel [1], Alexei D. Averin [1,2], Olga A. Maloshitskaya [1], Vitaly A. Roznyatovskiy [1], Evgenii N. Savelyev [3], Boris S. Orlinson [3], Ivan A. Novakov [3] and Irina P. Beletskaya [1,2,*]

1 Department of Chemistry, Lomonosov Moscow State University, Leninskie Gory, 1-3, 119991 Moscow, Russia; alisa-harlamova@mail.ru (A.D.K.); antonabel@list.ru (A.S.A.); alexaveron@yandex.ru (A.D.A.); maloshitskaya@mail.ru (O.A.M.); Vit.Rozn@nmr.chem.msu.su (V.A.R.)

2 Frumkin Institute of Physical Chemistry and Electrochemistry, Russian Academy of Sciences, Leninsky Pr. 31, 119071 Moscow, Russia

3 Volgograd State Technical University, 28 Lenina prosp., 400131 Volgograd, Russia; savelyev_en@vstu.ru (E.N.S.); orlinson@vstu.ru (B.S.O.); president@vstu.ru (I.A.N.)

* Correspondence: beletska@org.chem.msu.ru; Tel.: +7-495-939-11-39

† Dedicated to Prof. Christian Bruneau for his outstanding contribution to catalysis.

**Abstract:** *N*-heteroaryl substituted adamantane-containing amines are of substantial interest for their perspective antiviral and psychotherapeutic activities. Chlorine atom at alpha-position of *N*-heterocycles has been substituted by the amino group using convenient nucleophilic substitution reactions with a series of adamantylalkylamines. The prototropic equilibrium in these compounds was studied using NMR spectroscopy. The introduction of the second amino substituent in 4-amino-6-chloropyrimidine, 2-amino-chloropyrazine, and 1-amino-3-chloroisoquinoline was achieved using Pd(0) catalysis.

**Keywords:** amines; adamantane; Pd catalysis; amination; pyrimidine; isoquinoline; pyrazine

## 1. Introduction

Amino substituted pyrimidines, pyrazines, and isoquinolines attract the researchers' interest due to their versatile biological activities stemming from the ability to form hydrogen bonds with various biomolecules, like nucleobases. Some derivatives of aminopyrimidine were found to act as inhibitors of various ferments: 1-phosphatidylinositol-3-phosphate 5-kinase (FAB1B) (e.g., bacimethrin) [1–3], 1-acyl-*sn*-glycerol-3-phosphate acyltransferase (plsC) [4], [Pyruvate dehydrogenase (acetyl-transferring)] kinase isozyme 1 (PDHA1) (e.g., 6′-((6-aminopyrimidin-4-yl)amino)-8′-methyl-2′*H*-spiro[cyclohexane-1,3′-imidazo[1,5-a]pyridine]-1′,5′-dione) [5], and perform as multitarget RET (rearranged during transfection) inhibitors [6]. In particular, substituted 4,6-diaminopyrimidines are capable of blocking epidermal growth factor receptor (EGFR), what make them perspective for the lung cancer treatment [7]. The last five years have demonstrated that aminopyrazine derivatives constitute an important platform for the creation of the inhibitors of mutant isocitrate dehydrogenase 1 (IDH1) [8], mitogen-activated protein kinase-interacting kinases 1 and 2 (MNK1/2) [9], and serine/threonine kinase (BRAF) (e.g., 1-{4-[6-(3,4,5-Trimethoxyphenylamino)-pyrazin-2-yl]phenyl}-3-phenyl urea) [10]. 2,6-Diaminopyrazine may serve as a backbone for the creating Nav1.7 antagonists [11], while substituted aminoisoquinolines (*N*-Methyl-3-(4-methylpiperazin-1-yl)isoquinolin-1-amine) bind to the receptor 5-HT3 [12].

Adamantane group helps to increase the lipophilicity of the molecules assuring their penetration through the biological membranes. Due to this ability adamantane derivatives demonstrate a wide range of biological activities [13]. The derivatives of adamantane-containing amines are known as the remedies against the Parkinson's disease (e.g., 1-adamantylamine) [14,15], they exhibit antitumor [16] and anti-HIV activities [16, 17], and are widely renowned as influenza viral inhibitors [18]. An imposing array of the peptide derivatives containing adamantaneamines demonstrate a wide scope of biological activities [19]. The derivatives of the heterocyclic compounds bearing adamantaneamine moieties are of special interest as psychotropic agents (e.g., 2-(1-adamantyl)-*N*-1*H*-indazol-5-ylacetamide) [16,20,21], they act as 11β-HSD1 (11β-Hydroxysteroid dehydrogenase type 1) inhibitors [22–24], are able to elicit anti-nicotine antibodies [25], and show antiviral and antimicrobial activities [26].

In order to search for novel perspective biologically active compounds on the basis of amino substituted heterocycles a convenient method for the synthesis of ample series of such molecule bearing versatile groups is needed. Known approaches are often limited by harsh reaction conditions, thus diminishing the scope of available substrates, e.g., unsymmetrical 4,6-diaminopyrimidines were obtained using Pd-catalyzed reactions in low yields (5–27%) [11]. Another study revealed the formation of many by-products in these processes and a strong demand for a fine adjustment of the reaction conditions [27]. The methods for 1,3-diaminoisoquinolines preparation are also limited. One of the best methods envisages α-cyano-o-tolunitrile cyclization by the action of organolithium compounds [28]. They can be also synthesized by a two-step non-catalytic amination of 1,3-dichloroisoquinoline under harsh conditions, which provides quite moderate yields (up to 31%) [12]. Fluorescent 1-morpholinoisoquinoline-3-amines were synthesized from 1-bromoisoquinoline-3-amine by heating with excess morpholine [29]. Recently, an original approach has been proposed for diamino derivatives of isoquinoline and pyrimidine, consisting of the catalytic cyclization of cyanamides and ynamides in the presence of gold complexes [30].

For the aforementioned reasons, the aim of this work is the elaboration of the approach to adamantane-containing 4,6-diaminopyrimidines, 2,6-diaminopyrazines, and 1,3-diaminoisoquinolines. Selective monoamination of the corresponding dichloroheteroarenes can be accomplished in high yields under catalyst-free conditions [31]. Non-catalytic introduction of the second amino group is seriously hindered by the electron donor effect of the first amino group. It is rational to use the Pd-catalyzed amination at the second step as it is depicted on Scheme 1. Earlier we demonstrated Pd-catalyzed diamination to be useful in one-step syntheses of symmetrical adamantane-containing diamino derivatives of pyridines [32], quinolines [33], and 1,10-phenanthrolines [34].

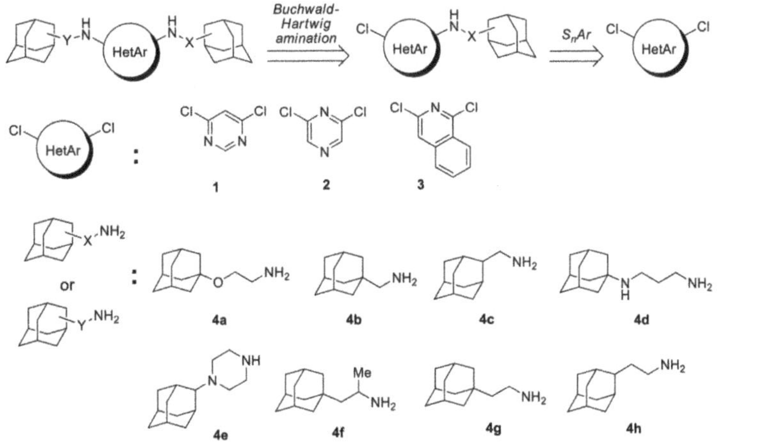


**Scheme 1.** A two-step approach to adamantane-containing diamino heteroarenes studied in this work.

## 2. Results and Discussion

In the present study, we employed commercially available 3,6-dichloropyrimidine **1**, 2,6-dichloropyrazine **2**, and 1,3-dichloroisoquinoline **3** and a set of adamantane-containing amines differing by the substituents at the amino group (Scheme 1). At first, the catalyst-free monoamination of 4,6-dichloropyrimidine **1** was undertaken, and the reactions were conducted under earlier optimized conditions (4 equiv. $K_2CO_3$, DMF, 140 °C) (Scheme 2).

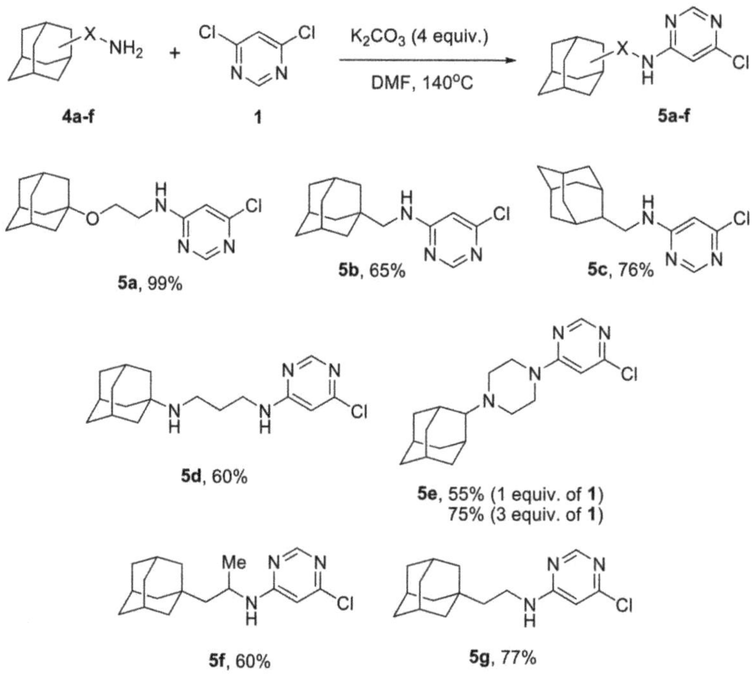


**Scheme 2.** Monoamination of 4,6-dichloropyrimidine with adamantane-containing amines.

The heteroarylation of a sterically unhindered amine **4a** proceeded smoothly and resulted in almost quantitative yield of the product **5a**. Amines **4c,g** with a closer position of the adamantane core to the amino group produced the target compounds in 76 and 77% yields, respectively. An increase in the steric hindrances in **4b,f** resulted in lower yields of the amination products **5b,f** (65 and 60%). The diamine **4d** reacted selectively and not surprisingly only the primary amino group participated in the heteroarylation affording compound **5d** in 60% yield. Initially, 55% yield was obtained in the reaction with the secondary amine **5e**, but the result was improved (75%) by taking 3 equiv. 4,6-dichloropyrimidine.

Catalyst-free monoamination of 2,6-dichloropyrazine **2** and 1,3-dichloroisoquinoline **3** with a wide scope of adamantane-containing amines was studied earlier [31]. The known protocol [31] was employed for the synthesis of *N*-(2-(1-adamantyloxy)ethyl)-6-chloropyrazin-2-amine **6** and *N*-[2-(1-adamantyloxy)ethyl]-3-chloroisoquinolin-1-amine **7** in 82 and 89% yields (Scheme 3) for further studies of the substitution of the chlorine in these compounds.

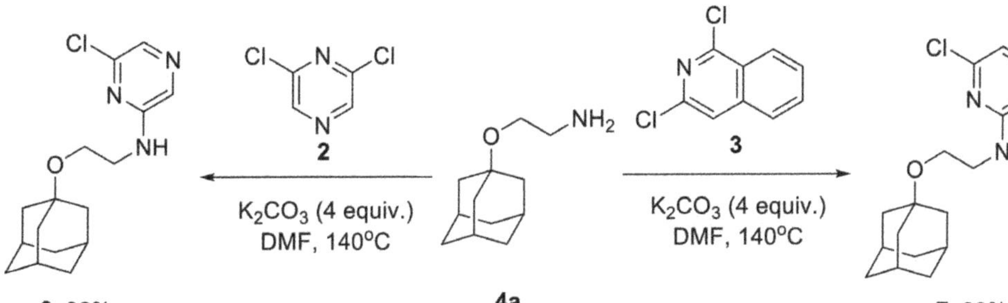


**Scheme 3.** Monoamination of 2,6-dichloropyrazine and 1,3-dichloroisoquinoline.

The synthesis of adamantane-containing 4,6-diaminopyrimidines was studied using a model compound **5a** with $Pd(dba)_2$ as a precatalyst (Scheme 4, Table 1). Classical phosphine ligands, like BINAP (2,2′-bis(diphenylphosphino)-1,1′-binaphthyl) and DavePhos (2-Dicyclohexylphosphino-2′-(*N,N*-dimethylamino)biphenyl) [35], were studied, as well as Ph-JosiPhos and Cy-JosiPhos (CyPF-$^t$Bu), which were shown to be efficient in the amination of halosubstituted heterocycles [36,37], were also tested. Other donor phosphine ligands with bulky substituents (SPhos, XPhos, RuPhos BrettPhos) were not studied in this reaction as they earlier had been shown to be much less efficient in the heteroarylation of adamantane-containing amines with 2-bromopyridines [38]. The reaction of **5a** with 1 equiv. of amine **4a** in the presence of Pd(0)/BINAP (Table 1, entry 1) produced a complex mixture of compounds. The $^1$H NMR signals in the range of 4.0–4.5 ppm (attributed to the signals of $CH_2N(HetAr)_2$ groups) suggest the formation of various products of *N,N*-diheteroarylation including oligomeric ones. MALDI-TOF mass spectra revealed the presence of the oligomers comprising 2–3 pyrimidine units combined with 3 or 4 amine fragments which could not be separated by column chromatography (e.g., **(4a)$_3$Het$_2$**, $[M + H]^+$ 738.48 and **(4a)$_4$Het$_3$**, $[M + H]^+$ 1009.59, Scheme 4). *N,N*-diheteroarylation was observed to be typical in the amination of 2-halosubstituted 6-membered heterocycles (pyridine and quinoline) [32,33,39,40].

**Table 1.** Pd-catalyzed amination of 4-amino-6-chloropyrimidine **5a**.

| Entry | Amine | Equiv. of Amine | Ligand | $Pd(dba)_2$/L, mol% | Product, Yield, % |
|---|---|---|---|---|---|
| 1 | **4a** | 1 | BINAP | 4/4.5 | **8a**, oligomers [1] |
| 2 | **4a** | 2 | Cy-JosiPhos | 2/2.5 | **8a**, oligomers [1] |
| 3 | **4a** | 2 | DavePhos | 4/4.5 | **8a**, oligomers [1] |
| 4 | **4a** | 2 | Ph-JosiPhos | 4/4.5 | **8a**, oligomers [1] |
| 5 | **4a** | 4 | DavePhos | 4/4.5 | **8a**, 60 |
| 6 | **4a** | 4 | BINAP | 8/9 | **8a**, 61 |
| 7 | **4b** | 4 | DavePhos | 4/4.5 | **8b**, 40 |
| 8 | **4f** | 4 | DavePhos | 4/4.5 | **8f**, 46 |

[1] Side products were observed in $^1$H NMR spectra of the reaction mixtures and confirmed by MALDI-TOF mass spectroscopy.

The use of bulky ligands (DavePhos, Ph-JosiPhos, and Cy-JosiPhos) did not lead to an increase in the product yield even in the presence of 2 equiv. amine (entries 2–4). The use of 4 equiv. amine allowed to obtain the target product in 60% yield (entry 5). The use of BINAP in this case gave the same yield, but with higher catalyst loading (entry 6). The reaction of more sterically hindered amines **4b** and **4f** with **5a** in the presence of Pd(0)/DavePhos catalyst led to the formation of the unsymmetrical products **8b** (40%) and **8f** (46%), respectively (entries 7, 8). *N,N*-diheteroarylation was also observed in all cases; however, corresponding products were always obtained as mixtures and could not be isolated in pure state.

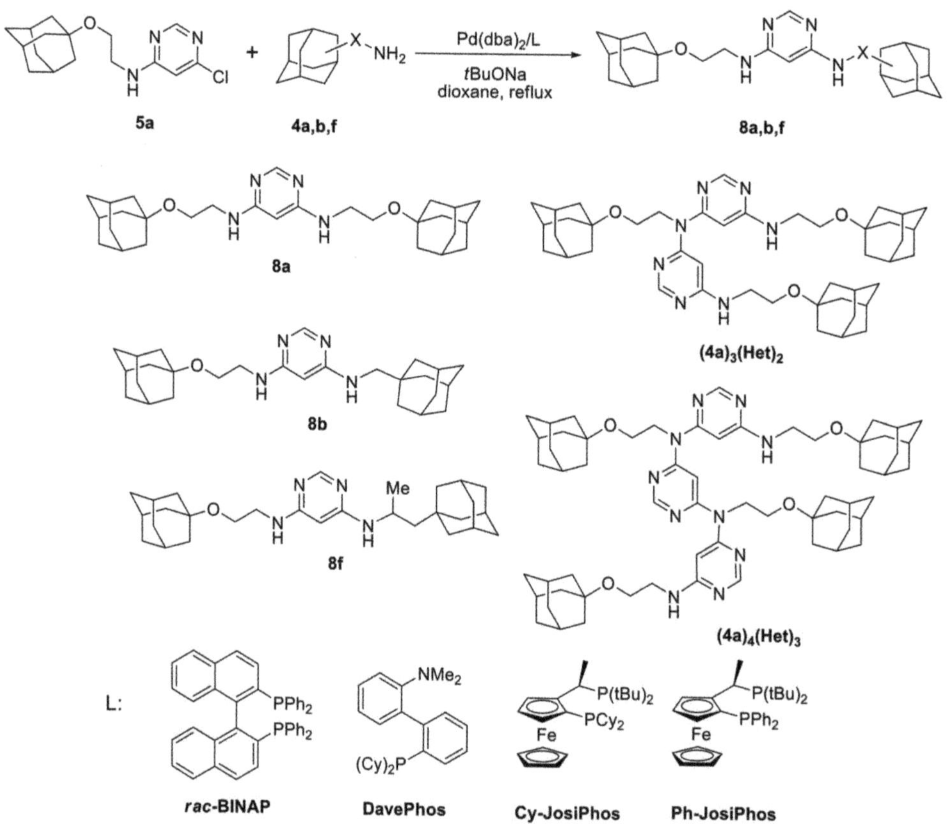


**Scheme 4.** Synthesis of adamantane-containing 4,6-diaminopyrimidines.

Such propensity for the diheteroarylation can be explained by the fact that 4-amino-6-chloropyrimidines exist as two tautomers **A** and **B** in equilibrium (Scheme 5). It may increase the NH-Het proton mobility and result in a faster *N,N*-diheteroarylation. Tautomeric equilibria of amine-imine type are natural for 2-aminoheterocycles and have been under investigation as it is a common form of isomerism for nucleobases. This phenomenon governs the ability of the heterocycles to form hydrogen bonds [41] and participate in redox processes [42].

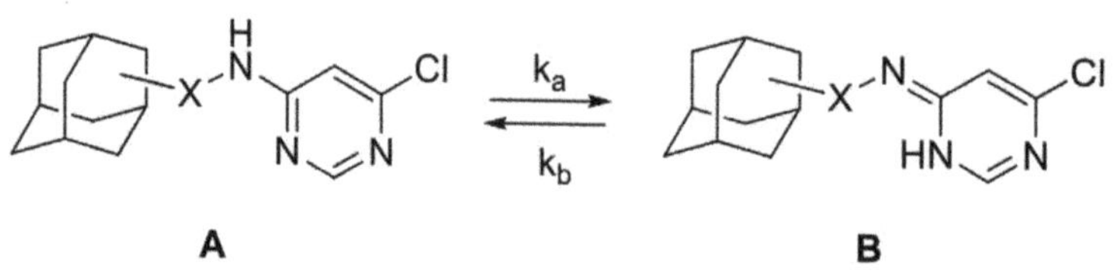


**Scheme 5.** Prototropic equilibrium in 4-amino-6-chloropyrimidines.

In the case of the pyrimidine derivatives **5**, the tautomers were observed in the $^1$H NMR spectra. Line broadening was notable for NH, aliphatic CHN protons, as well for the protons of the heterocyclic ring. To get a deeper insight in the phenomenon, the influence of the steric hindrances at the amino group on the tautomerism was studied for the compounds **5b**, **5c**, **5f**, and **5g**. NMR spectra of these compounds were registered in $CDCl_3$ at different temperatures in the range 223–323 K to get activation energy characteristics presented in Table 2.

**Table 2.** The activation energy characteristics of prototropic equlibrium of **5b,c,f,g**.

| Entry | Compound | X | Reaction | $K_{273}$ | $\Delta H^{\neq}$, kcal/mol | $\Delta S^{\neq}$, cal/mol × K | $\Delta G^{\neq}_{(273\ K)}$, kcal/mol |
|---|---|---|---|---|---|---|---|
| 1 | **5g** | 1-$CH_2CH_2$ | A→B | 0.45 | 17.84 | 13.58 | 14.24 |
| 2 | **5g** | 1-$CH_2CH_2$ | B→A | | 16.89 | 12.65 | 13.81 |
| 3 | **5b** | 1-$CH_2$ | A→B | 0.495 | 19.30 | 17.51 | 14.67 |
| 4 | **5b** | 1-$CH_2$ | B→A | | 18.46 | 15.81 | 14.29 |
| 5 | **5c** | 2-$CH_2$ | A→B | 0.54 | 16.31 | 7.38 | 14.48 |
| 6 | **5c** | 2-$CH_2$ | B→A | | 15.42 | 5.30 | 14.15 |
| 7 | **5f** | 1-$CH_2CH(CH_3)$ | A→B | 0.575 | 17.36 | 11.90 | 14.26 |
| 8 | **5f** | 1-$CH_2CH(CH_3)$ | B→A | | 16.69 | 10.59 | 13.96 |

The spectra were fitted using WinDNMR software and tautomers ratio was calculated (see Supplementary Materials). Reaction rate constants sum ($k = k_a + k_b$) and equilibrium constant ($K = k_a/k_b = [B]/[A]$) were determined for each temperature. The activation energy characteristics ($\Delta H^{\neq}$ and $\Delta S^{\neq}$) were calculated from the experiments using Eyring equation and are given in Table 2. While enthalpy and entropy of the activation of the processes differ substantially, the Gibbs energy does not show significant dependence on the structure of the compounds. With elevating the temperature, an increase in the imine ratio is observed and reaches 40% at 351–325 K. This could explain an easy formation of the palladium amide **I** complex from the imine form and, consequently, the tendency of the monoarylated product to participate in the second arylation step forming the *N,N*-diaryl derivative (Scheme 6). As it is known, the deprotonation of the palladium amine complex with its transformation into the amide complex is a rate-determining step of the catalytic cycle, and, in the present case, formation of the amide complex **I** is faster than amide complex **II** because of equilibrium between **A** and **B** forms.

The amination of 2-amino-6-chloropyrazine **6** (Scheme 7) using 1 equiv. of **4a** also led to a complex mixture of oligomers (Table 3, entries 1, 2), preventing the isolation of the target compound **9a** in a pure state. The application of 2 equiv. amine in the presence of Pd(0)/Cy-JosiPhos catalytic system afforded **9a** in 30% yield (entry 3) and the use of 4 equiv. amine with Ph-JosiPhos allowed the isolation of **9a** in 90% yield (entry 4). Under analogous conditions, **9b**, **9g**, and **9h** were synthesized in moderate yields 36–48% (entries 5, 7, 8). Indeed, the target products were obtained in much better yields in the reaction mixtures, but the losses during the separation from the oligomeric products badly decreased the isolated yields. Compound **9f** could not be isolated in a pure state due to such problem; its yield was estimated as 47% by $^1$H NMR spectrum (entry 6).

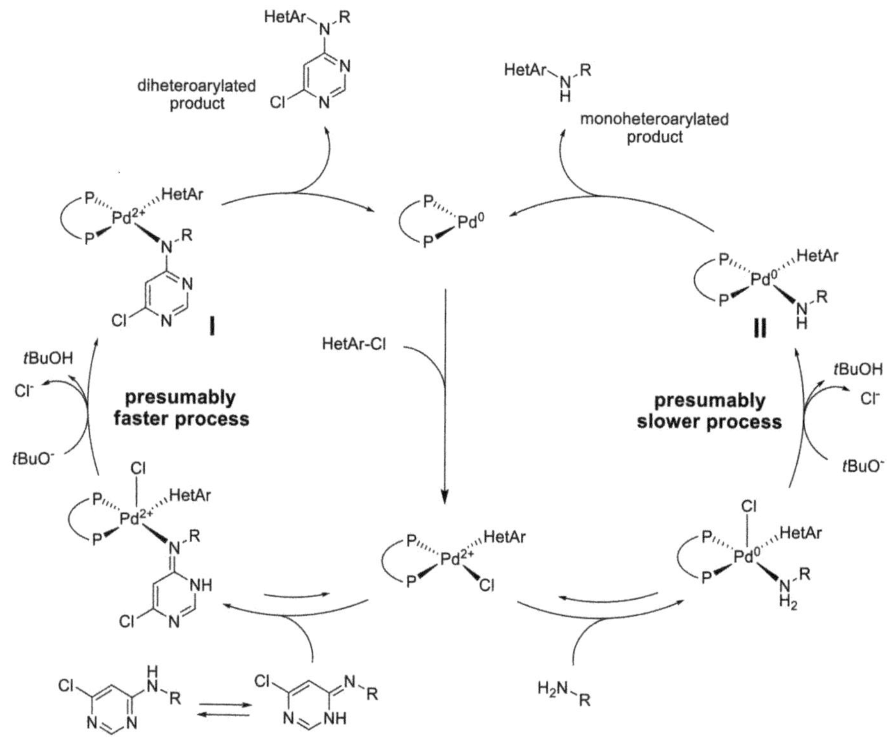


**Scheme 6.** Proposed mechanism of the formation of mono- and di-heteroarylated products.

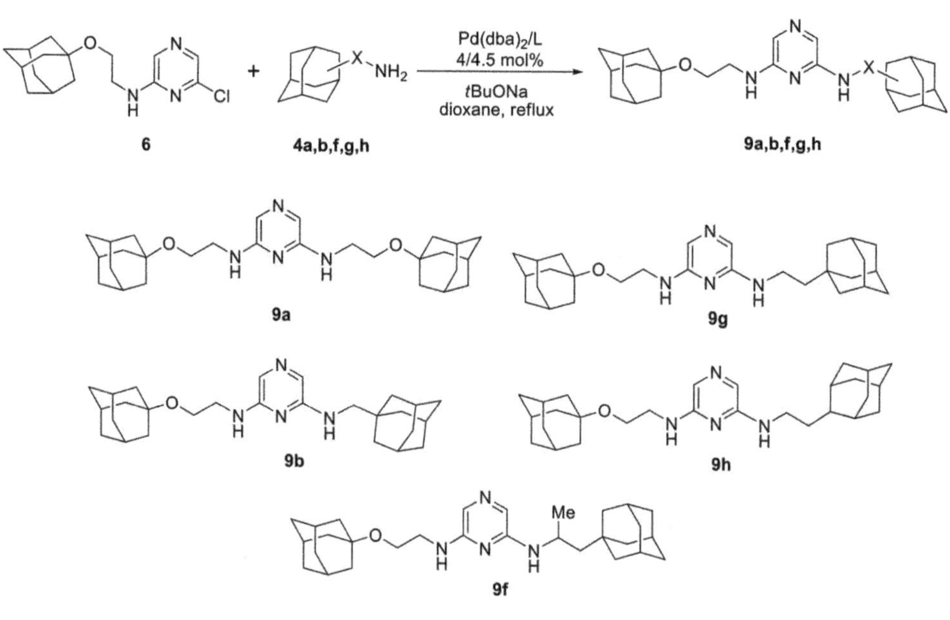


**Scheme 7.** Synthesis of adamantane-containing 2,6-diaminopyrazines.

**Table 3.** Pd-catalyzed amination of 2-amino-6-chloropyrazine **6**.

| Entry | Amine | Equiv. of Amine | Ligand | Product, Yield (%) |
|---|---|---|---|---|
| 1 | **4a** | 1 | BINAP | **9a**, oligomers [a] |
| 2 | **4a** | 1 | DavePhos | **9a**, oligomers [a] |
| 3 | **4a** | 2 | Cy-JosiPhos | **9a**, 30 |
| 4 | **4a** | 4 | Ph-JosiPhos | **9a**, 90 |
| 5 | **4b** | 4 | Ph-JosiPhos | **9b**, 42 |
| 6 | **4f** | 4 | Ph-JosiPhos | **9f**, (47) [b] |
| 7 | **4g** | 4 | Ph-JosiPhos | **9g**, 48 |
| 8 | **4h** | 4 | Ph-JosiPhos | **9h**, 36 |

[a] Side products were observed in $^1$H NMR spectra of the reaction mixtures and confirmed by MALDI-TOF mass spectroscopy (**(4a)$_3$Het$_2$**, $[M + H]^+$ 738.48 and **(4a)$_4$Het$_3$**, $[M + H]^+$ 1009.61). [b] Yield was determined by $^1$H NMR spectrum of the reaction mixture.

The amination of 2-amino-3-chloroisoquinoline **7** (Scheme 8) is also complicated by the formation of oligomers; however, in this case, it is somewhat less prominent, presumably due to more steric hindrances at the NH group. The application of 2 equiv. amine in the presence of Pd(0)/Cy-JosiPhos and Pd(0)/DavePhos catalytic systems gave only a mixture of oligomers (Table 4, entries 1,2). In the first case, the formation of the product **11** of C-Cl bond reduction was observed (entry 1). The use of 4 equiv. amine in the presence of Pd(0)/DavePhos afforded the desired compound **10a** in 77% yield (entry 3). The test of the BINAP ligand, even at greater catalyst loading, did not lead to an increase in the product yield (entry 4). Under optimized conditions, 1,3-diaminoisoquinolines **10b**, **10f** and **10g** were obtained in 43–67% yields (entries 5–7).

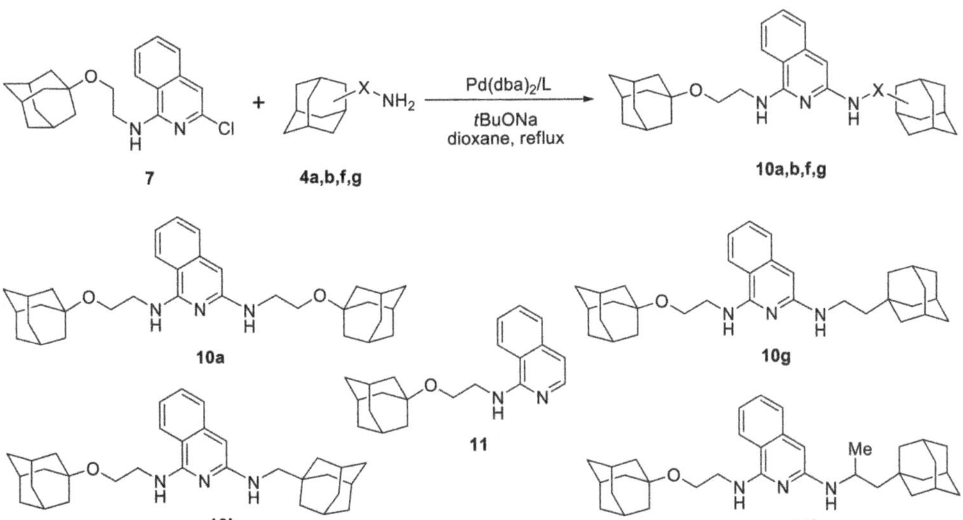


**Scheme 8.** Synthesis of adamantane-containing 1,3-diaminoisoquinolines.

**Table 4.** Pd-catalyzed amination of 1-amino-3-chloroisoquinoline **7**.

| Entry | Amine | Equiv. of Amine | Ligand | $Pd(dba)_2$/L, mol% | Product, Yield |
|---|---|---|---|---|---|
| 1 | **4a** | 2 | Cy-JosiPhos | 4/4.5 | **10a**, **11** [a] |
| 2 | **4a** | 2 | DavePhos | 4/4.5 | **10a**, oligomers [a] |
| 3 | **4a** | 4 | DavePhos | 4/4.5 | **10a**, 77% |
| 4 | **4a** | 4 | BINAP | 8/9 | **10a**, 76% |
| 5 | **4b** | 4 | DavePhos | 4/4.5 | **10b**, 62% |
| 6 | **4f** | 4 | DavePhos | 4/4.5 | **10f**, 67% |
| 7 | **4g** | 4 | DavePhos | 4/4.5 | **10g**, 43% |

[a] Side products were observed in NMR spectra of the reaction mixtures and confirmed by MALDI-TOF mass spectroscopy (e.g., $(\mathbf{4a})_3\mathbf{Het}_2$, $[M + H]^+$ 836.52).

## 3. Materials and Methods

NMR spectra were registered using a Bruker Avance 400 spectrometer (Bruker Daltonics, Germany), MALDI-TOF spectra were obtained with a Bruker Autoflex II spectrometer (Bruker Daltonics, Germany) using 1,8,9-trihydroxyanthracene as a matrix and polyethylene glycols (PEGs) as internal standards. Dichloropyrimidine, dichloropyrazine, dichloroisoquinoline, BINAP, DavePhos and JosiPhos ligands, sodium *tert*-butoxide, and potassium carbonate were purchased from Aldrich (Daltonics, Germany) and Acros (Morris Plains, NJ, USA) and used without further purification. Amines **4a** and **4b** were prepared according to reported procedures of References [43,44], respectively. Amines **4c** and **4e,g,h**, were obtained according to a method described in Reference [45], amines **4d** and **4f** were obtained according to methods described in References [39,46]. $Pd(dba)_2$ was synthesized from $PdCl_2$ according to a known procedure [47]. Dioxane was distilled over NaOH followed by the distillation over sodium under argon. Dimethylformamide was distilled over sodium hydride under reduced pressure. Dichloromethane and methanol were used freshly distilled.

### 3.1. N-(Heteroaryl)-Substituted Adamantane-Containing Amines 5–7 (General Procedure)

A corresponding chlorosubstituted heteroarene (0.5–2 mmol), finely powdered anhydrous $K_2CO_3$ (1.25–8 mmol), DMF (1–4 mL), and a corresponding adamantane-containing amine **4** (0.5–2 mmol) were placed into a glass vial equipped with a magnetic stirrer and screw tap, and the reaction mixture was stirred for 24 h at 140 °C. On the reaction completion, the mixture was cooled to room temperature, dichloromethane (5 mL) was added, an inorganic precipitate was filtered off and additionally washed with dichloromethane (5 mL), the combined organic filtrates were concentrated in vacuo, and the residues were analyzed by NMR spectroscopy. The products were purified by chromatography on silica gel, using the following sequence of eluents: hexanes—$CH_2Cl_2$ (4:1–1:4), $CH_2Cl_2$, $CH_2Cl_2$—MeOH (200:1–50:1).

*N-[2-(1-Adamantyloxy)ethyl]-6-chloropyrimidin-4-amine* (**5a**). Obtained from dichloropyrimidine **1** (298 mg), amine **4a** (390 mg) in the presence of $K_2CO_3$ (1.12 g) in 4 mL of DMF. Yield 608 mg (99%), white amorphous powder, m.p. 136–137 °C. $^1$H-NMR ($CDCl_3$) δ 1.55–1.64 (m, 6H, Ad), 1.69–1.70 (m, 6H, Ad), 2.10 (s, 3H, Ad), 3.41 (br. s, 2H, $CH_2$(NH)), 3.55 (br.t, 2H, $^3J_{obs}$ = 4.9 Hz, CH2(O)), 5.73 (br. s., 1H, NH), 6.35 (s, 1H, H5), 8.29 (s, 1H, H2). $^{13}$C-NMR($CDCl_3$) δ 30.2 (3C, Ad), 36.1 (3C, Ad), 41.2 (3C, Ad), 41.6 (1C, $CH_2$(NH)), 57.9 (1C, $CH_2$(O)), 72.4 (1C, $C_{quat}$(O)), 103.8 (1C, C5), 158.1 (2C, C2, C4), 163.1 (1C, C6). HRMS (MALDI-TOF): $m/z$ $[M + H]^+$ calcd for $C_{16}H_{23}ClN_3O$: 308.1524; observed: 308.1481.

*N-[(1-Adamantyl)methyl]-6-chloropyrimidin-4-amine* (**5b**). Obtained from dichloropyrimidine (75 mg), amine **5b** (83 mg) in the presence of $K_2CO_3$ (276 mg) in 1 mL of DMF. Yield 90 mg (65%), yellowish viscous oil. $^1$H-NMR ($CDCl_3$) δ 1.44–1.75 (m, 12H, Ad), 1.99 (s, 3H, Ad), 2.92 (br. s., 2H, $CH_2$(NH)), 5.84 (br. s., 1H, NH), 6.33 (s, 1H, H5), 8.28

(s, 1H, H2). $^{13}$C-NMR($CDCl_3$) δ 28.1 (3C, Ad), 34.1 (1C, $C_{quat}$), 36.8 (3C, Ad), 40.3 (3C, Ad), 53.5 (1C, $CH_2$(NH)), 100.3 (1C, C5), 158.2 (2C, C2, C4), 159.1 (1C, C4), 163.9 (1C, C6). HRMS (MALDI-TOF): $m/z$ [M + H]$^+$ calcd for $C_{15}H_{21}ClN_3$: 278.1419; observed: 278.1399.

*N-[(2-Adamantyl)methyl]-6-chloropyrimidin-4-amine* (**5c**). Obtained from $K_2CO_3$ (276 mg) in 1 mL of DMF. Yield 105 mg (76%), yellowish viscous oil. $^1$H-NMR ($CDCl_3$) δ 1.55 (d, 2H, $^3J$ = 11.8 Hz, Ad), 1.67–1.71 (m, 4H, Ad), 1.77–1.90 (m, 9H, Ad), 3.35 (br. s, 2H, $CH_2$(NH)), 5.84 (br. s., 1H, NH), 6.33 (s, 1H, H5), 8.28 (s, 1H, H2). $^{13}$C-NMR($CDCl_3$) δ 27.9 (1C, Ad), 28.0 (1C, Ad), 30.0 (2C, Ad), 31.6 (2C, Ad), 37.9 (1C, Ad), 38.6 (2C, Ad), 43.9 (2C, $CH_2$(NH), Ad), 100.4 (1C, C5), 153.5 (2C, C2, C4), 163.4 (1C, C6). HRMS (MALDI-TOF): $m/z$ [M + H]$^+$ calcd for $C_{15}H_{21}ClN_3$: 278.1419; observed: 278.1463.

*N-(6-chloropyrimididin-4-yl)-N′-(1-Adamantyl)propan-1,3-diamine* (**5d**). Obtained from dichloropyrimidine (75 mg), amine **4d** (104 mg) in the presence of $K_2CO_3$ (276 mg) in 1 mL of DMF. Yield 96 mg (60%), brownish viscous oil. $^1$H-NMR ($CDCl_3$) δ 1.52–1.66 (m, 14H, $CH_2$, Ad), 2.18 (s, 3H, Ad), 3.20–3.39 (m, 5H, NH, $CH_2$(NH)), 6.51 (s, 1H, H5), 8.34 (s, 1H, H2). $^{13}$C-NMR($CDCl_3$) δ 29.3 (3C, Ad), 29.8 (1C, $CH_2$), 35.8 (3C, Ad), 36.7 (1C, $CH_2$(NH)), 38.7 (1C, $CH_2$(NH)), 42.2 (3C, Ad), 56.7 (1C, $C_{quat}$), 104.9 (1C, C2), 156.8 (1C, C4), 161.9 (1C, C6), 162.2 (1C, C5). HRMS (MALDI-TOF): $m/z$ [M + H]$^+$ calcd for $C_{17}H_{26}ClN_4$: 321.1841; observed: 321.1834.

*N-[4-(2-Adamantyl)piperazin-1-yl]-6-chloropyrimidine* (**5e**). Obtained from dichloropyrimidine (224 mg), amine **4e** (113 mg) in the presence of $K_2CO_3$ (276 mg) in 1 mL of DMF. Yield 125 mg (75%), brownish viscous oil. $^1$H-NMR ($CDCl_3$) δ 1.43 (d, 2H, $^3J$ = 12.1 Hz, Ad), 1.55–1.62 (m, 4H, Ad), 1.71–1.79 (m, 4H, Ad), 2.06 (s, 5H, Ad), 2.39–2.43 (m, 4H, $CH_2$(N)), 3.62 (br. s, 4H, $CH_2$(N)), 6.47 (s, 1H, H5), 8.35 (s, 1H, H2). $^{13}$C-NMR($CDCl_3$) δ 27.0 (1C, Ad), 27.3 (1C, Ad), 28.8 (2C, Ad), 31.1 (2C, Ad), 36.9 (2C, Ad), 37.5 (1C, Ad), 44.2 (2C, $CH_2$(N)), 48.8 (2C, $CH_2$(N)), 67.0 (1C, Ad(N)), 101.0 (1C, C2), 157.8 (1C, C5), 159.7 (1C, C4), 162.0 (1C, C6). HRMS (MALDI-TOF): $m/z$ [M + H]$^+$ calcd for $C_{18}H_{26}ClN_4$: 333.1841; observed: 333.1866.

*N-[2-(1-Adamantyl)propan-2-yl]-6-chloropyrimidin-4-amine* (**5f**). Obtained from dichloropyrimidine (75 mg), amine **4f** (98 mg) in the presence of $K_2CO_3$ (276 mg) in 1 mL of DMF. Yield 92 mg (60%), yellowish viscous oil. $^1$H-NMR ($CDCl_3$) δ 1.15 (d, 3H, $^3J$ = 6.3 Hz, $CH_3$), 1.26–1.29 (m, 2H, $CH_2$(Ad)), 1.43–1.50 (m, 6H, Ad), 1.54–1.66 (m, 6H, Ad), 1.89 (s, 3H, Ad), 3.68 (br. s, 1H, CHN), 5.51 (br. s, 1H, NH), 6.27 (s, 1H, H5), 8.28 (s, 1H, H2). $^{13}$C-NMR($CDCl_3$) δ 23.0 (1C, $CH_3$), 28.4 (3C, Ad), 32.4 (1C, $C_{quat}$), 36.8 (3C, Ad), 42.8 (4C, Ad, $CH_2$(Ad)), 52.0 (1C, $CH_2$(NH)), 100.1 (1C, C5), 158.4 (2C, C2, C4), 161.9 (1C, C6). HRMS (MALDI-TOF): $m/z$ [M + H]$^+$ calcd for $C_{17}H_{25}ClN_3$: 306.1732; observed: 306.1757.

*N-[2-(1-Adamantyl)ethyl]-6-chloropyrimidin-4-amine* (**5g**). Obtained from dichloropyrimidine (75 mg), amine **4g** (90 mg) in the presence of $K_2CO_3$ (276 mg) in 1 mL of DMF. Yield 112 mg (77%), yellowish glassy compound. $^1$H-NMR ($CDCl_3$) δ 1.35–1.38 (m, 2H, $CH_2$(Ad)), 1.48–1.55 (m, 6H, Ad), 1.57–1.73 (m, 6H, Ad), 1.95 (s, 3H, Ad), 3.22 (br. s, 2H, $CH_2$N), 5.62 (br. s, NH), 6.29 (s, 1H, H5), 8.29 (s, 1H, H2). $^{13}$C-NMR($CDCl_3$) δ 28.6 (3C, Ad), 32.0
(1C, $CH_2$(Ad)), 36.7 (1C, $C_{quat}$ (Ad)), 37.0 (3C, Ad), 42.5 (3C, Ad), 43.5 (1C, Ad, $CH_2$(NH)), 103.3 (1C, C5), 155.4 (1C, C4), 158.4 (1C, C2), 163.4 (1C, C6). HRMS (MALDI-TOF): $m/z$ [M + H]$^+$ calcd for $C_{16}H_{23}ClN_3$: 292.1575; observed: 292.1540.

Syntheses of *N*-(2-(1-Adamantyloxy)ethyl)-6-chloropyrazin-2-amine (**6**) and *N*-[2-(1-Adamantyloxy)ethyl]-3-chloroisoquinolin-1-amine (**7**) were previously reported in ref. [31].

### *3.2. Palladium-Catalyzed Amination of Chloroheterocycles—General Procedure*

A two-neck flask equipped with a condenser and a magnetic stirrer, flushed with dry argon, was charged with corresponding chloroheterocycle (0.2 mmol), Pd(dba)$_2$ (2.5–12 mg, 2–8 mol%), phosphine ligand (2.5–9 mol%), and absolute dioxane (2 mL). The mixture was stirred for 2–3 min, then corresponding amine **4** (0.2–0.8 mmol) and *t*BuONa (0.375 mmol) were added, and the reaction mixture was refluxed for 24 h. After cooling it down to ambient temperature, the reaction mixture was diluted with $CH_2Cl_2$, the solution filtered and evaporated in vacuo, and the residue was chromatographed on silica gel using a sequence of eluents: hexanes, hexanes–$CH_2Cl_2$ 2:1–1:1, $CH_2Cl_2$, $CH_2Cl_2$/MeOH 200:1–3:1.

*N,N′-bis[2-(1-adamantyloxy)ethyl]pyrimidine-4,6-diamine* (**8a**). Obtained from chloroheterocycle **5a** (61.5 mg), amine **4a** (156 mg) in the presence of Pd(dba)$_2$ (5 mg), DavePhos (3.5 mg) and *t*BuONa (29 mg). Eluent $CH_2Cl_2$/MeOH 50:1. Yield 57 mg (61%), yellowish viscous oil. $^1$H-NMR ($CDCl_3$) δ 1.55–1.64 (m, 12H, Ad), 1.72 (s, 12H, Ad), 2.14 (s, 6H, Ad), 3.32–3.34 (m, 4H, $CH_2$(NH))), 3.57 (t, 4H, $^3J$ = 5.1 Hz, $CH_2$(O)), 5.14 (br. s, 2H, NH), 5.29 (s, 1H, H5), 8.07 (s, 1H, H2). $^{13}$C-NMR($CDCl_3$) δ 30.4 (6C, Ad), 36.3 (6C, Ad), 41.5 (6C, Ad), 41.5 (2C, $CH_2$(NH)), 58.2 (2C, $CH_2$(O)), 72.5 (2C, $C_{quat}$(O)), 80.2 (1C, C5), 157.5 (1C, C2), 162.7 (2C, C4, C6). HRMS (MALDI-TOF): *m*/*z* [M + H]$^+$ calcd for $C_{28}H_{43}N_4O_2$: 467.3381; observed: 467.3344.

*N-[2-(1-adamantyloxy)ethyl]-N′-[(1-adamantyl)methyl]pyrimidine-4,6-diamine* (**8b**). Obtained from chloroheterocycle **5a** (61.5 mg), amine **4b** (132 mg) in the presence of Pd(dba)$_2$ (5 mg), DavePhos (3.5 mg) and *t*BuONa (29 mg). Eluent $CH_2Cl_2$/MeOH 50:1. Yield 35 mg (40%), yellowish viscous oil. $^1$H-NMR ($CDCl_3$) δ 1.52–1.71 (m, 24H, Ad), 1.97 (s, 3H, Ad), 2.12 (s, 3H, Ad), 2.83 (d, 2H, $^3J$ = 5.9 Hz, $CH_2$(NH)), 3.35 (q, 2H, $^3J$ = 5.1 Hz, $CH_2$(NH)), 3.57 (t, 2H, $^3J$ = 5.9 Hz, $CH_2$(O)), 5.20 (br. s, NH), 5.27 (s, 1H, H5), 8.00 (s, 1H, H2). $^{13}$C-NMR($CDCl_3$) δ 28.2 (3C, Ad), 30.4 (3C, Ad), 36.3 (3C, Ad), 36.8 (3C, Ad), 40.4 (3C, Ad), 41.5 (3C, Ad), 42.0 (1C, $CH_2$(NH)), 53.6 (1C, $CH_2$(NH)), 58.2 (1C, $CH_2$(O)), 72.5 (1C, $C_{quat}$(O)), 79.3 (1C, C5), 156.6 (1C, C2), 162.6 (2C, C4, C6). HRMS (MALDI-TOF): *m*/*z* [M + H]$^+$ calcd for $C_{27}H_{40}N_4O$: 437.3275; observed: 437.3255.

*N-[2-(1-adamantyloxy)ethyl]-N′-[2-(1-adamantyl)propan]pyrimidine-4,6-diamine* (**8f**). Obtained from chloroheterocycle **5a** (61.5 mg), amine **4f** (155 mg) in the presence of Pd(dba)$_2$ (5 mg), DavePhos (3.5 mg) and *t*BuONa (29 mg). Eluent $CH_2Cl_2$/MeOH 50:1. Yield 43 mg (46%), yellowish viscous oil.$^1$H-NMR ($CDCl_3$) δ 1.14 (d, 3H, $^3J$ = 6.3 Hz, $CH_3$), 1.49–1.51 (m, 6H, Ad, $CH_2$), 1.55–1.67 (m, 14H, Ad, $CH_2$), 1.70–1.73 (m, 6H, Ad), 1.90 (s, 3H, Ad), 2.12 (s, 3H, Ad), 3.32–3.36 (q, 2H, $^3J$ = 5.3 Hz, $CH_2$(NH)), 3.56–3.60 (m, 3H, CH(NH), $CH_2$(O)), 5.23 (s, 1H, H5), 8.04 (s, 1H, H2), NH protons were not unambiguously attributed.$^{13}$C-NMR($CDCl_3$) δ 23.2 (1C, $CH_3$), 28.2 (3C, Ad), 30.4 (3C, Ad), 32.4 (1C, $C_{quat}$(Ad)), 36.3 (3C, Ad), 36.9 (3C, Ad), 41.5 (3C, Ad), 42.0 (1C, $CH_2$(Ad)), 42.6 (1C, $CH_2$(NH)), 42.9 (3C, Ad), 52.3 (1C, $CH_2$(NH)), 58.2 (1C, $CH_2$(O)), 72.4 (1C, $C_{quat}$(O)), 79.6 (1C, C5), 157.7 (1C, C2), 161.3 (1C, C4), 162.8 (1C, C6). HRMS (MALDI-TOF): *m*/*z* [M + H]$^+$ calcd for $C_{29}H_{44}N_4O$: 465.3588; observed: 465.3603.

*N,N′-bis[2-(1-adamantyloxy)ethyl]pyrazine-2,6-diamine*(**9a**). Obtained from chloroheterocycle **6** (61.5 mg), amine **4a** (156 mg) in the presence of Pd(dba)$_2$ (5 mg), Ph-JosiPhos (5 mg) and *t*BuONa (29 mg). Eluent $CH_2Cl_2$/MeOH 50:1. Yield 84 mg (90%), yellowish viscous oil. $^1$H-NMR ($CDCl_3$) δ 1.56–1.65 (m, 12H, Ad), 1.72 (s, 12H, Ad), 2.13 (s, 6H, Ad), 3.39–3.43 (m, 4H, $CH_2$(NH)), 3.56–3.59 (m, 4H, $CH_2$(O)), 4.68 (s, 2H, NH), 7.17 (s, 2H, H3, H5). $^{13}$C-NMR($CDCl_3$) δ 30.5 (6C, Ad), 36.4 (6C, Ad), 41.6 (6C, Ad), 41.9 (2C, $CH_2$(NH)), 58.5 (2C, $CH_2$(O)), 72.4 (2C, $C_{quat}$(O)), 118.4 (2C, C3, C5), 153.4 (2C, C2, C6). HRMS (MALDI-TOF): *m*/*z* [M + H]$^+$ calcd for $C_{28}H_{43}N_4O_2$: 467.3381; observed: 467.3419.

*N-[2-(1-adamantyloxy)ethyl]-N′-[(1-adamantyl)methyl]pyrazine-2,6-diamine* (**9b**). Obtained from chloroheterocycle **6** (61.5 mg), amine **4b** (132 mg) in the presence of Pd(dba)$_2$ (5 mg), Ph-JosiPhos (5 mg) and *t*BuONa (29 mg). Eluent $CH_2Cl_2$/MeOH 100:1. Yield 37 mg (42%), yellowish viscous oil. $^1$H-NMR ($CDCl_3$) δ 1.52–1.72 (m, 24H, Ad), 1.96 (s, 3H, Ad), 2.12 (s, 3H, Ad), 2.95 (d, 2H, $^3J$ = 6.7 Hz, $CH_2$(NH)), 3.39 (q, 2H, $^3J$ = 5.5 Hz, $CH_2$(NH)), 3.57 (t, 2H, $^3J$ = 5.5 Hz, $CH_2$(O)), 4.36 (t, 1H, $^3J$ = 5.9 Hz, NH), 4.66 (t, 1H, $^3J$ = 5.5 Hz, NH), 7.12 (s, 1H, H5), 7.15 (s, 1H, H3). $^{13}$C-NMR($CDCl_3$) δ 28.2 (3C, Ad), 30.4 (3C, Ad), 34.1 (1C, $C_{quat}$), 36.3 (3C, Ad), 36.9 (3C, Ad), 40.4 (3C, Ad), 41.5 (3C, Ad), 41.9 (1C, $CH_2$(NH)), 53.2 (1C, $CH_2$(Ad)), 58.4 (1C, $CH_2$(O)), 72.4 (1C, $C_{quat}$(O)), 115.4 (1C, C3), 115.7 (1C, C5),

153.6 (1C, C2), 154.3 (1C, C6). HRMS (MALDI-TOF): *m/z* $[M + H]^+$ calcd for $C_{27}H_{41}N_4O$: 437.3275; observed: 437.3261.

*N-[2-(1-adamantyloxy)ethyl]-N′-[2-(1-adamantyl)ethan]pyrazine-2,6-diamine* (**9g**). Obtained from chloroheterocycle **6** (61.5 mg), amine **4g** (143 mg) in the presence of $Pd(dba)_2$ (5 mg), Ph-JosiPhos (5 mg) and *t*BuONa (29 mg). Eluent $CH_2Cl_2$/MeOH 50:1. Yield 43 mg (48%), yellowish viscous oil. $^1$H-NMR ($CDCl_3$) δ 1.50–1.84 (m, 26H, Ad, $CH_2$(Ad)), 2.13 (s, 6H, Ad), 3.20–3.25 (m, 2H, $CH_2$(NH)), 3.39 (q, 2H, $^3J$ = 5.4 Hz, $CH_2$(NH)), 3.56 (t, 2H, $^3J$ = 5.3 Hz, $CH_2$(O)), 4.30 (t, 1H, $^3J$ = 5.4, NH), 4.68 (t, 1H, $^3J$ = 5.6 Hz, NH), 7.14 (s, 1H, H3), 7.17 (s, 1H, H5). $^{13}$C-NMR($CDCl_3$) δ 27.9 (1C, $CH_2$(Ad)), 30.4 (3C, Ad), 31.5 (3C, Ad), 31.6 (3C, Ad), 31.8 (1C, $C_{quat}$), 36.4 (3C, Ad), 38.2 (1C, $CH_2$(NH)), 39.0 (3C, Ad), 41.5 (3C, Ad), 41.8 (1C, $CH_2$(NH)), 58.5 (1C, $CH_2$(O)), 72.3 (1C, $C_{quat}$(O)), 117.6 (1C, C3), 118.6 (1C, C5), 153.4 (2C, C2, C6). HRMS (MALDI-TOF): *m/z* $[M + H]^+$ calcd for $C_{28}H_{43}N_4O$: 451.3431; observed: 451.3454.

*N-[2-(1-adamantyloxy)ethyl]-N′-[2-(2-adamantyl)ethan]pyrazine-2,6-diamine* (**9h**). Obtained from chloroheterocycle **6** (61.5 mg), amine **4h** (143 mg) in the presence of $Pd(dba)_2$ (5 mg), Ph-JosiPhos (5 mg) and *t*BuONa (29 mg). Eluent $CH_2Cl_2$/MeOH 50:1. Yield 32 mg (36%), yellowish viscous oil. $^1$H-NMR ($CDCl_3$) δ 1.51–1.94 (m, 29H, Ad, $CH_2$(Ad)), 2.14 (s, 3H, Ad), 3.22–3.26 (m, 2H, $CH_2$(NH)), 3.37–3.42 (m, 2H, $CH_2$(NH)), 3.57 (t, 2H, $^3J$ = 5.4 Hz, $CH_2$(O)), 4.17 (s, 1H, NH), 4.69 (s, 1H, NH), 7.13 (s, 1H, H3), 7.18 (s, 1H, H5). $^{13}$C-NMR($CDCl_3$) δ 28.5 (1C, Ad), 28.6 (1C, Ad), 30.4 (3C, Ad), 36.3 (1C, Ad), 36.4 (3C, Ad), 36.9 (2C, Ad), 37.0 (2C, Ad), 41.5 (3C, Ad), 41.9 (1C, $CH_2$(Ad)), 42.0 (1C, $CH_2$(NH)), 42.4 (1C, Ad), 42.5 (2C, Ad), 44.0 (1C, $CH_2$(NH)), 58.5 (1C, $CH_2$(O)), 72.3 (1C, $C_{quat}$(O)), 117.6 (1C, C3), 118.7 (1C, C5), 153.4 (1C, C6), 153.5 (1C, C2). HRMS (MALDI-TOF): *m/z* $[M + H]^+$ calcd for $C_{28}H_{43}N_4O$: 451.3431; observed: 451.3430.

*N,N′-bis[2-(1-adamantyloxy)ethyl]isoquinoline-1,3-diamine* (**10a**). Obtained from chloroheterocycle **7** (71.5 mg), amine **4a** (156 mg) in the presence of $Pd(dba)_2$ (5 mg), DavePhos (3.5 mg) and *t*BuONa (29 mg). Eluent $CH_2Cl_2$/MeOH 50:1. Yield 79 mg (77%), yellowish viscous oil. $^1$H-NMR ($CDCl_3$) δ 1.57–1.65 (m, 12H, Ad), 1.76 (s, 12H, Ad), 2.15 (s, 6H, Ad), 3.37 (t, 2H, $^3J$ = 5.6 Hz, $CH_2$(NH)), 3.63–3.67 (m, 4H, $CH_2$(NH), $CH_2$(O)), 3.70–3.72 (m, 2H, $CH_2$(O)), 4.62 (br. s., 1H, NH), 5.65 (s, 1H, NH), 5.87 (s, 1H, H4), 7.04 (ddd, 1H, $^3J$ = 8.2, $^3J$ = 6.4, $^4J$ = 1.7 Hz, H7), 7.33–7.39 (m, 2H, H5, H6), 7.54 (d, 1H, $^3J$ = 8.3 Hz, H8). $^{13}$C-NMR($CDCl_3$) δ 30.4 (6C, Ad), 36.3 (6C, Ad), 41.5 (3C, Ad), 41.6 (3C, Ad), 41.7 (1C, $CH_2$(NH)), 43.3 (1C, $CH_2$(NH)), 58.6 (1C, $CH_2$(O)), 58.9 (1C, $CH_2$(O)), 72.2 (2C, $C_{quat}$(O)), 85.7 (1C, C4), 113.1 (1C, C8a), 120.6 (1C, C5), 121.6 (1C, C8), 125.1 (1C, C7), 129.5 (1C, C6), 140.5 (1C, C4a), 154.3 (1C, C1), 154.8 (1C, C3). HRMS (MALDI-TOF): *m/z* $[M + H]^+$ calcd for $C_{33}H_{46}N_3O_2$: 516.3584; observed: 516.3587.

*N$^3$-(1-adamantylmethyl)-N$^1$-[2-(1-adamantyloxy)ethyl]isoquinoline-1,3-diamine* (**10b**). Obtained from chloroheterocycle **7** (71.5 mg), amine **4b** (132 mg) in the presence of $Pd(dba)_2$ (5 mg), DavePhos (3.5 mg) and *t*BuONa (29 mg). Eluent $CH_2Cl_2$/MeOH 200:1. Yield 61 mg (62%), green viscous oil. $^1$H-NMR ($CDCl_3$) δ 1.62–1.77 (m, 24H, Ad), 2.00 (s, 3H, Ad), 2.16 (s, 3H, Ad), 2.91 (s, 2H, $CH_2$(NH)), 3.67–3.76 (m, 4H, $CH_2$(NH), $CH_2$(O)), 4.27 (br. s, 1H, NH), 5.82 (s, 1H, H4), 7.00–7.04 (m, 1H, H7), 7.32-7.37 (m, 2H, H5, H6), 7.51 (d, 1H, $^3J$ = 8.4 Hz, H8), 1 NH proton was not unambiguously attributed. $^{13}$C-NMR($CDCl_3$) δ 28.4 (3C, Ad), 30.5 (3C, Ad), 33.9 (1C, $C_{quat}$(Ad)), 36.4 (3C, Ad), 37.1 (3C, Ad), 40.7 (3C, Ad), 41.7 (4C, Ad, $CH_2$(Ad)), 55.2 (1C, $CH_2$(NH)), 58.9 (1C, $CH_2$(O)), 72.4 (1C, $C_{quat}$(O)), 84.9 (1C, C4), 113.0 (1C, C8a), 120.4 (1C, C5), 121.6 (1C, C8), 125.1 (1C, C7), 129.5 (1C, C6), 140.7 (1C, C4a), 154.7 (1C, C1), 155.1 (1C, C3). HRMS (MALDI-TOF): *m/z* $[M + H]^+$ calcd for $C_{32}H_{44}N_3O$: 486.3479; observed: 486.3506.

*N$^3$-[2-(1-adamantyl)-1-methylethyl]-N$^1$-[2-(1-adamantyloxy)ethyl]isoquinoline-1,3-diamine* (**10f**). Obtained from chloroheterocycle **7** (71.5 mg), amine **4f** (155 mg) in the presence of $Pd(dba)_2$ (5 mg), DavePhos (3.5 mg) and *t*BuONa (29 mg). Eluent $CH_2Cl_2$/MeOH 200:1. Yield 69 mg (67%), green viscous oil. $^1$H-NMR ($CDCl_3$) δ 1.23 (d, 3H, $^3J$ = 6.2 Hz, $CH_3$), 1.58–1.69 (m, 20H, Ad, $CH_2$), 1.76–1.77 (m, 6H, Ad), 1.93 (s, 3H, Ad), 2.15 (s, 3H, Ad), 3.68–3.78 (m, 5H, $CH_2$(NH), CH(NH), $CH_2$(O)), 4.17 (br. s, 1H, NH), 5.81 (s, 1H,

H4), 7.00–7.05 (m, 1H, H7), 7.33–7.38 (m, 2H, H5, H6), 7.52 (d, 1H, $^3J$ = 8.3 Hz, H8), 1 NH proton was not unambiguously attributed. $^{13}$C-NMR(CDCl$_3$) δ 23.4 (1C, $CH_3$), 28.7 (3C, Ad), 30.5 (3C, Ad), 32.6 (1C, $C_{quat}$(Ad)), 36.4 (3C, Ad), 37.0 (3C, Ad), 41.7 (4C, Ad, CH), 42.9 (3C, Ad), 43.3 (1C, $CH_2$(NH)), 52.7 (1C, $CH_2$(NH)), 58.7 (1C, $CH_2$(O)), 72.4 (1C, $C_{quat}$(O)), 85.1 (1C, C4), 112.9 (1C, C8a), 120.2 (1C, C5), 121.7 (1C, C8), 125.0 (1C, C7), 129.5 (1C, C6), 140.7 (1C, C4a), 153.2 (1C, C1), 154.4 (1C, C3). HRMS (MALDI-TOF): $m/z$ [M + H]$^+$ calcd for $C_{34}H_{48}N_3O$: 514.3792; observed: 514.3806.

*$N^3$-[2-(1-adamantyl)ethyl]-$N^1$-[2-(1-adamantyloxy)ethyl]isoquinoline-1,3-diamine* (**10g**). Obtained from chloroheterocycle **7** (71.5 mg), amine **4g** (143 mg) in the presence of Pd(dba)$_2$ (5 mg), DavePhos (3.5 mg) and *t*BuONa (29 mg). Eluent $CH_2Cl_2$/MeOH 150:1. Yield

43 mg (43%), green viscous oil. $^1$H-NMR (CDCl$_3$) δ 1.57–1.77 (m, 26H, Ad, $CH_2$), 1.98 (s, 3H, Ad), 2.15 (s, 3H, Ad), 3.17–3.21 (m, 2H, $CH_2$(NH)), 3.65–3.71 (m, 4H, $CH_2$(NH), $CH_2$(O)), 5.69 (br. s, 1H, NH), 5.81 (s, 1H, H4), 7.04 (m, 1H, $^3J$ = 8.1 Hz, H7), 7.34–7.40 (m, 2H, H5, H6), 7.51-7.54 (m, 1H, H8), 1 NH proton was not unambiguously attributed HRMS (MALDI-TOF): $m/z$ [M + H]$^+$ calcd for $C_{33}H_{46}N_3O$: 500.3635; observed: 500.3653.

## 4. Conclusions

To sum up, we have investigated a synthetic approach to adamantane-containing 4,6-diaminopyrimidine, 2,6-diaminopyrazine, and 1,3-diaminoisoquinoline based on consequent substitution of chlorine atoms in the corresponding dichloroheterocycle by means of convenient nucleophilic substitution and Pd-catalyzed amination, respectively. Selective monoamination of 4,6-diaminopyrimidine proceeds under catalyst-free conditions with products yields from good to excellent. Synthesis of 4,6-diaminopyrimidine, 2,6-diaminopyrazine and 1,3-diaminoisoquinoline by Pd-catalyzed amination of aminochloroderivatives is complicated by *N,N*-diarylation, leading to formation of oligomers; therefore, to suppress the side products formation, 4-fold excess of amine is required. Adamantane-containing 4,6-dialkylaminopyrimidines and 1,3-dialkylaminoisoquinolines have been obtained in moderate to good yields (40–60%) using DavePhos as a ligand while the use of Ph-JosiPhos ligand is necessary for the synthesis of adamantylated 2,6-diaminopyrazines. It has been shown that adamantane-containing 6-chloro-4-aminopyrimidines exhibit prototropic tautomerism, which was observed and quantitatively characterized by NMR-spectroscopy. Tautomerism between amine and imine forms of the *N*-heteroarylated derivatives of adamantaneamines is held responsible to the formation of *N,N*-diarylated species.

**Supplementary Materials:** The following are available online. Experimental details of studies of prototropic equilibria.

**Author Contributions:** Conceptualization, I.P.B. and A.D.A., Methodology, A.S.A. and A.D.K., Investigation, A.D.K., A.S.A., and O.A.M., Resources, E.N.S., B.S.O., and I.A.N., Data curation, V.A.R., Writing—Original draft preparation, A.S.A., Writing—Review and editing, I.P.B. and A.D.A., Visualization, A.S.A., Supervision, I.P.B., Project administration, A.D.A., Funding acquisition, A.D.A. and I.P.B. All authors have read and agreed to the published version of the manuscript.

**Funding:** This research was funded by the RFBR, grant number 17-03-00888.

**Data Availability Statement:** The data presented in this study are available in Supplementary Materials or on request from the corresponding author.

**Acknowledgments:** The study of prototropic equlibria was fulfilled using an Agilent 400-MR NMR spectrometer purchased by the MSU Development Program.

**Conflicts of Interest:** The authors declare no conflict of interest. The funders had no role in the design of the study, in the collection, analyses, or interpretation of data, in the writing of the manuscript or in the decision to publish the results.

**Sample Availability:** Samples of the compounds are not available from the authors.

## References


1. Reddick, J.J.; Saha, S.; Lee, J.-M.; Melnick, J.S.; Perkins, J.; Begley, T.P. The mechanism of action of bacimethrin, a naturally occurring thiamin antimetabolite. *Bioorg. Med. Chem. Lett.* **2001**, *11*, 2245–2248. [CrossRef]
2. Liang, X.; Wang, B.; Chen, C.; Wang, A.; Hu, C.; Zou, F.; Yu, K.; Liu, Q.; Li, F.; Hu, Z.; et al. Discovery of N-(4-(6-Acetamidopyrimidin-4-yloxy)phenyl)-2-(2-(trifluoromethyl)phenyl)acetamide (CHMFL-FLT3-335) as a Potent FMS-like Tyrosine Kinase 3 Internal Tandem Duplication (FLT3-ITD) Mutant Selective Inhibitor for Acute Myeloid Leukemia. *J. Med. Chem.* **2019**, *62*, 875–892. [CrossRef]
3. Manz, T.D.; Sivakumaren, S.C.; Yasgar, A.; Hall, M.D.; Davis, M.I.; Seo, H.-S.; Card, J.D.; Ficarro, S.B.; Shim, H.; Marto, J.A.; et al. Structure–Activity Relationship Study of Covalent Pan-phosphatidylinositol 5-Phosphate 4-Kinase Inhibitors. *ACS Med. Chem. Lett.* **2020**, *11*, 346–352. [CrossRef] [PubMed]
4. Gong, B.; Hong, F.; Kohm, C.; Jenkins, S.; Tulinsky, J.; Bhatt, R.; de Vries, P.; Singer, J.W.; Klein, P. Synthesis, SAR, and antitumor properties of diamino-C,N-diarylpyrimidine positional isomers: Inhibitors of lysophosphatidic acid acyltransferase-β. *Bioorg. Med. Chem. Lett.* **2004**, *14*, 2303–2308. [CrossRef] [PubMed]
5. Reich, S.H.; Sprengeler, P.A.; Chiang, G.G.; Appleman, J.R.; Chen, J.; Clarine, J.; Eam, B.; Ernst, J.T.; Han, Q.; Goel, V.K.; et al. Structure-based Design of Pyridone–Aminal eFT508 Targeting Dysregulated Translation by Selective Mitogen-activated Protein Kinase Interacting Kinases 1 and 2 (MNK1/2) Inhibition. *J. Med. Chem.* **2018**, *61*, 3516–3540. [CrossRef] [PubMed]
6. Mologni, L.; Dalla Via, M.; Chilin, A.; Palumbo, M.; Marzaro, G. Discovery of wtRET and V804MRET Inhibitors: From Hit to Lead. *ChemMedChem* **2017**, *12*, 1390–1398. [CrossRef]
7. Zhang, Y.; Lv, H.; Luo, L.; Xu, Y.; Pan, Y.; Wang, Y.; Lin, H.; Xiong, J.; Guo, P.; Zhang, J.; et al. Design, synthesis and pharmacological evaluation of N4,N6-disubstituted pyrimidine-4,6-diamine derivatives as potent EGFR inhibitors in non-small cell lung cancer. *Eur. J. Med. Chem.* **2018**, *157*, 1300–1325. [CrossRef] [PubMed]
8. Ma, T.; Zou, F.; Pusch, S.; Yang, L.; Zhu, Q.; Xu, Y.; Gu, Y.; von Deimling, A.; Zha, X. Design, synthesis and biological activity of 3-pyrazine-2-yl-oxazolidin-2-ones as novel, potent and selective inhibitors of mutant isocitrate dehydrogenase 1. *Biorg. Med. Chem.* **2017**, *25*, 6379–6387. [CrossRef]
9. Yuan, X.; Wu, H.; Bu, H.; Zheng, P.; Zhou, J.; Zhang, H. Design, synthesis and biological evaluation of pyridone–aminal derivatives as MNK1/2 inhibitors. *Biorg. Med. Chem.* **2019**, *27*, 1211–1225. [CrossRef]
10. Niculescu-Duvaz, I.; Roman, E.; Whittaker, S.R.; Friedlos, F.; Kirk, R.; Scanlon, I.J.; Davies, L.C.; Niculescu-Duvaz, D.; Marais, R.; Springer, C.J. Novel Inhibitors of the v-raf Murine Sarcoma Viral Oncogene Homologue B1 (BRAF) Based on a 2,6-Disubstituted Pyrazine Scaffold. *J. Med. Chem.* **2008**, *51*, 3261–3274. [CrossRef]
11. Bregman, H.; Nguyen, H.N.; Feric, E.; Ligutti, J.; Liu, D.; McDermott, J.S.; Wilenkin, B.; Zou, A.; Huang, L.; Li, X.; et al. The discovery of aminopyrazines as novel, potent Nav1.7 antagonists: Hit-to-lead identification and SAR. *Bioorg. Med. Chem. Lett.* **2012**, *22*, 2033–2042. [CrossRef]
12. Verheij, M.H.P.; Thompson, A.J.; van Muijlwijk-Koezen, J.E.; Lummis, S.C.R.; Leurs, R.; de Esch, I.J.P. Design, Synthesis, and Structure–Activity Relationships of Highly Potent 5-HT3 Receptor Ligands. *J. Med. Chem.* **2012**, *55*, 8603–8614. [CrossRef]
13. Wanka, L.; Iqbal, K.; Schreiner, P.R. The Lipophilic Bullet Hits the Targets: Medicinal Chemistry of Adamantane Derivatives. *Chem. Rev.* **2013**, *113*, 3516–3604. [CrossRef]
14. Gilligan, B.S.; Veale, J.; Wodak, J. Amantadine hydrochloride in the treatment of Parkinson's disease. *Med. J. Aust.* **1970**, *2*, 634–637. [CrossRef]
15. Hunter, K.R.; Stern, G.M.; Laurence, D.R.; Armitage, P. Amantadine in Parkinsonism. *Lancet* **1970**, *295*, 1127–1129. [CrossRef]
16. Da Settimo, A.; Marini, A.M.; Primofiore, G.; Da Settimo, F. Synthesis and evaluation of aminoadamantane derivatives for in vitro anti-HIV and antitumor activities. *Farmaco* **1995**, *50*, 321–326.
17. Danilenko, G.I.; Rybalko, S.L.; Maksimov, Y.N.; Baklan, V.F.; Guzhova, S.V. Adamantane-1- and norbornane-2-carboxylic acid hydrazides as HIV inhibitors. *Pharm. Chem. J.* **2000**, *34*, 23–24. [CrossRef]
18. Chayrov, R.; Parisis, N.A.; Chatziathanasiadou, M.V.; Vrontaki, E.; Moschovou, K.; Melagraki, G.; Sbirkova-Dimitrova, H.; Shivachev, B.; Schmidtke, M.; Mitrev, Y.; et al. Synthetic Analogues of Aminoadamantane as Influenza Viral Inhibitors—In Vitro, in Silico and QSAR Studies. *Molecules* **2020**, *25*, 3989. [CrossRef]
19. Grillaud, M.; Bianco, A. Multifunctional adamantane derivatives as new scaffolds for the multipresentation of bioactive peptides. *J. Pept. Sci.* **2015**, *21*, 330–345. [CrossRef]
20. Avdyunina, N.I.; Morqzov, I.S.; Bol'shakova, R.F.; Militareva, N.A.; Klimova, N.V.; Bykov, N.P.; Pyatin, B.M.; Khranilov, A.A.; Dvalishvili, É.G. Synthesis and pharmacological properties of benzimidazoline-3-acetic acid n-adamantylamides. *Pharm. Chem. J.* **1988**, *22*, 543–546. [CrossRef]
21. Baxter, A.; Bent, J.; Bowers, K.; Braddock, M.; Brough, S.; Fagura, M.; Lawson, M.; McInally, T.; Mortimore, M.; Robertson, M.; et al. Hit-to-Lead studies: The discovery of potent adamantane amide P2X7 receptor antagonists. *Bioorg. Med. Chem. Lett.* **2003**, *13*, 4047–4050. [CrossRef]
22. Sorensen, B.; Rohde, J.; Wang, J.; Fung, S.; Monzon, K.; Chiou, W.; Pan, L.; Deng, X.; Stolarik, D.; Frevert, E.U.; et al. Adamantane 11-β-HSD-1 inhibitors: Application of an isocyanide multicomponent reaction. *Bioorg. Med. Chem. Lett.* **2006**, *16*, 5958–5962. [CrossRef] [PubMed]

23. Rohde, J.J.; Pliushchev, M.A.; Sorensen, B.K.; Wodka, D.; Shuai, Q.; Wang, J.; Fung, S.; Monzon, K.M.; Chiou, W.J.; Pan, L.; et al. Discovery and Metabolic Stabilization of Potent and Selective 2-Amino-N-(adamant-2-yl) Acetamide 11β-Hydroxysteroid Dehydrogenase Type 1 Inhibitors. *J. Med. Chem.* **2007**, *50*, 149–164. [CrossRef] [PubMed]
24. Ryu, J.H.; Kim, S.; Han, H.Y.; Son, H.J.; Lee, H.J.; Shin, Y.A.; Kim, J.-S.; Park, H.-G. Synthesis and biological evaluation of picolinamides as potent inhibitors of 11β-hydroxysteroid dehydrogenase type 1 (11β-HSD1). *Bioorg. Med. Chem. Lett.* **2015**, *25*, 695–700. [CrossRef]
25. Collins, K.C.; Janda, K.D. Investigating Hapten Clustering as a Strategy to Enhance Vaccines against Drugs of Abuse. *Bioconjugate Chem.* **2014**, *25*, 593–600. [CrossRef]
26. Stankova, I.; Chuchkov, K.; Chayrov, R.; Mukova, L.; Galabov, A.; Marinkova, D.; Danalev, D. Adamantane Derivatives Containing Thiazole Moiety: Synthesis, Antiviral and Antibacterial Activity. *Int. J. Pept. Res. Ther.* **2020**, *26*, 1781–1787. [CrossRef]
27. Samson, D.; Daltrozzo, E. Synthesis of Diheteroarylamine Ligands by Palladium-Catalyzed Mono- and Diamination of Dichloroheteroarenes with Heteroarenamines. *Helv. Chim. Acta* **2011**, *94*, 46–60. [CrossRef]
28. Wang, A.; Zhang, H.; Biehl, E.R. Preparation of N1-alkyl- and N1,N1-dialkylisoquinoline-1,3-diamines and 1-alkyl- and 1-phenylisoquinolin-3-amines from the reaction of α-cyano- o-tolunitrile with lithium amides, alkyllithiums, and phenyllithium. *Heterocycles* **2000**, *53*, 291–300. [CrossRef]
29. Balog, J.; Riedl, Z.; Hajós, G.; Miskolczy, Z.; Biczók, L. New fluorescent isoquinoline derivatives. *Tetrahedron Lett.* **2011**, *52*, 5264–5266. [CrossRef]
30. Dubovtsev, A.Y.; Shcherbakov, N.V.; Dar'in, D.V.; Kukushkin, V.Y. The Dichotomy of Gold-catalyzed Interplay between Cyanamides and Ynamides: Controllable Switch from [2+2+2] to [4+2] Cycloaddition. *Adv. Synth. Catal.* **2020**, *362*, 2672–2682. [CrossRef]
31. Abel, A.S.; Grigorova, O.K.; Averin, A.D.; Maloshitskaya, O.A.; Butov, G.M.; Savelyev, E.N.; Orlinson, B.S.; Novakov, I.A.; Beletskaya, I.P. Amination of chloro-substituted heteroarenes with adamantane-containing amines. *Russ. Chem. Bull.* **2016**, *65*, 1820–1828. [CrossRef]
32. Abel, A.S.; Averin, A.D.; Buryak, A.K.; Savelyev, E.N.; Orlinson, B.S.; Novakov, I.A.; Beletskaya, I.P. The Palladium-Catalyzed Heteroarylation of Adamantylalkyl Amines with Dihalogenopyridines: Scope and Limitations. *Synthesis* **2017**, *49*, 5067–5080.
33. Abel, A.S.; Averin, A.D.; Maloshitskaya, O.A.; Savelyev, E.N.; Orlinson, B.S.; Novakov, I.A.; Beletskaya, I.P. Palladium-Catalyzed Amination of Dichloroquinolines with Adamantane-Containing Amines. *Molecules* **2013**, *18*, 2096–2109. [CrossRef]
34. Abel, A.S.; Zenkov, I.S.; Averin, A.D.; Cheprakov, A.V.; Bessmertnykh-Lemeune, A.G.; Orlinson, B.S.; Beletskaya, I.P. Tuning the Luminescent Properties of Ruthenium(II) Amino-1,10-Phenanthroline Complexes by Varying the Position of the Amino Group on the Heterocycle. *ChemPlusChem* **2019**, *84*, 498–503. [CrossRef] [PubMed]
35. Hartwig, J.F.; Shaughnessy, K.H.; Shekhar, S.; Green, R.A. Palladium-catalyzed amination of aryl halides. *Org. React.* **2019**, *100*, 853–958.
36. Hooper, M.W.; Utsunomiya, M.; Hartwig, J.F. Scope and Mechanism of Palladium-Catalyzed Amination of Five-Membered Heterocyclic Halides. *J. Org. Chem.* **2003**, *68*, 2861–2873. [CrossRef]
37. Shen, Q.; Hartwig, J.F. [(CyPF-tBu)PdCl2]: An Air-Stable, One-Component, Highly Efficient Catalyst for Amination of Heteroaryl and Aryl Halides. *Org. Lett.* **2008**, *10*, 4109–4112. [CrossRef]
38. Lyakhovich, M.S.; Murashkina, A.V.; Averin, A.D.; Abel, A.S.; Maloshitskaya, O.A.; Savelyev, E.N.; Orlinson, B.S.; Beletskaya, I.P. Arylation of Adamantanamines: X. Palladium- and Copper-Catalyzed Heteroarylation of Adamantane-Containing Amines with Bromopyridines. *Russ. J. Org. Chem.* **2019**, *55*, 737–747. [CrossRef]
39. Averin, A.D.; Ranyuk, E.R.; Golub, S.L.; Buryak, A.K.; Savelyev, E.N.; Orlinson, B.S.; Novakov, I.A.; Beletskaya, I.P. Synthesis of a New Family of Adamantylpyridin-2-amines by Palladium-Catalyzed Amination. *Synthesis* **2007**, *2007*, 2215–2221. [CrossRef]
40. Grigorova, O.K.; Averin, A.D.; Abel, A.S.; Maloshitskaya, O.A.; Kovalev, V.V.; Savelev, E.N.; Orlinson, B.S.; Novakov, I.A.; Beletskaya, I.P. Arylation of adamantanamines: IV. Palladium-catalyzed arylation of amines of adamantane series with isomeric chloroquinolines. *Russ. J. Org. Chem.* **2012**, *48*, 1391–1406. [CrossRef]
41. Raczyńska, E.D.; Kosińska, W.; Ośmiałowski, B.; Gawinecki, R. Tautomeric Equilibria in Relation to Pi-Electron Delocalization. *Chem. Rev.* **2005**, *105*, 3561–3612. [CrossRef]
42. Raczyńska, E.D.; Kolczyńska, K.; Stępniewski, T.M. Consequences of one-electron oxidation and one-electron reduction for 4-aminopyrimidine—DFT studies. *J. Mol. Model.* **2012**, *18*, 3523–3533. [CrossRef]
43. Plakhotnik, V.M.; Kovtun, V.Y.; Krasutskii, P.A.; Novikova, M.I.; Prokhorov, A.B. Derivatives of Adamantane. I. 2-Hydroxyethylamino Derivatives of Adamantane. *J. Org. Chem. USSR* **1981**, *17*, 1287–1290.
44. Novakov, I.A.; Kulev, I.A.; Radchenko, S.S.; Birznieks, K.A.; Boreko, E.I.; Vladyko, G.V.; Korobchenko, L.V. Synthesis and antiviral activity of the hydrochlorides of alicyclic mono- and diamines. *Pharm. Chem. J.* **1987**, *21*, 287–291. [CrossRef]
45. Novakov, I.A.; Orlinson, B.S.; Savel'ev, E.N.; Potaenkova, E.A.; Shilin, A.K. Method of Produging 2-(2-Amino) Alkyladamantanes. Patent number RU2495020C1, 10 October 2013. Available online: https://patents.google.com/patent/RU2495020C1/ru (accessed on 25 March 2021).
46. Joubert, J.; Dyk, S.V.; Green, I.R.; Malan, S.F. Synthesis, evaluation and application of polycyclic fluorescent analogues as N-methyl-d-aspartate receptor and voltage gated calcium channel ligands. *Eur. J. Med. Chem.* **2011**, *46*, 5010–5020. [CrossRef]
47. Ukai, T.; Kawazura, H.; Ishii, Y.; Bonnet, J.J.; Ibers, J.A. Chemistry of dibenzylideneacetone-palladium(0) complexes: I. Novel tris(dibenzylideneacetone)dipalladium(solvent) complexes and their reactions with quinones. *J. Organomet. Chem.* **1974**, *65*, 253–266. [CrossRef]

molecules

MDPI

Article

# Site-Selective Modification of a Porpholactone—Selective Synthesis of 12,13- and 17,18-Dihydroporpholactones

**Ana F. R. Cerqueira [1], Gustautas Snarskis [1], Jonas Zurauskas [1], Samuel Guieu [1,2], Filipe A. Almeida Paz [2] and Augusto C. Tomé [1,*]**

1 LAQV-REQUIMTE, Department of Chemistry, University of Aveiro, 3810-193 Aveiro, Portugal; anacerqueira@ua.pt (A.F.R.C.); gustautass@gmail.com (G.S.); jonas.zurauskas@gmail.com (J.Z.); sguieu@ua.pt (S.G.)

2 CICECO–Aveiro Institute of Materials, Department of Chemistry, University of Aveiro, 3810-193 Aveiro, Portugal; filipe.paz@ua.pt

* Correspondence: actome@ua.pt; Tel.: +351-234-370-712

Academic Editor: Maged Henary

Received: 20 May 2020; Accepted: 4 June 2020; Published: 6 June 2020

**Abstract:** The reaction of *meso*-tetrakis(pentafluorophenyl)porpholactone with azomethine ylides and nitrones affords pyrrolidine-fused and isoxazolidine-fused dihydroporpholactones that display, respectively, isobacteriochlorin- and chlorin-type UV–Vis spectra. These reactions are site-selective, yielding, respectively, 17,18- or 12,13-dihydroporpholactones. The crystal and molecular features of pyrrolidine-fused and isoxazolidine-fused dihydroporpholactones were unveiled from single-crystal X-ray diffraction studies.

**Keywords:** porpholactones; dihydroporpholactones; 1,3-dipolar cycloadditions; pyrrolidines; isoxazolidines

## 1. Introduction

Pyrrole-modified porphyrins have attracted considerable attention in recent years. This group of compounds comprises a large diversity of porphyrin analogues where one or more pyrrolic units of the porphyrin macrocycle are replaced by non-pyrrolic units. The synthesis, reactivity, structural features, optical properties, and applications of these compounds have been comprehensively reviewed [1–6]. In short, these compounds may be prepared by two complementary routes: by constructing the porphyrin macrocycle using adequate pyrrolic and non-pyrrolic building blocks or by chemical modification of already existing porphyrins. The latter route has been extensively used by the group of Brückner that, by using the "breaking and mending of porphyrins" approach [7], was able to produce a large diversity of pyrrole-modified porphyrins [2]. Focusing on their optical properties, these porphyrinoids may display porphyrin-, chlorin-, isobacteriochlorin-, or bacteriochlorin-like spectra, which is an important feature for a range of applications, including biological (photodynamic therapy (PDT) of cancer or multimodal imaging contrast agents) and technical ones (catalysis or optical sensors) [3,8–12].

Porpholactones, a class of pyrrole-modified porphyrins in which a pyrrolic unit is formally replaced by an oxazolone unit, can be conveniently obtained from *meso*-tetraarylporphyrins in a two-step procedure (osmium tetroxide-mediated dihydroxylation of the porphyrin followed by $KMnO_4$-induced cleavage of 2,3-dihydroxychlorin) [13] or simply by oxidation of a *meso*-tetraarylporphyrin with Oxone® in the presence of a catalytic amount of $RuCl_3$ [14].

In the late 1990s, the group of Cavaleiro reported that the porphyrin macrocycle can participate as a dienophile in Diels–Alder reactions (D–A) [15] or as a dipolarophile in 1,3-dipolar cycloadditions

(1,3-DC) [16]. The resulting monoadducts are heterocycle-fused chlorins, while bisadducts are bacteriochlorins or isobacteriochlorins. Concerning the 1,3-DC, the reaction of porphyrins with various types of 1,3-dipoles [17], namely, azomethine ylides [16,18,19] and nitrones [20,21], just to refer to the two types used in this work, has been reported. This is, effectively, an excellent and selective route to porphyrin derivatives with adequate optical properties for biological applications. Considering that 1,3-DC have also been successfully used for the peripheral functionalization of other porphyrin-type macrocycles, namely, tetraazaporphyrins [22], *N*-confused porphyrins [23], octaphyrins [24], and triply linked diporphyrins [25], the rarity of studies concerning the use of pyrrole-modified porphyrins as dipolarophiles is surprising [26]. In this article, we report the reaction of a porpholactone with two azomethine ylides and two nitrones. Since the porpholactone macrocycle is not symmetric, some site selectivity in these 1,3-DC reactions governed by the lactone unit was expected.

Porpholactones display porphyrin-like UV–Vis spectra, which indicates that the lactone moiety mimics very well the electronic properties of a β–β′ bond [27]. However, the reactivity of the three remaining β–β′ bonds is influenced differently by the lactone unit. This influence is observed, for instance, when porpholactone **1** reacts with Woollins' reagent and $PhMe_2SiH$ [28,29] to afford, selectively, a compound with a hydrogenated pyrrole unit adjacent to the lactone moiety (**A**, Figure 1) or when porpholactones react with hydrazine [30] (or tosylhydrazide) [31] to give compounds with a hydrogenated β–β′ bond opposite to the lactone moiety (**B**). The selective formation of *opp*-porphodilactones [32] and 12,13-dihydroxyporpholactone osmate esters (**C**) [11] from porpholactones are other examples of the orientation effect of the lactone unit. These observations prompted us to investigate the effect of the lactone unit on the reactivity of porpholactones with azomethine ylides and nitrones and, specifically, to find if it induces site selectivity and, eventually, regioselectivity. In these studies, we used *meso*-tetrakis(pentafluorophenyl)porpholactone (**1**) that was prepared by Zhang's method [14].

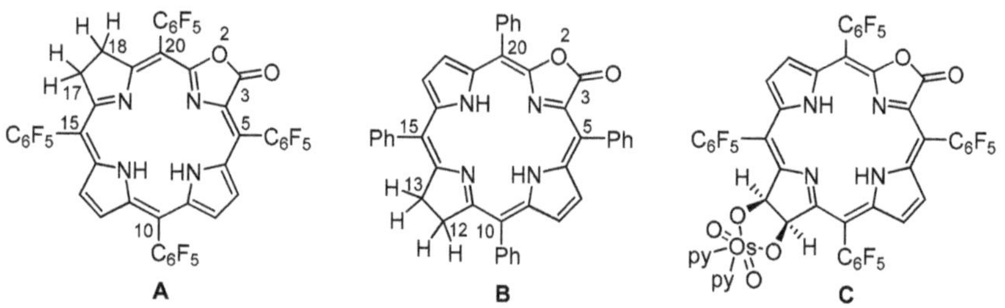

**A** **B** **C**

**Figure 1.** Known dihydroporpholactones structurally related to cycloadducts **3** and **6**/**7** [11,28,30].

## 2. Results and Discussion

The reaction of porpholactone **1** with azomethine ylide **2a** (generated in situ from *N*-methylglycine and paraformaldehyde) was performed under the same reaction conditions applied to *meso*-tetrakis(pentafluorophenyl)porphyrin [16] (Scheme 1). Interestingly, a single monoadduct was formed, indicating clearly that the reaction was site-selective. A similar reaction with azomethine ylide **2b** (generated in situ from *N*-benzylglycine and paraformaldehyde) also afforded a single monoadduct. Both cycloadducts displayed isobacteriochlorin-type UV–Vis spectra (Figure 2 and Supplementary Materials) similar to that reported for dihydroporpholactone **A** [28], signifying that the cycloadditions occurred selectively at one of the pyrrolic units adjacent to the lactone moiety (i.e., they should have structures **3** or **4**). Their emission spectra were also similar to that of an isobacteriochlorin [28], with a main band around 580 nm and a shoulder around 630 nm. The quantum yields were determined to be 0.59 and 0.69 for **3a** and **3b**, respectively. These values also correlate well with the quantum yields reported for isobacteriochlorins. Their $^1H$ NMR spectra revealed the signals of the NH protons at 3.58 and 4.50 ppm (for the *N*-methyl derivative) and at 3.58 and 4.60 ppm (for the *N*-benzyl derivative).

These signals disappeared after shaking with $D_2O$. $^1H$ NMR spectra of porphyrin derivatives with NH signals at such low fields are typical of isobacteriochlorins [15,18,21,33,34], and the same pattern is also observed in isobacteriochlorin-type structures such as compound **A** [28].

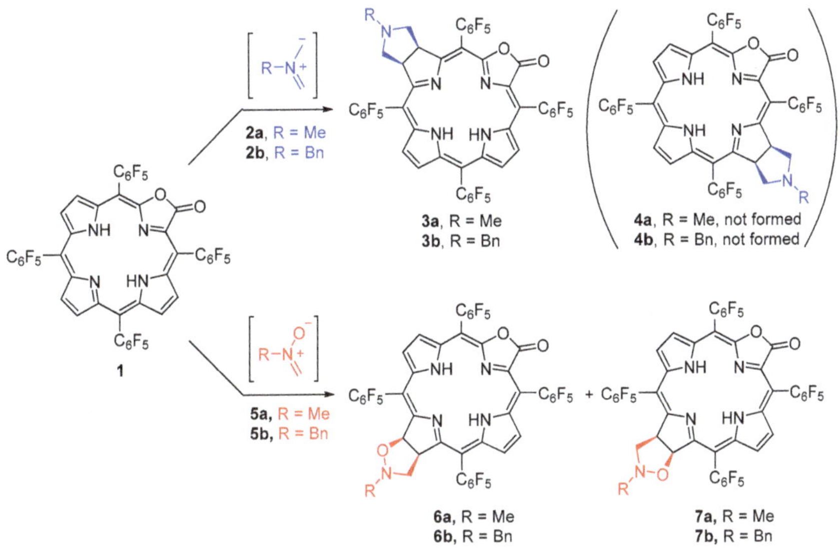


**Scheme 1.** Reaction of porpholactone **1** with azomethine ylides **2a**, **b** and nitrones **5a**, **b**.

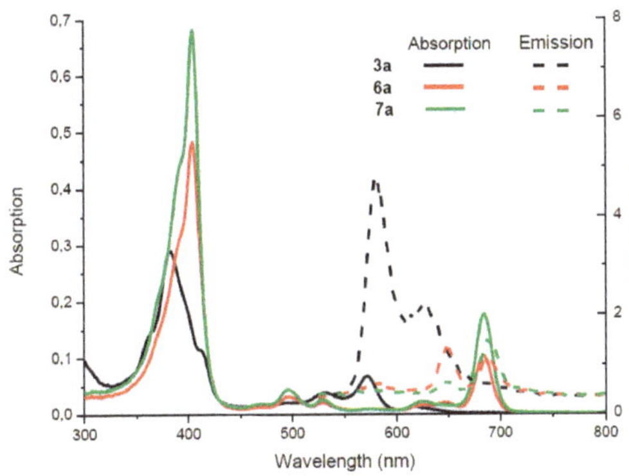


**Figure 2.** Absorption spectra of compounds **3a**, **6a**, and **7a** in chloroform (c = ~$2 \times 10^{-6}$ mol.L$^{-1}$).

The *N*-benzyl cycloadduct led to the isolation of poor crystals, which could be, nevertheless, investigated using single-crystal X-ray diffraction studies. The crystallographic studies performed revealed that the material crystallized in the centrosymmetric *P*-1 triclinic space group, with the asymmetric unit being composed of two disordered halves of two independent molecular units. A full disclosure of the structure of the cycloadduct was instead achieved by solving and refining the structure in the *P*1 triclinic space group (by discarding the center of inversion). With this procedure, it was possible to unequivocally confirm that the cycloadduct has structure **3b** (and not **4b**, see Scheme 1 and Figure 3). Though the X-ray diffraction reliability factors were high (due to the poor diffraction of the crystal), the disclosed structural features were in perfect agreement with those obtained from additional characterization techniques, namely, NMR and UV–Vis spectroscopy.

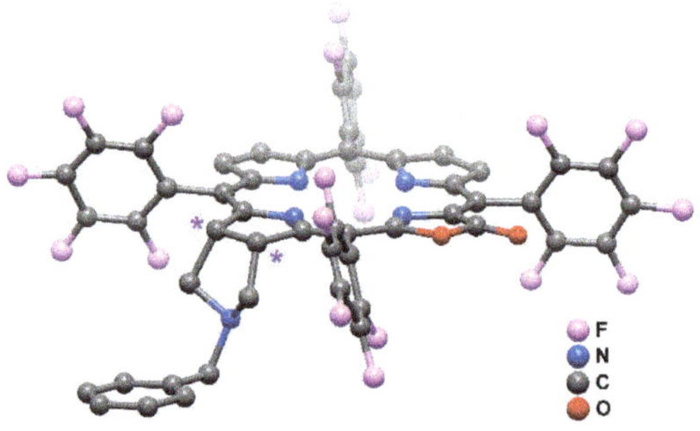


**Figure 3.** Ball-and-stick representation of the pyrrolidine-fused porpholactone derivative **3b**. The chiral centers are indicated by an asterisk. Hydrogen atoms were omitted for clarity reasons.

The reaction of porpholactone **1** with nitrone **5a** (generated in situ from *N*-methylhydroxylamine hydrochloride and paraformaldehyde in the presence of potassium carbonate) was performed under the same reaction conditions applied to *meso*-tetrakis(pentafluorophenyl)porphyrin [21]. TLC analysis of the reaction mixture showed one spot corresponding to porpholactone **1** and two very close spots corresponding to new compounds. The unreacted porpholactone and the two products could be separated by preparative TLC (silica gel) using a 1:1 mixture of $CH_2Cl_2$/hexane as the eluent. Similarly, when nitrone **5b** was used (generated in situ from *N*-benzylhydroxylamine hydrochloride and paraformaldehyde in the presence of potassium carbonate), two products with similar $R_f$ were also obtained. The UV–Vis spectra of the new compounds were identical to that of 12,13-dihydroxyporpholactone osmate ester **C**,[11] showing Q bands at $\lambda_{max}$ 682 nm (Figure 2). These spectra clearly indicate that the cycloadditions occurred selectively at the pyrrolic unit opposite to the lactone moiety. Consequently, the cycloadducts are regioisomers **6** and **7** [35]. The mass spectra of these products indicated that they are all monoadducts, showing the protonated molecular peaks $(M + H)^+ = 1052$ for **6a** and **7a** and $(M + H)^+ = 1128$ for **6b** and **7b**. Each pair of regioisomers was obtained in a ratio of ca. 2.4:1, indicating that cycloaddition, besides being site-selective, was also regioselective. A slow crystallization of the main cycloadduct formed in the reaction with nitrone **5a** allowed obtaining crystals adequate for single-crystal X-ray diffraction studies. These studies revealed that it has structure **6a** (Figure 4) and, therefore, the minor isomer has structure **7a**.

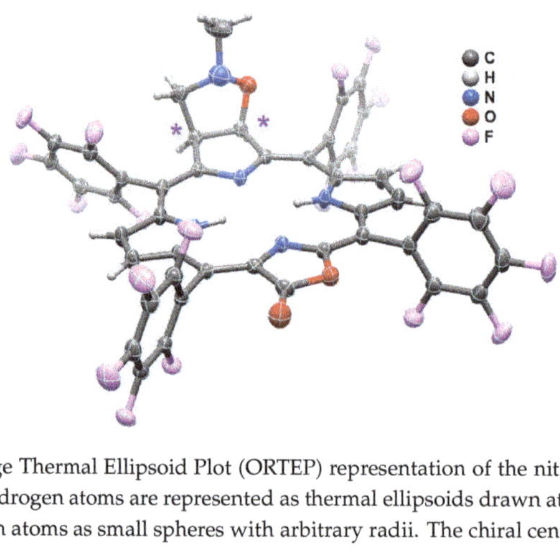


**Figure 4.** Oak Ridge Thermal Ellipsoid Plot (ORTEP) representation of the nitrone cycloadduct **6a** derivative. Non-hydrogen atoms are represented as thermal ellipsoids drawn at the 50% probability level, and hydrogen atoms as small spheres with arbitrary radii. The chiral centers are indicated by an asterisk.

The emission spectra of adducts **6** and **7** presented two bands around 650 nm and 690 nm and quantum yields between 0.14 and 0.23, which were much smaller than those for adducts **3** (Table S1, SM). The $^{1}$H NMR spectra of compounds **6** and **7** were markedly different from those of compounds **3a**/**3b**, particularly at the chemical shifts of the signals of the NH protons: −1.53 and −1.19 ppm for **6a**, −1.67 and −1.36 ppm for **7a**, −1.68 and −1.31 ppm for **6b**, and −1.73 and −1.43 ppm for **7b**. The $^{13}$C and $^{19}$F NMR spectra of the cycloadducts discussed above are also compatible with the proposed structures, displaying various sets of peaks as expected for porpholactone derivatives with reduced symmetry. In contrast to azomethine adducts **3**, nitrone cycloadducts **6** and **7** revealed to be unstable in solution at room temperature, affording, slowly, porpholactone **1**. This transformation, probably via retrocycloaddition, was easily observed by TLC and was also detected in the $^{13}$C NMR spectra of the cycloadducts that showed a signal corresponding to the carbonyl group of the adduct and a small one due to the carbonyl group of porpholactone **1**.

In a previous work [21], we have shown that the addition of an azomethine ylide to a chlorin results in the formation of an isobacteriochlorin, while the addition of a nitrone to a chlorin leads to the formation of a bacteriochlorin. Although being electronically related to porphyrins (and not to chlorins), porpholactones react with azomethine ylides and nitrones with site selectivity identical to that expected for a chlorin, and this is a noteworthy observation. The reason for the site selectivity observed in the reaction of 1,3-DC with chlorins was elucidated by a DFT study [36]: while the addition of an azomethine ylide is irreversible and kinetically controlled, the addition of a nitrone is reversible, pointing to a thermodynamic control of the reaction. Experimental observations in this work, namely, the retrocycloaddition observed with nitrone cycloadducts, suggest that a similar reaction control also operates with porpholactones.

In conclusion, this study showed that the reactions of *meso*-tetrakis(pentafluorophenyl) porpholactone with 1,3-dipoles are site-selective and, depending on the type of 1,3-dipole used, the resulting cycloadducts are 12,13- or 17,18-dihydroporpholactones, which display, respectively, chlorin- or isobacteriochlorin-type UV–Vis spectra. Considering that a large diversity of substituents may be linked to these cycloadducts by nucleophilic substitutions at the pentafluorophenyl groups [37,38], the reaction of porpholactone **1** with 1,3-dipoles may be an excellent route to a myriad of compounds for biological or technical applications.

## 3. Materials and Methods

### 3.1. Chemicals and Instrumentation

$^{1}$H, $^{13}$C and $^{19}$F NMR spectra were recorded on Bruker AVANCE 300 or Bruker AVANCE 500 spectrometers. $CDCl_3$ was used as solvent, and tetramethylsilane (TMS) as an internal reference. The chemical shifts are expressed in δ (ppm), and the coupling constants (*J*) in hertz (Hz). UV–Vis spectra were recorded on a Shimadzu UV-2501PC spectrophotometer using $CHCl_3$ as the solvent. Fluorescence emission spectra were recorded with a Jobin Yvon FluoroMax-3 spectrofluorometer using $CHCl_3$ as the solvent. Fluorescence quantum yields $\Phi_F$ were determined using 5,10,15,20-tetraphenylporphyrin (TPP) in chloroform ($\Phi_F = 0.11$) as the fluorescence standard. Mass spectra were recorded using a Micromass Q-TOF-2$^{TM}$ mass spectrometer and $CHCl_3$ as the solvent. Preparative thin-layer chromatography was carried out on 20 × 20 cm glass plates coated with silica gel (1 mm thick, Merck, Kenilworth, NJ, USA). Analytical TLC was carried out on sheets precoated with silica gel (Merck 60, 0.2 mm thick). Solvents were purified or dried according to the literature procedures. Compound **1** was prepared according to a published procedure [14].

## 3.2. *Synthesis*

### 3.2.1. General Procedure for the Synthesis of Cycloadducts **3**.

A solution of porpholactone **1** (50.0 mg, 0.05 mmol), N-substituted glycine (0.45 mmol), and paraformaldehyde (33.8 mg, 1.1 mmol) in toluene (25 mL) was heated at reflux under a nitrogen atmosphere for 4 h. Then, new portions of the N-substituted glycine (0.45 mmol) and paraformaldehyde (33.8 mg, 1.1 mmol) were added, and the mixture was refluxed for additional 4 h. The solvent was evaporated, and the compounds were separated by preparative TLC using dichloromethane/hexane as the eluent. The compound with higher $R_f$ corresponded to unreacted porpholactone (~10%), and the fraction running immediately below it corresponded to the expected cycloadduct. Isolated yields: **3a** = 85%; **3b** = 43%.

Adduct **3a**: (45.2 mg, 85% yield), $^1$H NMR (300 MHz, $CDCl_3$): δ 2.23 (s, 3H, $CH_3$), 2.44–2.54 (m, 2H, pyrrolidine-*H*), 2.84–2.98 (m, 2H, pyrrolidine-*H*), 3.58 (s, 1H, NH), 4.48–4.71 (m, 3H, NH and β-H [C (sp$^3$)]), 7.32 (dd, 1H, *J* = 4.8 and 1.4 Hz, β-H), 7.59 (d, 2H, *J* = 1.4 Hz, β-H), 7.77 (d, 1H, *J* = 4.8 Hz, β-H). $^{13}$C NMR (75 MHz, $CDCl_3$): δ 40.9, 47.6, 48.8, 62.0, 62.2, 83.2, 95.7, 109.3, 110.2, 110.6, 112.5, 113.7, 114.1, 122.0, 123.3, 134.7, 135.6, 135.9, 137.0, 138.5, 139.0, 141.2, 143.2, 144.1, 144.8, 145.4, 146.1, 146.6, 147.3, 151.2, 154.1, 157.6, 159.1, 162.2, 164.6. $^{19}$F NMR (282 MHz, $CDCl_3$): δ −158.0 to −155.9 (m, 8H, *m*-F), −148.3 to −147.2 (m, 4H, *p*-F), −135.6 to −132.0 (m, 8H, *o*-F). UV-Vis ($CHCl_3$): $\lambda_{max}$ (log ε) 382 (5.23), 531 (4.38), 572 (4.60), 617 (3.93). MS (ESI): *m/z* 1050.5 [M + H]$^+$.

Adduct **3b**: (24.2 mg, 43% yield), $^1$H NMR (300 MHz, $CDCl_3$): δ 2.53–2.60 (m, 2H, pyrrolidine-*H*), 2.84 (t, *J* = 8.7 Hz, 2H, pyrrolidine-*H*), 3.46 (s, 2H, $PhCH_2$), 3.58 (s, 1H, NH), 4.45–4.63 (m, 3H, NH and β-H [C (sp$^3$)]), 7.06–7.09 (m, 2H, Bn-H), 7.15–7.18 (m, 1H, Bn-H), 7.28–7.30 (m, 3H, Bn-H and β-H), 7.59 (d, 2H, *J* = 1.6 Hz, β-H), 7.77 (d, 1H, *J* = 4.8 Hz, β-H). $^{13}$C NMR (125 MHz, $CDCl_3$): δ 47.0, 48.2, 59.1, 59.7, 59.9, 83.1, 95.7, 109.4, 110.2, 110.5, 112.5, 114.0, 122.0, 123.2, 125.3, 127.7, 128.2, 128.4, 128.8, 129.05, 129.11, 134.8, 135.6, 135.8, 136.8, 138.8, 141.0, 143.2, 144.0, 144.5, 145.2, 146.0, 146.4, 146.8, 147.3, 151.3, 154.1, 157.6, 159.1, 162.3, 164.6. $^{19}$F NMR (282 MHz, $CDCl_3$): δ −158.0 to −155.9 (m, 8H, *m*-F), −148.3 to −147.3 (m, 4H, *p*-F), −135.7 to −131.8 (m, 8H, *o*-F). UV-Vis ($CHCl_3$): $\lambda_{max}$ (log ε) 382 (5.21), 532 (4.34), 572 (4.59), 629 (3.56). MS (ESI): *m/z* 1126.1 [M + H]$^+$.

### 3.2.2. General Procedure for the Synthesis of Cycloadducts **6** and **7**.

To a solution of porpholactone **1** (50.0 mg, 0.05 mmol) in toluene (5 mL), *N*-substituted hydroxylamine hydrochloride (0.20 mmol), paraformaldehyde (15.1 mg, 0.50 mmol), and $K_2CO_3$ (55.7 mg, 0.40 mmol) were added. The mixture was heated at 60 °C under a nitrogen atmosphere for 12 h, and then additional portions of *N*-substituted hydroxylamine hydrochloride, paraformaldehyde, and $K_2CO_3$ were added to the reaction mixture, which was heated for a total of 30 h. The reaction mixture was washed with $H_2O$ and then was purified by preparative TLC using dichloromethane/hexane (1:1) as the eluent. The fraction with higher $R_f$ corresponded to unreacted porpholactone (~60%), the following one was the major cycloadduct, and the third one the minor cycloadduct. Isolated yields: **6a** = 19% (48% yield based on consumed porpholactone **1**), **7a** = 8% (19% yield based on consumed porpholactone **1**); **6b** = 22% (43% yield based on consumed porpholactone **1**), **7b** = 9% (18% yield based on consumed porpholactone **1**).

Adduct **6a**: $^1$H NMR (300 MHz, $CDCl_3$): δ −1.53 (s, 1H, NH), −1.19 (s, 1H, NH), 2.57 (s, 3H, $CH_3$), 2.86–2.95 (m, 1H, isoxazolidine-H), 3.35–3.43 (m, 1H, isoxazolidine-H), 5.14–5.19 (m, 1H, β-H [C (sp$^3$)]), 6.65 (d, 1H, *J* = 6.8 Hz, β-H [C (sp$^3$)]), 8.19 (s, 1H, β-H), 8.48–8.52 (m, 2H, β-H), 8.64 (d, 1H, *J* = 4.0 Hz, β-H). $^{13}$C NMR (75 MHz, $CDCl_3$): δ 44.0, 55.4, 64.0, 85.0, 89.7, 98.7, 102.3; 105.5, 105.8, 110.7, 111.4, 114.5; 122.9, 125.3, 126.8, 127.9, 128.1, 128.2, 128.3, 134.7, 137.5, 138.2, 138.9, 140.9, 141.6, 143.5, 145.1, 147.1, 148.9, 152.6, 162.9, 165.8. $^{19}$F NMR (282 MHz, $CDCl_3$): δ −158.2 to −155.7 (m, 8H, *m*-F), −148.3 to −146.7 (m, 4H, *p*-F), −136.0 to −131.1 (m, 8H, *o*-F). UV-vis ($CHCl_3$): $\lambda_{max}$ (log ε) 404 (5.30), 497 (4.07), 530 (3.86), 625 (3.75), 684 (4.61). MS (ESI): *m/z* 1052.5 [M + H]$^+$.

Adduct **7a**: $^1$H NMR (300 MHz, $CDCl_3$): δ −1.67 (s, 1H, NH), −1.36 (s, 1H, NH), 2.57 (s, 3H, $CH_3$), 2.90–2.95 (m, 1H, isoxazolidine-H), 3.39–3.44 (m, 1H, isoxazolidine-H), 5.21–5.23 (m, 1H, β-H [C ($sp^3$)]), 6.66 (d, 1H, *J* = 7.4 Hz, β-H [C ($sp^3$)]), 8.33 (d, 1H, *J* = 4.5 Hz, β-H), 8.40 (d, 1H, *J* = 4.4 Hz, β-H), 8.56 (d, 1H, *J* = 4.4 Hz, β-H), 8.66 (d, 1H, *J* = 4.5 Hz, β-H). $^{19}$F NMR (282 MHz, $CDCl_3$): δ −158.4 to −155.6 (m, 8H, *m*-F), −148.7 to −146.1 (m, 4H, *p*-F), −136.3 to −131.2 (m, 8H, *o*-F). UV-vis ($CHCl_3$): $\lambda_{max}$ (log ε) 404 (5.44), 496 (4.20), 530 (3.97), 625 (3.90), 684 (4.83). MS (ESI): *m/z* 1052.2 $[M + H]^+$.

Adduct **6b**: $^1$H NMR (300 MHz, $CDCl_3$): δ −1.68 (s, 1H, NH), −1.31 (s, 1H, NH), 3.25 (s, 2H, isoxazolidine-*H*), 3.81 (s, 2H, $PhCH_2$), 5.24–5.25 (m, 1H, isoxazolidine-*H*), 6.65 (d, 1H, *J* = 7.4 Hz, β-H [C ($sp^3$)]), 7.00–7.02 (m, 2H, Bn-H), 7.19–7.22 (m, 3H, Bn-H), 8.22 (d, 1H, *J* = 3.2 Hz, β-H), 8.46 (d, 1H, *J* = 4.1 Hz, β-H), 8.55 (d, 1H, *J* = 4.1 Hz, β-H), 8.66 (d, 1H, *J* = 3.2 Hz, β-H). $^{13}$C NMR (125 MHz, $CDCl_3$): δ 44.0, 53.9, 64.6, 86.1, 89.3, 99.6, 101.0, 105.8, 110.7, 112.7, 113.7, 115.3, 122.3, 125.4, 127.3, 128.3, 136.8, 137.5, 138.9, 139.3, 139.4, 141.2, 141.6, 143.3, 143.7, 144.8, 145.2, 146.9, 152.9, 163.0, 165.8. $^{19}$F NMR (282 MHz, $CDCl_3$): δ −158.2 to −155.8 (m, 8H, *m*-F), −148.2 to −146.7 (m, 4H, *p*-F), −135.7 to −130.1 (m, 8H, *o*-F). UV-vis ($CHCl_3$): $\lambda_{max}$ (log ε) 404 (5.92), 496 (4.66), 529 (4.46), 623 (4.35), 646 (4.33), 682 (5.24). MS (ESI): *m/z* 1128.4 $[M + H]^+$.

Adduct **7b**: $^1$H NMR (300 MHz, $CDCl_3$): δ −1.73 (s, 1H, NH), −1.43 (s, 1H, NH), 3.31 (s, 2H, isoxazolidine-*H*), 3.85 (s, 2H, $PhCH_2$), 5.33–5.37 (m, 1H, isoxazolidine-*H*), 6.67 (d, 1H, *J* = 7.8 Hz, β-H [C ($sp^3$)]), 7.02–7.06 (m, 2H, Bn-H), 7.19–7.23 (m, 3H, Bn-H), 8.30 (d, 1H, *J* = 5.10 Hz, β-H), 8.42 (d, 1H, *J* = 4.2 Hz, β-H), 8.57 (d, 1H, *J* = 4.2 Hz, β-H), 8.68 (d, 1H, *J* = 5.1 Hz, β-H). $^{19}$F NMR (282 MHz, $CDCl_3$): δ −158.3 to 155.5 (m, 8H, *m*-F), −148.3 to −146.1 (m, 4H, *p*-F), −136.3 to −130.0 (m, 8H, *o*-F). UV-vis ($CHCl_3$): $\lambda_{max}$ (log ε) 404 (5.57), 497 (4.30), 529 (4.06), 626 (3.97), 643 (4.05), 684 (4.87). MS (ESI): *m/z* 1128.3 $[M + H]^+$.

CCDC 1832879, 1832880, and 1985131 contain the supplementary crystallographic data for this paper. These data can be obtained free of charge via www.ccdc.cam.ac.uk/data_request/cif, by emailing data_request@ccdc.cam.ac.uk, or by contacting The Cambridge Crystallographic Data Centre, 12 Union Road, Cambridge CB2 1EZ, UK; fax: +44 1223 336033.

**Supplementary Materials:** The following are available online. $^1$H, $^{13}$C and $^{19}$F NMR spectra, mass spectra, absorption, and emission spectra for the new compounds. Details of the crystal data collection, solution, and refinement of compounds **3b** and **6a**. Crystal structures in CIF format (CIF).

**Author Contributions:** Conceptualization, A.C.T.; synthesis of the porpholactone derivatives, A.F.R.C., G.S., J.Z.; single-crystal X-ray diffraction studies, S.G., F.A.A.P. All authors have read and agreed to the published version of the manuscript.

**Funding:** This research was funded by Fundação para a Ciência e a Tecnologia (FCT), through project PTDC/QEQ-QOR/6160/2014 and research units UID/QUI/00062/2019, UIDB/50006/2020, and UIDB/50011/2020.

**Acknowledgments:** Thanks are due to Fundação para a Ciência e a Tecnologia (FCT) for the financial support to project PTDC/QEQ-QOR/6160/2014, QOPNA research unit (FCT UID/QUI/00062/2019), the LAQV-REQUIMTE (UIDB/50006/2020), and CICECO (UIDB/50011/2020), financed through national funds and where applicable co-financed by FEDER, within the PT2020 Partnership Agreement, and also to the Portuguese NMR Network. S. Guieu acknowledges financial support from the pAge project (Centro-01-0145-FEDER-000003). Ana Cerqueira thanks FCT for her doctoral grant (SFRH/BD/135597/2018).

**Conflicts of Interest:** The authors declare no conflict of interest.

## References

1. Brückner, C.; Akhigbe, J.; Samankumara, L.P. Porphyrin analogs containing non-pyrrolic heterocycles. In *Handbook of Porphyrin Science*; Kadish, K.M., Smith, K.M., Guilard, R., Eds.; World Scientific: River Edge, NY, USA, 2014; Volume 31, pp. 1–276.
2. Brückner, C. The breaking and mending of *meso*-tetraarylporphyrins: Transmuting the pyrrolic building blocks. Acc. *Chem. Res.* **2016**, *49*, 1080–1092. [CrossRef] [PubMed]
3. Costa, L.D.; Costa, J.I.T.; Tomé, A.C. Porphyrin macrocycle modification: Pyrrole ring-contracted or -expanded porphyrinoids. *Molecules* **2016**, *21*, 320. [CrossRef] [PubMed]

4. Taniguchi, M.; Lindsey, J.S. Synthetic chlorins, possible surrogates for chlorophylls, prepared by derivatization of porphyrins. *Chem. Rev.* **2017**, *117*, 344–535. [CrossRef] [PubMed]
5. Chatterjee, T.; Shetti, V.S.; Sharma, R.; Ravikanth, M. Heteroatom-containing porphyrin analogues. *Chem. Rev.* **2017**, *117*, 3254–3328. [CrossRef]
6. Ning, Y.; Jin, G.-Q.; Zhang, J.-L. Porpholactone chemistry: An emerging approach to bioinspired photosensitizers with tunable near-infrared photophysical properties. *Acc. Chem. Res.* **2019**, *52*, 2620–2633. [CrossRef]
7. Akhigbe, J.; Samankumara, L.P.; Brückner, C. The breaking and mending of porphyrins: Reductive coupling of secochlorin bisaldehydes. *Tetrahedron Lett.* **2012**, *53*, 3524–3526. [CrossRef]
8. Ke, X.-S.; Ning, Y.; Tang, J.; Hu, J.-Y.; Yin, H.-Y.; Wang, G.-X.; Yang, Z.-S.; Jie, J.; Liu, K.; Meng, Z.-S.; et al. Gadolinium(III) porpholactones as efficient and robust singlet oxygen photosensitizers. *Chem. Eur. J.* **2016**, *22*, 9676–9686. [CrossRef]
9. Ning, Y.; Tang, J.; Liu, Y.-W.; Jing, J.; Sun, Y.; Zhang, J.-L. Highly luminescent, biocompatible ytterbium (III) complexes as near-infrared fluorophores for living cell imaging. *Chem. Sci.* **2018**, *9*, 3742–3753. [CrossRef]
10. Yang, Z.-S.; Ning, Y.; Yin, H.-Y.; Zhang, J.-L. Lutetium (III) porphyrinoids as effective triplet photosensitizers for photon upconversion based on triplet-triplet annihilation (TTA). *Inorg. Chem. Front.* **2018**, *5*, 2291–2299. [CrossRef]
11. Hewage, N.; Daddario, P.; Lau, K.S.F.; Guberman-Pfeffer, M.J.; Gascón, J.A.; Zeller, M.; Lee, C.O.; Khalil, G.E.; Gouterman, M.; Brückner, C. Bacterio- and isobacteriodilactones by stepwise or direct oxidations of *meso*-tetrakis(pentafluorophenyl)porphyrin. *J. Org. Chem.* **2019**, *84*, 239–256. [CrossRef]
12. Jin, G.-Q.; Ning, Y.; Geng, J.-X.; Jiang, Z.-F.; Wang, Y.; Zhang, J.-L. Joining the journey to near infrared (NIR) imaging: The emerging role of lanthanides in the designing of molecular probes. *Inorg. Chem. Front.* **2020**, *7*, 289–299. [CrossRef]
13. McCarthy, J.R.; Jenkins, H.A.; Brückner, C. Free base *meso*-tetraaryl-morpholinochlorins and porpholactone from *meso*-tetraaryl-2,3-dihydroxy-chlorin. *Org. Lett.* **2003**, *5*, 19–22. [CrossRef] [PubMed]
14. Yu, Y.; Lv, H.; Ke, X.; Yang, B.; Zhang, J.-L. Ruthenium-catalyzed oxidation of the porphyrin β,β′-pyrrolic ring: A general and efficient approach to porpholactones. *Adv. Synth. Catal.* **2012**, *354*, 3509–3516. [CrossRef]
15. Tomé, A.C.; Lacerda, P.S.S.; Neves, M.G.P.M.S.; Cavaleiro, J.A.S. *meso*-Arylporphyrins as dienophiles in Diels–Alder reactions: A novel approach to the synthesis of chlorins, bacteriochlorins and naphthoporphyrins. *Chem. Commun.* **1997**, 1199–1200. [CrossRef]
16. Silva, A.M.G.; Tomé, A.C.; Neves, M.G.P.M.S.; Silva, A.M.S.; Cavaleiro, J.A.S. *meso*-Tetraarylporphyrins as dipolarophiles in 1,3-dipolar cycloaddition reactions. *Chem. Commun.* **1999**, 1767–1768. [CrossRef]
17. Tomé, A.C.; Neves, M.G.P.M.S.; Cavaleiro, J.A.S. Porphyrins and other pyrrolic macrocycles in cycloaddition reactions. *J. Porphyrins Phthalocyanines* **2009**, *13*, 408–414. [CrossRef]
18. Silva, A.M.G.; Tomé, A.C.; Neves, M.G.P.M.S.; Silva, A.M.S.; Cavaleiro, J.A.S. 1,3-Dipolar cycloaddition reactions of porphyrins with azomethine ylides. *J. Org. Chem.* **2005**, *70*, 2306–2314. [CrossRef]
19. Silva, A.M.G.; Tomé, A.C.; Neves, M.G.P.M.S.; Cavaleiro, J.A.S.; Perrone, D.; Dondoni, A. Porphyrins in 1,3-dipolar cycloadditions with sugar azomethine ylides. Synthesis of pyrrolidinoporphyrin glycoconjugates. *Synlett* **2005**, 857–859. [CrossRef]
20. Aguiar, A.; Leite, A.; Silva, A.M.N.; Tomé, A.C.; Cunha-Silva, L.; Castro, B.; Rangel, M.; Silva, A.M.G. Isoxazolidine-fused *meso*-tetraarylchlorins as key tools for the synthesis of mono- and bis-annulated chlorins. *Org. Biomol. Chem.* **2015**, *13*, 7131–7135. [CrossRef]
21. Almeida, J.; Aguiar, A.; Leite, A.; Silva, A.M.N.; Cunha-Silva, L.; Castro, B.; Rangel, M.; Barone, G.; Tomé, A.C.; Silva, A.M.G. 1,3-Dipolar cycloadditions with *meso*-tetraarylchlorins – site selectivity and mixed bisadducts. *Org. Chem. Front.* **2017**, *4*, 534–544. [CrossRef]
22. Silva, A.M.G.; Lacerda, P.S.S.; Tomé, A.C.; Neves, M.G.P.M.S.; Silva, A.M.S.; Cavaleiro, J.A.S.; Makarova, E.A.; Lukyanets, E.A. Porphyrins in 1,3-dipolar cycloaddition reactions. Synthesis of new porphyrin-chlorin and porphyrin-tetraazachlorin dyads. *J. Org. Chem.* **2006**, *71*, 8352–8356. [CrossRef] [PubMed]
23. Li, X.; Liu, B.; Yu, X.; Yi, P.; Yi, R.; Chmielewski, P.J. 1,3-Dipolar cycloaddition of 2,6-dichlorobenzonitrile oxide to 2-methyl-N-confused porphyrin. Regio- and stereoselective synthesis and structural characterization of 2-aza-21-carbabacteriochlorin and resolution of 2-aza-21-carbachlorin enantiomers. *J. Org. Chem.* **2012**, *77*, 2431–2440. [CrossRef] [PubMed]

24. Hata, H.; Kamimura, Y.; Shinokubo, H.; Osuka, A. Synthesis of pyrrolidine-fused [34]- and [36]octaphyrins via 1,3-dipolar cycloaddition. *Org. Lett.* **2006**, *8*, 1169–1172. [CrossRef] [PubMed]
25. Tanaka, T.; Nakamura, Y.; Aratani, N.; Osuka, A. Regioselective [3+4] cycloaddition of an azomethine ylide to *meso–meso*, β−β, β′−β′ triply linked diporphyrins. *Tetrahedron Lett.* **2008**, *49*, 3308–3311. [CrossRef]
26. Yao, Y.; Rao, Y.; Liu, Y.; Jiang, L.; Xiong, J.; Fan, Y.-J.; Shen, Z.; Sessler, J.L.; Zhang, J.-L. Aromaticity versus regioisomeric effect of β-substituents in porphyrinoids. *Phys. Chem. Chem. Phys.* **2019**, *21*, 10152–10162. [CrossRef] [PubMed]
27. Brückner, C.; Ogikubo, J.; McCarthy, J.R.; Akhigbe, J.; Hyland, M.A.; Daddario, P.; Worlinsky, J.L.; Zeller, M.; Engle, J.T.; Ziegler, C.J.; et al. *meso*-Arylporpholactones and their reduction products. *J. Org. Chem.* **2012**, *77*, 6480–6494. [CrossRef]
28. Yu, Y.; Furuyama, T.; Tang, J.; Wu, Z.-Y.; Chen, J.-Z.; Kobayashi, N.; Zhang, J.-L. Stable iso-bacteriochlorin mimics from porpholactone: Effect of a β-oxazolone moiety on the frontier π-molecular orbitals. *Inorg. Chem. Front.* **2015**, *2*, 671–677. [CrossRef]
29. Wu, Z.-Y.; Wang, T.; Meng, Y.-S.; Rao, Y.; Wang, B.-W.; Zheng, J.; Gao, S.; Zhang, J.-L. Enhancing the reactivity of nickel(II) in hydrogen evolution reactions (HERs) by β-hydrogenation of porphyrinoid ligands. *Chem. Sci.* **2017**, *8*, 5953–5961. [CrossRef]
30. Akhigbe, J.; Haskoor, J.; Zeller, M.; Brückner, C. Porpholactams and chlorolactams: Replacement of a β, β′-double bond in *meso*-tetraphenyl-porphyrin and -chlorin by a lactam moiety. *Chem. Commun.* **2011**, *47*, 8599–8601. [CrossRef]
31. Akhigbe, J.; Haskoor, J.; Krause, J.A.; Zeller, M.; Brückner, C. Formation, structure, and reactivity of *meso*-tetraarylchlorolactones, -porpholactams, and -chlorolactams, porphyrin and chlorin analogues incorporating oxazolone or imidazolone moieties. *Org. Biomol. Chem.* **2013**, *11*, 3616–3628. [CrossRef]
32. Ke, X.-S.; Chang, Y.; Chen, J.-Z.; Tian, J.; Mack, J.; Cheng, X.; Shen, Z.; Zhang, J.-L. Porphodilactones as synthetic chlorophylls: Relative orientation of β-substituents on a pyrrolic ring tunes NIR absorption. *J. Am. Chem. Soc.* **2014**, *136*, 9598–9607. [CrossRef] [PubMed]
33. Chang, C.K. Synthesis and characterization of alkylated isobacteriochlorins, models of siroheme and sirohydrochlorin. *Biochemistry* **1980**, *19*, 1971–1976. [CrossRef] [PubMed]
34. Stolzenberg, A.M.; Spreer, L.O.; Holm, R.H. Octaethylisobacteriochlorin, a model of the sirohydrochlorin ring-system of siroheme enzymes - preparation and spectroscopic and electrochemical properties of the free base and its Zn(II) complex. *J. Am. Chem. Soc.* **1980**, *102*, 364–370. [CrossRef]
35. A mixture of isomers **6a/7a** was analyzed by HPLC: The two compounds show retention times at 32.15 min (**7a**, minor isomer) and 33.62 min (**6a**, major isomer) (see Supp. mat.)
36. Jimenez-Oses, G.; Garcia, J.I.; Silva, A.M.G.; Santos, A.R.N.; Tomé, A.C.; Neves, M.G.P.M.S.; Cavaleiro, J.A.S. Mechanistic insights on the site selectivity in successive 1,3-dipolar cycloadditions to *meso*-tetraarylporphyrins. *Tetrahedron* **2008**, *64*, 7937–7943. [CrossRef]
37. Costa, J.I.T.; Tomé, A.C.; Neves, M.G.P.M.S.; Cavaleiro, J.A.S. 5,10,15,20-tetrakis(pentafluorophenyl)porphyrin: A versatile platform to novel porphyrinic materials. *J. Porphyrins Phthalocyanines* **2011**, *15*, 1116–1133. [CrossRef]
38. Worlinsky, J.L.; Halepas, S.; Brückner, C. PEGylated *meso*-arylporpholactone metal complexes as optical cyanide sensors in water. *Org. Biomol. Chem.* **2014**, *12*, 3991–4001. [CrossRef]


**Sample Availability:** Samples of the compounds are available from the authors.

*molecules*

MDPI

*Article*

# Synthesis of Novel Tryptamine Derivatives and Their Biological Activity as Antitumor Agents

Giorgia Simonetti [1], Carla Boga [2,*], Joseph Durante [3], Gabriele Micheletti [2], Dario Telese [2], Paolo Caruana [2], Andrea Ghelli Luserna di Rorà [1], Fabio Mantellini [3], Samantha Bruno [4], Giovanni Martinelli [1] and Natalia Calonghi [5,*]

1 Biosciences Laboratory, IRCCS Istituto Romagnolo per lo Studio dei Tumori "Dino Amadori"—IRST S.r.l., 47014 Meldola (FC), Italy; giorgia.simonetti@irst.emr.it (G.S.); andrea.ghellilusernadirora@irst.emr.it (A.G.L.d.R.); giovanni.martinelli@irst.emr.it (G.M.)
2 Department of Industrial Chemistry "Toso Montanari", Alma Mater Studiorum—Università di Bologna, Viale del Risorgimento 4, 40136 Bologna, Italy; gabriele.micheletti3@unibo.it (G.M.); dario.telese2@unibo.it (D.T.); paolo.caruana@gidi.it (P.C.)
3 Department of Biomolecular Sciences, University of Urbino "Carlo Bo", Via I Maggetti 24, 61029 Urbino (PU), Italy; jdurante6@gmail.com (J.D.); fabio.mantellini@uniurb.it (F.M.)
4 Department of Experimental, Diagnostic and Specialty Medicine, Institute of Hematology and Medical Oncology "L. and A. Seràgnoli", University of Bologna, 40138 Bologna, Italy; samantha.bruno2@unibo.it
5 Department of Pharmacy and Biotechnology, University of Bologna, 40121 Bologna, Italy
* Correspondence: carla.boga@unibo.it (C.B.); natalia.calonghi@unibo.it (N.C.); Tel.: +39-051-209-3616 (C.B.); +39-051-209-1231 (N.C.)

**Abstract:** We synthesized five novel tryptamine derivatives characterized by the presence of an azelayl chain or of a 1,1,1-trichloroethyl group, in turn connected to another heterocyclic scaffold. The combination of tryptamin-, 1,1,1-trichloroethyl- and 2-aminopyrimidinyl- moieties produced compound **9** identified as the most active compound in hematological cancer cell lines ($IC_{50}$ = 0.57–65.32 μM). Moreover, keeping constant the presence of the tryptaminic scaffold and binding it to the azelayl moiety, the compounds maintain biological activity. Compound **13** is still active against hematological cancer cell lines and shows a selective effect only on HT29 cells ($IC_{50}$ = 0.006 μM) among solid tumor models. Compound **14** loses activity on all leukemic lines, while showing a high level of toxicity on all solid tumor lines tested ($IC_{50}$ 0.0015–0.469 μM).

**Keywords:** cancer; tryptamine; leukemias; chloral; pyrimidine

## 1. Introduction

The indole nucleus (**1**) belongs to many natural heterocyclic compounds and is of interest in many applied fields, such as industrial, agricultural and medicinal chemistry [1]. In many natural molecules and synthetic or semi-synthetic drugs this scaffold represents a pharmacophoric group fundamental for the interaction with receptors. Among the plethora of indole derivatives present in the animal and vegetal realm, a great importance has been recognized to tryptamine (**2**). The tryptamine is a biosynthetic precursor of many natural alkaloids [2,3] and is frequently used as chemical building block in the total synthesis of biologically active and pharmaceutically important compounds [4,5]. In Figure 1 are shown some examples of natural tryptamine derivatives with important biological roles such as L-tryptophan, serotonin, melatonin, besides the tryptane drugs sumatripan, rizatripan and the anticancer agents vincristine, vinblastine and panobinostat.

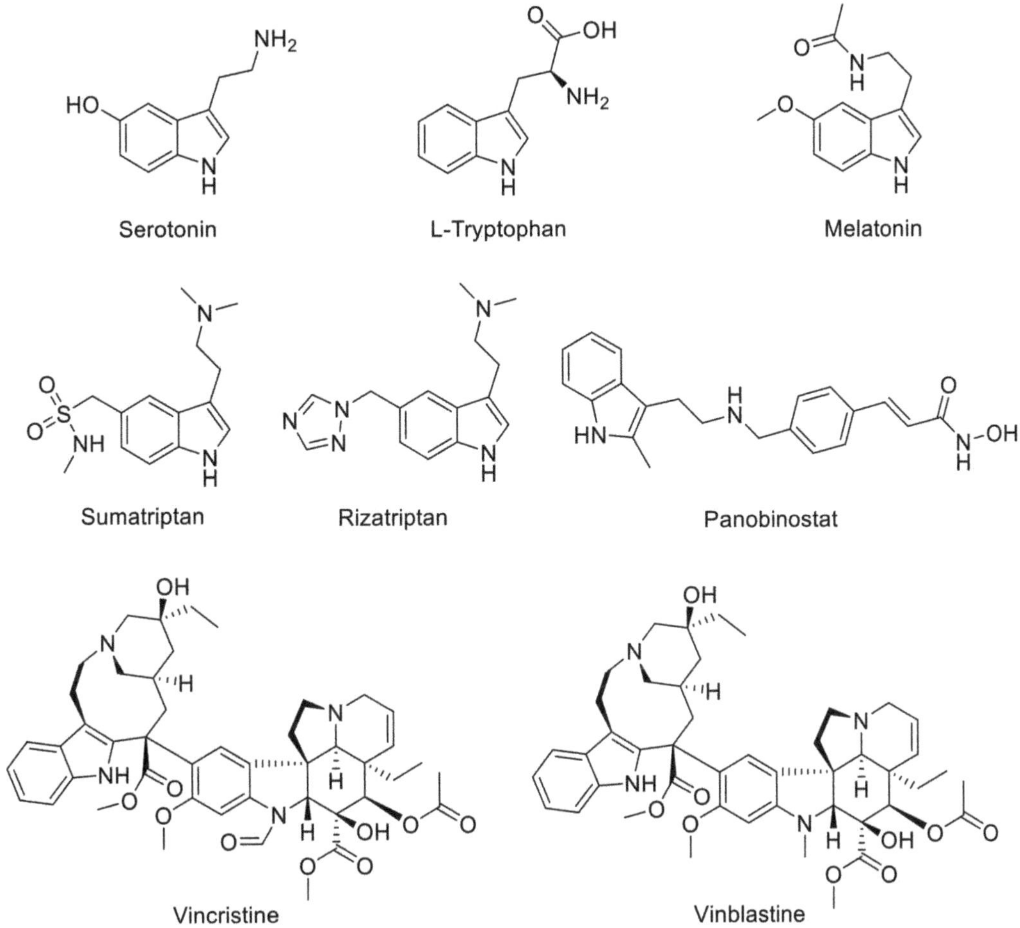


**Figure 1.** Natural products and pharmaceuticals containing tryptamine subunit.

The latter is active against multiple myeloma with a mechanism involving inhibition of histone deacetylase (HDAC-6) [6], as well as recently patented [7] structures containing an aliphatic chain ending with a hydroxamic acid and an amide group involving a tryptamine subunit (compound **SP-1-163**, Figure 2A).

Recently, we synthesized a series of compounds with structural analogy with compound **SP-1-163** (Figure 2A). We prepared structural hybrids between azelaic acid methyl ester and several amino-aza-heterocycles (Figure 2B,D). The azelayl moiety recalls part of 9-hydroxystearic acid, a cellular lipid showing antiproliferative activity toward cancer cells with HDAC as the molecular target [8–16]. Actually, we found that some derivatives belonging to series in Figure 2B–D behave as selective histone deacetylase inhibitors (HDACi): benzothiazole-based series (Figure 2B) is active against HT29 human colon cancer cells line [17] whereas, among the series containing pyridinyl (or piperidinyl, benzimidazolyl, benzotriazolyl) groups (Figure 2C,D), two aminopyrimidinyl and the benzimidazolyl derivatives showed specific activity on osteosarcoma cells [18]. The two latter moieties, aminopyrimidyl- and imidazolyl- one are also present in Apcin, (Figure 2E) a small molecule that blocks the interaction between APC/C and Cdc20 [19]. A recently published patent reported the synthesis and biological tests of many derivatives of Apcin-A (Figure 2F) [20]. However, in none of the above cited articles, the tryptamine moiety is present.

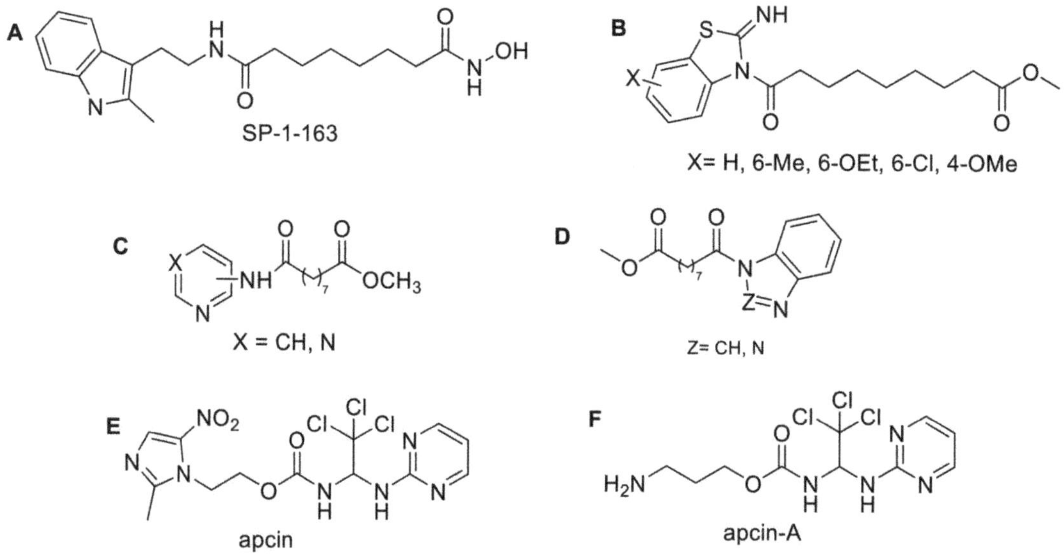


**Figure 2.** Biologically active compounds bearing (**A**) indole-, (**B**) thiazole-, (**D**) triazole-, (**C**) pyridinyl- and (**E**,**F**) pyrimidinyl-scaffolds.

Due to the importance of both, trichloromethyl and aminopyrimidyl group, in influencing the biological activity of some above cited compounds, we centred our attention towards the synthesis of novel tryptamine derivatives bearing both these structural motifs and structural hybrids connecting one tryptamine moiety an azelayl one. Herein we report the synthesis and the results obtained on the biological activity of the novel compounds towards a panel of solid and hematological cancer cell lines.

## 2. Results and Discussion

### 2.1. Chemistry

#### 2.1.1. Synthesis of Ureido Derivatives 4 and 5, Bearing Tryptamine and Trichloromethyl Moieties

First, we synthesized compounds **4** and **5**, bearing both tryptamine and trichloromethyl moieties. The reaction of tryptamine with potassium cyanate gave the ureido derivative **2** that, by reaction with chloral hydrate under different experimental conditions, produced compound **4** or compound **5** bearing, respectively, one and two tryptamine moieties (Scheme 1). Compounds **4** and **5** have been obtained, after purification by column chromatography on silica gel, in 93% and 50% yield, respectively and have been fully characterized.

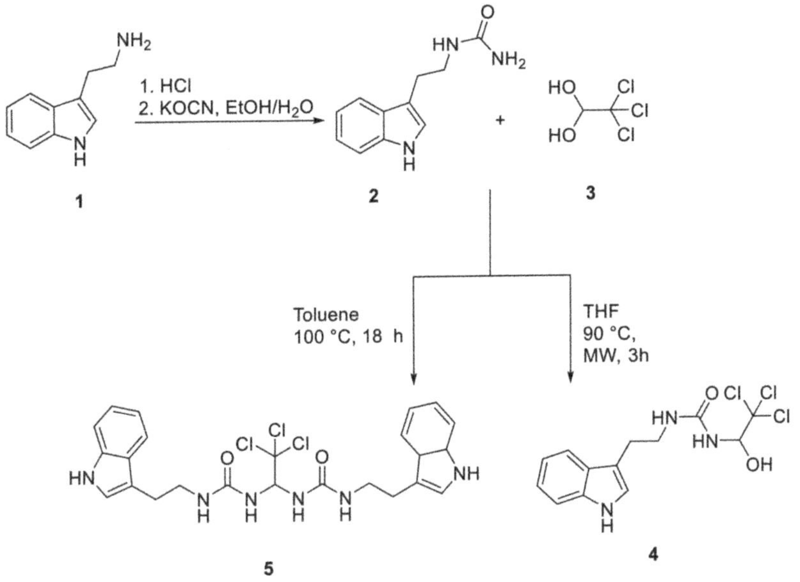

**Scheme 1.** Synthetic pathway to obtain compounds **4** and **5**.

2.1.2. Synthesis of *N*-(2-(1*H*-indol-3-yl)ethyl)-2,2,2-trichloro-*N*′-(pyrimidin-2yl)etan-1,1-diamine (**9**)

Compound **9**, contemporarily bearing tryptamine, pyrimidine and trichloromethyl moieties, was obtained through the multistep procedure shown in Scheme 2.

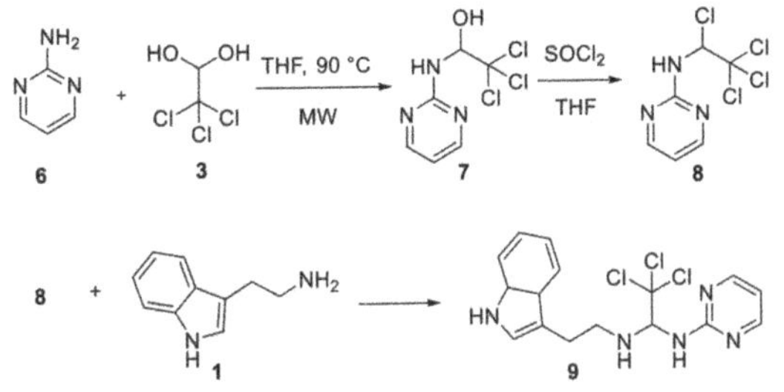

**Scheme 2.** Synthetic route to compound **9**.

2-Aminopyrimidine (**6**) was reacted with chloral hydrate (**3**) in THF under microwaves irradiation giving the hemiaminal (**7**) in 84% yield. The latter was subjected to chlorination by treatment with $SOCl_2$ at room temperature in anhydrous THF and under nitrogen flow, in order to remove hydrochloric acid produced during the reaction. Intermediate compound **8** was then reacted without purification with tryptamine (**1**) and the reaction course was monitored by $^1$H NMR of a sample of concentrated crude reaction mixture until to reveal a conversion of about 80%. Compound **9** was recovered, after chromatography on neutral alumina, with purity > 99% even if in only 23% yield; the reason of the low yield might be due to the decomposition of the product during the purification step. We tried also the reaction between compounds **8** and **2** but no product was detected, probably because of the low nucleophilicity of the nitrogen amide atom of compound **2**. Compound **9** was subjected to biological essays, as well as compound **7**, chosen with the aim to compare their activities.

2.1.3. Synthesis of Hybrids Containing Tryptamine and Azelaoyl Moieties

Based on literature reports on the biological activity of compounds bearing different heterocyclic moieties bound to an azelayl chain through an amide bond [17,18], we planned to synthesize compounds **13** and **14**, bearing a tryptamine group.

The synthetic approach, shown in Scheme 3, is based on the formation of the amide (**13**) under Schotten-Bauman like conditions. Thus, we first prepared the acyl chloride derivative (**12**) by reaction between the commercially available azelaic acid monomethyl ester (**10**) and oxalyl chloride (**11**). Then, we reacted this activated azelaoyl moiety with tryptamine. The ester bond of compound **13** was further selectively and almost quantitatively hydrolysed to free acid (**14**) in order to check the biological activity of both, the acid and the ester. The novel compounds have been purified and fully characterized.

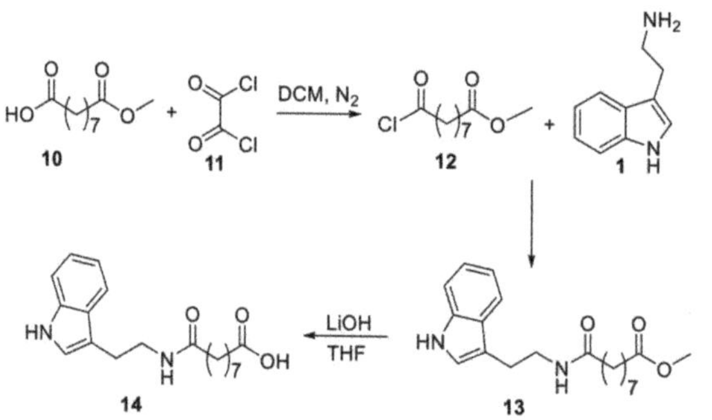


**Scheme 3.** Synthesis of compounds **13** and **14**.

## 2.2. *Biological Activity*

Effect of Compounds on Cells Viability

To investigate whether the compounds have an antitumor activity, we performed in vitro preclinical assays. In vitro growth inhibitory concentration was determined by incubating the cells with increasing concentrations (0.01–250 μM) of the compounds for 24 h. Data obtained from cell growth assays were elaborated to assess the concentration of each compound required for 50% inhibition of cell viability ($IC_{50}$) and the results are shown in Table 1. All the newly synthesized compounds showed a biological activity. However, we observed striking differences in the models response.

**Table 1.** $IC_{50}$ (μM) values of the new compounds in the analyzed tumor cell lines [a].

| | 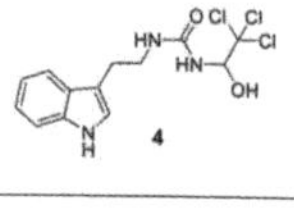 | 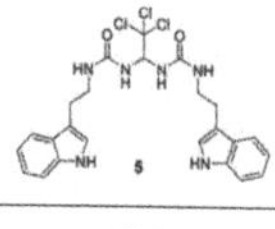 | 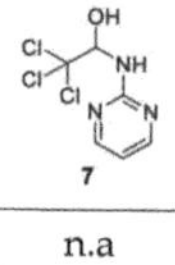 | 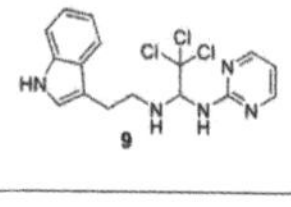 | 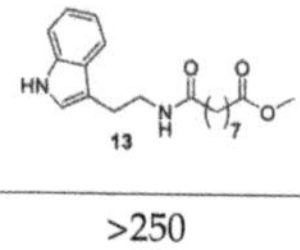 | 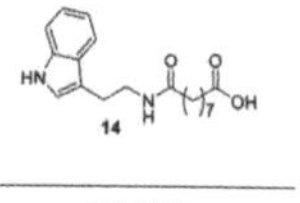 |
|---|---|---|---|---|---|---|
| A431 | n.a | n.a | n.a | n.a | >250 | 0.0072 |
| HT29 | 0.0115 | 212 | n.a | n.a | 0.006 | 0.096 |
| IGROV1 | >250 | n.a | n.a | n.a | >250 | 0.0015 |
| U2OS | 22.54 | n.a | 0.383 | 235 | 222 | 0.469 |
| KG-1 | n.a | n.a | n.a | n.a | 32.44 | n.a |
| MV-4-11 | n.a | n.a | n.a | 28.95 | 102.50 | n.a |
| REH | n.a | n.a | n.a | 65.32 | 29.32 | n.a |
| Jurkat 6 | n.a | n.a | 61.12 | 0.570 | n.a | n.a |

[a] n.a—not active.

Compound **9**, that is characterized by 2-aminopyrimidyl- and trichloroethyl- moieties, similarly to those in Apcin, was active against 3 out of 4 hematological models (MV-4-11, REH and, in particular, the T-cell acute lymphoblastic leukemia cell line Jurkat 6). However, this compound showed poor biological activity when tested in solid tumor models. Indeed, it was able to reduce cell growth only in the osteosarcoma U2OS cell line at high doses ($IC_{50}$ = 235 μM).

Apcin interferes with the biological activity of Cdc20, that functions as an oncogenic factor in tumorigenesis: it is upregulated across several cancer types, including ovarian/uterine, colon and colorectal cancer, oral squamous cell carcinoma [21] and in aneuploid compared with euploid acute myeloid leukemia [22]. Moreover, its overexpression is associated with poor prognosis in colorectal cancer [23], oral squamous cell carcinoma [24] and serous epithelial ovarian cancer [25], among the tumor types analyzed in the present manuscript. The binding site of Apcin on Cdc20 has been identified [19] and a study on SAR has revealed that the pyrimidine ring and aminal nitrogens, together with the hydrophobic trichloromethyl group, are important structural motifs; in contrast, the elimination of the nitro-imidazole moiety produces little effect. Apcin showed preclinical activity against multiple myeloma [26], prostate cancer [27], glioblastoma [28] and osteosarcoma [29] cells. Very recently, during the current investigation, the synthesis and the in vitro evaluation in a panel of solid tumor cells [MCF-7, A375, A549, HepG2, Hela, Ovcar-3 and Caov-3) of a series of 2,2,2-trichloro-1-aryl carbamate derivatives in which Apcin was modified by changing the pyrimidinyl or the 1-(2-methoxyethyl)-2-methyl-5-nitro-1H-imidazolyl moiety, has been reported [30]. Few studies are currently available on acute leukemias [31]. Withaferin A, a compound inducing degradation of the Mad2-Cdc20 complex was shown to reduce cell viability in acute myeloid and lymphoblastic models [32–34].

Since compound **9** showed a selective activity against leukemic cell lines, we then investigated whether the tryptaminic and 2-aminopyrimidyl moieties of compound **9** were effective against solid tumor models, when tested separately. We observed that the trichloro-1-(pyrimidin-2-ylamino)ethyl group (compound **7**) maintained some activity against Jurkat 6 cells and was more active against U2OS cells, while solely the presence of tryptaminyl and trichloroethyl groups (connected through an ureido moiety) (as in compound **4**), produced the total loss of activity against hematological models, while being effective against U2OS and the colon cancer cell line HT29. Moreover, the dimeric form of compound **4**, with symmetry with respect to the trichloroethyl group, (compound **5**) showed a further activity reduction, being able to reduce cell growth in a single cell line and at very high doses that hamper any preclinical development. Overall, these data suggest that both the triptaminyl and the pyrimidinyl moieties connected through the trichloroehtyl group (compound **9**) are relevant to the compound effectiveness against acute leukemia models, while showing a modest and selective activity in solid cancers.

Therefore, we sought to identify novel compounds able to target solid tumors. Keeping constant the presence of the tryptaminic scaffold and binding it to the azelayl moiety (compound **13**), we maintained a biological activity against acute myeloid and B-cell acute lymphoblastic leukemia cell lines and observed a selective effect in HT29 cells, against solid cancer models. Conversely, solid tumor models displayed a specific vulnerability towards compound **14** (the acid free form of the ester of compound **13**), that was not effective against hematological cell lines. Of note, compounds **13** and **14** were both active against HT29 cells, in line with previous observations on similar compounds [17]. Moreover, these compounds recall the structure of HDAC inhibitors, that showed modest efficacy as single agent in acute leukemias [35,36].

## 3. Materials and Methods

### 3.1. Chemical Syntheses

The reagents used, unless stated otherwise, were purchased from Sigma-Aldrich (Milan, Italy). $CH_2Cl_2$ was dried by distillation over $P_2O_5$. Anhydrous THF was freshy

When the conversion resulted quantitative, the solvent was removed and the white solid obtained was characterized and used without further purification. m.p.: 116.3–118.8 °C; $^1$H-NMR (300 MHz, DMSO-$d_6$, 25 °C) δ, ppm = 8.45 (d, *J* = 4.6 Hz, 2 H), 7.74 (d, *J* = 9.5 Hz, 1 H, NH), 6.84 (t, *J* = 4.6 Hz, 1 H), 6.21 (d, *J* = 9.5 Hz, 1 H, C<u>H</u>CCl$_3$); $^{13}$C-NMR (150 MHz, DMSO-$d_6$, 25 °C) δ, ppm = 160.2, 158.0 (CH), 112.4 (CH), 102.9, 82.4 (CH); GC-MS (*m/z*): 189 (18, M-70), 154 (100, M-105), 119 (10, M-140), 79 (20); ESI-MS$^+$ (*m/z*): 224 [M − Cl]$^+$.

#### 3.1.6. 2,2,2-Trichloro-*N*-(2-(3a,7a-dihydro-1*H*-indol-3-yl)ethyl)-*N*′-(pyrimidin-2-yl)ethane-1,1-diamine (Compound **9**)

Tryptamine (compound **1**, 0.200 g, 1.25 mmol) in anhydrous THF (5 mL) was added to a solution of compound **8** (0.120 mg, 0.5 mmol) in anhydrous THF (5 mL). The reaction mixture was heated at 50 °C overnight. After removal of the solvent, the crude was subjected to FC on neutral alumina (changing gradient eluent from *n*-hexane/ethyl acetate 1/1 until pure ethyl acetate) and 44.2 mg (0.115 mmol, 23% yield) of pure compound **9**, as waxy brown solid was obtained. m.p.: 132.5–134.5 °C; $^1$H-NMR (400 MHz, DMSO-$d_6$, 25 °C) δ, ppm = 10.76 (br. s, 1 H, NH indole), 8.37 (d, *J* =4.7 Hz, 2 H), 7.56 (d, *J* = 9.1 Hz, 1 H), 7.39 (d, *J* = 7.8 Hz, 1 H), 7.30 (dt, $J_1$ = 8.0, $J_2$ = 0.8 Hz, 1 H), 7.11 (d, *J* = 2.3 Hz, 1 H), 7.03 (ddd, *J* = 8.0 Hz, *J* = 7.0 Hz, *J* = 1.2 Hz, 1 H), 6.91 (ddd, *J* = 7.8 Hz, *J* = 7.0 Hz, *J* = 1.0 Hz, 1 H), 6.73 (t, *J* = 4.7 Hz, 1 H), 5.70 (dd, $J_1$ = 10.8, $J_2$ = 9.1 Hz, 1 H, C<u>H</u>CCl$_3$), 3.04–2.76 (m, 4 H); $^{13}$C-NMR (100 MHz, DMSO-$d_6$, 25 °C) δ, ppm = 162.0, 158.1 (CH), 157.9, 136.1, 127.1 (CH), 122.6 (CH), 120.8 (CH), 118.1 (CH), 111.9, 111.8 (CH), 111.3 (CH), 103.8, 76.3 (CH), 47.3 (CH$_2$), 25.5 (CH$_2$); ATR-IR: (cm$^{-1}$): 3411, 3221, 1584, 1444, 1415, 798, 784, 740; ESI-MS$^+$ (*m/z*): 384 [M + H]$^+$, 406 [M+Na]$^+$, 424 [M + K]$^+$; ESI-HRMS$^+$ (*m/z*): for $C_{16}H_{16}Cl_3N_5Na^+$ Calc. 406.03690, found 406.0369.

#### 3.1.7. Methyl 9-((2-(1*H*-indol-3-yl)ethyl)amino)-9-oxononanoate (Compound **13**)

Tryptamine (compound **1**, 320.5 mg, 2 mmol) was added to a magnetically stirred solution of crude freshly prepared compound **12** (1 mmol) [17,18]. After 3 h at room temperature, $^1$H-NMR analysis of a sample revealed disappearance of the signals belonging to **12**. After removal of the solvent in vacuo and purification through FC (eluent: DCM/MeOH 9.5/0.5) 199.5 mg (0.58 mmol, 58%) of pure **13** was obtained as a light brown solid: m.p.:56.5–58.0 °C; $^1$H-NMR (300 MHz, CDCl$_3$, 25 °C) δ, ppm = 8.60 (s, 1 H, NH), 7.59 (d, *J* = 7.8 Hz, 1 H), 7.37 (d, *J* = 8.1 Hz, 1 H), 7.19 (t, *J* = 7.0 Hz, 1 H), 7.11 (t, *J* = 7.2 Hz, 1 H), 7.00 (s, 1 H), 5.65 (br.s, 1 H, NH), 3.67 (s, 3 H), 3.59 (q, *J* = 6.4 Hz, 2 H, CH$_2$C<u>H$_2$</u>NH), 2.97 (t, *J* = 6.4 Hz, 2 H), 2.29 (t, *J* = 7.3 Hz, 2 H, C<u>H$_2$</u>COOCH$_3$), 2.08 (t, *J* = 7.3 Hz, 2 H), 1.65–1.50 (m, 4 H), 1.26 (br.s, 6 H); $^{13}$C-NMR (100 MHz, CDCl$_3$, 25 °C) δ, ppm = 174.4, 173.5, 136.4, 127.3, 122.1 (CH), 122.0 (CH), 119.3 (CH), 118.5 (CH), 112.6, 111.3 (CH), 51.5 (CH$_3$), 39.7 (CH$_2$), 36.5 (CH$_2$), 34.0 (CH$_2$), 28.9 (CH$_2$, 2 signals overlapped), 28.8 (CH$_2$), 25.6 (CH$_2$), 25.2 (CH$_2$), 24.7 (CH$_2$); ATR-IR: (cm$^{-1}$): 3390, 3272, 1730, 1633, 737; ESI-MS$^+$ (*m/z*): 345 [M + H]$^+$, 367 [M + Na]$^+$, 383 [M + K]$^+$; ESI-HRMS$^+$ (*m/z*): for $C_{20}H_{28}N_2NaO_3^+$ Calc. 367.19976, found 367.1998.

#### 3.1.8. 9-((2-(1*H*-Indol-3-yl)ethyl)amino)-9-oxononanoic Acid (Compound **14**)

LiOH·H$_2$O (25 mg, 0.6 mmol) was added to a solution of compound **13** (0.172 g, 0.5 mmol) in 25 mL of a 20% *v/v* solution of THF in H$_2$O and the mixture was stirred at room temperature for 3 h. After acidification with 10% aq. HCl, EtOAc and H$_2$O were added to the mixture. The extracted organic layer was dried over anhydrous MgSO$_4$ and concentrated and pure compound **14** was recovered in 86% yield (142 mg, 0.41 mmol) as pale grey solid: m.p.: 88.0–91.4 °C; $^1$H-NMR (300 MHz, CDCl$_3$, 25 °C) δ, ppm = 8.42 (br.s, 1 H, NH), 7.58 (d, *J* = 7.8 Hz, 1 H), 7.37 (d, *J* = 7.8 Hz, 1 H), 7.19 (dt, $J_1$ = 7.8 Hz, $J_2$ = 1.2 Hz 1 H), 7.11 (dt, $J_1$ = 7.8 Hz, $J_2$ = 1.2 Hz 1 H), 7.01 (d, *J* = 1.9 Hz, 1 H), 5.63 (br.s, 1 H, NH), 3.60 (q, *J* = 6.2 Hz, 2 H), 2.96 (t, *J* = 7.0 Hz, 2 H), 2.38–2.28 (m, 4 H), 2.09 (t, *J* = 6.2, 2H) 1.69–1.48 (m, 6 H), 1.39–1.29 (br.s, 2 H); $^{13}$C NMR (75 MHz, CDCl$_3$, 25 °C) δ, ppm = 179.0, 173.5, 173.4, 127.3, 122.2 (CH), 122.1 (CH), 119.4 (CH), 118.6 (CH),

112.7, 111.3 (CH), 39.6 ($CH_2$), 36.7 ($CH_2$), 33.9 ($CH_2$), 30.3 ($CH_2$), 28.8 ($CH_2$), 28.7 ($CH_2$), 25.5 ($CH_2$), 25.2 ($CH_2$), 24.6 ($CH_2$); $^1$H-NMR (600 MHz, $CD_3CN$, 25 °C) δ, ppm = 9.17 (br.s, 1 H, NH), 7.59 (d, $J$ = 8.0 Hz, 1 H), 7.40 (d, $J$ = 8.2 Hz, 1 H), 7.14 (t, $J$ = 8.2 Hz, 1 H), 7.09 (d, $J$ = 1.6 Hz, 1 H), 7.06 (t, $J$ = 8.0 Hz, 1 H), 6.53 (br.s, 1 H, NH), 3.46 (q, $J$ = 7.0 Hz, 2 H), 2.91 (t, $J$ = 7.2 Hz, 2 H), 2.27 (t, $J$ = 7.6, 2H), 2.09 (t, $J$ = 7.7 hZ, 2H), 1.60–1.48 (m, 4 H) 1.34–1.20 (m, 6 H); $^{13}$C-NMR (150 MHz, $CD_3CN$, 25 °C) δ, ppm = 175.4, 174.1, 137.5, 128.5, 123.5 (CH), 122.3 (CH), 119.7 (CH), 119.4 (CH), 113.4, 112.2 (CH), 40.5 ($CH_2$), 36.8 ($CH_2$), 34.2 ($CH_2$), 29.60 ($CH_2$), 29.58 ($CH_2$), 29.54 ($CH_2$), 26.4 ($CH_2$), 26.0 ($CH_2$), 25.5 ($CH_2$); ATR-IR: ($cm^{-1}$): 3388, 3269, 1710, 1631; ESI-MS$^+$ ($m/z$): 331 $[M + H]^+$, 353 $[M + Na]^+$, 369 $[M + K]^+$; ESI-HRMS$^+$ ($m/z$): for $C_{19}H_{26}N_2NaO_3{}^+$ Calc. 353.18411, found 353.1841.

### 3.2. *Cell Culture and Treatments*

#### 3.2.1. Cell Culture

The squamous carcinoma (A431), human colon cancer (HT29), human bone osteosarcoma (U2OS), a human T-cell acute lymphoblastic leukemia (Jurkat 6) and acute myeloid leukemia (MV-4-11) cell lines were purchased from American Type Culture Collection (ATCC, Manassas, VA). Two additional human cell lines, a B-cell acute lymphoblastic leukemia (REH) and an acute myeloid leukemia (KG-1) model were obtained from Leibniz-Institut DSMZ-Deutsche Sammlung von Mikroorganismen und Zellkulturen GmbH (Germany) and the human ovarian cancer cell line (IGROV1) has been kindly provided by Istituto Nazionale Tumori (IRCCS, Milan, Italy). Cells were cultured in RPMI 1640 medium (Labtek Eurobio, Milan, Italy), supplemented with 10% heat-inactivated fetal bovine serum (Thermo Fisher Scientific, Waltham, MA, USA) or fetal calf serum (Euroclone, Milan, Italy), 100 U/mL penicillin, 100 µg/mL streptomycin (GE Healthcare, Chicago, IL, USA) and 2mM L-glutamine (Sigma-Aldrich, Milan, Italy), at 37 °C and 5% $CO_2$ atmosphere. The compounds were dissolved in DMSO (Sigma-Aldrich, Milan, Italy) in a stock solution.

#### 3.2.2. Cell Viability Assays

To evaluate the compounds activity, the cells were treated for 24 h with vehicle (DMSO, as control) or with the test samples at concentrations between 0.01 µM and 250 µM. Cell growth was assessed by the luminescence-based RealTime-Glo MT Cell Viability Assay (Promega, Madison, WI, USA) or the colorimetric 3-(4,5-dimethylthiazolyl-2)-2,5-diphenyltetrazolium bromide assay (MTT, Sigma-Aldrich, Milan, Italy). RealTime-Glo MT Cell Viability Assay was performed according to manufacturer instructions and luminescence was quantified by using GloMax 96 Microplate Luminometer (Promega, Madison, WI, USA). As for MTT assays, the culture medium was removed and cells incubated with 0.1 mL of MTT dissolved in PBS at the concentration of 0.2 mg/mL following Micheletti et.al. [16]. The absorbance at 570 nm was measured using a multiwell plate reader (Tecan, Männedorf, Switzerland). The $IC_{50}$ was determined from the dose-response curve by using Graph Pad software v.6.0.

## 4. Conclusions

We synthesized five novel derivatives characterized by the tryptamine nucleus as the common structural motif. This heterocycle was bound to an azelayl chain through an amide bond or to a 1,1,1-trichloroethyl group, in turn connected to another heterocyclic scaffold. In particular, ureido derivatives **4** and **5** bearing one and two tryptamine groups, respectively, were prepared by reaction of 1-(2-(1*H*-indol-3-yl)ethyl)urea with chloral hydrate. Reaction of 2-aminopyrimidine with chloral hydrate gave compound **7** that, after treatment with thionyl chloride and subsequent nucleophilic attack by tryptamine, produced compound **9**. The combination of tryptamine and azelaoyl scaffolds under Schotten-Baumann like conditions produced structural hybrids compounds **13** and **14**, a methyl ester and its free acid form, respectively, whose structures recall those of compounds behaving as HDAC inhibitors.

Additionally, the biological activity of these compounds was investigated on a panel of solid and hematological cancer cell lines and the data reported suggest that their cellular toxicity could be related to different mechanisms involved in different biological targets.

Compound **9** shows a marked cytotoxicity on leukemic cell lines tested, with $IC_{50}$ values comprised from 28.5 μM for MV-4-11 to 0.570 μM for Jurkat 6; was inactive only in KG-1. In all solid tumor lines tested it is inactive, except for the U2OS cell line where it induces cytotoxic effect at high concentrations ($IC_{50}$ = 235 μM).

The binuclear compound **5** loses activity in leukemic and solid tumor cell lines, acting only in HT29 at high concentrations ($IC_{50}$ = 212 μM).

Compound **4** loses activity in all leukemic lines, while in solid tumors shows a cytotoxic effect only in HT29 ($IC_{50}$ = 0.0115 μM) and in U2OS ($IC_{50}$ = 22.54 μM).

These data confirm that both the triptaminyl and the pyrimidinyl moieties connected through the trichloroehtyl group (compound **9**) are relevant to the compound effectiveness against acute leukemia models, while showing a modest and selective activity in solid cancers.

Interestingly, keeping constant the presence of the tryptaminic scaffold and binding it to the azelayl moiety, the compounds maintain a biological activity.

Compound **13** is active against KG-1 ($IC_{50}$ = 32.44 μM), MV-4-11 ($IC_{50}$ = 102.50 μM), REH ($IC_{50}$ = 29.32 μM) and a selective effect only against HT29 cells ($IC_{50}$ = 0.006 μM), among solid tumor models.

Compound **14** loses activity on all leukemic lines, while showing a marked cytotoxicity on all solid tumor lines tested, with $IC_{50}$ values of 0.0072 μM for A431, 0.096 μM for HT29, 0.0015 for IGROV1 and 0.469 for U2OS.

Studies addressing the clarification and/or identification of additional biological targets as well as the deepen investigation of structure–activity relationships are currently ongoing in our laboratories.

**Supplementary Materials:** The following are available online, Figures S1–S31: $^{1}$H-, $^{13}$C-NMR and ESI-Ms spectra.

**Author Contributions:** Conceptualization, G.S., C.B. and N.C.; methodology, A.G.L.d.R., S.B., N.C., J.D., G.M. (Gabriele Micheletti), F.M.; data analysis, A.G.L.d.R., G.S., N.C., C.B.; investigation, J.D., D.T., G.M. (Giovanni Martinelli), N.C., P.C.; writing—original draft preparation, G.S., C.B. and N.C.; writing—review and editing, A.G.L.d.R., G.M. (Giovanni Martinelli), C.B., N.C. All authors have read and agreed to the published version of the manuscript.

**Funding:** This research was funded by University of Bologna, Alma Idea Junior Research Grant (to G.S.) and RFO (ex60%) funds (N.C. and C.B.).

**Data Availability Statement:** Not applicable.

**Acknowledgments:** We are grateful to Lanfranco Masotti for the helpful discussion. The authors thank Luca Zuppiroli for running the mass spectra.

**Conflicts of Interest:** The authors declare no conflict of interest.

**Sample Availability:** Samples of compounds **7** and **13** are available from the authors.

## References

1. Gribble, G.W. *Heterocyclic Scaffolds II: Reactions and Applications of Indoles in Topics in Heterocyclic Chemistry*; Springer: Berlin/Heidelberg, Germany, 2010; Volume 26.
2. O'Connor, S.E. *Comprehensive Natural Products II*; Mander, L., Liu, H.-W., Eds.; Elsevier: Amsterdam, The Netherlands, 2010; Volume 1, p. 977.
3. Aniszewski, T. *Alkaloids Chemistry, Biology, Ecology and Applications*, 2nd ed.; Elsevier: Amsterdam, The Netherlands, 2015.
4. Han, S.; Movassaghi, M.J. Concise total synthesis and stereochemical revision of all (−)-Trigonoliimines. *Am. Chem. Soc.* **2011**, *133*, 10768–10771. [CrossRef]

5. Jones, S.B.; Simmons, B.; Mastracchio, A.; MacMillan, D.W.C. Collective synthesis of natural products by means of organocascade catalysis. *Nature* **2011**, *475*, 183–188. [CrossRef]
6. Eleutherakis-Papaiakovou, E.; Kanellias, N.; Kastritis, E.; Gavriatopoulou, M.; Terpos, E.; Dimopoulos, M.A. Efficacy of Panobinostat for the Treatment of Multiple Myeloma. *J. Oncol.* **2020**, *2020*, 1–11. [CrossRef]
7. Grindrod, S.; Jung, M.; Brown, M.; Dritschilo, A. *Dual Function Molecules for hIstone Deacetylase Inhibition and Ataxia Telangiectasia Mutated Activation and Methods of Use Thereof*; US 2016/0257649 Al; Shuttle Pharmaceuticals, LLC.: Rockville, MD, USA, 2016.
8. Bertucci, C.; Hudaib, M.; Boga, C.; Calonghi, N.; Cappadone, C.; Masotti, L. Gas chromatography/mass apectrometry assay of endogenous cellular lipid peroxidation products: Quantitative analysis of 9- and 10-hydroxystearic acids. *Rapid Commun. Mass Spectrom.* **2002**, *16*, 859–864. [CrossRef]
9. Calonghi, N.; Cappadone, C.; Pagnotta, E.; Farruggia, G.; Buontempo, F.; Boga, C.; Brusa, G.; Santucci, M.; Masotti, L. 9-Hydroxystearic acid upregulates p21WAF1 in HT29 cancer cells. *Biochem. Biophys. Res. Commun.* **2004**, *314*, 138–142. [CrossRef]
10. Calonghi, N.; Cappadone, C.; Pagnotta, E.; Boga, C.; Bertucci, C.; Fiori, J.; Tasco, G.; Casadio, R.; Masotti, L. Histone deacetylase 1: a target of 9-hydroxystearic acid in the inhibition of cell growth in human colon cancer. *J. Lipid Res.* **2005**, *46*, 1596–1603. [CrossRef]
11. Calonghi, N.; Pagnotta, E.; Parolin, C.; Tognoli, C.; Boga, C.; Masotti, L. 9-Hydroxystearic acid interferes with EGF signalling in a human colon adenocarcinoma. *Biochem. Biophys. Res. Commun.* **2006**, *342*, 585–588. [CrossRef]
12. Calonghi, N.; Pagnotta, E.; Parolin, C.; Molinari, C.; Boga, C.; Piaz, F.D.; Brusa, G.; Santucci, M.; Masotti, L. Modulation of apoptotic signalling by 9-hydroxystearic acid in osteosarcoma cells. *Biochim. et Biophys. Acta (BBA) Mol. Cell Biol. Lipids* **2007**, *1771*, 139–146. [CrossRef]
13. Parolin, C.; Calonghi, N.; Presta, E.; Boga, C.; Caruana, P.; Naldi, M.; Andrisano, V.; Masotti, L.; Sartor, G. Mechanism and stereoselectivity of HDAC I inhibition by (R)-9-hydroxystearic acid in colon cancer. *Biochim. Biophys. Acta (BBA) Mol. Cell Biol. Lipids* **2012**, *1821*, 1334–1340. [CrossRef]
14. Boanini, E.; Torricelli, P.; Boga, C.; Micheletti, G.; Cassani, M.C.; Fini, M.; Bigi, A. (9R)-9-Hydroxystearate-Functionalized Hydroxyapatite as Anti-Proliferative and Cytotoxic Agent towards Osteosarcoma Cells. *Langmuir* **2016**, *32*, 188–194. [CrossRef]
15. Busi, A.; Aluigi, A.; Guerrini, A.; Boga, C.; Sartor, G.; Calonghi, N.; Sotgiu, G.; Posati, T.; Corticelli, F.; Fiori, J.; et al. Unprecedented Behavior of (9R)-9-Hydroxystearic Acid-Loaded Keratin Nanoparticles on Cancer Cell Cycle. *Mol. Pharm.* **2019**, *16*, 931–942. [CrossRef] [PubMed]
16. Calonghi, N.; Boga, C.; Telese, D.; Bordoni, S.; Sartor, G.; Torsello, C.; Micheletti, G. Synthesis of 9-Hydroxystearic Acid Derivatives and Their Antiproliferative Activity on HT 29 Cancer Cells. *Molecules* **2019**, *24*, 3714. [CrossRef]
17. Boga, C.; Micheletti, G.; Orlando, I.; Strocchi, E.; Vitali, B.; Verardi, L.; Sartor, G.; Calonghi, N. New Hybrids with 2-aminobenzothiazole and Azelayl Scaffolds: Synthesis, Molecular Docking and Biological Evaluation. *Curr. Org. Chem.* **2018**, *22*, 1649–1660. [CrossRef]
18. Micheletti, G.; Calonghi, N.; Farruggia, G.; Strocchi, E.; Palmacci, V.; Telese, D.; Bordoni, S.; Frisco, G.; Boga, C. Synthesis of Novel Structural Hybrids between Aza-Heterocycles and Azelaic Acid Moiety with a Specific Activity on Osteosarcoma Cells. *Molecules* **2020**, *25*, 404. [CrossRef] [PubMed]
19. Sackton, K.L.; Dimova, N.; Zeng, X.; Tian, W.; Zhang, M.; Sackton, T.B.; Meaders, J.L.; Pfaff, K.L.; Sigoillot, F.D.; Yu, H.; et al. Synergistic blockade of mitotic exit by two chemical inhibitors of the APC/C. *Nat. Cell Biol.* **2014**, *514*, 646–649. [CrossRef] [PubMed]
20. Wan, Y.; Zhou, Z.; Chi, J.; Schiltz, G. *Bifunctional Compounds Comprising Apcin-a and Their Use in the Treatment of Cancer*; WO 2020/214555 A1; Northwestern University: Evanston, IL, USA, 2020.
21. Simonetti, G.; Bruno, S.; Padella, A.; Tenti, E.; Martinelli, G. Aneuploidy: Cancer strength or vulnerability? *Int. J. Cancer* **2019**, *144*, 8–25. [CrossRef]
22. Simonetti, G.; Padella, A.; Valle, I.F.D.; Fontana, M.C.; Fonzi, E.; Bruno, S.; Baldazzi, C.; Guadagnuolo, V.; Manfrini, M.; Ferrari, A.; et al. Aneuploid acute myeloid leukemia exhibits a signature of genomic alterations in the cell cycle and protein degradation machinery. *Cancer* **2018**, *125*, 712–725. [CrossRef]
23. Wu, W.-J.; Hu, K.-S.; Wang, D.-S.; Zeng, Z.-L.; Zhang, D.; Chen, D.-L.; Bai, L.; Xu, R. CDC20 overexpression predicts a poor prognosis for patients with colorectal cancer. *J. Transl. Med.* **2013**, *11*, 142. [CrossRef]
24. Moura, I.M.B.; Delgado, M.L.; Silva, P.M.A.; Lopes, C.A.; Amaral, J.B.D.; Monteiro, L.S.; Bousbaa, H. High CDC20 expression is associated with poor prognosis in oral squamous cell carcinoma. *J. Oral Pathol. Med.* **2013**, *43*, 225–231. [CrossRef]
25. Ouellet, V.; Guyot, M.-C.; Le Page, C.; Filali-Mouhim, A.; Lussier, C.; Tonin, P.N.; Provencher, D.; Mes-Masson, A.-M. Tissue array analysis of expression microarray candidates identifies markers associated with tumor grade and outcome in serous epithelial ovarian cancer. *Int. J. Cancer* **2006**, *119*, 599–607. [CrossRef]
26. Lub, S.; Maes, A.; Maes, K.; De Veirman, K.; De Bruyne, E.; Menu, E.; Fostier, K.; Kassambara, A.; Moreaux, J.; Hose, D.; et al. Inhibiting the anaphase promoting complex/cyclosome induces a metaphase arrest and cell death in multiple myeloma cells. *Oncotarget* **2015**, *7*, 4062–4076. [CrossRef] [PubMed]
27. Wu, F.; Dai, X.; Gan, W.; Wan, L.; Li, M.; Mitsiades, N.; Wei, W.; Ding, Q.; Zhang, J. Prostate cancer-associated mutation in SPOP impairs its ability to target Cdc20 for poly-ubiquitination and degradation. *Cancer Lett.* **2017**, *385*, 207–214. [CrossRef] [PubMed]

28. De, K.; Grubb, T.M.; Zalenski, A.A.; Pfaff, K.E.; Pal, D.; Majumder, S.; Summers, M.K.; Venere, M. Hyperphosphorylation of CDH1 in Glioblastoma Cancer Stem Cells Attenuates APC/CCDH1 Activity and Pharmacologic Inhibition of APC/CCDH1/CDC20 Compromises Viability. *Mol. Cancer Res.* **2019**, *17*, 1519–1530. [CrossRef] [PubMed]
29. Gao, Y.; Zhang, B.; Wang, Y.; Shang, G. Cdc20 inhibitor apcin inhibits the growth and invasion of osteosarcoma cells. *Oncol. Rep.* **2018**, *40*, 841–848. [CrossRef] [PubMed]
30. Huang, P.; Le, X.; Huang, F.; Yang, J.; Yang, H.; Ma, J.; Hu, G.; Li, Q.; Chen, Z. Discovery of a Dual Tubulin Polymerization and Cell Division Cycle 20 Homologue Inhibitor via Structural Modification on Apcin. *J. Med. Chem.* **2020**, *63*, 4685–4700. [CrossRef]
31. Di Rorà, A.G.L.; Martinelli, G.; Simonetti, G. The balance between mitotic death and mitotic slippage in acute leukemia: A new therapeutic window? *J. Hematol. Oncol.* **2019**, *12*, 1–16. [CrossRef]
32. Oh, J.H.; Lee, T.-J.; Kim, S.H.; Choi, Y.H.; Lee, S.-H.; Lee, J.M.; Kim, Y.-H.; Park, J.-W.; Kwon, T.K. Induction of apoptosis by withaferin A in human leukemia U937 cells through down-regulation of Akt phosphorylation. *Apoptosis* **2008**, *13*, 1494–1504. [CrossRef]
33. Okamoto, S.; Tsujioka, T.; Suemori, S.; Kida, J.; Kondo, T.; Tohyama, Y.; Tohyama, K. Withaferin A suppresses the growth of myelodysplasia and leukemia cell lines by inhibiting cell cycle progression. *Cancer Sci.* **2016**, *107*, 1302–1314. [CrossRef]
34. Sanchez-Martin, M.; Ambesi-Impiombato, A.; Qin, Y.; Herranz, D.; Bansal, M.; Girardi, T.; Paietta, E.; Tallman, M.S.; Rowe, J.M.; De Keersmaecker, K.; et al. Synergistic antileukemic therapies inNOTCH1-induced T-ALL. *Proc. Natl. Acad. Sci. USA* **2017**, *114*, 2006–2011. [CrossRef]
35. Garcia-Manero, G.; Yang, H.; Bueso-Ramos, C.; Ferrajoli, A.; Cortes, J.; Wierda, W.G.; Faderl, S.; Koller, C.; Morris, G.; Rosner, G.; et al. Phase 1 study of the histone deacetylase inhibitor vorinostat (suberoylanilide hydroxamic acid [SAHA]) in patients with advanced leukemias and myelodysplastic syndromes. *Blood* **2008**, *111*, 1060–1066. [CrossRef]
36. Abaza, Y.; Kadia, T.; Jabbour, E.J.; Konopleva, M.Y.; Borthakur, G.; Ferrajoli, A.; Estrov, Z.; Wierda, W.G.; Alfonso, A.; Chong, T.H.; et al. Phase 1 dose escalation multicenter trial of pracinostat alone and in combination with azacitidine in patients with advanced hematologic malignancies. *Cancer* **2017**, *123*, 4851–4859. [CrossRef] [PubMed]
37. Aillaud, I.; Barber, D.M.; Thompson, A.L.; Dixon, D.J. Enantioselective Michael Addition/Iminium Ion Cyclization Cascades of Tryptamine-Derived Ureas. *Org. Lett.* **2013**, *15*, 2946–2949. [CrossRef] [PubMed]
38. Nelson, W.J.; Edwards, L.D.; Christian, E.J.; Jenkins, G.L. The Study, Testing and Synthesis of Certain Organic Compounds for Rodenticidal Activity. *J. Am. Pharm. Assoc.* **1947**, *36*, 349–352. [CrossRef] [PubMed]

*molecules*

MDPI

*Communication*

# Hybrid Quinoline-Sulfonamide Complexes ($M^{2+}$) Derivatives with Antimicrobial Activity

**Dumitrela Diaconu [1,2], Violeta Mangalagiu [2,*], Dorina Amariucai-Mantu [1], Vasilichia Antoci [1], Cristian Levente Giuroiu [3,*] and Ionel I. Mangalagiu [1,2,*]**

1 Faculty of Chemistry, Alexandru Ioan Cuza University of Iasi, 11 Carol Bvd, 700506 Iasi, Romania; cucu.dumitrela@yahoo.com (D.D.); dorinaiasi@yahoo.com (D.A.-M.); vasilichia2004@yahoo.com (V.A.)
2 Institute of Interdisciplinary Research—CERNESIM Center, Alexandru Ioan Cuza University of Iasi, 11 Carol Bvd, 700506 Iasi, Romania
3 Endodontics, Faculty of Dental Medicine, Grigore T. Popa University of Medicine and Pharmacy, 16 Universităţii Street, 700115 Iasi, Romania
* Correspondence: violeta.mangalagiu@uaic.ro (V.M.); giuroiu.cristian@umfiasi.ro (C.L.G.); ionelm@uaic.ro (I.I.M.)

Academic Editor: Maged Henary
Received: 14 May 2020; Accepted: 24 June 2020; Published: 26 June 2020

**Abstract:** Two new series of hybrid quinoline-sulfonamide complexes ($M^{2+}$: $Zn^{2+}$, $Cu^{2+}$, $Co^{2+}$ and $Cd^{2+}$) derivatives (**QSC**) were designed, synthesized and tested for their antimicrobial activity. The synthesis is straightforward and efficient, involving two steps: acylation of aminoquinoline followed by complexation with metal acetate ($Cu^{2+}$, $Co^{2+}$ and $Cd^{2+}$) or chloride ($Zn^{2+}$). The synthesized **QSC** compounds were characterized by FTIR and NMR spectroscopy and by X-ray diffraction on single crystal. The **QSC** compounds were preliminary screened for their antibacterial and antifungal activity and the obtained results are very promising. In this respect, the hybrid *N*-(quinolin-8-yl)-4-chloro-benzenesulfonamide cadmium (II), considered as leading structure for further studies, has an excellent antibacterial activity against *Staphylococcus aureus ATCC25923* (with a diameters of inhibition zones of 21 mm and a minimum inhibitory concentration (MIC) of $19.04 \times 10^{-5}$ mg/mL), a very good antibacterial activity against *Escherichia coli ATCC25922* (with a diameters of inhibition zones of 19 mm and a MIC of $609 \times 10^{-5}$ mg/mL), and again an excellent antifungal activity against *Candida albicans ATCC10231* (with a diameters of inhibition zones of 25 mm and a MIC of $19.04 \times 10^{-5}$ mg/mL).

**Keywords:** hybrid quinoline-sulfonamide complexes; small-molecule drugs; antimicrobial activity

## 1. Introduction

Despite of the significant advances in the antimicrobial therapy accomplished in the last few decades, infectious diseases caused by microorganisms (bacteria, fungus, viruses, *Mycobacterium tuberculosis*, etc.) represent seriously threaten of modern medicine and global public health. Drug resistance, multi-drug resistance and extensively-drug-resistance are the leading cause of these drawbacks, but some other causes could be also taken into consideration [1–3]. Quinoline based compounds are small molecules of huge importance from pharmacological point of view, having a wide range of biological activities such as antiplasmodial and antimalarial, antibacterial, antifungal, antitubercular, anti-HIV, antiviral (including against COVID-19), etc. [4–16]. A special class of quinoline derivatives which pay a particularly attention on scientific community, are quinoline-sulfonamide complexes (**QSC**), studied especially for their fotoluminiscent (mostly fluorescent) properties [17–23]. As far for biological activity, these compounds were tested mostly as antiprotozoals [24,25] and very few data was found for their antibacterial and antifungal activity [26]. The antibacterial activity of azaheterocycles sulfonamides is well known [1,2].

Encouraged by our recent results in the field of (di)azine with antimicrobial activity [11,15,27–40], we report here the design, synthesis, antibacterial and antifungal evaluation of some newly hybrid quinoline-sulfonamide complexes.

## 2. Results and Discussion

### 2.1. Design and Chemistry

Having in view the biological potential of quinoline and sulfonamide scaffolds (especially antimicrobial) [9–15], as well as those one of quinoline-sulfonamide combined scaffold (especially anti-HIV-1) [16], we decide to combine the pharmacophoric properties of these core scaffolds with the complementary biological properties of counter cation $M^{2+}$ ($M^{2+}$: $Zn^{2+}$, $Cu^{2+}$, $Co^{2+}$ and $Cd^{2+}$), with the final goal of obtaining better biological activity and better pharmacokinetic properties for our compounds. In this respect, we design two new classes of hybrid quinoline-sulfonamide complexes, namely *N*-(quinolin-8-yl)-4-R-*benzene* sulfonamide metal (II) (**QBSC**) and *N*-(quinolin-8-yl)-quinoline -8-sulfonamide metal (II) (**QQSC**), Scheme 1.

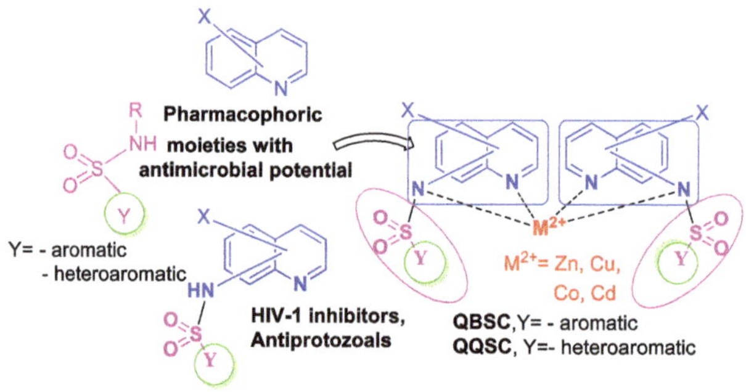


**Scheme 1.** Design in the class of hybrid quinoline-sulfonamide complexes derivatives.

As in related cases [21–24], the general route to obtain the desired compounds involves a simple and efficient two-step procedure. The first step consist in the acylation of (3, 4 or 8)amino-quinoline with variously 4-R-benzenesulfonyl chlorides (R = Cl, $NO_2$, OMe) and quinolylsulfonyl chlorides, when the corresponding ligands quinoline-sulfonamide type **3** are obtained. The second step consist in the complexation of ligands **3** with metal acetate ($Cu^{2+}$, $Co^{2+}$, $Cd^{2+}$) or chloride ($Zn^{2+}$). In this way, we obtained the two classes of compounds desired: **QBSC** type **4–6** and **QQSC** type **7**. The procedure is depicted in Scheme 2 for the complexes derived from 8-aminoquinoline.

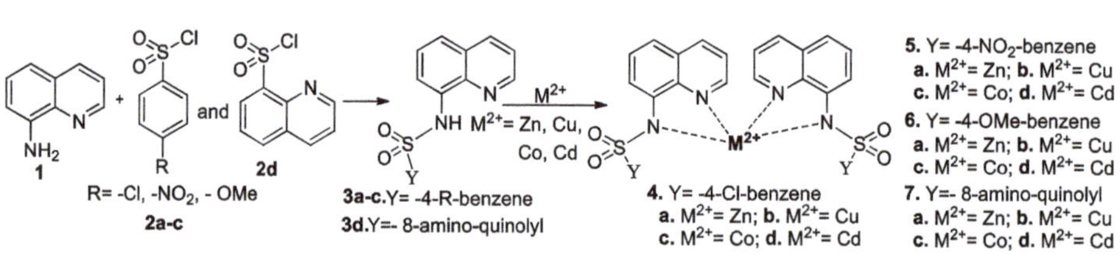


**Scheme 2.** Reaction pathways to obtain hybrid quinoline-sulfonamide complexes derivatives.

The structures of **QSC** compounds were proved by elemental and spectral analysis (FT-IR, $^1$H-NMR, $^{13}$C{$^1$H}-NMR, and two-dimensional experiments 2D-COSY, HMQC, HMBC), and single crystal X-ray structure determination. If we consider the $M^{2+}$[*N*-(quinolin-8-yl)-4-chloro-benzenesulfonamide]$_2$

derivatives **QBSC 4a–d** as representative for the hybrid **QSC**, the spectral analysis reveal strong evidence for the proposed structures.

In the FT-IR spectra of sulfonamide ligand **3a** and its complexes **QBSC 4a–d** (Figure 1), the most representative bands, together with their assignments, are given in Table 1.

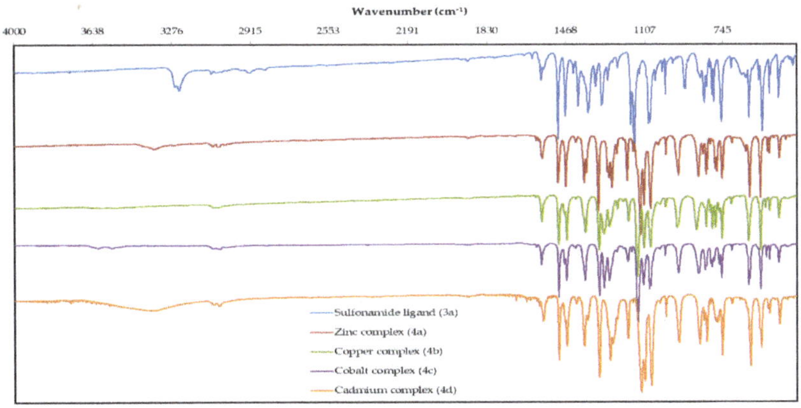


**Figure 1.** FT-IR spectra of sulfonamide ligand 3a, zinc (II) complex (4a), copper (II) complex (4b), cobalt (II) complex (4c) and cadmium (II) complex (4d).

**Table 1.** Representative bands of sulfonamide ligand **3a** and its complexes with divalent ions $Zn^{2+}$, $Cu^{2+}$, $Co^{2+}$ and $Cd^{2+}$.

| $\nu$ (cm$^{-1}$) | Sulfonamide Ligand (3a) | Zinc Complex (4a) | Copper Complex (4b) | Cobalt Complex (4c) | Cadmium Complex (4d) |
|---|---|---|---|---|---|
| $\nu_{N\text{-}H}$ | 3267 (m) | - | - | - | - |
| $\nu_{asSO2}$ | 1372 (s-m) | 1389 (s-m) | 1385 (s-m) | 1386 (s-m) | 1392 (s-m) |
| $\nu_{symSO2}$ | 1177 (s) | 1138 (s) | 1155 (s) | 1151 (s) | 1136 (s) |
| $\nu_{C\text{-}N}$ | 1584 (m) | 1583 (m) | 1583 (m) | 1584 (m) | 1578 (m) |
| $\nu_{S\text{-}N}$ | 927 (m) | 954 (m) | 954 (m) | 961 (m) | 957 (m) |
| $\nu_{C\text{-}S}$ | 624 (s) | 624 (s) | 629 (s) | 624 (s) | 621 (s) |

$\nu$—stretching; s—strong; m—medium; w—weak; as—asymmetric; sym—symmetric.

The band from 3267 cm$^{-1}$ (medium intensity), which is corresponding to the N–H stretching vibration in the free ligand, is missing in the spectra of the complexes, confirming deprotonation of the nitrogen atom of the sulfonamide and its coordination to the metal ion. The bands corresponding to the asymmetric and symmetric stretching vibration of the sulfonyl group in ligand appear at 1372 cm$^{-1}$ respectively at 1177 cm$^{-1}$, while in spectra of the complexes are shifted with ≈20 cm$^{-1}$ to higher wave numbers respectively ≈40 cm$^{-1}$ to lower wave numbers; this is because in the free ligand a larger double bond character of the SO bonds could be incriminated. The band due to the sulfonyl group is split in the spectra of the complexes, because of the different spatial orientation of these groups, as the X-ray show. We also notice a similar shift with ≈20 cm$^{-1}$ to higher wave numbers for the S–N stretching vibration in the spectra of the complexes, probably because the N atom is involved in the bonding to the metal atom. The remaining bands appear at wave numbers in accordance with the proposed structures both in the free ligand and complexes.

The $^{1}$H-NMR and $^{13}$C{1H}-NMR spectra of the sulfonamide ligand and its complexes shows characteristic chemical shifts that are in agreement to the proposed structure. The most significant signal in the $^{1}$H-NMR spectra (Figure 2), corresponding of the hydrogen atom from sulfonamide group **$H_9$** and, appear in the free ligand at a chemical shift of 10.20 ppm. This signal is missing in the spectra of **QBSC** complexes, which is a solid prove for the complexation with the metal ion. We could also notice that the signals of hydrogen atoms near the metal ion $\mathbf{H_2}$, $\mathbf{H_3}$, $\mathbf{H_4}$ (from pyridine ring), are deshielded in **QBSC** complexes with about 0.30 ppm due to the powerful deshielding effect of the metal ion, a electron density transfer from the ligand to the metal ion being responsible for this.

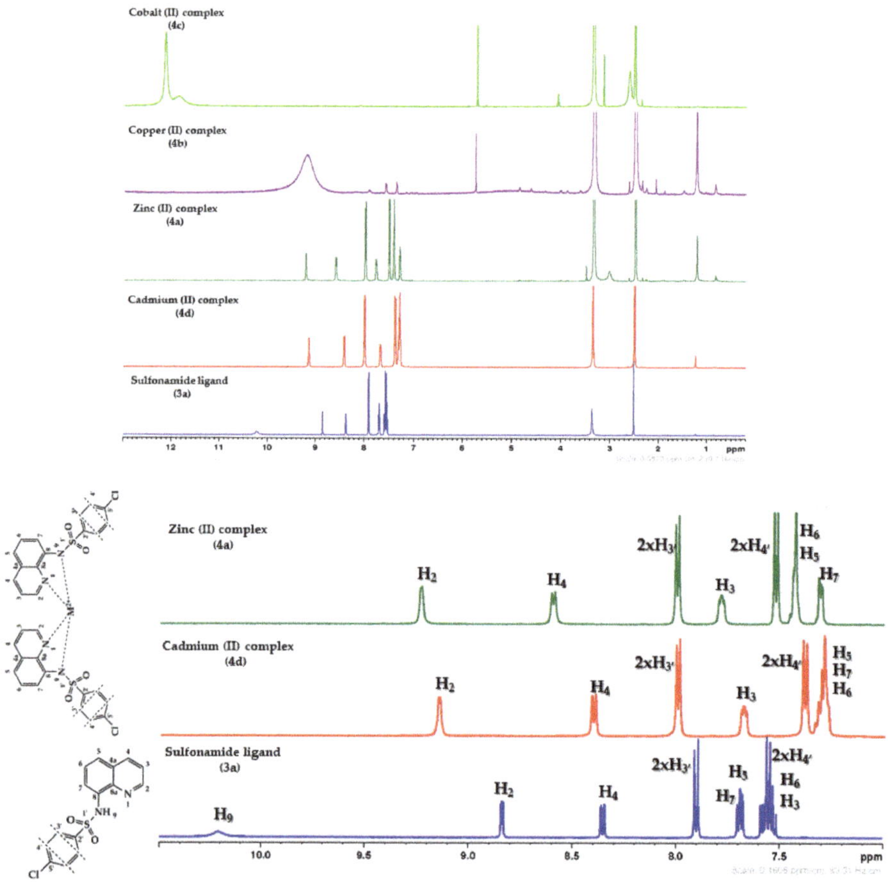


**Figure 2.** [1]H-NMR spectra for sulfonamide ligand (**3a**) and its complexes (**4a–d**). At the bottom part of the image is represented a detail of aromatic zone (7–11 ppm).

Similar considerations could be done for $^{13}C\{^1H\}$-NMR spectra, Figure 3. The most relevant signals in the $^{13}C\{^1H\}$-NMR spectra, correspond to the carbon atoms $\mathbf{C_{2'}}$, $\mathbf{C_8}$, $\mathbf{C_5}$ and $\mathbf{C_7}$. In **QBSC** complexes, the $\mathbf{C_{2'}}$ carbons (*ipso*-sulfonamide) appear to a chemical shift of about 142 ppm due to the powerful deshielding effect of sulfonamide group and the metal ion, while $\mathbf{C_8}$ (carbon from attached benzene ring of quinoline) appear to a chemical shift of about 141 ppm, the same reasons being incriminated. Comparative with the free ligand, in **QBSC** complexes, these carbons are deshielded with about 8 ppm for $\mathbf{C_8}$, respectively, with about 4 ppm for $\mathbf{C_{2'}}$, due to the powerful deshielding effect of the metal ion. The most shielded carbons are $\mathbf{C_5}$ and $\mathbf{C_7}$. In **QBSC** complexes, these carbons appear to a chemical shift of about 117 ppm for $\mathbf{C_5}$, respectively, 115 ppm for $\mathbf{C_7}$, being shielded comparative with the free ligand with about 20 ppm for $\mathbf{C_5}$ respectively with about 2 ppm for $\mathbf{C_7}$. As far for the NMR spectra of $Cu^{2+}$ and $Co^{2+}$ complexes, the spectra are broad because of their different magnetic properties (paramagnetic).

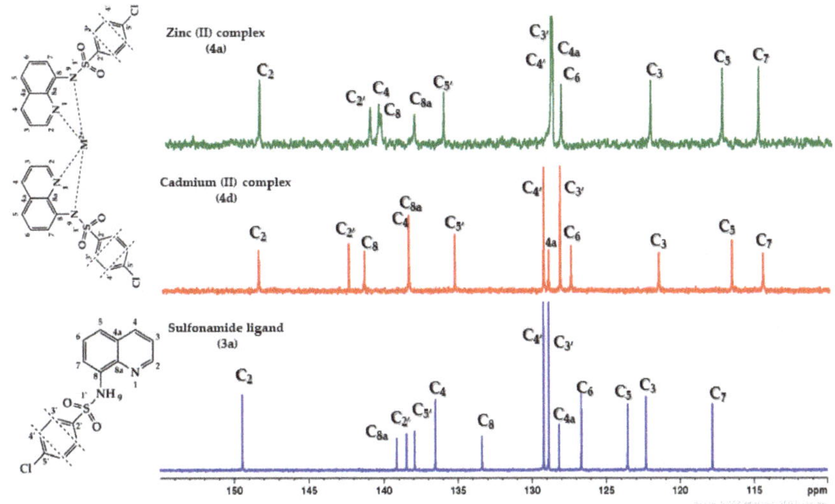

**Figure 3.** $^{13}C\{^1H\}$-NMR spectra detail (110–160 ppm) for sulfonamide ligand (**3a**), Zn (II) and Cd (II) complexes.

In the case of compounds **4b** and **4c,** the structure of compounds was assigned unambiguously by single-crystal X-ray investigation (for **4a** and **4d**, we did not obtained yet proper crystals), Figure 4A,B.

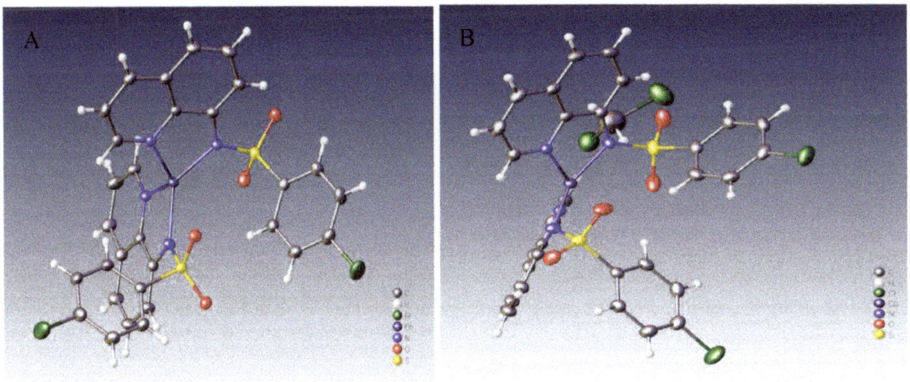

**Figure 4.** (**A**) Molecular structure of [Co(*N*-(quinoline-8-yl)-4-chloro-benzenesulfonamide)$_2$] **4c** complex. (**B**) Molecular structure of [Cu(*N*-(quinoline-8-yl)-4-chloro-benzenesulfonamide)$_2$] **4b** complex.

The structure of **QBSC** cobalt complex **4c** was resolved by direct methods and refined in the monoclinic $P_{21}$/n space group type. Molecular information's shows a tetrahedral coordination of cobalt with the bidentate ligand trough Co-Nquinoline and Co-Nsulfonamide bonds. The Co-Nquinoline bond lengths (2.038 and 2.029 Å) are slightly larger than Co-Nsulfonamide bonds (1.970 and 1.983 Å) but in an acceptable range as reported by other papers for similar complexes. The structure of **QBSC** copper complex **4b** was resolved by direct methods and refined in the monoclinic $I_2$/a space group type. Molecular information's shows a tetrahedral coordination of copper with the bidentate ligand trough Cu-Nquinoline and Cu-Nsulfonamide bonds. The Cu-Nquinoline bond lengths (1.980 and 1.991 Å) are slightly larger than Cu-Nsulfonamide bonds (1.960 and 1.944 Å) but in an acceptable range as reported by other papers for similar complexes. Copies of NMR spectra of ligand and **QBSC** complexes and checkCIF files for X-ray data of **QBSC** complex **4b** and **4c** are presented to Supplementary Materials.

### *2.2. Antimicrobial Assay*

The in vitro antimicrobial activity of ligand **3** and **QSC** compounds **4a–d** was determined by the Kirby–Bauer disk diffusion method [41] using nutrient agar medium (Mueller Hinton agar for antibacterial tests and Sabouraud agar for antifungal tests). The antibacterial activity was evaluated against two strains bacteria (Gram-positive *Staphylococcus aureus ATCC 25923* and Gram-negative *Escherichia coli ATCC 25922*) and the antifungal activity against fungus *Candida albicans ATCC 10231*. As positive control (C+) was used, Penicillin 10 IU for *Staphylococcus aureus*, Carbenicillin 100 μg/mL for *Escherichia coli* and Nystatin 500,000 IU for *Candida albicans*; the negative control (C−) consist in sterile filter paper disks with no antimicrobial compounds. The more susceptible were the germs, the larger the diameter (mm) of the inhibition zones is. The obtained results are expressed as diameters of inhibition zones (mm) and, for ligand **3**, and **QBSC 4a–d** compounds, are presented in Table 2 and Figure 5A–C.

**Table 2.** The antibacterial and antifungal activity for ligand **3a** and **QBSC 4a–d** compounds.

| Strain | Diameter of Inhibition Zone | | | | |
|---|---|---|---|---|---|
| | [a] 3a | [a] 4a (Zn) | [a] 4b (Cu) | [a] 4c (Co) | [a] 4d (Cd) |
| *S. aureus ATCC 25923* | 18 ± 1.73 | 11 ± 1.73 | 16 ± 1 | 17 ± 2 | **21** ± 2 |
| *E. coli ATCC 25922* | 0 | 12 ± 2 | 14.5 ± 2 | 10.7 ± 2 | 19 ± 1.73 |
| *C. albicans ATCC 10231* | **26.5** ± 1.80 | 12 ± 2 | 0 | 11 ± 1 | **25** ± 1.15 |

All values represented in the table are average of results of five separately conducted experiments. Underline means active and bold and underline means very active. [a] Diameter of inhibition zone (mm), [a] X ± SD, mean of five measurements ± standard deviation.

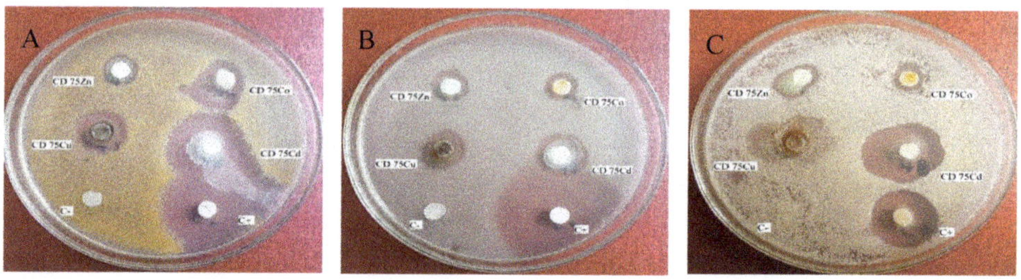


**Figure 5.** (**A**) The antibacterial activity for **QBSC** compounds **4a** (CD 75Zn), **4b** (CD 75Cu), **4c** (CD 75Co) and **4d** (CD 75Cd) against *S. aureus* (C+: positive control; C−: negative control). (**B**) The antibacterial activity for **QBSC** compounds **4a** (CD 75Zn), **4b** (CD 75Cu), **4c** (CD 75Co) and **4d** (CD 75Cd) against *E. coli* (C+: positive control; C−: negative control). (**C**) The antifungal activity for **QBSC** compounds **4a** (CD 75Zn), **4b** (CD 75Cu), **4c** (CD 75Co) and **4d** (CD 75Cd) against *C. albicans* (C+: positive control; C−: negative control).

From the data presented in Table 2 and Figure 5A–C, we may notice that some of our **QBSC** compounds demonstrated to be effective against the tested strain. Against bacterial strain *Staphylococcus aureus* one compound **QBSC 4d** is very active (having a diameter of inhibition zone of 21 mm) and three others compounds are active: **QBSC 4c**, **QBSC 4b** and the ligand **3a** (with the diameter of inhibition zone of 17, 16 and 18 mm). Against bacteria *Escherichia coli* one compound **QBSC 4d** is active (19 mm) while against fungus *Candida albicans* two compounds are very active: **QBSC 4d** and the ligand **3a** (25 respectively 26.5 mm).

The compounds which exhibited significant antimicrobial activity were later tested using the standardized broth microdilution assay procedure to determine the minimum inhibitory concentration (MIC) of the compounds under investigation against the reference microorganisms [42]. The resulted MIC value is defined as the lowest concentration of the antimicrobial agent under investigation, which prevents visible growth of the tested microorganism. The obtained results are listed in Table 3.

**Table 3.** The minimum inhibitory concentration (MIC) for ligand **3a** and **QBSC 4a–d** compounds (mg/mL).

| Strain | MIC (mg/mL) | | | | |
|---|---|---|---|---|---|
| | 3a | 4a (Zn) | 4b (Cu) | 4c (Co) | 4d (Cd) |
| *S. aureus ATCC 25923* | 12.5 | 25 | 0.04875 | 12.5 | 0.00019 |
| *E. coli ATCC 25922* | - | 25 | 0.04875 | 12.5 | 0.00609 |
| *C. albicans ATCC 10231* | 12.5 | 12.5 | - | 12.5 | 0.00019 |

As we may notice from Table 3, Cd complex (**QBSC 4d**) is active to a very low concentration, having a MIC of 19.04 × $10^{-5}$ mg/mL in the case of *Staphylococcus aureus* and *Candida albicans*, respectively 609 × $10^{-5}$ mg/mL in the case of *Escherichia coli*. Significant results was obtained also for Cu complex (**QBSC 4b**) which have MIC value of 4875 × $10^{-5}$ mg/mL in the case of bacterial streams *Staphylococcus aureus* and *Escherichia coli*.

The diameter of inhibition zone and MIC data reveal that our **QBSC** compounds (except the Zn complexes) have a quasi-nonselective activity against bacteria *Staphylococcus aureus*. Against *Escherichia coli* only Cd complex (**QBSC 4d**) have a significant activity, while against fungus *Candida albicans* Cd complex (**QBSC 4d**) and quinoline sulfonamide ligand (**3a**) present a strong activity. The above presented results also reveal a clear influence of the metal cation, the Cd complex (**QBSC 4d**) being far away the most active tested compound, having a quasi-nonselective antibacterial and antifungal activity. The activity of cadmium complexes are higher the most probable because of a better synergism ligand cadmium.

As to the mechanism of action of our **QBSC** compounds, we may presume that they could act as carbonic anhydrase inhibitors, as the literature describe for related compounds [26,43].

## 3. Experimental

### 3.1. Chemistry

All the reagents and solvents were purchased from commercial sources and used without further purification. Melting points were recorded on a Electrothermal MEL-TEMP II (Barnstead International, Dubuque, IA, USA) apparatus in open capillary tubes and are uncorrected. Analytical thin-layer chromatography (TLC) was performed with commercial Merck silica gel 60 $F_{254}$ plates and visualized with UV light ($\lambda_{max}$ = 254 or 365 nm). The NMR spectra were recorded on a Bruker Avance III 500 MHz spectrometer (Bruker Vienna, Austria) operating at 500 MHz for $^{1}$H and 125 MHz for $^{13}$C. Chemical shifts were reported in delta (δ) units, part per million (ppm) and coupling constants (*J*) in Hz. The following abbreviations were used to designate chemical shift multiplicities: s = singlet, d = doublet, ad = apparent doublet, t = triplet, q = quartet, aq = apparent quartet, m = multiplet. Infrared (IR) data were recorded as films on potassium bromide (KBr) pellets on a FT-IR VERTEX 70 Bruker spectrophotometer. In order to determine the structure of complexes, a crystal of each complex was selected, mounted on a hair thread and inserted into the four-circle SuperNova single crystal diffraction instrument. Data acquisition was made at 100 °K (−173.15 °C) using CuKa radiation. A number of 5608 reflections from a total of 33212 acquired in $2.8345 < \theta < 70.8363$ range were used for refinement and structure solution.

Compound **3a**, which have already been reported in literature, showed spectral data in agreement to the reported data [16,17,20].

3.1.1. General Procedure for the Synthesis of Sulfonamide Ligand **3a** and its Complexes **4a–d**

Synthesis of the Ligand

*4-chloro-N-(quinolin-8-yl)benzenesulfonamide* (**3a**), 1 mmol of 8-aminoquinoline was dissolved in minimum volume of dichloromethane $CH_2Cl_2$, then was added to a stirred solution of 4-chlorobenzenesulfonyl chloride (1.1 mmol) and pyridine. The crude product was washed with HCl (1 M), then with a solution of saturated $NaHCO_3$. The organic extract was dried on $Na_2SO_4$ and the solvent was removed in vacuum. The solid obtained was purified on column chromatography ($CH_2Cl_2$/AcOEt = 70/30) giving the white solid 4-chloro-*N*-(quinolin-8-yl)benzenesulfonamide.

Synthesis of the Complexes

The complexes were prepared by direct reaction between the sulfonamide ligand and Zn(II), Cu(II), Co(II) and Cd(II) salts.

*[Zn(N-(quinoline-8-yl)-4-chloro-benzenesulfonamide)2]* (**4a**), 2 mmol of sulfonamide ligand **3a** were dissolved in 70 mL MeOH and 2 mL $NH_4OH$ were added. 1 mmol of $ZnCl_2$ dissolved in 50 mL methanol were added dropwise while solution was magnetically stirred. When addition is completed, a yellow precipitate is formed, which is separated by filtration. Addition of a base for deprotonating the nitrogen from amine was necessary to prepare the zinc complex. [21]

*[Cu(N-(quinoline-8-yl)-4-chloro-benzenesulfonamide)$_2$],[Co(N-(quinoline-8-yl)-4-chloro-benzenesulfonamide)$_2$], [Cd(N-(quinoline-8-yl)-4-chloro-benzenesulfonamide)$_2$]* (**4b–d**), on a methanolic solution of metal (Cu, Co and Cd) (II) acetate (1 mmol) was added dropwise 80 mL of a solution containing 2 mmol of sulfonamide-ligand **3a**. After overnight stirring at room temperature, crystals were formed and they were separated by filtration [23].

*4-chloro-N-(quinolin-8-yl)benzenesulfonamide* (**3a),** White solid; yield: 87%; mp 129–130 °C; IR (KBr), $\nu_{max}$ 3267, 1584, 1506, 1372, 1177, 1094, 927, 755, 624, 562 $cm^{-1}$; $^1$H NMR (500 MHz, DMSO-$d_6$) δ 7.54 (4H, m, 2 × H-4′, H-6, H-3), 7.68 (2H, m, H-7, H-5), 7.89 (2H, d, *J* = 8.5 Hz, 2 × H-3′), 8.35 (1H, dd, *J* = 8.5 Hz, *J* = 1.5 Hz, H-4), 8.84 (1H, dd, *J* = 4.5 Hz, *J* = 1.5 Hz, H-2), 10.20 (1H, s, H-9); $^{13}$C{1H} NMR (125 MHz, DMSO-$d_6$) δ 117.79 (C-7), 122.33 (C-3), 123.57 (C-5), 126.66 (C-6), 128.17 (C-4a), 128.88 (2 × C-3′), 129.23 (2 × C-4′), 133.38 (C-8), 136.52 (C-4), 137.91 (C-5′), 138.47 (C-2′), 139.14 (C-8a), 149.45 (C-2); Anal. Calcd. for $C_{15}H_{11}ClN_2O_2S$ C, 56.52; H, 3.48; N, 8.79. Found C, 56.47; H, 3.51; N, 8.74.

*[Zn(N-(quinoline-8-yl)-4-chloro-benzenesulfonamide)$_2$]* (**4a**), Yellowish green crystals; yield 92%; IR (KBr), $\nu_{max}$ 3390, 1583, 1507, 1471, 1389, 1196, 1138, 954, 753, 624, 572 $cm^{-1}$; $^1$H NMR (500 MHz, DMSO-$d_6$) δ 7.30 (2H, dd, *J* = 6.0 Hz, *J* = 2.5 Hz, 2 × H-7), 7.43 (4H, ad, *J* = 6.0 Hz, 2 × H-6, 2 × H-5), 7.52 (4H, d, *J* = 8.5 Hz, 4 × H-4′), 7.78 (2H, aq, *J* = 6.5 Hz, 2 × H-3), 8.00 (4H, d, *J* = 8.5 Hz, 4 × H-3′), 8.59 (2H, d, *J* = 7.5 Hz, 2 × H-4), 9.23 (2H, ad, *J* = 3.0 Hz, 2 × H-2); $^{13}$C{1H} NMR (125 MHz, DMSO-*d6*) δ 115.07 (2 × C-7), 117.52 (2 × C-5), 122.38 (2 × C-3), 128.38 (2 × C-6), 128.94 (2 × C-4a), 129.01 (4 × C-3′), 129.07 (4 × C-4′), 136.32 (2 × C-5′), 138.30 (2 × C-8a), 140.55 (2 × C-8), 140.70 (2 × C-4), 141.26 (2 × C-2′), 148.65 (2 × C-2); Anal. Calcd. for $C_{30}H_{20}C_{12}N_4O_4S_2Zn$ C, 51.41; H, 2.88; N, 7.99. Found C, 51.47; H, 2.81, N 8.04.

*[Cu(N-(quinoline-8-yl)-4-chloro-benzenesulfonamide)$_2$]* (**4b**), Dark brown crystals; yield 85%; IR (KBr), $\nu_{max}$ 1583, 1507, 1467, 1385, 1155, 954, 753, 624, 572 $cm^{-1}$; Anal. Calcd. for $C_{30}H_{20}Cl_2CuN_4O_4S_2$ C, 51.54; H, 2.88; N, 8.01. Found C, 51.59; H, 2.80, N 8.06.

*[Co(N-(quinoline-8-yl)-4-chloro-benzenesulfonamide)$_2$]* (**4c**), Brick-red crystals; yield 87%; IR (KBr), $\nu_{max}$ 1584, 1502, 1468, 1386, 1195, 1151, 961, 755, 624, 572 $cm^{-1}$; Anal. Calcd. for $C_{30}H_{20}Cl_2CoN_4O_4S_2$ C, 51.89; H, 2.90; N, 8.07. Found C, 51.94; H, 2.86, N 8.11.

*[Cd(N-(quinoline-8-yl)-4-chloro-benzenesulfonamide)2]* (**4d**), Beige crystals; yield 79%; IR (KBr), $\nu_{max}$ 1578, 1503, 1468, 1323, 1275, 1136, 957, 859, 753, 621, 568 $cm^{-1}$; $^1$H NMR (500 MHz, DMSO-$d_6$) δ 7.30 (6H, m,

2 × H-7, 2 × H-6, 2 × H-5), 7.38 (4H, d, *J* = 8.5 Hz, 4 × H-4′), 7.78 (2H, aq, *J* = 8.0 Hz, 2 × H-3), 8.00 (4H, d, *J* = 8.0 Hz, 4 × H-3′), 8.40 (2H, d, *J* = 8.0 Hz, 2 × H-4), 9.15 (2H, ad, *J* = 4.5 Hz, 2 × H-2); $^{13}C\{1H\}$ NMR, (125 MHz, DMSO-*d6*) δ 114.53(2 × C-7), 116.63 (2 × C-5), 121.61 (2 × C-3), 127.51 (2 × C-6), 128.24 (4 × C-3′), 129.04 (2 × C-4a), 129.38 (4 × C-4′), 135.57 (2 × C-5′), 138.46 (2 × C-8a, 2 × C-4), 141.43 (2 × C-8), 142.48 (2 × C-2′), 148.50 (2 × C-2); Anal. Calcd. for $C_{30}H_{20}CdCl_2N_4O_4S_2$ C, 48.18; H, 2.70; N, 7.49. Found C, 48.10; H, 2.78, N 7.42.

### 3.2. Antimicrobial Assay

#### 3.2.1. Disk-Diffusion Method

For inoculum preparation, reference microbial cultures of bacteria (*Staphylococcus aureus ATCC 25923, Escherichia coli ATCC 25922*) and fungi (*Candida albicans ATCC 10231*) were employed. A number of approximately 5 colonies from each type of culture were used to inoculate 10 mL of Mueller Hinton (MH) agar (for antibacterial tests) and Sabouraud agar (for antifungal tests). Using a Beckman Coulter DU 730 spectrophotometer (λ = 600 nm), the turbidity of the inoculum was adjusted to a 0.5 McFarland standard (1–2 × $10^8$ CFU/mL for bacteria and 1–5 × $10^6$ CFU/mL for *Candida*), and the inoculum was transferred, in a 1 mL volume, onto the surface of the growth media specific for bacteria (MH) and fungi (Sabouraud). Once the inoculum was absorbed, sterile paper disks of approximately 6 mm in diameter and impregnated with 10 μL of antibacterial compound (dissolved in DMSO 3%) were placed on the surface of the culture media; for all the tested compounds, the concentration used was 25 mg/mL. Following incubation at the optimal temperatures for bacteria and fungi, of 37 °C and 28 °C, respectively, for 24 h (bacteria) and 72 h (fungi), the diameters of the inhibition zones were measured using a ruler. The controls were prepared in the same growth conditions (i.e., C+: sterile filter paper disks impregnated with antibiotics inducing sensitivity in the organisms under investigation, namely Penicillin 10 IU for *Staphylococcus aureus*, Carbenicillin 100 μg/mL for *Escherichia coli* and Nystatin 500,000 IU for *Candida albicans*, and C−: sterile filter paper disks with no antimicrobial compounds).

#### 3.2.2. Broth Microdilution Method

The working technique involves the use of a 96-well microtiter plate (microdilution). In each well of the plate, 80 μL of growth medium MH, 10 μL of microbial inoculum (*Staphylococcus aureus ATCC 25923, Escherichia coli ATCC 25922, or Candida albicans ATCC 10231*) prepared in the same manner as in the diffusion test (i.e., by diluting the standardized microbial suspension adjusted to a 0.5 McFarland standard), and 100 μL of antimicrobial substance to be tested were transferred by pipetting, in different concentrations. To this purpose, double dilutions of the antimicrobial agent were made in the DMSO 3%, starting with the 25 mg/mL dilution (e.g., 12.5 mg/mL, 6.25 mg/mL, 3.12 mg/mL, 1.56 mg/mL, 0.78 mg/mL and so on). For each tested microorganism, a positive control C+ (containing 80 μL of MH growth medium and 10 μL of antimicrobial compound) and a negative one C- (containing 80 μL of MH growth medium and 10 μL of diluted microbial culture) were prepared. Following the incubation of the microplates at 37 °C for 24 h (for *Staphylococcus aureus ATCC 25923* and *Escherichia coli ATCC 25922*) and at 28 °C for 72 h (for *Candida albicans ATCC 10231*), 10 μL of resazurin were added in each well. The samples were incubated once again at the temperature optimal for each microorganism for one hour. The color of the indicator turned from purple to pink. Resazurin is a colorimetric indicator for cell viability widely applied for monitoring cell proliferation. The redox dye, resazurin, enters the cytosol in the oxidized form (purple–blue) and is converted to the reduced form, resorufin (pink).

## 4. Conclusions

Two new series of hybrid quinoline-sulfonamide complexes ($M^{2+}$: $Zn^{2+}$, $Cu^{2+}$, $Co^{2+}$ and $Cd^{2+}$) derivatives were designed, synthesized and tested for their antimicrobial activity. The synthesis is straight and efficient, involving two steps: acylation of aminoquinoline followed by complexation with metal acetate ($Cu^{2+}$, $Co^{2+}$ and $Cd^{2+}$) or chloride ($Zn^{2+}$). The synthesized compounds were characterized by FTIR, NMR spectroscopy and by X-ray diffraction on single crystal. The Co (II) complex crystallize in the monoclinic $P2_1/n$ space group type, with a tetrahedral coordination of cobalt with the bidentate ligand trough Co-$N_{quinoline}$ and Co-$N_{sulfonamide}$ bonds. The **QSC** compounds were preliminary in vitro screened for their antibacterial and antifungal activity and the obtained results are very promising. Against bacterial strain *Staphylococcus aureus* one compound have an excellent antibacterial activity **QBSC 4d** ($\Phi$ = 21 mm, MIC = $19.04 \times 10^{-5}$ mg/mL) and three others compounds are active: **QBSC 4c, QBSC 4b** and the quinoline sulfonamide ligand **3a** ($\Phi$ of 17, 16 and 18 mm). Against bacteria *Escherichia coli* only one compound **QBSC 4d** present activity (19 mm, MIC of $609 \times 10^{-5}$ mg/mL). Against fungus *Candida albicans* again the **QBSC 4d** complex have an excellent antibacterial activity ($\Phi$ = 25 mm, MIC = $9.04 \times 10^{-5}$ mg/mL) and also the ligand **3a** have an excellent antibacterial activity ($\Phi$ = 26.5 mm) but to a relatively high concentration (MIC = 12.5 mg/mL). These results reveal a clear influence of the metal cation, the Cd complex (**QBSC 4d**) being far away the most active tested compound, having a quasi-nonselective antibacterial and antifungal activity. The activity of cadmium complexes are higher the most probable because of a better synergism ligand cadmium.

**Supplementary Materials:** The following are available online: $^1$H- and $^{13}$C-NMR of compounds **3a, 4a, 4d** (pages 1–4), chechCIF reports for compounds **4b** and **4c** (pages 5–11).

**Author Contributions:** Design, conception and writing: V.M. and I.I.M.; Synthesis, structure elucidation and biological data analysis: D.D., V.M., D.A.-M., V.A., C.L.G. and I.I.M. All authors also reviewed and approved the final version. All authors have read and agreed to the published version of the manuscript.

**Funding:** This research received no external funding.

**Acknowledgments:** Authors are thankful to CERNESIM, for NMR and X-ray experiments. The authors gratefully acknowledge Simona Dunca for her help in biological assay and senior researcher Tiberiu Roman in X-ray experiments.

**Conflicts of Interest:** The authors declare no conflict of interest.

## References

1. Brunton, L.; Knollmann, B.; Hilal-Dandan, R. *Goodman & Gilman's the Pharmacological Basis of Therapeutics*, 13th ed.; McGraw-Hill: New York, NY, USA, 2013; ISBN 9781259584732.
2. Silverman, R.B.; Holladay, M.W. *The Organic Chemistry of Drug Design and Drug Action*, 3rd ed.; Academic Press: Cambridge, MA, USA, 2014; ISBN 9780123820303.
3. WHO Global Strategy for Containment of Antimicrobial Resistance. Available online: https://www.who.int/drugresistance/WHO_Global_Strategy_English.pdf (accessed on 14 June 2020).
4. Guarner, J. Three Emerging Coronaviruses in Two Decades the Story of SARS, MERS, and Now COVID-19. *Am. J. Clin. Pathol.* **2020**, *153*, 420–421. [CrossRef] [PubMed]
5. Xiao, C.; Li, X.; Liu, S.; Gao, S.J.; Gao, F. HIV-1 did not contribute to the 2019-nCoV genome. *Emerg. Infect. Dis.* **2020**, *9*, 378–381. [CrossRef] [PubMed]
6. Kandeel, M.; Al-Nazawi, M. Virtual screening and repurposing of FDA approved drugs against COVID-19 main protease. *Life Sci.* **2020**, *251*, 117627. [CrossRef] [PubMed]
7. Vellingiri, B.; Jayaramayya, K.; Iyer, M.; Kumar, N.S.; Subramaniam, M.D. COVID-19: A promising cure for the global panic. *Sci. Total Environ.* **2020**, *725*, 138277. [CrossRef] [PubMed]
8. Yan, R.; Zhang, Y.; Li, Y.; Xia, L.; Guo, Y.; Zhou, Q. Structural basis for the recognition of SARS-CoV-2 by full-length human ACE2. *Science* **2020**, *367*, 1444–1448. [CrossRef] [PubMed]
9. Kumari, L.S.; Mazumder, A.; Kumar, V.; Gupta, S. Synthesis and biological potentials of quinoline analogues: A review of literature. *Mini-Rev. Org. Chem.* **2019**, *16*, 653–688. [CrossRef]
10. Zhang, J.; Wang, S.; Ba, Y.; Xu, Z. 1,2,4-Triazole-quinoline/quinolone hybrids as potential anti-bacterial agents. *Eur. J. Med. Chem.* **2019**, *174*, 1–8. [CrossRef]
11. Al Matarneh, C.; Sardaru, M.; Apostu, M.; Rosca, I.; Ciobanu, C.; Mangalagiu, I.I.; Danac, R. Synthesis and antibacterial evaluation of new pyrrolo[3′,4′:3,4]pyrrolo[1,2-a]quinoline and pyrrolo[3′,4′:3,4]pyrrolo[1,2-a]isoquinoline derivatives. *Studia UBB Chem.* **2019**, *64*, 67–80. [CrossRef]

12. Kalaria, P.N.; Karad, S.C.; Raval, D.K. A review on diverse heterocyclic compounds as the privileged scaffolds in antimalarial drug discovery. *Eur. J. Med. Chem.* **2018**, *158*, 917–936. [CrossRef]
13. Ajani, O.O.; Iyaye, K.T.; Audu, O.Y.; Kuye, A.O.; Olanrewaju, I.O. Microwave Assisted Synthesis and Antimicrobial Potential of Quinoline-Based 4-Hydrazide-Hydrazone Derivatives. *J. Heterocycl. Chem.* **2018**, *55*, 302–312. [CrossRef]
14. Hu, Y.Q.; Gao, C.; Zhang, S.; Xu, L.; Xu, Z.; Feng, L.S.; Wu, X.; Zhao, F. Quinoline hybrids and their antiplasmodial and antimalarial activities. *Eur. J. Med. Chem.* **2017**, *139*, 22–47. [CrossRef]
15. Mantu, D.; Antoci, V.; Moldoveanu, C.; Zbancioc, G.; Mangalagiu, I.I. Hybrid imidazole (benzimidazole)/pyridine (quinoline) derivatives and evaluation of their anticancer and antimycobacterial activity. *J. Enz. Inhib. Med. Chem.* **2016**, *31*, 96–103. [CrossRef] [PubMed]
16. Zhong, F.; Geng, G.; Chen, B.; Pan, T.; Li, Q.; Zhang, H.; Bai, C. Identification of benzenesulfonamide quinoline derivatives as potent HIV-1 replication inhibitors targeting Rev protein. *Org. Biomol. Chem.* **2015**, *13*, 1792–1799. [CrossRef] [PubMed]
17. Sen, C.; Sahoo, T.; Singh, H.; Suresh, E.; Ghosh, S.C. Visible light-promoted photocatalytic C-5 carboxylation of 8-aminoquinoline amides and sulfonamides via a single electron transfer pathway. *J. Org. Chem.* **2019**, *84*, 9869–9896. [CrossRef] [PubMed]
18. Pascual-Álvarez, A.; Topala, T.; Estevan, F.; Sanz, F.; Alzuet-Piña, G. Photoinduced and self-activated nuclease activity of copper(II) complexes with *N*-(quinolin-8-yl)quinolin-8-sulfonamide-DNA and bovine serum albumin binding. *Eur. J. Inorg. Chem.* **2016**, *2016*, 982–994. [CrossRef]
19. Meeusen, J.W.; Tomasiewicz, H.; Nowakowski, A.; Petering, D.H. TSQ (6-methoxy-8-p-toluenesulfonamido-quinoline), a common fluorescent sensor for cellular zinc, images zinc proteins. *Inorg. Chem.* **2011**, *50*, 7563–7573. [CrossRef]
20. Rouffet, M.; De Oliveira, C.A.F.; Udi, Y.; Agrawal, A.; Sagi, I.; McCammon, J.A.; Cohen, S.M. From sensors to silencers: Quinoline- and benzimidazole-sulfonamides as inhibitors for zinc proteases. *J. Am. Chem. Soc.* **2010**, *132*, 8232–8233. [CrossRef]
21. Macías, B.; García, I.; Villa, M.V.; Borrás, J.; Castineiras, A.; Sanz, F. Synthesis and structural characterization of zinc complexes with sulfonamide containing 8-aminoquinoline. *Z. Anorg. Allg. Chem.* **2003**, *629*, 255–260. [CrossRef]
22. Fahrni, C.J.; O'Halloran, T.V. Aqueous coordination chemistry of quinoline-based fluorescence probes for the biological chemistry of zinc. *J. Am. Chem. Soc.* **1999**, *121*, 11448–11458. [CrossRef]
23. Da Silva, L.E.; de Sousa, P.T., Jr.; Joussef, A.C.; Piovezan, C.; Neves, A. Synthesis, structure and physicochemical properties of zinc and copper complexes based on sulfonamides containing 8-aminoquinoline ligands. *Quim. Nova* **2008**, *31*, 1161–1164. [CrossRef]
24. Da Silva, L.E.; Joussef, A.C.; Pacheco, L.K.; Da Silva, D.G.; Steindel, M.; Rebelo, R.A.; Schmidt, B. Synthesis and in vitro evaluation of leishmanicidal and trypanocidal activities of *N*-quinolin-8-yl arylsulfonamides. *Bioorg. Med. Chem.* **2007**, *15*, 7553–7560. [CrossRef]
25. Da Silva, L.E.; de Sousa, P.T., Jr.; Maciel, E.N.; Numes, R.K.; Eger, I.; Steindel, M.; Rebelo, R.A. In vitro antiprotozoal evaluation of zinc and copper complexes based on sulfonamides containing 8-aminoquinoline ligands. *Lett. Drug Des. Discov.* **2010**, *7*, 679–685. [CrossRef]
26. Diaz, J.R.A.; Baldo, M.F.; Echeverría, G.; Baldoni, H.; Vullo, D.; Soria, D.B.; Supuran, C.T.; Cami, G.E. A substituted sulfonamide and its Co (II), Cu (II), and Zn (II) complexes as potential antifungal agents. *J. Enz. Inhib. Med. Chem.* **2016**, *31*, 51–62. [CrossRef] [PubMed]
27. Antoci, V.; Cucu, D.; Zbancioc, G.; Moldoveanu, C.; Mangalagiu, V.; Amariucai-Mantu, D.; Aricu, D.; Mangalagiu, I.I. Bis-(imidazole/benzimidazole)-pyridine derivatives: Synthesis, structure and antimycobacterial activity. *Future Med. Chem.* **2020**, *12*, 207–222. [CrossRef] [PubMed]
28. Olaru, A.M.; Vasilache, V.; Danac, R.; Mangalagiu, I.I. Antimycobacterial activity of nitrogen heterocycles derivatives: 7-(pyridine-4-yl)-indolizine derivatives. Part VII. *J. Enz. Inhib. Med. Chem.* **2017**, *32*, 1291–1298. [CrossRef] [PubMed]
29. Mantu, D.; Antoci, V.; Nicolescu, A.; Delenu, C.; Vasilache, V.; Mangalagiu, I.I. Synthesis, stereochemical studies and antimycobacterial activity of new acetyl-hydrazines pyridazinone. *Curr. Org. Synth.* **2017**, *14*, 112–119. [CrossRef]

30. Al Matarneh, C.M.; Shova, S.; Mangalagiu, I.I.; Danac, R. Synthesis, structure, antimycobacterial and anticancer evaluation of new pyrrolo-(phenanthroline) derivatives. *J. Enz. Inhib. Med. Chem.* **2016**, *31*, 470–480. [CrossRef]
31. Aricu, A.; Ciocarlan, A.; Lungu, L.; Barba, A.; Shova, S.; Zbancioc, G.; Mangalagiu, I.I.; D'Ambrosio, M.; Vornicu, N. Synthesis of new antibacterial and antifungal drimane sesquiterpenoids with azaheterocyclic units. *Med. Chem. Res.* **2016**, *25*, 2316–2323. [CrossRef]
32. Al Matarneh, C.; Ciobanu, C.I.; Mangalagiu, I.I.; Danac, R. Design, synthesis and antimycobacterial activity of some new azaheterocycles: 4,7-phenanthroline with p-halogeno-benzoyl skeleton. Part VI. *J. Serb. Chem. Soc.* **2016**, *81*, 133–140.
33. Danac, R.; Al Matarneh, C.M.; Shova, S.; Daniloaia, T.; Balan, M.; Mangalagiu, I.I. New indolizines with phenanthroline skeleton: Synthesis, structure, antimycobacterial and anticancer evaluation. *Bioorg. Med. Chem.* **2015**, *23*, 2318–2327. [CrossRef]
34. Danac, R.; Daniloaia, T.; Antoci, V.; Vasilache, V.; Mangalagiu, I.I. Design, synthesis and antimycobacterial activity of some new azaheterocycles: Phenanthroline with p-halo-benzoyl skeleton. Part, V. *Lett. Drug Des. Discov.* **2015**, *12*, 14–19. [CrossRef]
35. Balan, A.M.; Miron, A.; Tuchilus, C.; Rotinberg, P.; Mihai, C.T.; Mangalagiu, I.I.; Zbancioc, G. Synthesis and in vitro analysis of novel dihydroxyacetophenone derivatives with antimicrobial and antitumor activities. *Med. Chem.* **2014**, *10*, 476–483.
36. Kuchkova, K.; Aricu, A.; Barba, A.; Vlad, P.; Shova, S.; Secara, E.; Ungur, N.; Tuchilus, C.; Zbancioc, G.; Mangalagiu, I.I. Design, syntheses and antimicrobial activity of some novel homodrimane sesquiterpenoids with diazine skeleton. *Med. Chem. Res.* **2014**, *23*, 1559–1568. [CrossRef]
37. Tucaliuc, R.; Cotea, V.; Niculaua, M.; Tuchilus, C.; Mantu, D.; Mangalagiu, I.I. New pyridazine–fluorine derivatives: Synthesis, chemistry and biological activity. Part II. *Eur. J. Med. Chem.* **2013**, *67*, 367–372. [CrossRef] [PubMed]
38. Mantu, D.; Antoci, V.; Mangalagiu, I.I. Design, synthesis and antituberculosis activity of some new pyridazine derivatives: Bis-pyridazine. Part IV. *Infect. Disord. Drug Targets* **2013**, *13*, 344–351. [CrossRef] [PubMed]
39. Mantu, D.; Luca, M.C.; Moldoveanu, C.; Zbancioc, G.; Mangalagiu, I.I. Synthesis and antituberculosis activity of some new pyridazine derivatives. Part II. *Eur. J. Med. Chem.* **2010**, *45*, 5164–5168. [CrossRef]
40. Balan, A.M.; Florea, O.; Moldoveanu, C.; Zbancioc, G.; Iurea, D.; Mangalagiu, I.I. Diazinium salts with dihydroxyacetophenone skeleton: Syntheses and antimicrobial activity. *Eur. J. Med. Chem.* **2009**, *44*, 2275–2279. [CrossRef]
41. CLSI Document M07-A11. *Methods for Dilution Antimicrobial Susceptibility Tests for Bacteria That Grow Aerobically; Approved Standard*, 11th ed.; Clinical and Laboratory Standards Institute: Wayne, PA, USA, 2018; Available online: https://clsi.org/media/1928/m07ed11_sample.pdf (accessed on 14 June 2020).
42. Kavanagh, A.; Ramu, S.; Gong, Y.; Copper, M.A.; Blaskovich, M.A.T. Effects of microplate type and broth additives on microdilution MIC susceptibility assays. *Antimicrob. Agents Ch.* **2019**, *63*, 1–17. [CrossRef]
43. Supuran, C.T. Carbonic anhydrases: Novel therapeutic applications for inhibitors and activators. *Nat. Rev. Drug Discov.* **2008**, *7*, 168–181. [CrossRef]

**Sample Availability:** Samples of the compounds are available from the authors.

molecules

MDPI

Article

# Synthesis and Spectroscopic Analysis of Piperine- and Piperlongumine-Inspired Natural Product Scaffolds and Their Molecular Docking with IL-1β and NF-κB Proteins

**Gabriel Zazeri [1,2], Ana Paula R. Povinelli [1,2], Cécile S. Le Duff [3], Bridget Tang [3], Marinonio L. Cornelio [1,*] and Alan M. Jones [2,*]**

1 Departamento de Física–IBILCE, Rua Cristovão Colombo, 2265 CEP 15054-000 São José do Rio Preto–São Paulo, Brazil; gabriel.zazeri@unesp.br (G.Z.); ana.povinelli@unesp.br (A.P.R.P.)
2 School of Pharmacy, University of Birmingham, Edgbaston B15 2TT, UK
3 School of Chemistry, University of Birmingham, Edgbaston B15 2TT, UK; C.S.LeDuff@bham.ac.uk (C.S.L.D.); B.Tang@bham.ac.uk (B.T.)
* Correspondence: m.cornelio@unesp.br (M.L.C.); a.m.jones.2@bham.ac.uk (A.M.J.)

Academic Editor: Maged Henary
Received: 19 May 2020; Accepted: 16 June 2020; Published: 19 June 2020

**Abstract:** Inspired by the remarkable bioactivities exhibited by the natural products, piperine and piperlongumine, we synthesised eight natural product-inspired analogues to further investigate their structures. For the first time, we confirmed the structure of the key cyclised dihydropyrazolecarbothioamide piperine analogues including the use of two-dimensional (2D) $^{15}$N-based spectroscopy nuclear magnetic resonance (NMR) spectroscopy. Prior investigations demonstrated promising results from these scaffolds for the inhibition of inflammatory response via downregulation of the IL-1β and NF-κB pathway. However, the molecular interaction of these molecules with their protein targets remains unknown. Ab initio calculations revealed the electronic density function map of the molecules, showing the effects of structural modification in the electronic structure. Finally, molecular interactions between the synthesized molecules and the proteins IL-1β and NF-κB were achieved. Docking results showed that all the analogues interact in the DNA binding site of NF-κB with higher affinity compared to the natural products and, with the exception of **9a** and **9b**, have higher affinity than the natural products for the binding site of IL-1β. Specificity for the molecular recognition of **3a**, **3c** and **9b** with IL-1β through cation–π interactions was determined. These results revealed **3a**, **3c**, **4a**, **4c** and **10** as the most promising molecules to be evaluated as IL-1β and NF-κB inhibitors.

**Keywords:** molecular docking; piperine; piperlongumine

## 1. Introduction

Nature is a creative machine for the design of bioactive molecules with the potential to become efficient drugs for the treatment of several diseases. In recent decades, such creative scaffolds have driven the design of new molecules with pharmacological potential, including the concept of diversity-oriented synthesis (DOS) [1,2]. In recent years, both piperine and piperlongumine have been explored because of their wide spectrum of biological activity [3–8].

Piperine is an alkaloid found in piper species such as *Piper nigrum* (black pepper) and *Piper longum* (long pepper). Piperine is not only used as a seasoning but also in various preparations of traditional medicine, including the oldest medical science, practiced in India since ancient times (Ayurveda) [9]. Piperine has been widely studied by the scientific community, because of its anti-inflammatory, anti-carcinogenic, immunomodulatory and hepatoprotective activities [3]. As an anti-inflammatory, piperine acts through the inhibition of IL-1β and NF-κB inflammation pathway, leading to the downregulation of pro-inflammatory proteins, such as iNOS and COX-2 [10–12].

Piperine-inspired molecules investigated in the present work have had their anti-inflammatory and anti-carcinogenic activity previously studied by Mathew et al. [13,14], with promising results. In particular, **4a** had a comparable anti-inflammatory effect to Diclofenac. Furthermore, **3c** and **4c** showed inhibitory effects on the HCT116 colon cancer cell line. However, their interactions with the IL-1β and NF-κB pathways have not been investigated.

Piperlongumine (PPL), is an alkaloid isolated from long pepper that is widely used in Indian traditional medicine [15]. The biological activities of PPL and its analogues include anti-inflammatory, anti-carcinogenic and anti-atherosclerotic activities, among others [6–8,16]. Similar to piperine, studies indicated that anti-inflammatory and anti-carcinogenic activities of PPL are a consequence of the inhibition of the NF-κB pathway [17–20].

PPL has been shown to bind to the unit p65 of NF-κB, inhibiting NF-κB/DNA binding activity and blocking the transcription of cytokines and other pro-inflammatory proteins [18].

Despite the investigations reported in the literature that show promising results of these natural-product-inspired analogues in the inhibition of inflammatory response via the downregulation of IL-1β and NF-κB pathway, the molecular interaction of these molecules with the protein targets are unknown.

Herein, we explored the binding environment of the synthesised analogues in NF-κB and IL-1β using molecular docking. For piperine-inspired molecules, we investigated the effect caused by the substitution of the piperidine for an aromatic ring in the piperine scaffold (**3a**), a nitroarene group (**3b**) and an aminoarene group (**3c**). We investigated the effect of the cyclisation of the piperine scaffold to form a dihydropyrazolecarbothioamide moiety (**4a** and **4c**). For PPL-inspired molecules, we investigated the effects of removing a Michael acceptor (**9a**), the conversion of a lactam to a ketone (**10**) and the influence of methoxy groups (**9b**).

We present an adapted synthesis of piperine- and PPL-inspired molecules including data from 2D $^{1}$H-$^{15}$N HSQC and HMBC spectra, computational characterization of the electronic structure of the analogues using *ab initio* calculations and molecular docking of the confirmed structures with the proteins IL-1β and NF-κB.

## 2. Results and Discussion

### 2.1. Spectroscopic Characterization of Natural Product Inspired Analogues

The synthesis of the piperine-inspired analogues began with a $MnO_2$-mediated oxidation of piperonyl alcohol to the corresponding aldehyde with a 97% yield (Scheme 1). Claisen–Schmidt condensation of **2** with a variety of acetophenones afforded **3a**–**3c** in excellent yields (80–90%) after crystallisation. The initial synthetic route to **4c** required the synthesis of the nitro derivative (**3b**) followed by cyclisation with thiosemicarbazide and reduction, as the free amine may undergo unwanted side reactions during the cyclisation step. Unfortunately, all attempts to react **3b** with thiosemicarbazide resulted in recovered starting material. However, for the parent unsubstituted compound (**3a**) a cyclised compound (**4a**) was formed with 60% yield. Pleasingly, the unprotected amine containing molecule **3c** was smoothly converted to the cyclised molecule **4c** with 60% yield, mitigating the need to pursue **3b** further.

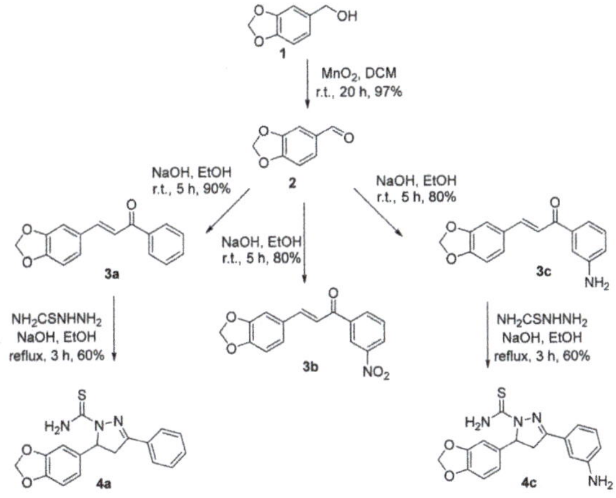


**Scheme 1.** Synthesis of piperine-inspired molecules.

The syntheses of piperine analogues have been reported by Mathew et al. [13] but with limited spectroscopic characterization ($^1$H NMR and IR spectroscopy) of molecules of type **4**. We therefore performed re-synthesis prior to the computational study to confirm the connectivity of the new ring system. There is a potential for either a five-membered product (**4a**), or a seven-membered ring system (**5**) to form (Scheme 2). Selected instructive 2D $^1$H-$^{13}$C HMBC and $^1$H-$^{15}$N HMBC NMR spectra connectivities are shown in Scheme 2, along with the $^{15}$N NMR chemical shifts. Critically, the results showed the correct connectivity for a five-membered dihydropyrazolecarbothioamide system product (**4a** not **5**). **4a** was found to slowly degrade upon standing in $CDCl_3$ at room temperature for an extended period of time.

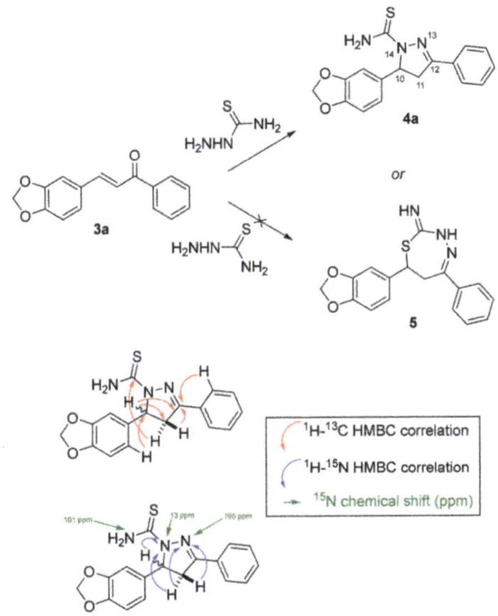


**Scheme 2.** Two potential cyclisation outcomes upon **3a** and the selected instructive NMR correlations for **4a** in the 2D $^1$H-$^{13}$C HMBC and 2D $^1$H-$^{15}$N HMBC spectra.

The synthesis of the PPL-inspired analogues (Scheme 3) used a one-pot Doebner-modified Knoevenagel condensation and concomitant decarboxylation, to prepare the key acrylic acids (**7a,b**) from the appropriate benzaldehydes. Reaction of the acrylic acids with thionyl chloride under Vilsmeier–Haack conditions gave the short-lived vinylogous acyl chlorides (**8a,b**) which were reacted with either sodium 2-oxopiperidin-1-ide (derived from δ-valerolactam) or with lithium cyclohex-1-en-1-olate (derived from cyclohexanone), to afford the final products **9a,b** and **10** with modest isolated yields.

Although **10a** has been reported in the literature, we identified a previously unobserved $^1$H NMR spectroscopic signal at 15.76 ppm (Supplementary Materials), indicative of an intramolecular hydrogen bond occurring through tautomerization to give the stabilized structure, **10**.

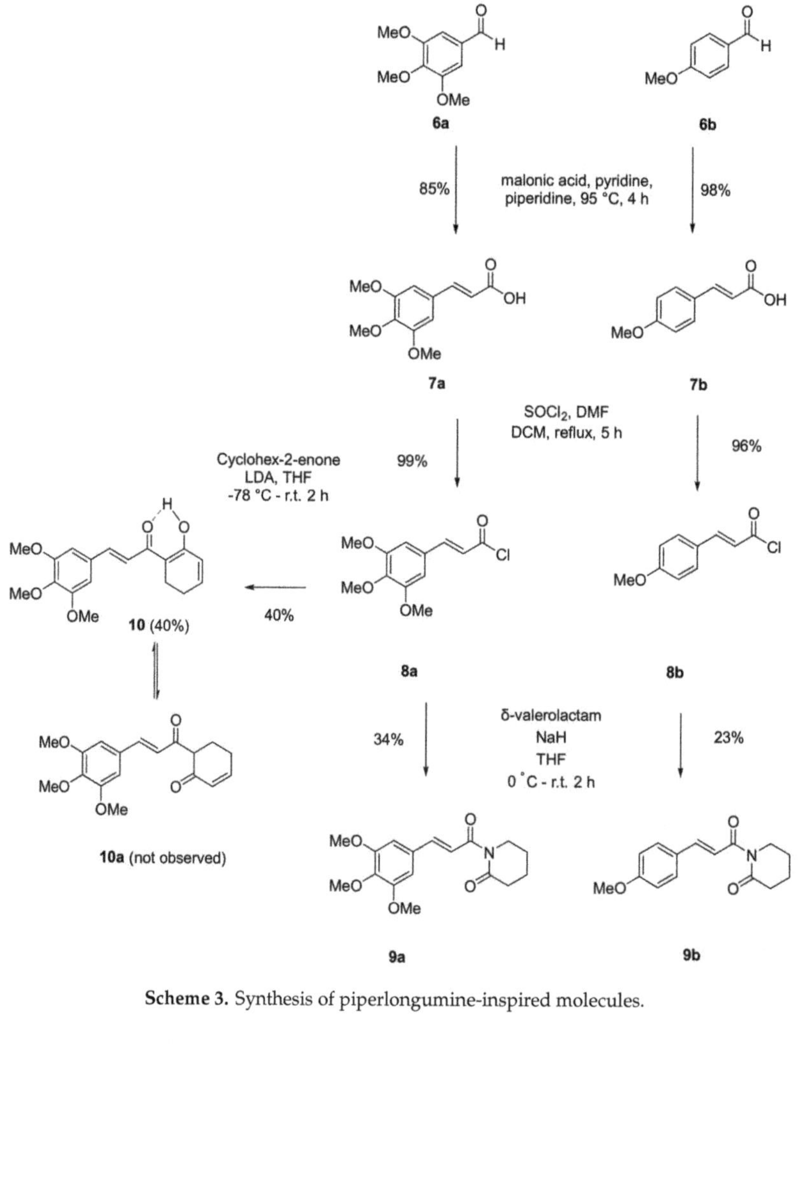


**Scheme 3.** Synthesis of piperlongumine-inspired molecules.

### 2.2. *Electronic Structures of Piperine and PPL-Inspired Molecules*

*Ab initio* calculations were performed to obtain the structural parameterisation to be used in the molecular docking calculations. In addition, these calculations provided information about the electronic structure that contributed to the characterisation of the compounds.

Figure 1 shows the structures resulting from *ab initio* calculations of their respective map of electrostatic potential (MEP). **3a,b,c** presented a planar structure due to the high number of conjugated double bonds. A similar result was found for piperine previously [21]. **3a,b,c** have the most negative charge density around oxygen atoms, while the most positive charge densities are concentrated on the extremities of the structures with the intermediate region being more neutral. As a special case, the nitro group in **3b** relocated the negative charges from the aromatic ring to the oxygen atoms, consequently the aromatic ring of **3b** became more positive when compared to **3a,c** and may explain its unreactivity to thiosemicarbazide. This relocation of negative charges caused **3b** to have high affinity for a microenvironment mainly composed by polar amino acids, which differs from **3a,c,** which preferred less polar microenvironments (see molecular docking). The MEP of **4a,c** indicated that the negative density charge was concentrated around the oxygen, nitrogen and the sulfur atoms, while the positive density charge was concentrated on the dihydropyrazole and 1,3-benzodioxole rings, with the neutral region being the aromatic ring.

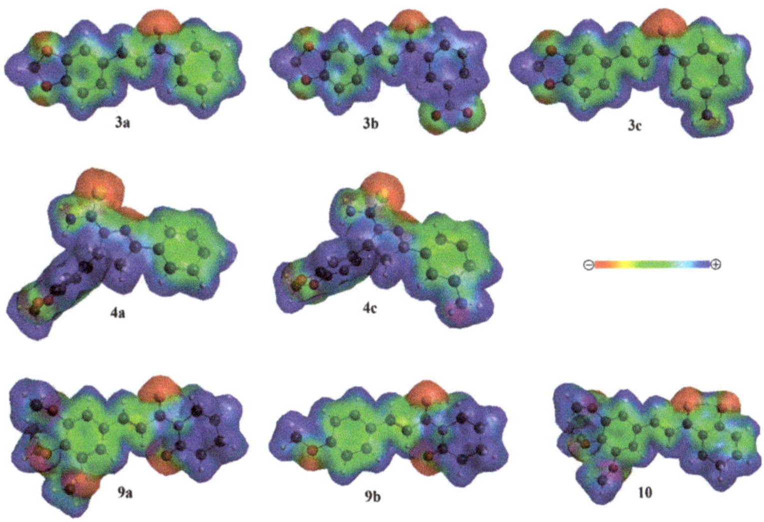


**Figure 1.** Map of electronic potential (MEP) of piperine and PPL-inspired molecules, where the scale is from negative density charge (represented by red) to positive density charge (represented by blue).

A minimal puckering of the five-membered ring system of **4a** modelled in $CDCl_3$ revealed a maximal torsional angle of +4.8° around C(10)-N(14)-N(13)-C(12) and a minimal torsional angle of −3.0° across the ring system. This deviation away from planarity may explain the low 15 ppm $^{15}N$ NMR signal observed in this ring system.

**9a, 10** and **9b** presented a planar structure, except for methoxy groups (see Figure S39, Supplementary Materials). $^{1}H$ NMR of **10** (Figure S38, Supplementary Materials) showed a resonance peak at 15.76 ppm, associated with the hydroxyl from cyclohexanone forming an intramolecular hydrogen bond with the adjacent carbonyl oxygen; consequently, this hydrogen is not exchangeable and the signal is observed in the $^{1}H$ NMR spectrum. According to *ab initio* calculations for **10**, the intramolecular hydrogen bond length is 1.55 Å. The planarity of the three structures are quite similar to the characteristics found in PPL [22]. According to MEP, the three structures presented a negative density charge concentrated around oxygen atoms, while the positive density distributed on the extremity of the molecule and the aromatic ring is a neutral part of the molecules. The negative density charge concentrated on the atoms identified plays a crucial role in the interaction of **10** with NF-κB, as the binding site is positively charged.

*2.3. Molecular Docking*

According to molecular docking results with IL-1β (Figure 2), piperine and analogues **3a**, **4a**, **3c** and **4c** bound to the same binding site with the binding energy scores of −6.08, −6.04, −7.18, −6.25 and −7.22 kcal/mol, respectively.

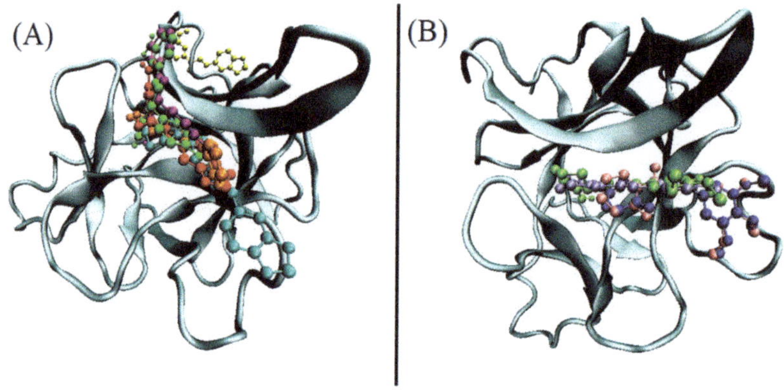


**Figure 2.** IL-1β (iceblue) binding environments to (**A**) piperine and analogues (Piperine-cyan, **3a**-orange, **4a**-purple, **3b**-yellow, **3c**-red, **4c**-green). (**B**) PPL and analogues (PPL-blue, **9a**-pink, **10**-lime, **9b**-iceblue).

Figure 3 and Table 1 show the amino acids that compose the microenvironment of each molecule with IL-1β. According to the docking results **4a**, **3c** and **4c** had a more negative binding energy than piperine; having a higher affinity for this environment when compared to piperine (Table 2). Most of the amino acids that composed the binding site are non-polar, with limited neutral and charged polar amino acids participating. The higher affinity of the analogues for the binding site revealed that the addition of an aromatic ring, and consequently the new electronic distribution, contributed to the increase in affinity. Moreover, the aromatic rings of **3a,c** exhibited cation–π interactions with the protonated amine group of Lys77 amino acid (see Supplementary Materials), which contributed to the high negative binding energy of these analogues to the protein. The cation–π interaction is caused by the molecular electron delocalization, reinforcing the importance of the increase in electron delocalization for the affinity at the IL-1β binding site.

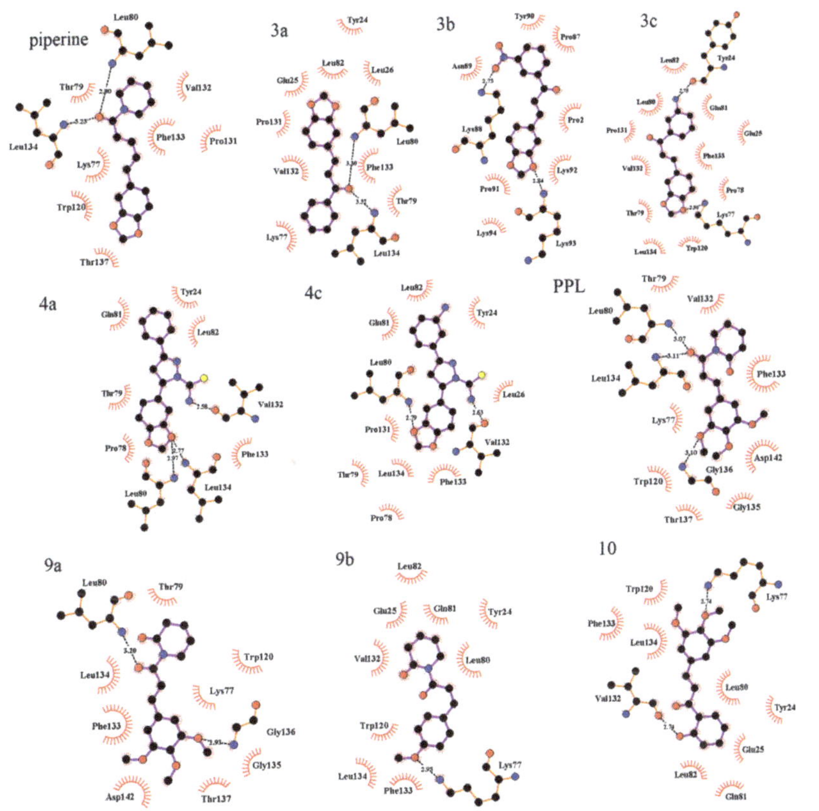


**Figure 3.** IL-1β binding microenvironments details for piperine and PPL analogues visualized with LigPlot.

**Table 1.** Amino acids that compose the microenvironment of the complex IL-1β/piperine and PPL analogues, obtained by molecular docking.

| Molecule | Amino Acids | | | |
|---|---|---|---|---|
| | Non-Polar | Positively Charged | Negatively Charged | Polar |
| Piperine | Leu80, Leu134, Val32, Phe133, Pro131, Trp120 | Lys77 | - | Thr137, Thr79 |
| **3a** | Leu82, Leu26, Leu80, Leu134, Phe133, Val132 and Pro131 | Lys77 | Glu25 | Thr79 |
| **4a** | Leu80,Leu82, Leu134,Val132, Phe133, Pro78 | - | - | Thr79, Gln81, Tyr24 |
| **3b** | Pro2, Pro87, Pro91 | Lys88, Lys92, Lys93, Lys94 | - | Asn89, Tyr90, |
| **3c** | Leu80, Leu82, Leu134, Phe133, Pro78, Trp120, Val132, Pro131 | Lys77 | Glu25 | Tyr24, Gln81 |
| **4c** | Leu26, Val132, Phe133, Pro78, Leu134, Leu82 Pro131, Leu80, | - | - | Gln81, Tyr24, Thr79 |

**Table 1.** *Cont.*

| Molecule | Amino Acids | | | |
|---|---|---|---|---|
| | Non-Polar | Positively Charged | Negatively Charged | Polar |
| PPL | Val132, Phe133, Gly135, Gly136, Trp120, Leu134, Leu80 | Lys77 | Asp142 | Thr79, Thr137 |
| **9a** | Leu80, Trp120, Gly136, Gly135, Phe133, Leu134 | Lys77 | Asp142 | Thr79, Thr137 |
| **10** | Trp120, Leu80, Leu82, Val32, Leu134, Phe133 | Lys77 | Glu25 | Tyr24, Gln81 |
| **9b** | Leu82, Leu80, Phe133, Leu134, Trp120, Val132 | Lys77 | Glu25, | Gln81, Tyr24 |

As a consequence of the new structural properties, **4a** and **4c** presented the best affinities to this binding site. Analogue **3b** bound with a binding energy of −7.44 kcal/mol to an orthosteric binding site, where the majority of amino acids are positive and neutral polar amino acids. The differences between **3a,c** and **3b** are due to the aromatic ring substitution, the nitro group in **3b** drove the interaction to a less hydrophobic environment, differently from the amino group (**3c**).

The binding site found by molecular docking for PPL and analogues was the same as the piperine binding site. Table 2 shows that PPL, **9a**, **10** and **9b** had binding scores of −5.83, −5.38, −6.19 and −5.62 kcal/mol, respectively. In the case of PPL analogues, **10** presented the most negative binding energy and highest affinity for the binding site. The results showed that the removal of two methoxy groups (**9b**) limited the possibility of performing multiple hydrogen bonds. Furthermore, **9b** exhibited a cation–$\pi$ interaction with the protonated amine of Lys77 (see Supplementary Materials), which contributed to the negative binding energy. Docking results also showed that the removal of the double bond in the cyclic ring (**9a**) resulted in higher binding energy (less negative) than the other molecules, which reinforced the importance of electron delocalization in the binding affinity.

**Table 2.** Binding energy scores obtained for the proteins IL-1β and NF-κB with Piperine, PPL and analogues.

| Molecules | Energy Score kcal/mol (IL-1B) | Energy Score kcal/mol (NF-KB) |
|---|---|---|
| Piperine | −6.08 | −6.08 |
| **3a** | −6.04 | −6.53 |
| **3b** | −7.44 | −6.24 |
| **3c** | −6.25 | −6.07 |
| **4a** | −7.18 | −6.64 |
| **4c** | −7.22 | −6.4 |
| PPL | −5.83 | −5.36 |
| **9a** | −5.38 | −5.85 |
| **10** | −6.19 | −5.72 |
| **9b** | −5.62 | −5.87 |

In the case of the interaction with NF-κB, all the piperine and piperlongumine analogues, with the exception of **3c**, presented a more negative binding energy (Table 2) than the natural products. Piperine, **4a**, **3b**, **3c**, **4c**, PPL, **9a**, **10** and **9b** all bound to the DNA binding site of NF-κB (Figure 4) [23]. Table 3 and Figure 5 show that the microenvironments of interaction of these molecules in NF-κB present a significant number of non-polar amino acids (except for **3b**), similar to the IL-1β binding site. However, in the case of the NF-κB binding site, there is also a greater number of positively charged amino acids. The interaction of the analogues with the positively charged amino acids may play an important role in the inhibition of the interaction NF-κB(p65)-DNA, as positively charged amino acids (including Lys122 and Lys123) stabilize the NF-κB(p65)-DNA complex *via* interaction with the negatively charged phosphates groups of the DNA [24].

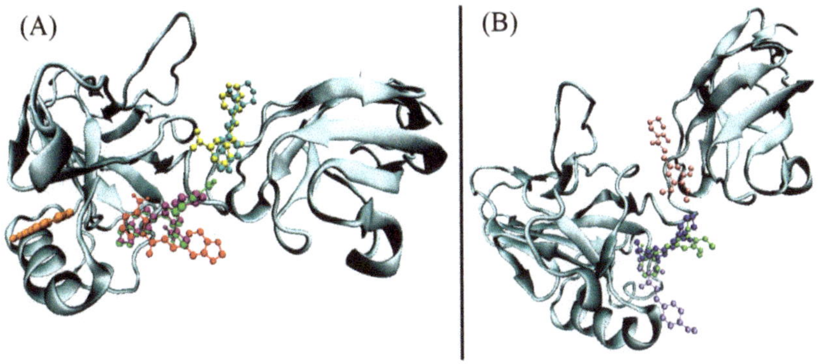


**Figure 4.** NF-κB (iceblue) binding environments to (**A**) Piperine and analogues (Piperine-cyan, **3a**-orange, **4a**-purple, **3b**-yellow, **3c**-red, **4c**-green). (**B**) PPL and analogues (PPL-blue, **9a**-pink, **10**-lime, **9b**-iceblue).

**Table 3.** Amino acids that compose the microenvironment of the complex NF-κB/piperine and PPL analogues, obtained by molecular docking.

| Molecules | Amino Acids | | | |
|---|---|---|---|---|
| | **Non-Polar** | **Positively Charged** | **Negatively Charged** | **Polar** |
| Piperine | Ala192, Leu194 | Lys195, Arg187, Lys218 | Glu193, Glu282, Asp217 | Asn186, |
| **3a** | Val121, Ala129, Cys38, Cys120 | Lys37, Lys122, Arg133 | Glu89 | Tyr36, Gln132 |
| **4a** | Ala188, Cys120, Leu154, Val121, Pro189 | Arg187, Lys122, Lys123, His88 | Asp185 | Tyr36, His88, Asn155 |
| **3b** | Ala192 | Arg33, Arg187, Lys195, Lys218 | Asp217, Glu193, | Asn186, |
| **3c** | Cys120, Leu154, Val121, Pro189, Ala188, Phe34 | His88, Lys123 | - | His88, Tyr36, Asn155, Gln220, Asn190, Asp185 |
| **4c** | Pro189, Leu154, His88, Val121, Cys120, Ala188 | Lys123, Lys122, Arg187 | - | Asp185, Tyr36, His88, Asn155, |
| PPL | Cys120, Phe34, Leu154, Ala188, Pro189 | Lys218, Arg187, His88 | Asp185, | Tyr36, Asn155 |
| **9a** | Ala188, Ala192, Pro189 | Lys218, Lys195, Arg33, Arg187, Lys194 | Asp217, Glu193 | Asn186, |
| **10** | Ala188, Phe34, Cys120, Leu154, Val121, Pro189 | Lys218, Arg187, His88 | Asp185 | Asn155, His88 |
| **9b** | Leu154, Cys120, Val121, | His88, Lys123, Lys122, Arg124 | Asp185 | Tyr36, Asn155 |

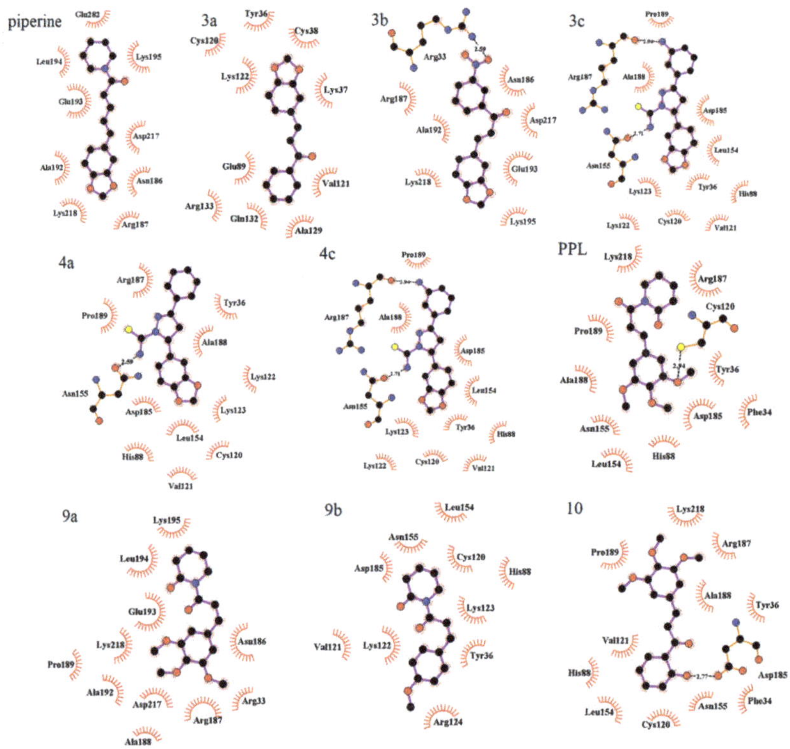


**Figure 5.** NF-κB binding microenvironments details for piperine and PPL analogues visualized with LigPlot.

Chen Y.Q. et al. [24] showed that the phenol ring of Tyr36 is anchored by a hydrogen bond to the phosphate backbone of DNA and makes van der Waals contacts with the methyl group of thymine at positions 1 and 2 of DNA, which makes **3a**, **4a**, **3c**, **4c** and **9b** good candidates to inhibit this interaction. Our molecular docking results revealed that Tyr36 was part of the binding microenvironment of these analogues and performed non-specific interactions.

Moreover, the side chain of Arg187 performs a hydrogen bond with the oxygen atom of thymine, and the side chain of Arg33 performs hydrogen bonds to oxygen and nitrogen atoms of guanine [24]. In this case, our molecular docking results showed that **3b** and **4c** perform hydrogen bonds with Arg33 and Arg187, indicating promising results for these compounds as inhibitors of this interaction between the arginine and DNA bases thymine and guanine.

It has been shown that the specificity of the interaction p65-DNA is likely due to the interactions between the G-C base pair and the side chains of Arg33 and Glu39 [24]. The amino acid Arg33, highlighted as being fundamental to DNA molecular recognition, is present in the microenvironments of the analogues **3b** and **9a** and performs a hydrogen bond with **3b**, which indicates that these analogues may shield the DNA recognition.

## 3. Materials and Methods

All reagents and solvents were obtained commercially from Sigma-Aldrich or Fischer Scientific and were used as supplied, with the exception of tetrahydrofuran (THF) and dichloromethane (DCM) which were treated with 3.0 Å molecular sieves (20% *m/v*) for a minimum of 48 h prior to use [25]. The progress of the syntheses was monitored by thin-layer chromatography (TLC). General procedures for the syntheses of PPL-inspired molecules were adapted from Sun Lan-Di et al. [18] For the syntheses of piperine-inspired molecules, the procedures were adapted from Mathew, A. et al. [13].

$^1$H and $^{13}$C NMR spectra were recorded either on a Bruker AVIII operating at 300 MHz for $^1$H and fitted with a 5mm BBFO probe or on a Bruker AVANCE NEO operating at 400 MHz for $^1$H fitted with a 5mm "smart" BBFO probe, respectively. $^1$H-$^1$H COSY, $^1$H-$^{13}$C and $^1$H-$^{15}$N HSQC, $^1$H-$^{13}$C and $^1$H-$^{15}$N HMBC NMR spectra were recorded on a Bruker AVANCE NEO console operating at 500 MHz for $^1$H and fitted with a nitrogen-cooled BBFO probe. Chemical shift data for $^1$H are reported in parts per million (ppm, δ scale) downfield from tetramethylsilane (TMS:δ 0.0) and referenced internally to the residual proton in the solvent. The deuterated solvents used for NMR analysis were: chloroform ($CDCl_3$: δH 7.26, δC 77.2), dimethyl sulfoxide (DMSO-$d_6$: δH 2.50, δC 39.5), and methanol ($CD_3OD$: δH 3.31, δC 49.0). Coupling constants (*J*) are given in hertz (Hz). The data are presented as follows: chemical shift, multiplicity (s = singlet, d = doublet, t = triplet, q = quartet, p = pentet, m = multiple, br = broad, app = apparent and combinations thereof), coupling constant and integration.

Mass spectra data were recorded using a Waters® Xevo G2-XS TOF using electro-spray ionization in positive (ESI+) mode.

### 3.1. *Synthesis of Piperine-Inspired Molecules*

#### Synthesis of Piperonal (**2**)

To a stirred solution of piperonyl alcohol (**1**) (152 mg, 1.0 mmol) in DCM (100 mL), manganese dioxide (1739 mg, 20.0 mmol) was added at a rate of 1.0 mmol/h until completion. The reaction mixture was filtered through a pad of Celite® and the filtrate was concentrated *in vacuo* to afford the desired compound as white crystals (148 mg, 97%). $^1$H NMR (300 MHz, $CDCl_3$) δ 9.81 (s, 1H), 7.41 (dd, *J* = 7.9, 1.5 Hz, 1H), 7.33 (d, *J* = 1.5 Hz, 1H), 6.93 (d, *J* = 7.9 Hz, 1H), 6.08 (s, 2H); $^{13}$C NMR (101 MHz, CDC13) δ 190.5, 153.3, 148.9, 132.1, 128.9, 108.5, 107.1, 102.3. Data were in accordance with the literature [26].

#### Synthesis of (*E*)-3-(Benzo[d][1,3]dioxol-5-yl)-1-phenylprop-2-en-1-one (**3a**)

Acetophenone (240 mg, 2.0 mmol), **2** (300 mg, 2.0 mmol), ethanol (95%, 1.0 mL) and sodium hydroxide solution (10% *w/w* in $H_2O$, 1.0 mL) were added to a round-bottom flask. The reaction mixture was stirred at room temperature for 5 h. The reaction mixture was washed with ethanol (100 mL) and filtered under vacuum. The solid was dried *in vacuo* to afford the desired compound as a yellow powder (270 mg, 90%). $^1$H NMR (300 MHz, $CDCl_3$) δ 8.06–7.95 (m, 2H), 7.74 (d, *J* = 15.6 Hz, 1H), 7.63–7.46 (m, 3H), 7.37 (d, *J* = 15.6 Hz, 1H), 7.19–7.08 (m, 2H), 6.85 (d, *J* = 8.0 Hz, 1H), 6.03 (s, 2H); $^{13}$C NMR (101 MHz, $CDCl_3$) δ 190.6, 150.1, 148.6, 144.9, 138.6, 132.8, 129.5, 128.8, 128.6, 125.5, 120.3, 108.9, 106.8, 101.8; LRMS (ES$^+$) *m/z*: 253.09 $[M + H]^+$; HRMS (ES$^+$) *m/z* calcd. $C_6H_{13}O_3$ $[M + H]^+$ = 253.0865; observed 253.0860 (−2.0 ppm).

#### Synthesis of (*E*)-3-(Benzo[d][1,3]dioxol-5-yl)-1-(3-nitrophenyl)prop-2-en-1-one (**3b**)

A round bottom flask was charged with 3-nitroacetophenone (330.3 mg, 2.0 mmol), **2** (300.3 mg, 2.0 mmol), ethanol (95%, 1.0 mL), and sodium hydroxide solution (10% *w/w* in $H_2O$, 1.0 mL). The mixture was stirred at room temperature for 5 h. The mixture was washed with ethanol (100 mL) and filtered under vacuum. The powder was recrystallized from hot ethanol and the product was afforded as orange crystals (240 mg, 80%). $^1$H NMR (400 MHz, $CDCl_3$) δ 8.82 (t, *J* = 1.9 Hz, 1H), 8.43 (ddd, *J* = 8.2, 2.3, 1.1 Hz, 1H), 8.33 (ddd, *J* = 7.8, 1.7, 1.1 Hz, 1H), 7.81 (d, *J* = 15.5 Hz, 1H), 7.71 (t, *J* = 8.0 Hz, 1H), 7.36 (d, *J* = 15.5 Hz, 1H), 7.21–7.14 (m, 2H), 6.87 (d, *J* = 8.0 Hz, 1H), 6.05 (s, 2H); $^{13}$C NMR (101 MHz, $CDCl_3$) δ 188.0, 150.7, 148.7, 148.6, 146.8, 139.9, 134.2, 130.0, 128.9, 127.10, 126.1, 123.4, 118.7, 108.9, 106.9, 102.0; LRMS (ES$^+$) *m/z*: 298.07 $[M + H]^+$; HRMS (ES$^+$) *m/z*: calcd. $C_{16}H_{12}NO_5$ $[M + H]^+$ = 298.0715; observed 298.0712 (1.0 ppm).

Synthesis of (*E*)-1-(3-Aminophenyl)-3-(benzo[d][1,3]dioxol-5-yl)prop-2-en-1-one (**3c**)

A round bottom flask was charged with 3-aminoacetophenone (270.3 mg, 2.0 mmol), **2** (300.3 mg, 2.0 mmol), ethanol (95%, 1.0 mL), and sodium hydroxide solution (10% *w/w* in $H_2O$, 1.0 mL). The mixture was stirred at room temperature for 5 h. The mixture was washed with ethanol (100 mL) and filtered under vacuum. The crude product was purified by column chromatography ($SiO_2$; EtOAc/hexane 1:1) to afford the product as a yellow powder (240.2 mg, 80%). $^1$H NMR (300 MHz, $CDCl_3$) δ 7.73 (d, *J* = 15.6 Hz, 1H), 7.39 (ddd, *J* = 7.7, 1.7, 1.1 Hz, 1H), 7.37–7.27 (m, 3H), 7.18–7.10 (m, 2H), 6.90 (ddd, *J* = 7.9, 2.5, 1.1 Hz, 1H), 6.85 (d, *J* = 8.0 Hz, 1H), 6.04 (s, 2H), 3.85 (s, 2H); $^{13}$C NMR (101 MHz, $CDCl_3$) δ 190.7, 150.01, 148.6, 147.0, 144.5, 139.7, 129.6, 129.6, 125.3, 120.6, 119.5, 118.9, 114.6, 108.8, 106.8, 101.8; LRMS (ES$^+$) *m/z*: 268.10 [M + H]$^+$; HRMS (ES$^+$) *m/z*: calcd. $C_{16}H_{14}NO_3$ [M + H]$^+$ = 268.0974; observed 268.0974 (0.0 ppm).

Synthesis of 5-(Benzo[d][1,3]dioxol-5-yl)-3-phenyl-4,5-dihydro-1H-pyrazole-1-carbothioamide (**4a**)

Ethanol (95%, 25 mL), NaOH (1.0 g, 0.025 mol), **3a** (2.52 g, 0.01 mol) and thiosemicarbazide (911 mg, 0.01 mol) were added to a round-bottom flask. The reaction mixture was stirred for 3 h at reflux. Upon completion, the reaction mixture was added to ice. The resulting precipitate was washed with diethyl ether (100 mL) and water (100 mL) under vacuum filtration. The white powder was recrystallized from hot ethanol to afford the desired product as white crystals (1.51 g, 60%). $^1$H NMR (300 MHz, $CDCl_3$) δ 7.79–7.66 (m, 2H), 7.52–7.37 (m, 3H), 7.09 (s, 1H), 6.86–6.57 (m, 3H), 6.31–5.76 (m, 4H), 3.81 (dd, *J* = 17.7, 11.4 Hz, 1H), 3.18 (dd, *J* = 17.8, 3.6 Hz, 1H); $^{13}$C NMR (126 MHz, $CDCl_3$) δ 176.9, 156.2, 148.3, 147.2, 135.9, 131.3, 130.8, 129.1, 127.1, 119.2, 108.7, 106.1, 101.3, 63.5, 43.4; $^{15}$N NMR (51 MHz, $CDCl_3$) δ 194.9; 101.3; 13.3; LRMS (ES$^+$) *m/z*: 326.10 [M + H]$^+$; HRMS (ES$^+$) *m/z*: calcd. $C_{17}H_{16}N_3O_2S$ [M + H]$^+$ = 326.0963; observed 326.0968 (1.5 ppm).

Synthesis of 3-(3-Aminophenyl)-5-(benzo[d][1,3]dioxol-5-yl)-4,5-dihydro-1H-pyrazole-1-carbothioamide (**4c**)

A round-bottom flask was charged with ethanol (95%, 25 mL) NaOH (1000 mg, 0.025mol,), **3c** (2673 mg 0.01 mol) and thiosemicarbazide (911 mg, 0.01 mol). The reaction mixture was stirred for 3 h at reflux. Upon completion, the reaction mixture was added to ice. The resulting solid was washed with diethyl ether and water, then filtered. The crude product was purified by column chromatography ($SiO_2$; EtOAc/hexane 7:3) to afford the desired compound as an off-yellow powder (1604 mg, 60%). $^1$H NMR (500 MHz, DMSO-$d_6$) δ 7.98 (s, 1H), 7.67 (s, 1H), 7.08 (app t, *J* = 7.8 Hz, 1H), 7.03 (d app t, *J* = 7.8, 1.1 Hz, 1H), 6.99 (app t, *J* = 2 Hz,1H), 6.83 (d, *J* = 8.0 Hz, 1H), 6.67 (ddd, *J* = 7.9, 2.3, 1.1 Hz, 1H), 6.63 (d, *J* = 1.7 Hz, 1H), 6.59 (dd, *J* = 8.1, 1.8 Hz, 1H), 5.99–5.95 (m, 2H), 5.81 (dd, *J* = 11.2, 3.1 Hz, 1H), 5.18 (s, 2H), 3.81 (dd, *J* = 17.9, 11.3 Hz, 1H), 2.98 (dd, *J* = 17.8, 3.2 Hz, 1H); $^{13}$C NMR (126 MHz, DMSO-$d_6$) δ 175.9, 155.8, 148.8, 147.2, 146.1, 136.9, 131.3, 129.1, 118.3, 116.2, 114.8, 112.0, 108.2, 105.8, 100.9, 62.4, 42.6; $^{15}$N NMR (51 MHz, $CDCl_3$) δ 192.6; 108.6; 60.9; 14.6; LRMS (ES$^+$) *m/z*: 341.11 [M + H]$^+$; HRMS (ES$^+$) *m/z*: calcd. $C_{17}H_{17}N_4O_2S$ [M + H]$^+$ = 341.1072; observed 341.1076 (1.2 ppm).

### 3.2. *Synthesis of PPL-Inspired Molecules*

Synthesis of (*E*)-3-(3,4,5-Trimethoxyphenyl)acrylic acid (**7a**)

Malonic acid (1.24 g, 12mmol) was added to a stirred solution of **6a** (1.94 g, 10 mmol), pyridine (6.0 mL) and piperidine (0.6 mL). The reaction was stirred at reflux for 4 h. The mixture was then cooled to room temperature and poured into a solution of HCl (10 M in $H_2O$, 80 mL) at 0 °C. The white solid that formed was recovered by filtration and washed with water (200 mL) to afford the title compound as yellow powder (1.65g, 85%). $^1$H NMR (300 MHz, $CDCl_3$) δ 7.71 (d, *J* = 15.8 Hz, 1H), 6.78 (s, 2H), 6.36 (d, *J* = 15.9 Hz, 1H), 3.90 (s, 6H), 3.89 (s, 3H). $^{13}$C NMR (101 MHz, $CDCl_3$) δ 172.4, 153.6, 147.3, 140.7, 129.7, 116.6, 105.7, 61.2, 56.4; LRMS (ES$^-$) *m/z*: 237.0763 [M-H]$^+$. Data was in accordance with the literature [27].

Synthesis of (*E*)-3-(4-Methoxyphenyl)acrylic acid (**7b**)

Malonic acid (1.24 g, 12 mmol) was added to a stirred solution of **6b** (1.36 g, 10 mmol), pyridine (6 mL) and piperidine (0.6 mL). The reaction was stirred at reflux for 4 h. The mixture was then cooled to room temperature and poured into a solution of HCl (10 M in $H_2O$, 80 mL) at 0 °C. The white solid that formed was recovered by filtration and washed with water (200 mL) to afford the title compound as white powder (1.33g, 98%). $^1H$ NMR (300 MHz, $CD_3OD$) δ 7.62 (d, *J* = 16.0 Hz, 1H), 7.58–7.47 (m, 2H), 7.01–6.88 (m, 2H), 6.33 (d, *J* = 15.9 Hz, 1H), 3.82 (s, 3H). Data were in accordance with the literature [28].

Synthesis of (*E*)-3-(3,4,5-Trimethoxyphenyl)acryloyl chloride (**8a**)

To a stirred solution of **7a** (714 mg, 3.0 mmol) in DCM (6.0 mL), thionyl chloride (0.65 mL, 9.0 mmol) and DMF (0.01 mL) were added. The reaction was stirred at reflux for 5 h under argon. The solvent was removed under reduced pressure and dried *in vacuo* to afford the title compound as a yellow powder (707 mg, 99%) and used immediately in the next step. $^1H$ NMR (300 MHz, $CDCl_3$) δ 7.75 (d, *J* = 15.4 Hz, 1H), 6.79 (s, 2H), 6.55 (d, *J* = 15.4 Hz, 1H), 3.91 (s, 3H), 3.91 (s, 6H).

Synthesis of (*E*)-3-(4-Methoxyphenyl)acryloyl chloride (**8b**)

To a stirred solution of **7b** (534 mg, 3.0 mmol) in DCM (6.0 mL), thionyl chloride (0.65 mL, 9.0 mmol) and DMF (0.01 mL) were added. The reaction was stirred at reflux for 5 h under argon. The solvent was removed under reduced pressure and dried *in vacuo* to afford the title compound as a yellow powder (513 mg, 96%) and used immediately in the next step. $^1H$ NMR (300 MHz, $CD_3OD$) δ 7.62 (d, *J* = 16.0 Hz, 1H), 7.58–7.47 (m, 2H), 7.00–6.89 (m, 2H), 6.33 (d, *J* = 15.9 Hz, 1H), 3.82 (s, 3H).

Synthesis of (*E*)-1-(3-(3,4,5-Trimethoxyphenyl)acryloyl)piperidin-2-one (**9a**)

To a stirred solution of δ-valerolactam (278 mg, 2.8 mmol) in THF (12 mL) at 0 °C, NaH (112 mg, 2.8 mmol, 60% *w/w* in oil) was added slowly. The reaction was warmed to room temperature and stirred for 2 h. The mixture was cooled to 0°C and **8a** (641 mg, 2.5mmol) was added. The reaction was stirred for 1 h at 0 °C and for a further 24 h at room temperature under argon. The solution was poured into ice water and stirred for 15 min. The organic phase was recovered by extraction with ethyl acetate (15 mL), washed with brine (30 mL) and NaOH (2.0 M in $H_2O$, 30 mL) and dried ($MgSO_4$). The organic phase was concentrated by rotary evaporation under reduced pressure. The crude product was purified by column chromatography ($SiO_2$; EtOAc/petroleum ether 1:1) to afford the title compound as a yellow powder (219 mg, 34%). $^1H$ NMR (300 MHz, $CDCl_3$) δ 7.63 (d, *J* = 15.5 Hz, 1H), 7.35 (d, *J* = 15.6 Hz, 1H), 6.78 (s, 2H), 3.88 (s, 6H), 3.86 (s, 3H), 3.79 (td, *J* = 5.1, 4.1, 2.7 Hz, 2H), 2.68–2.53 (m, 2H), 1.95–1.80 (m, 4H). Data were in accordance with the literature [18].

Synthesis of (*E*)-1-(3-(4-Methoxyphenyl)acryloyl)piperidin-2-one (**9b**)

To a stirred solution of δ-valerolactam (278 mg, 2.8 mmol) in THF (12 mL) at 0 °C, NaH (112 mg, 2.8 mmol, 60% *w/w* in oil) was added slowly. The reaction warmed to room temperature and stirred for 2 h. The mixture was cooled to 0 °C and **8b** (490 mg, 2.5mmol) was added. The reaction was stirred for 1 h at 0 °C and for a further 24 h at room temperature under argon. The solution was poured into ice water and stirred for 15 min. The organic phase was recovered by extraction with ethyl acetate (15 mL), washed with brine (30 mL) and NaOH (2.0 M in $H_2O$, 30 mL) and dried ($MgSO_4$). The organic phase was concentrated by rotary evaporation under reduced pressure. The crude product was purified by column chromatography ($SiO_2$; EtOAc/petroleum ether 1:1) to afford the title compound as a yellow powder (114 mg, 23%). $^1H$ NMR (300 MHz, $CDCl_3$) δ 7.69 (d, *J* = 15.6 Hz, 1H), 7.57–7.47 (m, 2H), 7.35 (d, *J* = 15.6 Hz, 1H), 6.95–6.81 (m, 2H), 3.83 (s, 3H), 3.79 (td, *J* = 5.2, 4.2, 2.3 Hz, 2H), 2.66–2.54 (m, 2H), 1.93–1.84 (m, 4H). Data were in accordance with the literature [29].

Synthesis (*E*)-6-(3-(3,4,5-Trimethoxyphenyl)acryloyl)cyclohex-2-en-1-one (**10**)

To a stirred solution of cyclohex-2-enone (577 mg, 6.0 mmol) in THF (15.0 mL) at −78 °C, lithium di*iso*propylamide (0.6 mL, 6.0 mmol) was added dropwise. The solution was stirred at −78 °C for 45 min under argon. A solution of **8a** (770 mg, 3.0 mmol) in THF (15 mL) was slowly added to the initial solution and stirred for a further 1 h at −78 °C, then 1 h at 0 °C. The organic phase was recovered by extraction with ethyl acetate (15 mL), washed with brine (30 mL), and dried ($MgSO_4$). The crude product was purified by column chromatography ($SiO_2$; EtOAc/petroleum ether 1:1) to afford the title compound as a yellow powder (228 mg, 40%). $^1H$ NMR (300 MHz, $CDCl_3$) δ 15.76 (t, *J* = 1.1 Hz, 1H), 7.55 (d, *J* = 15.5 Hz, 1H), 6.90–6.80 (m, 2H), 6.76 (s, 2H), 6.16 (dtd, *J* = 10.0, 2.0, 0.9 Hz, 1H), 3.90 (d, *J* = 1.0 Hz, 6H), 3.88 (d, *J* = 0.9 Hz, 3H), 2.75 (t, *J* = 7.2 Hz, 2H), 2.42 (qd, *J* = 5.3, 4.7, 2.6 Hz, 2H). Data were in accordance with the literature [29] except the signal at 15.76 ppm.

### 3.3. Electronic Structure Characterization

The molecular structures of the analogues Piperine and PPL were built in Avogadro software [30] and optimized by *ab initio* calculation. The calculations were performed using the Gamess2018 quantum mechanics package [31,32] with Hartree–Fock (HF) formalism [33] and density functional theory (DFT) [34]. 6-311+G(1d,1p) was used as the set of the bases and B3LYP as the functional [35]. The optimized geometries were determined with a Polarizable Continuum Model (PCM) solvent model [36] for $H_2O$ and **4a** was also optimized in $CHCl_3$. The optimizations were followed by harmonic frequency calculations to obtain the vibrational, the rotational, and the translational contributions to the free energy. The electrostatic potential map and the partial charges were determined using the geodesic method [37] along with the same functional base set and solvent model used for the optimization of the structure. The structure and the normal frequency modes analyses were visualized by wxMacMolPlt software [38] to assure that the result is not a structure in a transition state.

### 3.4. Molecular Docking

The optimized structures of each analogue were obtained from Section 3.3. IL-1β structure was obtained from chain A of PDB-1ITB and p65 unit of NF-κB was obtained from the chain A of PDB-2O61.

AutoDockTools [39] software of the MGL program Tools 1.5.4 was used to prepare the proteins by adding polar hydrogen atoms and Gasteiger charges. Blind docking was performed to explore the whole IL-1β protein. The maps were generated by AutoGrid 4.2 program with a spacing of 0.4583 Å, dimension of 126×126×108 points and grid center coordinates as being 41.028, −0.369 and 12.346 for x, y and z coordinates, respectively. The NF-κB maps were generated by AutoGrid 4.2 program [39] with a spacing of 0.375 Å, dimension of 90 × 82 × 92 points and grid center coordinates as being 21.573, −12.537 and −0.788 for x, y and z coordinates, respectively. AutoDock 4.2[39] was used to investigate the protein binding site using the Lamarckian Genetic Algorithm (LGA) with a population size of 150, maximum number of generations of 27000 and energy evaluations equal to 2.5 × $10^6$. The other parameters were selected as the software default. To generate different conformations, the total numbers of runs were set to 100. The final energy scores were calculated following the equation

$$\Delta G = \left(V_{bound}^{L-L} - V_{umbound}^{L-L}\right) + \left(V_{bound}^{P-P} - V_{umbound}^{P-P}\right) + \left(V_{bound}^{P-L} - V_{umbound}^{P-L}\right) + \Delta S_{conformation}. \quad (1)$$

The potentials utilized to perform the calculation were the following:

$$V\ (energy\ score) = I.\sum_{i,j}\left(\frac{A_{ij}}{r_{ij}^{12}} - \frac{B_{ij}}{r_{ij}^{6}}\right) + J.\sum_{i,j} E(t).\left(\frac{C_{ij}}{r_{ij}^{12}} - \frac{D_{ij}}{r_{ij}^{10}}\right) + K.\sum_{i,j}\frac{q_i.q_j}{\varepsilon.r_{ij}^2} + \Delta W \quad (2)$$

The weighting constants I, *J*, E(t) and K are those optimized to calibrate the empirical free energy based on a set of experimentally characterized complexes. The first term is the Lenard–Jones potential, in which parameters A and B are taken from the Amber force field. The second term refers to the hydrogen bond in which parameters C and D are obtained to ensure a minimum energy of 5.0 kcal/mol in 1.9 Å for O-H and N-H and 1.0 kcal/mol in 2.5 Å for S-H [40]. The function E(t) provides directionality based on the angle t of the geometry of an ideal hydrogen bond. The third term is a shielded Coulomb potential for electrostatic interaction. The last term is the desolvation potential based on the volume of the atoms surrounding a given atom and sheltering of the solvent [40]. The final conformations were chosen among the most negative energies that belong to the most representative cluster and visualized by visual molecular dynamics software (VMD) [41]. The binding microenvironment was generated by LigPlot [42].

## 4. Conclusions

In this study, we have confirmed the structure of some ambiguous complex natural product -likescaffolds from the literature through *de novo* synthesis, spectroscopic analysis including $^{15}$N NMR techniques, and *ab initio* calculations. With the definitive structures in hand, we used molecular docking to investigate the rationale for the promising biological results these molecules exhibit in the inhibition of the inflammatory response (*via* downregulation of IL-1β and NF-κB pathway). This work revealed **3a,c**, **4a,c** and **10** as the most promising molecules to be evaluated as IL-1β and NF-κB inhibitors in future studies.

**Supplementary Materials:** The following are available online, copies of $^{1}$H, $^{13}$C and 2D NMR spectra, and *ab initio* calculations of selected dihedral angles.

**Author Contributions:** Conceptualization, M.L.C. and A.M.J.; methodology, M.L.C., A.M.J., A.P.R.P. and G.Z.; software, A.P.R.P. and G.Z.; validation, B.T. and C.S.L.D., formal analysis, M.L.C., C.S.L.D., and A.M.J.; investigation, A.P.R.P., G.Z., B.T. and C.S.L.D.; resources, A.M.J., B.T. and C.S.L.D.; data curation, A.P.R.P., G.Z. and A.M.J.; writing—original draft preparation, A.P.R.P., G.Z. and A.M.J.; writing—review and editing, A.M.J., A.P.R.P., G.Z., M.L.C. and C.S.L.D.; visualization, A.P.R.P. and G.Z.; supervision, A.M.J. and M.L.C.; project administration, A.M.J; funding acquisition, M.L.C, A.M.J, A.P.R.P. and G.Z. All authors have read and agreed to the published version of the manuscript.

**Funding:** This study was financed in part by the Coordenação de Aperfeiçoamento de Pessoal de Nível Superior–Brasil (CAPES)–Finance Code 001 in the form of research scholarships for A.P.R.P. and G.Z. The APC was funded by Molecules, MDPI.

**Acknowledgments:** The computations described in this paper were performed using the University of Birmingham's BlueBEAR HPC service, which provides a High Performance Computing service to the University's research community. See http://www.birmingham.ac.uk/bear for more details.

**Conflicts of Interest:** The authors declare no conflict of interest.

## References

1. Collins, I.; Jones, A.M. Diversity-oriented synthetic strategies applied to cancer chemical biology and drug discovery. *Molecules* **2014**, *19*, 17221–17255. [CrossRef] [PubMed]
2. Newman, D.J. Natural products as leads to potential drugs: An old process or the new hope for drug discovery? *J. Med. Chem.* **2008**, *51*, 2589–2599. [CrossRef] [PubMed]
3. Srinivasan, K. Black pepper and its pungent principle-piperine: A review of diverse physiological effects. *Crit. Rev. Food Sci. Nutr.* **2007**, *47*, 735–748. [CrossRef] [PubMed]
4. Umadevi, P.; Deepti, K.; Venugopal, D.V.R. Synthesis, anticancer and antibacterial activities of piperine analogs. *Med. Chem. Res.* **2013**, *22*, 5466–5471. [CrossRef]
5. Venkatasamy, R.; Faas, L.; Young, A.R.; Raman, A.; Hider, R.C. Effects of piperine analogues on stimulation of melanocyte proliferation and melanocyte differentiation. *Bioorg. Med. Chem.* **2004**, *12*, 1905–1920. [CrossRef] [PubMed]
6. Bezerra, D.P.; Pessoa, C.; de Moraes, M.O.; Saker-Neto, N.; Silveira, E.R.; Costa-Lotufo, L.V. Overview of the therapeutic potential of piplartine (piperlongumine). *Eur. J. Pharm. Sci.* **2013**, *48*, 453–463. [CrossRef]
7. Adams, D.J.; Dai, M.; Pellegrino, G.; Wagner, B.K.; Stern, A.M.; Shamji, A.F.; Schreiber, S.L. Synthesis, cellular evaluation, and mechanism of action of piperlongumine analogs. *Proc. Natl. Acad. Sci. USA* **2012**, *109*, 15115–15120. [CrossRef]

8. Piska, K.; Gunia-Krzyżak, A.; Koczurkiewicz, P.; Wójcik-Pszczoła, K.; Pękala, E. Piperlongumine (piplartine) as a lead compound for anticancer agents – Synthesis and properties of analogues: A mini-review. *Eur. J. Med. Chem.* **2018**, *156*, 13–20. [CrossRef]
9. Meghwal, M.; Goswami, T.K. Piper nigrum and piperine: An update. *Phyther. Res.* **2013**, *27*, 1121–1130. [CrossRef]
10. Bang, J.S.; Oh, D.H.; Choi, H.M.; Sur, B.-J.; Lim, S.-J.; Kim, J.Y.; Yang, H.I.; Yoo, M.C.; Hahm, D.-H.; Kim, K.S. Anti-inflammatory and antiarthritic effects of piperine in human interleukin 1β-stimulated fibroblast-like synoviocytes and in rat arthritis models. *Arthritis Res. Ther.* **2009**, *11*, R49. [CrossRef]
11. Ying, X.; Chen, X.; Cheng, S.; Shen, Y.; Peng, L.; Xu, H. Piperine inhibits IL-β induced expression of inflammatory mediators in human osteoarthritis chondrocyte. *Int. Immunopharmacol.* **2013**, *17*, 293–299. [CrossRef] [PubMed]
12. Ying, X.; Yu, K.; Chen, X.; Chen, H.; Hong, J.; Cheng, S.; Peng, L. Piperine inhibits LPS induced expression of inflammatory mediators in RAW 264.7 cells. *Cell. Immunol.* **2013**, *285*, 49–54. [CrossRef] [PubMed]
13. Mathew, A.; Sheeja, M.T.L.; Kumar, K.; Radha, A.T. Design, synthesis and biological evaluation of pyrazole analogues of natural piperine. *Hygeia JD Med.* **2011**, *3*, 48–56.
14. Qu, H.; Lv, M.; Xu, H. Piperine: Bioactivities and structural modifications. *Mini Rev. Med. Chem.* **2015**, *15*, 145–156. [CrossRef]
15. Prasad, S.; Tyagi, A.K. Historical spice as a future drug: Therapeutic potential of piperlongumine. *Curr. Pharm. Des.* **2016**, *22*, 4151–4159. [CrossRef]
16. Wu, Y.; Min, X.; Zhuang, C.; Li, J.; Yu, Z.; Dong, G.; Yao, J.; Wang, S.; Liu, Y.; Wu, S. Design, synthesis and biological activity of piperlongumine derivatives as selective anticancer agents. *Eur. J. Med. Chem.* **2014**, *82*, 545–551. [CrossRef]
17. Ginzburg, S.; Golovine, K.V.; Makhov, P.B.; Uzzo, R.G.; Kutikov, A.; Kolenko, V.M. Piperlongumine inhibits NF-κB activity and attenuates aggressive growth characteristics of prostate cancer cells. *Prostate* **2014**, *74*, 177–186. [CrossRef]
18. Sun, L.-D.; Wang, F.; Dai, F.; Wang, Y.-H.; Lin, D.; Zhou, B. Development and mechanism investigation of a new piperlongumine derivative as a potent anti-inflammatory agent. *Biochem. Pharmacol.* **2015**, *95*, 156–169. [CrossRef]
19. Si, D.; Wang, Y.; Zhou, Y.-H.; Guo, Y.; Wang, J.; Zhou, H.; Li, Z.-S.; Fawcett, J.P. Mechanism of CYP2C9 inhibition by flavones and flavonols. *Drug Metab. Dispos.* **2009**, *37*, 629–634. [CrossRef]
20. Gu, S.M.; Lee, H.P.; Ham, Y.W.; Son, D.J.; Kim, H.Y.; Oh, K.W.; Han, S.-B.; Yun, J.; Hong, J.T. Piperlongumine improves lipopolysaccharide-induced amyloidogenesis by suppressing NF-KappaB pathway. *Neuromol. Med.* **2018**, *20*, 312–327. [CrossRef]
21. Zazeri, G.; Povinelli, A.P.R.; de Lima, F.M.; Cornélio, M.L. Experimental approaches and computational modeling of rat serum albumin and its interaction with piperine. *Int. J. Mol. Sci.* **2019**, *20*, 2856. [CrossRef] [PubMed]
22. Povinelli, A.P.R.; Zazeri, G.; de Freitas Lima, M.; Cornélio, M.L. Details of the cooperative binding of piperlongumine with rat serum albumin obtained by spectroscopic and computational analyses. *Sci. Rep.* **2019**, *9*, 1–11. [CrossRef] [PubMed]
23. Panne, D.; Maniatis, T.; Harrison, S.C. An atomic model of the interferon-β enhanceosome. *Cell* **2007**, *129*, 1111–1123. [CrossRef] [PubMed]
24. Chen, Y.-Q.; Ghosh, S.; Ghosh, G. A novel DNA recognition mode by the NF-κB p65 homodimer. *Nat. Struct. Biol.* **1998**, *5*, 67–73. [CrossRef] [PubMed]
25. Williams, D.B.G.; Lawton, M. Drying of organic solvents: Quantitative evaluation of the efficiency of several desiccants. *J. Org. Chem.* **2010**, *75*, 8351–8354. [CrossRef] [PubMed]
26. Bellardita, M.; Loddo, V.; Palmisano, G.; Pibiri, I.; Palmisano, L.; Augugliaro, V. Photocatalytic green synthesis of piperonal in aqueous TiO2 suspension. *Appl. Catal. B Environ.* **2014**, *144*, 607–613. [CrossRef]
27. Elamathi, P.; Chandrasekar, G.; Muthuraman, S.; Kolli, M.K. Pore size engineering of hexagonal mesoporous carbon nitride (HMCN) for high catalytic performance in the synthesis of α, β-unsaturated acid and its derivatives. *Appl. Surf. Sci.* **2019**, *463*, 481–491. [CrossRef]
28. Schmink, J.R.; Kormos, C.M.; Devine, W.G.; Leadbeater, N.E. Exploring the scope for scale-up of organic chemistry using a large batch microwave reactor. *Org. Process. Res. Dev.* **2010**, *14*, 205–214. [CrossRef]

29. Peng, S.; Zhang, B.; Meng, X.; Yao, J.; Fang, J. Synthesis of piperlongumine analogues and discovery of nuclear factor erythroid 2-related factor 2 (Nrf2) activators as potential neuroprotective agents. *J. Med. Chem.* **2015**, *58*, 5242–5255. [CrossRef]
30. Hanwell, M.D.; Curtis, D.E.; Lonie, D.C.; Vandermeersch, T.; Zurek, E.; Hutchison, G.R. Avogadro: An advanced semantic chemical editor, visualization, and analysis platform. *J. Cheminform.* **2012**, *4*, 17. [CrossRef]
31. Schmidt, M.W.; Baldridge, K.K.; Boatz, J.A.; Elbert, S.T.; Gordon, M.S.; Jensen, J.H.; Koseki, S.; Matsunaga, N.; Nguyen, K.A.; Su, S. General atomic and molecular electronic structure system. *J. Comput. Chem.* **1993**, *14*, 1347–1363. [CrossRef]
32. Gordon, M.S.; Schmidt, M.W. Advances in electronic structure theory: GAMESS a decade later. In *Theory and Applications of Computational Chemistry*; Elsevier: Amsterdam, The Netherlands, 2005; pp. 1167–1189.
33. Slater, J.C. A simplification of the Hartree-Fock method. *Phys. Rev.* **1951**, *81*, 385. [CrossRef]
34. Parr, R.G. Density functional theory of atoms and molecules. In *Horizons of Quantum Chemistry*; Springer: Boston, MA, USA, 1980; pp. 5–15.
35. Hertwig, R.H.; Koch, W. On the parameterization of the local correlation functional. What is Becke-3-LYP. *Chem. Phys. Lett.* **1997**, *268*, 345–351. [CrossRef]
36. Tomasi, J.; Mennucci, B.; Cammi, R. Quantum mechanical continuum solvation models. *Chem. Rev.* **2005**, *105*, 2999–3094. [CrossRef] [PubMed]
37. Spackman, M.A. Potential derived charges using a geodesic point selection scheme. *J. Comput. Chem.* **1996**, *17*, 1–18. [CrossRef]
38. Bode, B.M.; Gordon, M.S. A graphical user interface for GAMESS. *J. Mol. Graph. Model.* **1998**, *16*, 133–138. [CrossRef]
39. Morris, G.M.; Huey, R.; Lindstrom, W.; Sanner, M.F.; Belew, R.K.; Goodsell, D.S.; Olson, A.J. AutoDock4 and AutoDockTools4: Automated docking with selective receptor flexibility. *J. Comput. Chem.* **2009**, *30*, 2785–2791. [CrossRef]
40. Povinelli, A.P.R.; Zazeri, G.; Cornélio, M.L. Molecular Mechanism of Flavonoids Using Fluorescence Spectroscopy and Computational Tools. In *Flavonoids-A Coloring Model for Cheering up Life*; IntechOpen: London, UK, 2019.
41. Humphrey, W.; Dalke, A.; Schulten, K. VMD: Visual molecular dynamics. *J. Mol. Graph.* **1996**, *14*, 33–38. [CrossRef]
42. Wallace, A.C.; Laskowski, R.A.; Thornton, J.M. LIGPLOT: A program to generate schematic diagrams of protein-ligand interactions. *Protein Eng. Des. Sel.* **1995**, *8*, 127–134. [CrossRef]

**Sample Availability:** Samples of the compounds are available from the authors upon reasonable request.

*molecules*

MDPI

*Article*

# Rational Design, Synthesis, Characterization and Evaluation of Iodinated 4,4′-Bipyridines as New Transthyretin Fibrillogenesis Inhibitors

**Alessandro Dessì [1], Paola Peluso [1,*], Roberto Dallocchio [1], Robin Weiss [2], Giuseppina Andreotti [3], Mariateresa Allocca [3,4], Emmanuel Aubert [5], Patrick Pale [2], Victor Mamane [2,*] and Sergio Cossu [6]**

1 Institute of Biomolecular Chemistry ICB, CNR, Secondary Branch of Sassari, Traversa La Crucca 3, Regione Baldinca, Li Punti, 07100 Sassari, Italy; alessandro.dessi@cnr.it (A.D.); roberto.dallocchio@cnr.it (R.D.)

2 Strasbourg Institute of Chemistry, UMR CNRS 7177, Team LASYROC, 1 rue Blaise Pascal, University of Strasbourg, CEDEX, 67008 Strasbourg, France; robin.weiss@unistra.fr (R.W.); ppale@unistra.fr (P.P.)

3 Institute of Biomolecular Chemistry ICB, CNR, Via Campi Flegrei 34, 80078 Pozzuoli (NA), Italy; giuseppina.andreotti@icb.cnr.it (G.A.); mariateresa.allocca@gmail.com (M.A.)

4 Department of Environmental, Biological and Pharmaceutical Sciences and Technologies (DiSTABiF), University of Campania "Luigi Vanvitelli", Via Vivaldi, 43-81100 Caserta, Italy

5 Crystallography, Magnetic Resonance and Modelling (CRM2), UMR CNRS 7036, University of Lorraine, Bd des Aiguillettes, 54506 Vandoeuvre-les-Nancy, France; emmanuel.aubert@univ-lorraine.fr

6 Department of Molecular Science and Nanosystems DSMN, Venice Ca' Foscari University, Via Torino 155, 30172 Mestre Venezia, Italy; cossu@unive.it

* Correspondence: paola.peluso@cnr.it (P.P.); vmamane@unistra.fr (V.M.); Tel.: +39-079-2841218 (P.P.); +33-3-68851612 (V.M.)

Academic Editor: Maged Henary
Received: 16 April 2020; Accepted: 6 May 2020; Published: 8 May 2020

**Abstract:** The 3,3′,5,5′-tetrachloro-2-iodo-4,4′-bipyridine structure is proposed as a novel chemical scaffold for the design of new transthyretin (TTR) fibrillogenesis inhibitors. In the frame of a proof-of-principle exploration, four chiral 3,3′,5,5′-tetrachloro-2-iodo-2′-substituted-4,4′-bipyridines were rationally designed and prepared from a simple trihalopyridine in three steps, including a Cu-catalysed Finkelstein reaction to introduce iodine atoms on the heteroaromatic scaffold, and a Pd-catalysed coupling reaction to install the 2′-substituent. The corresponding racemates, along with other five chiral 4,4′-bipyridines containing halogens as substituents, were enantioseparated by high-performance liquid chromatography in order to obtain pure enantiomer pairs. All stereoisomers were tested against the amyloid fibril formation (FF) of wild type (WT)-TTR and two mutant variants, V30M and Y78F, in acid mediated aggregation experiments. Among the 4,4′-bipyridine derivatives, interesting inhibition activity was obtained for both enantiomers of the 3,3′,5,5′-tetrachloro-2′-(4-hydroxyphenyl)-2-iodo-4,4′-bipyridine. In silico docking studies were carried out in order to explore possible binding modes of the 4,4′-bipyridine derivatives into the TTR. The gained results point out the importance of the right combination of H-bond sites and the presence of iodine as halogen-bond donor. Both experimental and theoretical evidences pave the way for the utilization of the iodinated 4,4′-bipyridine core as template to design new promising inhibitors of TTR amyloidogenesis.

**Keywords:** bipyridines; docking; fibril formation; halogen bond; misfolding inhibition; transthyretin

## 1. Introduction

Human transthyretin (hTTR, prealbumin) is a homotetrameric protein (55 kDa) made up of four subunits (A-B-C-D, Figure 1a), each composed of 127 aminoacids [1–3]. The protein is mainly produced by the liver, but other sources of TTR, including the choroid plexus, the retinal pigment epithelium, and the α-cells of pancreatic islets are known. TTR is involved in the transport of thyroid hormones (thyroxine ($T_4$) and triiodothyronine ($T_3$)) (Figure 1b) in blood and cerebrospinal fluid. The tetrameric assembly of TTR contains a central hydrophobic channel with two symmetrical funnel-shaped $T_4$ binding pockets located at the energetically weaker dimer-dimer A-B/C-D interface [4], the other A-C/B-D interface being stabilized by interstrand hydrogen bonds (HBs).

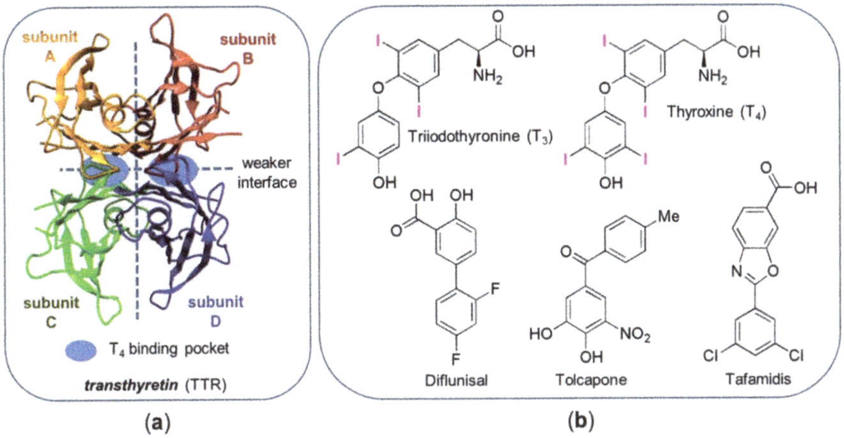


**Figure 1.** (**a**) Ribbon diagram picture of wild type (WT)-TTR (released from PDB ID 1ICT [2]); (**b**) structures of thyroxine ($T_4$), triiodothyronine ($T_3$), tafamidis and other ATTR drug candidates under clinical trials.

The presence of mutations in TTR results in destabilization of the tetramer and dissociation into amyloidogenic monomers, which misfold and self-aggregate into insoluble amyloid fibrils. TTR amyloidogenesis has been implicated to cause amyloid diseases (TTR amyloidosis, ATTR) [5,6]. Amyloid structures derived from wild-type (WT)-TTR can deposit in the heart and peripheral nerves causing senile systemic amyloidosis (SSA), whereas over 100 TTR mutants were shown to be implicated in three other groups of diseases, namely familial amyloidotic polyneuropathy (FAP), cardiomyopathy (FAC), and central nervous system selective amyloidosis (CNSA). Among known TTR mutants, the V30M [7] and the Y78F [8] are the most common FAP mutation and the most amyloidogenic, respectively. Moreover, the importance of TTR stability also concerns neurodegenerative disorders such as Parkinson's and Alzheimer's diseases [9,10].

In 1996 it was observed that $T_4$ is able to prevent amyloid fibril formation (FF), but with adverse side effects due to its hormonal activity [11]. However, this study proved that stabilization of the native TTR tetramer by small molecule binding to one or both of the $T_4$ binding pockets could be a rationale for the kinetic inhibition of TTR amyloidogenesis, tetramer dissociation being the rate-determining step in amyloid formation [12,13]. Indeed, TTR can bind molecules other than $T_4$ because more than 99% of $T_4$ binding sites are unoccupied due to the fact that two other carriers, albumin and thyroid-binding globulin, transport the majority of $T_4$ in the blood. Significantly, this observation paved the way for the development of an oral therapy as a valid alternative to more invasive approaches [14].

In the last decades, several small molecules have proven to be able to bridge neighbouring monomers of TTR via specific hydrophobic and electrostatic noncovalent interactions, to stabilize the tetramer, to inhibit the tetramer dissociation, and to reduce FF [3,15–28]. However, to date few structures possess the requirements to be drug candidates (Figure 1b), and the ATTR still lacks an effective therapy. So far, tafamidis [29] has been approved for clinical use in Europe and Japan for the treatment of early-stage FAP [30], but advanced disease responds poorly to tafamidis administration [31]. Then, recently the drug tolcapone, which was approved for the treatment of Parkinson's disease, has been repurposed for the treatment of ATTR [32]. Nonsteroidal anti-inflammatory drugs (NSAIDs) also inhibit formation of amyloidogenic monomers. Among them, diflunisal was shown to slow the progression of FAP over a period of 2 years, but adverse gastrointestinal effects limit its use [16,33]. In this regard, it is worth mentioning that small molecules should be selective for TTR and neither bind thyroid hormone receptors nor cyclooxygenase-1 (COX-1) to be effective clinical candidates [16,18].

Over time, a large number of SAR studies have been published in order to identify typical substructures which are shared by compounds that stabilize TTR tetramer [3,34–39]. In this field, the potential of iodine as substituent (iodination hypothesis) has been intensively explored through evaluating the inhibition ability of iodinated compounds with respect to non-iodinated analogues [10,11,17,36,40–43]. Among iodinated motifs, 2,4,6-triiodophenol proved to be one of the most potent TTR fibrillogenesis inhibitor known so far [11], and iododiflunisal was shown to stabilize TTR [17]. Nevertheless, in some cases iodination does not improve inhibition activity [17,42,44], the effectiveness of this strategy depending on inhibitor scaffold structure and location of iodine in the molecular framework [42]. In general, the real function of iodine in TTR binding and stabilization still remains unclear due to the fact that halogens as substituents can contribute to protein-ligand binding through multiple roles such as hydrophobic centres, HB acceptors and electrophilic halogen bond (XB) donors. In particular, XBs were found to have a relevant role in the binding of halogenated ligands with proteins [42,45], and short I···O contacts were found to underlie the selective binding of $T_4$ to TTR [46]. Despite the potential of iodine substituents to contribute to TTR stabilization, studies on iodinated compounds are reported in smaller degree compared to compounds containing fluorine, chlorine and bromine as substituents. Currently, the scarce availability of iodinated compounds has clearly limited the study of the iodine effect on TTR misfolding inhibition, reducing the possibility to gather conclusive information on iodine function.

In the last few years, our groups have reported the synthesis and characterization of halogenated 4,4′-bipyridines [47–50]. These molecules were shown to be efficient as XB donors in the solid state [48] and in solution [51,52]. On this basis, starting from the chemistry and properties of 4,4′-bipyridines **1–5** [48], we describe herein the design and synthesis of iodinated 4,4′-bipyridines **6–10** and their evaluation as TTR fibrillogenesis inhibitor (Figure 2a). Due to the atropisomeric geometry of their halogenated heteroaromatic scaffold, compounds **1–5** and **7–10** are chiral and exhibit (*M*)- and (*P*)-enantiomers (Figure 2b). Quantitative evaluation of the inhibition efficacy of both (*M*)- and (*P*)-enantiomers against TTR misfolding was performed through acid-mediated in vitro assays of WT-, V30M-, and Y78F-TTR aggregation. The relationship between chemical structures, inhibition activity, and binding mode was explored by molecular docking and electrostatic potential isosurfaces ($V_S$) analysis.

In particular, this study aims at gathering information on the potential role of substructures containing halogen σ-holes in TTR binding and stabilization. It is noteworthy that halogenated 4,4′-bipyridines derivatives have never been designed nor tested as TTR fibrillogenesis inhibitors.

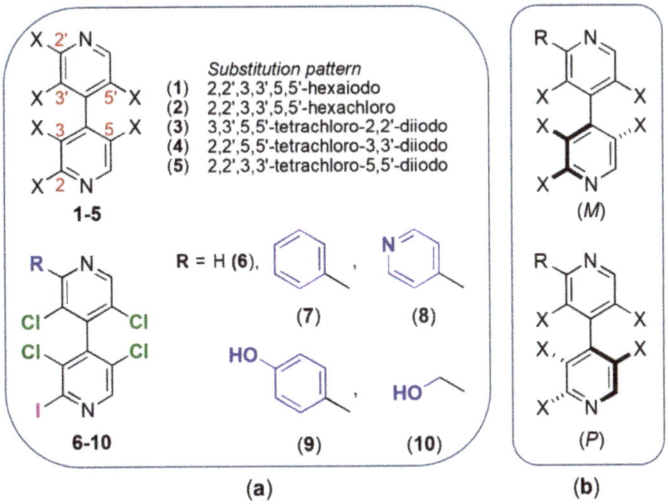


**Figure 2.** (**a**) Structures of halogenated 4,4′-bipyridines **1–10**; (**b**) (*M*) and (*P*) absolute configurations of the atropisomeric 4,4′-bipyridines **1–5** and **7–10**.

## 2. Results and Discussion

### 2.1. Rational Design

In the majority of the TTR:small molecule crystal structures reported to date [3], the molecule is bound to the $T_4$ binding site, with the exception of polyphenol (−)-epigallocatechin gallate (EGCG) which binds TTR molecular surface [19] and few other allosteric inhibitors [24,25]. Each $T_4$ binding pocket is composed of a small inner cavity (delimited by the pair $Ser_{117}/Se_{117'}$), and a large outer cavity (delimited by the pair $Lys_{15}/Lys_{15'}$), with three pairs of symmetric hydrophobic depressions named halogen binding pockets (hBPs) (Figure 3) where the iodine atoms of $T_4$ are located.

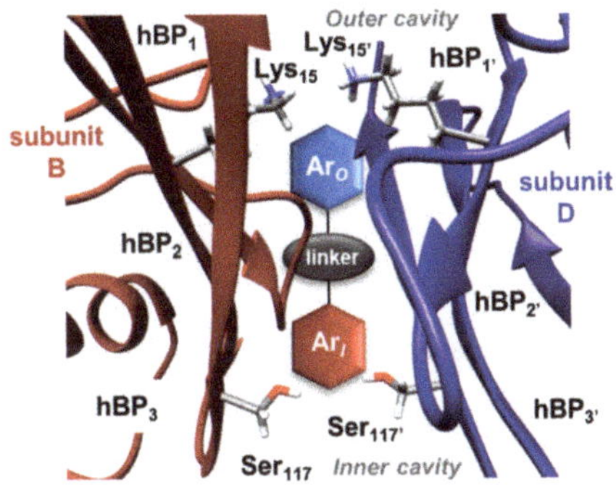


**Figure 3.** Expanded schematic view of one of the two $T_4$ binding pockets (dimer BD), where $hBP_1$ is located between the side chains of $Lys_{15/15'}$, $Leu_{17/17'}$, $Thr_{106/106'}$ and $Val_{121/121'}$, $hBP_2$ between the side chains of $Leu_{17/17'}$, $Ala_{108/108'}$, $Ala_{109/109'}$ and $Leu_{110/110'}$ and $hBP_3$ between the side chains of $Ser_{117/117'}$, $Thr_{119/119'}$, $Ala_{108/108'}$ and $Leu_{110/110'}$.

As reported by Kelly and co-workers [53], typical inhibitors are characterized by two aryl rings ($Ar_O$ and $Ar_I$) connected directly or through a linker. The binding ability of this kind of molecules can be modulated by tuning structure and substitution pattern of the three substructures, namely $Ar_O$, $Ar_I$ and linker. Scaffolds bearing halogen substituents on one ring, and a HB centre on the other ring, which is able to interact with $Lys_{15}$ ε-$NH_3^+$ group, represent the typical motif of most inhibitors reported so far. In general, TTR can accommodate small molecules with different orientations. Indeed, in the forward binding mode, the phenyl ring substituted with halogens prefers the inner cavity, whereas in the reverse binding mode it is located in the outer cavity [3,15,16].

### 2.1.1. Conceptual Basis

As reported [3,42,46], the possibility of XB formation emerges from the crystallographic analysis of complexes between TTR and some of the halogenated ligands reported so far. Indeed, contacts ranging from 2.8 to 3.5 Å have been observed between halogen substituents of small molecules and $Ala_{109}$, $Ser_{117}$, and $Thr_{119}$ carbonyls in TTR, acting as XB acceptors. The XB is a noncovalent interaction which originates from the anisotropic charge distribution of bound halogens, generating an area of lower electron density, the electrophilic σ-hole, located on the elongation of the covalent bond (Figure 4a) [54].

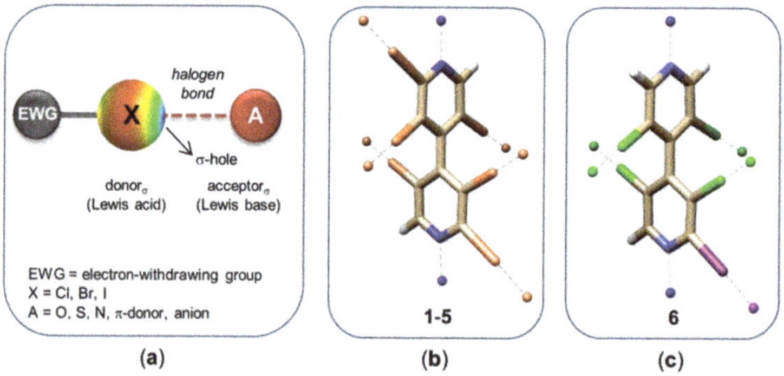


**Figure 4.** (**a**) Schematic description of XB. On X surface, electrostatic potential ($V_S$) > 0 (lower electron density) and $V_S$ < 0 (higher electron density) are indicated in blue and red, respectively. Intermediate values are in orange, yellow, and green; (**b**) and (**c**) positions of nitrogen $V_{S,min}$ regions (blue) and $V_{S,max}$ in the structure of halogenated 4,4′-bipyridines **1–5** and **6** (hydrogen, white). $V_{S,max}$ colors: halogen, coral; chlorine, green; iodine, purple.

From this perspective, the electrostatic potential ($V$) is a useful tool for understanding molecular interactive capability. In particular, the calculated positive $V$ on the isodensity surface near the halogen σ-hole, the $V_{S,max}$, is advantageously used to assess σ-hole depth which, in turn, has been found to be related to the strengths of XB [55,56]. On this basis, the $V_S$ values on a 0.002 au molecular isosurface of polyhalogenated 4,4′-bipyridines **1–6**, bearing iodines and chlorines as substituents, were calculated in order to localize regions of higher (negative $V_{S,min}$) and lower (positive $V_{S,max}$) electron charge density, and to profile the binding capability of diverse halogenated 4,4′-bipyridyl scaffolds as templates for the design of new TTR stabilizers (Figure 4b,c). Several key structural aspects in halogenated 4,4′-bipyridines highlight the interest of studying this family of molecules:

(i) 4,4′-Bipyridines **1–6** consist of two linked heteroaromatic rings that accommodate six (**1–5**) and five (**6**) (Figure 4b,c) highly oriented halogens as substituents. 4,4′-Bipyridyl derivatives have been almost unexplored in the field of TTR stabilization to date, and only the 5-cyano-2-methyl-3,4′-bipyridin-6(1*H*)-one milrinone was found to be a strong competitive inhibitor of $T_4$ binding to TTR [57];

(ii) The two electron-poor bipyridyl rings are characterized by positive $V_{S,max}$ ranging from 72.06 to 96.58 kJ/mol (Supplementary Materials, Table S1), similar to the values calculated for tafamidis, which contains an electron-poor substructure centred on the oxazole ring (98.49; 98.88 kJ/mol) (Table S2);

(iii) The presence of four 3,3′,5,5′-substituents induces chirality by restricted rotation around the 4,4′-bond (atropisomerism), introducing stereochemical features that could be fruitfully exploited to improve binding efficacy and selectivity toward TTR. So far, few studies considered chiral inhibitors and their stereochemical properties [35]. Moreover, the atropisomeric structure of the 3,3′,5,5′-tetrasubstituted-4,4′-bipyridyl ring mimics the skewed conformation of $T_4$;

(iv) The two pyridyl nitrogens can work as HB acceptors, exhibiting $V_{S,min}$ values ranging from −122.43 to −117.07 kJ/mol (Supplementary Materials, Table S1). Furthermore, nitrogen is known to be a high-impact design element because substitution of a CH group with a N atom, in aromatic and heteroaromatic ring frameworks, often improves the pharmacological profile of a molecular structure at different levels [58];

(v) Iodine is considered a powerful XB donor due to its polarizability, in particular when it is bound to electron-withdrawing groups (EWGs). $T_4$ presents multiple iodine atoms which are accommodated in the hBPs of the $T_4$ binding site of TTR. For $T_4$, we calculated $V_{S,max}$ ranging from 109.11 to 143.05 kJ/mol (Supplementary Materials, Table S2). In compounds **1** and **3–6**, iodine substituents are activated as XB donors due to the EWG effect exerted by the tetrachlorinated heteroaromatic scaffold, with $V_{S,max}$ values ranging from 133.42 to 167.06 kJ/mol (Table S1). In this regard, it is worth mentioning that in our previous studies [48–52,59], the function of compounds **1–5** as XB donors was demonstrated by theoretical calculations, and HPLC, NMR, and X-ray diffraction (XRD) analysis involving oxygen and nitrogen as XB acceptors. On the other hand, iodine is able to fill the hBPs better than other halogens due to its volume, so optimizing the strength of van der Waals interactions [42];

(vi) In compounds **2–6**, the chlorine substituents could also function as potential XB donors, even if lower $V_{S,max}$ values ranging from 70.96 to 98.81 kJ/mol were calculated (Supplementary Materials, Table S1) due to the lower polarizability and the higher electronegativity of chlorine with respect to iodine. Moreover, COX-1 being characterized by smaller hydrophobic binding pockets with respect to TTR [34,35], the presence of bulkier chlorines, with respect to hydrogens, might reduce binding affinity of the small molecule towards COX-1, thus increasing selectivity in TTR binding;

(vii) Since compounds **3–5** contain the same type and number of halogenated substituents but a different substitution pattern, it is possible to evaluate the scaffold effect on iodine properties and activity. Recently, Boeckler and co-workers demonstrated by theoretical calculations that the attachment position of a halogen within a heteroaromatic scaffold can influence size and shape of the σ-hole and, in turn, the strength of the XB [56];

(viii) All halogens can also act as hydrophobic sites and HB acceptors due to a belt of higher electron density located around the σ-hole (Figure 4a).

### 2.1.2. Molecular Docking of Polyhalogenated 4,4′-Bipyridines 1–6 in the TTR Tetramer

Molecular docking is one of the most popular computational approaches in structure-based drug design [60]. This technique can be used either to identify the correct conformation of the ligand within the target binding pocket or to estimate the interaction energy between a target and a ligand [61,62]. Molecular dynamics (MD) simulations can be also advantageously used to evaluate the molecular flexibility of ligands and receptors [63]. However, as some conformational changes occur in the time scale of only dozens of nanoseconds, this aspect could compromise the MD simulation viability for virtual screening studies. Moreover, computational cost of MD simulations is generally high. Therefore, a useful theoretical strategy is to select promising conformations from the docking study. In this regard, it is worth mentioning that different programs and theoretical methods are available for docking purposes, and each docking program shows advantages and limitations to carry out docking studies and docking-based virtual screening [64–67]. On the other hand, Hou and co-worker recently illustrated that no single docking program has dominative advantages than other programs [60,67].

Herein, due to the novelty of the 4,4′-bipyridyl motif in this field, a blind docking [21] exploration was performed in order to inspect the disposition of all enantiomers (*M*) and (*P*) of compounds **1–5** and the achiral **6** into the whole TTR, focusing on the binding capability toward the $T_4$ pockets. Despite the fact that flexible docking is frequently used to model ligand-receptor complexes accounting for molecular flexibility [64,65], we do not consider protein flexibility herein, rather focusing on the capability of the new compounds to insert in the same $T_4$ binding cavity hosting $T_4$, as derived from the selected crystal complex. For this purpose, the released crystal structure of TTR complex (PDB ID: 1ICT, chains ABCD) [2] from the RCSB protein databank (www.rcbs.org) was used. AutoDock 4.2.6 was employed as docking program [68,69], and the software Chimera 1.13.1 [70] for the graphical representation of the poses derived from the docking calculation. Moreover, due to the atropisomeric features of the selected compounds, ligand flexibility is rather limited in this case. With the aim to assess the electrophilic behaviour of the halogens, the extra point [71,72] or explicit σ-hole (ESH) (Supplementary Materials, Table S7) [73,74] concept was used to model the XB [51] in TTR/4,4′-bipyridine complexes. In the context of drug design, the use of the ESH correction to model XB in drug-receptor or drug-enzyme interactions has been recently reported [75].

For both enantiomers of **1**, (*P*)-**4** and (*M*)-**5**, all poses laid outside the $T_4$ binding pockets, and on the surface of only one monomer. 4,4′-Bipyridines **2**, **3**, **6** and the enantiomers (*M*)-**4** and (*P*)-**5** were found in the $T_4$ pockets with docking score percentages lower than 21% and binding energy ranging from −6.14 to −4.93 kcal/mol. In particular, among all sites emerged from the blind docking procedure, the $T_4$ pockets were found to be the lowest energy sites for all compounds (Supplementary Materials, Table S8). By comparing the clustering of the docking poses of the (*M*) series, it could be observed a clear preference of **3** for the $T_4$ pockets compared to compounds **4** and **5** (Figure 5a). Indeed, 21% of docking poses of (*M*)-**3** laid inside the $T_4$ binding pockets, whereas lower percentages resulted for **2** and **4** (8% and 5%, respectively), these poses anchoring the side chains of the amino acid residues which identify the three hBPs (Supplementary Materials, Table S8 and Figure S2). The lowest binding energy values (Figure 5b) were observed for all poses of compounds **3** and **6** in the $T_4$ pockets, thus the 3,3′,5,5′-tetrachloro-2-iodo-4,4′-bipyridine motif showed higher binding capability for the $T_4$ pocket with respect to the other halogenated scaffolds. With the aim to confirm the docking results, all compounds **1–6** were tested in a first series of TTR FF assays.

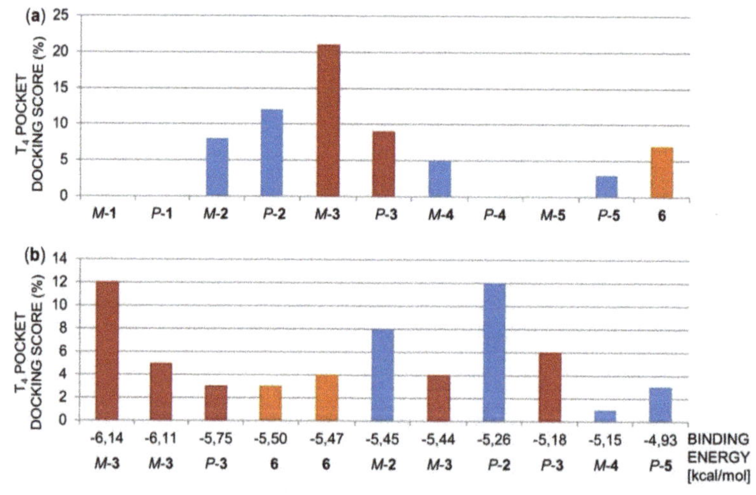


**Figure 5.** (**a**) Blind docking scores for the enantiomers of compounds **1–5** and the achiral **6** in the $T_4$ pockets; (**b**) docking score and binding energies of each pose of **1–6** laying in the $T_4$ pockets.

### 2.1.3. Acid-Mediated TTR FF Assay for Compounds **1–6** and Structure-Activity Relationships

Simulating the conditions found in the lysosome, the treatment of transparent solutions of tetrameric TTR with acids induces FF and precipitation that can be observed in vitro [15]. As FF is proportional to the turbidity degree of the parent solution, the inhibition capability of small molecules tested as fibrillogenesis inhibitors can be derived from turbidimetry analysis [76]. On this basis, the enantiomers of compounds **1–5** and the 2-iodinated-4,4′-bipyridine **6** were tested in this acid-mediated TTR fibrillogenesis assay in order to evaluate their capability to inhibit FF and precipitation. Both WT- and the mutant Y78F-TTR [8,77] were used as assay proteins. Thus, the compounds under evaluation were first incubated for 30 min with TTR at neutral pH (36 °C). The pH was then lowered to give the maximal rate of FF for a given variant (4.4 for WT, 5.0 for Y78F), and the samples were incubated for 72 h at 36 °C. For each sample, the degree of FF was determined by comparing its turbidity at 400 nm to that of a sample of TTR without test compound. On this basis, FF percentage (FF%) characterizes compound activity. Thus, the capability of compounds **1–6** in terms of FF% are summarized in Table 1. The assays were carried out at two inhibitor concentrations, namely 7.2 μM (TTR/inhibitor ratio 1:2) and 3.6 μM which is equal to the TTR concentration in plasma. diflunisal was used as the positive control, whereas TTR under acidic conditions, without inhibitor, was fixed as a negative control (100% FF mark). On this basis, 10% FF corresponds to a compound inhibiting 90% of TTR fibrillogenesis.

**Table 1.** Inhibition of WT- and Y78F-TTR amyloid fibril formation under acidic denaturation condition in the presence of diflunisal, pure enantiomers of derivatives **1–5**, and achiral **6**.

| Compound | FF% [1] (WT-TTR) | | FF% [1] (Y78F-TTR) | |
|---|---|---|---|---|
| | 7.2 μM | 3.6 μM | 7.2 μM | 3.6 μM |
| Diflunisal | 6 | 18 | 18 | 43 |
| (*M*)-**1** | 99 | 100 | 100 | 100 |
| (*P*)-**1** | 100 | 100 | 100 | 100 |
| (*M*)-**2** | 93 | 98 | 89 | 94 |
| (*P*)-**2** | 95 | 97 | 87 | 93 |
| (*M*)-**3** | 94 | 94 | 72 | 62 |
| (*P*)-**3** | 96 | 100 | 85 | 87 |
| (*M*)-**4** | 96 | 97 | 87 | 91 |
| (*P*)-**4** | 96 | 99 | 95 | 95 |
| (*M*)-**5** | 90 | 97 | 85 | 91 |
| (*P*)-**5** | 98 | 98 | 100 | 94 |
| **6** | 91 | 95 | 73 | 82 |

[1] Fibril formation (FF)% represents the extent of amyloidogenic TTR FF in the presence of inhibitors (7.2 μM or 3.6 μM inhibitor, 3.6 μM TTR, pH 4.4 (WT) or 5.0 (Y78F), 36 °C, 72 h), compared to untreated TTR (100% fibril formation). The experiments were performed in triplicate and the average values are reported in the Table. The standard deviations were in the range 5–10.

With WT-TTR, high degree of fibrillogenesis was observed for compounds **1–6** with FF% ranging from 90 to 100%, whereas with the mutant variant Y78F slightly lower values were found in almost all cases. In accord with the docking evaluations, in general the (*M*)-enantiomers were found to be slightly more effective than the (*P*)-enantiomers, whereas both enantiomers of compound **1** showed no inhibition activity against fibrillogenesis. Interestingly, compounds (*M*)-**3** and **6** proved to be the best inhibitors against Y78F-TTR fibrillogenesis with values ranging from 62 to 82%.

Compounds **1–6** were also docked in the $T_4$ pocket at the BD interface in order to derive the respective estimated free energy of binding (EFEB) (Supplementary Materials, Table S9). The crystallographic $T_4$ structure [2] was used as benchmark ligand to validate the docking procedure (Supplementary Materials, Figure S3). The predictive success of the EFEB values was verified by linear regression.

For enantiomers **1–5** and compound **6**, the results of fitting a simple linear regression model to describe the relationship between FF% and EFEB, as an independent variable, is reported in Figure 6 for Y78F at 7.2 μM (Supplementary Materials, Figure S4 for the plots of WT-TTR and Y78F at 3.6 μM). In all cases, the *P*-values of the considered independent variable are lower than the statistical benchmark value of 0.05.

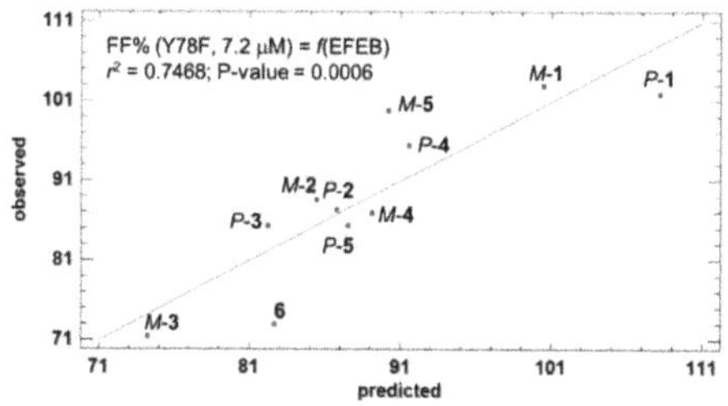


**Figure 6.** Linear regression analysis describing the relationships between FF% (Y78F-TTR, inhibitor concentration = 7.2 μM) and calculated EFEB by docking in the $T_4$ pocket (BD).

It is worth mentioning that no statistical correlation was found between FF% and the EFEB values calculated without the application of the ESH parametrization for halogens ($0.1199 \leq P\text{-value} \leq 0.9871$).

The complete inactivity of compound **1** could be related to the six bulky iodine substituents which prevent the accommodation of the molecule in the $T_4$ pocket. From a comparative analysis of the structure-activity relationships, it seems that the presence of iodine substituents at positions 3,3′,5,5′ (compounds **1**, **4**, **5**) is detrimental for both binding and inhibition activity, whereas 2- and 2′-iodine substitutions exhibit a beneficial effect on 4,4′-bipyridine activity.

From these results, the 3,3′,5,5′-tetrachloro-2-iodo-4,4′-bipyridyl substructure (iodine $V_{S,max}$ values: 140.8 kJ/mol for **3**, 136.8 kJ/mol for **6**) has been identified as the most interesting scaffold for elaborating more specific compounds. On this basis, compounds **7–10** were prepared by focused procedures to introduce a phenyl, a 4-pyridyl, a 4-hydroxyphenyl and a hydroxymethyl as a 2′-substituent, respectively. These substituents were selected to probe how subtle structural changes at position 2′ can influence the inhibition activity.

## 2.2. Chemistry

### 2.2.1. Syntheses of 4,4′-Bipyridines 1–10

The synthesis of chiral hexahalogenated 4,4′-bipyridines **1–5** was previously reported by our groups, exploiting convergent or divergent strategies depending on halogen type and position on the heteroaromatic scaffold [47,48]. These methodologies proved to be extremely versatile and allowed to introduce Cl, Br, and I at any position of the 4,4′-bipyridyl scaffold [48].

3,3′,5,5′-Tetrachloro-2,2′-diiodo-4,4′-bipyridine (**3**) was prepared in two steps from the commercially available 2-bromo-3,5-dichloropyridine (**11**). First, a lithium diisopropylamide (LDA)-mediated dimerization afforded 3,3′,5,5′-tetrachloro-2,2′-dibromo-4,4′-bipyridine (**12**), and then the bromine atoms in 2,2′-positions were exchanged for iodines through a diaminocopper-catalyzed Finkelstein reaction. Along with the expected 4,4′-bipyridine **3**, careful chromatographic purification allowed obtaining in small quantity the 3,3′,5,5′-tetrachloro-2-iodo- 4,4′-bipyridine **6** (Scheme 1).

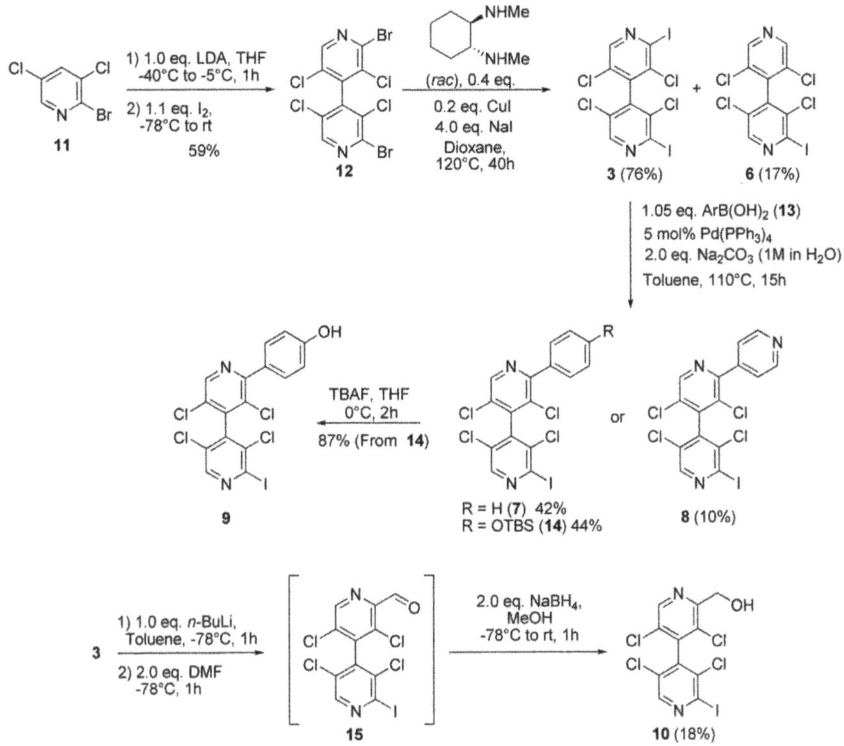

**Scheme 1.** Synthesis of bipyridines **6–10**.

For 4,4′-bipyridines **7–9**, the aromatic ring in 2-position was introduced through a Suzuki coupling reaction involving 4,4′-bipyridine **3** and one equivalent of the respective boronic acid **13**. The use of phenyl- and 4-pyridylboronic acids **13a,b** afforded 3,3′,5,5′-tetrachloro-2-iodo-2′-phenyl-4,4′-bipyridine (**7**) and 3,3′,5,5′-tetrachloro-2-iodo-2′-(4- pyridyl)-4,4′-bipyridine (**8**), respectively.

The direct synthesis of the 3,3′,5,5′-tetrachloro-2-iodo-2′-(4-hydroxyphenyl)-4,4′-bipyridine (**9**) by coupling of **3** with 4-hydroxyphenylboronic acid (**13c**) failed under Suzuki coupling conditions. Therefore, compound **9** was obtained in two steps by using the *tert*-butyldimethylsilyl (TBS)-protected 4-hydroxyphenylboronic acid **13d**. After the cross-coupling reaction between compounds **3** and **13d**, 3,3′,5,5′-tetrachloro-2-iodo-2′-(4-*tert*-butyldimethylsilyloxyphenyl)- 4,4′-bipyridine (**14**) was isolated, and the TBS-protecting group was subsequently removed by using a tetrahydrofuran solution of tetrabutylammonium fluoride ($n$-Bu$_4$NF), affording 4,4′-bipyridine **9**. Finally, 3,3′,5,5′-tetrachloro-2-iodo-2′-hydroxymethyl-4,4′-bipyridine (**10**) was obtained in a one-pot two-step process starting from 4,4′-bipyridine **3**. After iodine-lithium exchange with one equivalent of $n$-butyllithium ($n$-BuLi) in toluene, the lithiated species was quenched with dimethylformamide (DMF) to give the aldehyde intermediate **15** which was directly reduced with sodium borohydride ($NaBH_4$) to afford bipyridine **10**.

### 2.2.2. Enantioseparation of 4,4′-Bipyridines 7–10 on Chiral Stationary Phases

*Rac*-4,4′-bipyridines **1–5** were enantioseparated at multimilligram scale on polysaccharide-based chiral stationary phases, as previously reported by our groups [48,59]. Pure enantiomers (>95% ee) of 3,3′,5,5′-tetrachloro-2-iodo-2′-substituted-4,4′-bipyridines **7–10** were obtained in good amounts by means of HPLC multimilligram enantioseparation under normal phase elution conditions (Supplementary Materials, Table S10). In particular, the enantiomers of compounds **7** and **9** were recovered by using Chiralpak IA (immobilized amylose tris(3,5-dimethyl- phenylcarbamate)) as a chiral column, whereas the Chiralcel OD-H (cellulose tris(3,5-dimethylphenylcarbamate)) was used for the enantioseparations of compounds **8** and **10**. Recorded in ethanol, the ECD spectra of the four enantiomer pairs **7–10** showed the expected opposite traces for the two atropisomers (Supplementary Materials, Figures S21–S24).

#### 2.2.3. Absolute Configuration Assignment of **7–10**

The absolute configuration of HPLC-separated enantiomers of bipyridines **1** and **2** was previously assigned through XRD analysis by using the anomalous dispersion of heavy atoms [48,59]. However, for the enantiomers of bipyridines **3–5**, which could not be crystallized, the absolute configuration was determined by electronic circular dichroism (ECD) coupled with time-dependent density functional theory (TD-DFT) calculations [59]. Analogously, the absolute configurations assignment of enantiomers of the newly synthesized bipyridines **7–10** was performed by comparing the measured ECD spectra with the ones calculated by TD-DFT. The calculation of the ECD spectra was performed considering all the possible conformers arising from the rotation of the substituent in 2′-position with respect to the pyridine ring [78] (see Supplementary Materials, S6 for details). For each compound, except a systematic shift of about 15 nm between the measured and calculated spectra [50,78], a very good match was obtained allowing unambiguous absolute configuration assignment of all enantiomers (Supplementary Materials, Table S10 and Figures S25–S28).

### 2.3. *Biological Evaluation of Compounds* **7–10** *and Structure-Activity Relationships*

The enantiomers of compounds **7–10** were tested by using the acid-mediated TTR FF assays described above, in order to evaluate their capability to inhibit fibrillogenesis as soluble TTR is treated with acidic medium. WT- and the mutants Y78F- [8], and V30M-TTR [7] were used as assay proteins, whose stability order is WT > V30M > Y78F [7,8]. The results are reported in Table 2.

**Table 2.** Inhibition of WT-, Y78F-, and V30M-TTR amyloid fibril formation under acidic denaturation condition in the presence of diflunisal, and pure enantiomers of derivatives **7–10**.

| Compound | FF% [1] (WT-TTR) | | FF% [1] (Y78F-TTR) | | FF% [1] (V30M-TTR) | |
|---|---|---|---|---|---|---|
| | 7.2 μM | 3.6 μM | 7.2 μM | 3.6 μM | 7.2 μM | 3.6 μM |
| Diflunisal | 6 | 18 | 18 | 43 | 36 | 33 |
| (*M*)-**7** | 96 | 100 | 82 | 84 | nd | nd |
| (*P*)-**7** | 88 | 95 | 71 | 88 | nd | nd |
| (*M*)-**8** | 58 | 72 | 79 | 82 | 50 | 58 |
| (*P*)-**8** | 42 | 67 | 51 | 67 | 38 | 43 |
| (*M*)-**9** | 16 | 49 | 44 | 71 | 38 | 40 |
| (*P*)-**9** | 17 | 49 | 44 | 72 | 39 | 41 |
| (*M*)-**10** | 62 | 79 | 80 | 88 | 59 | 75 |
| (*P*)-**10** | 80 | 89 | 85 | 91 | 67 | 72 |

[1] Fibril formation (FF)% represents the extent of amyloidogenic TTR FF in the presence of inhibitors (7.2 μM or 3.6 μM inhibitor, 3.6 μM TTR, pH 4.4 (WT) or 5.0 (V30M and Y78F), 36 °C, 72 h), compared to untreated TTR (100% fibril formation). The experiments were performed in triplicate and the average values are reported in the Table. The standard deviations were in the range 5–10; nd, not determined.

Among the three TTR forms, the FF% values were higher against V30M and Y78F than WT-TTR. On the basis of the turbidimetric assay results, the inhibition activity trend was shown to be **9** > **8** > **10** > **7**, with few exceptions. Again, the (*M*) enantiomers were found to be more active than the (*P*)-enantiomers for compounds **9** and **10**, whereas the (*P*)-enantiomers proved to be more effective for **7** and **8**. For both enantiomers of compound **9**, amyloid fibrillogenesis was significantly suppressed on WT-TTR at 7.2 μM of inhibitor concentration (FF% 16 and 17). Both (*M*)-**9** and (*P*)-**9** were also tested at different concentrations ranging from 0 to 15 μM using diflunisal for comparison (Supplementary

Information, Figure S29). As reported for other known TTR stabilizers, compound **9** dose-dependently inhibited WT-TTR amyloidogenesis.

Structure-activity relationships revealed that a HB centre on one pyridyl ring contributes to increase the inhibition activity, moderately for compounds **8** and **10**, more for compound **9**. In compound **7**, the presence of the hydrophobic phenyl, as distinctive substituent, appears to be detrimental for the inhibition activity. Molecular docking carried out targeting the $T_4$ pocket showed that compounds **7–10** could be accommodated in the hormone-binding site. Focusing on the four (*M*)-enantiomers, the following observations emerged (Figure 7):

(i) Compound (*M*)-**9** (Figure 7a) fully occupies the $T_4$ pocket (molecular length 13.2 Å, $V_S$ isosurface enclosed volume 367.0 Å$^3$), where the 4-hydroxyphenyl group is oriented toward B:Thr$_{106}$ and B:Val$_{121}$ (hBP$_1$) and the four chlorines at the 3,3,5,5′-positions of the heteroaromatic ring anchor the residues B:Ala$_{108}$ and D:Ala$_{108'}$ (hBP$_2$). Moreover, the $N'_{pyr}$ ($V_{S,min}$ = -128.3 kJ/mol) forms a HB with the ε-ammonium group of D:Lys$_{15'}$ (2.6 Å), and 2-iodine ($V_{S,max}$ = 129.8 kJ/mol) showed a short contact with the side chain oxygen of D:Ser$_{117''}$ (3.2 Å) (hBP$_3$). Interestingly, the comparison of the respective $V_S$ isosurface evidences for compound **9** a shape similarity to both $T_4$ and tafamidis (Supplementary Information, Figure S1);

(ii) Compound **10** (Figure 7b) is the smallest molecule of the series with a molecular length of about 9.80 Å and a volume of 303.1 Å$^3$, therefore it is not able to fully occupy the $T_4$ pocket, 2-iodine showing a longer contact with B:Ser$_{117}$ (4.4 Å) despite a positive $V_{S,max}$ value (141.6 kJ/mol). Moreover, the best conformation of compound **10** is characterized by an intramolecular HB involving the hydroxyl group and $N'_{pyr}$ ($V_{S,min}$ = −29.12 kJ/mol). The latter is therefore less prone to interact with the side chain of D:Lys$_{15'}$;

(iii) For both compounds **7** and **8** (Figure 7c), reverse binding modes were found by molecular docking, with the $N_{pyr}$ interacting with D:Lys$_{15'}$ in all cases. The basic difference between the two compounds, which could justify the different inhibition activity, lies in the presence of a $N_{pyr}$, as a HB acceptor, at the 2′-position of compound **8** which makes possible an interaction with B:Ser$_{117}$, thus anchoring the two monomers B and D.

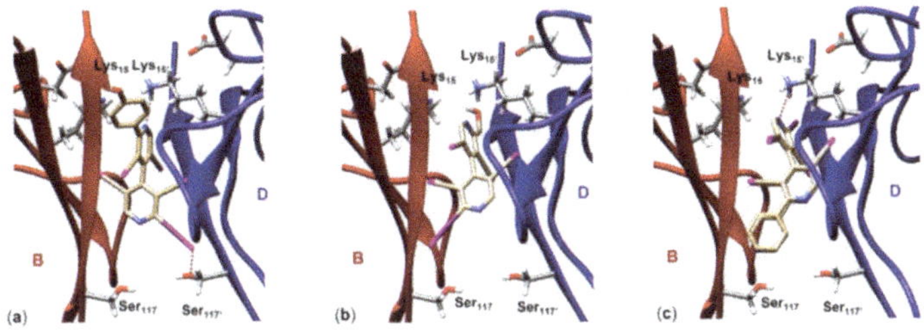


**Figure 7.** Docking modes into the $T_4$ binding pocket (BD) for the (*M*)-enantiomers of **9** (**a**), **10** (**b**) and the pair **7**/**8** (superimposed structures) (**c**).

## 3. Materials and Methods

### 3.1. Chemistry

#### 3.1.1. General Information

Proton ($^1$H-NMR) and carbon ($^{13}$C-NMR) nuclear magnetic resonance spectra were recorded on Bruker Avance III instruments operating at 500 MHz (Bruker Corporation, Billerica, MA, USA). The chemical shifts are given in parts per million (ppm) on the delta scale. The solvent peak was used as reference values for $^1$H-NMR ($CDCl_3$ = 7.26 ppm) and for $^{13}$C-NMR ($CDCl_3$ = 77.16 ppm). Data are presented as follows: chemical shift, multiplicity (s= singlet, d= doublet, t= triplet, q= quartet, quint= quintet, m= multiplet, b= broad), integration, and coupling constants (*J*/Hz). High-resolution mass spectra (HRMS) data were recorded on a Bruker micrOTOF spectrometer equipped with an orthogonal electrospray interface (ESI). Melting points were measured on Stuart SMP3 apparatus from Cole Parmer (London, UK) and are uncorrected. Analytical thin layer chromatography (TLC plates from Merck KGaA, Darmstadt, Germany) was carried out on silica gel 60 F254 plates with visualization by ultraviolet light. Reagents and solvents were purified using standard means. Tetrahydrofuran (THF) was distilled from sodium metal/benzophenone and stored under an argon atmosphere. Anhydrous reactions were carried out in flame-dried glassware and under an argon atmosphere. 2,2′,3,3′,5,5′-Hexaiodo-4,4′-bipyridine (**1**), 2,2′,3,3′,5,5′-hexachloro-4,4′-bipyridine (**2**), 3,3′,5,5′-tetrachloro-2,2′-diiodo-4,4′-bipyridine (**3**), 2,2′,5,5′-tetrachloro-3,3′- diiodo-4,4′-bipyridine (**4**), 2,2′,3,3′-tetrachloro-5,5′-diiodo-4,4′-bipyridine (**5**) and 3,3′,5,5′-tetra- chloro-2,2′-dibromo-4,4′-bipyridine (**12**) were prepared according to the literature [48]. All other chemicals were used as received. CD spectra were recorded on a J-810 instrument from Jasco (JASCO International Co. Ltd., Tokyo, Japan) at room temperature using 0.15–0.30 mM samples in ethanol and a 1 mm quartz cell, with the following conditions: 100 nm/min scanning speed, 1 nm data pitch, 4.0 nm bandwidth, 1 s response time.

#### 3.1.2. Syntheses of 3,3′,5,5′-Tetrachloro-2,2′-diiodo-4,4′-bipyridine (3) and 3,3′,5,5′-tetrachloro-2-iodo-4,4′-bipyridine (6)

In a dry Schlenk tube were placed 2,2′-dibromo-tetrahalo-4,4′-bipyridine (800 mg, 1.77 mmol), NaI (1.06 g, 7.08 mmol), CuI (50 mg, 0.35 mmol), and (*rac*)-*trans*-*N*,*N*-dimethyl- cyclohexane-1,2-diamine (64 mg, 0.71 mmol). The Schlenk tube was evacuated and filled with argon before addition of degassed dioxane (5 mL). The mixture was heated at 120 °C for 60 h. After cooling to room temperature, $NH_4OH$ (7 mL) and $H_2O$ (8 mL) were added. Then, the product was extracted with dichloromethane (4 × 40 mL). After drying over $Na_2SO_4$, filtration, and concentration, the mixture was purified by chromatography on silica gel (pentane/dichloromethane 7/3) to give bipyridine **3** [48] (white powder, 733 mg, 76%, $R_f$ = 0.27) and bipyridine **6** (white powder, 126 mg, 17%, $R_f$ = 0.15). Mp: 126–127 °C; $^1$H-NMR (500 MHz, $CDCl_3$) δ 8.67 (s, 2H), 8.46 (s, 1H). $^{13}$C-NMR (126 MHz, $CDCl_3$) δ 148.0; 147.8; 140.6; 140.3; 137.3; 131.2; 130.9; 119.5. HRMS (ESI-TOF) $[M + H]^+$ *m*/*z*: Calcd. for $C_{10}H_3Cl_4IN_2$ 418.8168, found: 418.8152.

#### 3.1.3. General Procedure for the Synthesis of Bipyridines 7, 8 and 14

In a dry Schlenk tube were placed bipyridine **6** (0.28–0.72 mmol) and tetrakis(triphenylphosphine) palladium (10 mol%). The Schlenk tube was evacuated and filled with argon before addition of degassed toluene (2–5 mL). Then a boronic acid solution (1 eq.) in methanol (0.5–1.0 mL) was added and after 10 min of stirring, at room temperature, a sodium carbonate solution (2 eq.) in distilled water (0.5–1.0 mL) was added. The mixture was heated at 110 °C for 20 h. After cooling to room temperature, brine (10 mL) was added. Then, the product was extracted with dichloromethane (3 × 15 mL). After drying over $Na_2SO_4$, filtration, and concentration, the products were purified by chromatography on silica gel.

3,3′,5,5′-Tetrachloro-2-iodo-2′-phenyl-4,4′-bipyridine (7)

Compound **7** was obtained as colorless solid (85 mg, 62%) using the following conditions: **6** (150 mg, 0.28 mmol), tetrakis(triphenylphosphine)palladium (32 mg, 0.028 mmol), phenylboronic acid (34 mg, 0.28 mmol), sodium carbonate (59 mg, 0.55 mmol). Chromatography on silica gel (cyclohexane/ethyl acetate 95/5). Mp: 105–106 °C; $^1$H-NMR (500 MHz, $CDCl_3$) δ 8.76 (s, 1H), 8.49 (s, 1H), 7.78–7.71 (m, 2H), 7.53–7.46 (m, 3H). $^{13}$C-NMR (126 MHz, $CDCl_3$) δ 156.2, 147.8, 147.5, 141.9, 141.3, 137.3, 137.1, 131.2, 129.6, 129.5, 129.1, 128.7, 128.4, 119.5. HRMS (ESI-TOF) $[M + H]^+$ *m*/*z*: Calcd. for $C_{16}H_8Cl_4N_2$ 495.8481, found: 494.8509.

3,3′,5,5′-Tetrachloro-2-iodo-2′-(4-pyridyl)-4,4′-bipyridine (8)

Compound **8** was obtained as a viscous wax (49 mg, approx. 75% purity according to $^{1}$H-NMR after chromatography on silica gel with eluent: cyclohexane/ethyl acetate/triethylamine 85/10/5) using the following conditions: **6** (150 mg, 0.28 mmol), tetrakis(triphenylphosphine)palladium (22 mg, 0.019 mmol), 4-pyridinylboronic acid (35 mg, 0.29 mmol), sodium carbonate (59 mg, 0.55 mmol). A pure sample (13.3 mg, 10% yield) was obtained after HPLC purification on a Chiralpak IA column (*n*-hexane/2-propanol 90:10, 0.8 mL/min). $^{1}$H-NMR (500 MHz, $CDCl_3$) δ 8.79 (m, 3H), 8.50 (s, 1H), 7.71 (d, *J* = 5.0 Hz, 2H). $^{13}$C-NMR (126 MHz, $CDCl_3$) δ 153.3, 150.1, 148.0, 147.9, 144.6, 142.4, 140.8, 137.2, 131.1, 130.7, 129.1, 124.0, 119.5. HRMS (ESI-TOF) $[M + H]^+$ *m*/*z*: Calcd. for $C_{15}H_7Cl_4IN_3$ 495.8433, found: 494.8400.

3,3′,5,5′-Tetrachloro-2-iodo-2′-(4-((tert-butyldimethylsilyl)oxy)phenyl)-4,4′-bipyridine (14)

Compound **14** was obtained as viscous oil (199 mg, 44%) using the following conditions: **6** (324 mg, 0.72 mmol), tetrakis(triphenylphosphine)palladium (58 mg, 0.0150 mmol), 4-(*tert*-butyldimethylsilyloxy)-phenylboronic acid (190 mg, 0.753 mmol), sodium carbonate (152 mg, 1.43 mmol). Chromatography on silica gel (cyclohexane/ethyl acetate 95/5). $^{1}$H-NMR (500 MHz, $CDCl_3$) δ 8.72 (s, 1*H*), 8.48 (s, 1*H*), 7.68 (d, *J* = 8.7 Hz, 2H), 6.94 (d, *J* = 8.7 Hz, 2H), 1.00 (s, 9H), 0.24 (s, 6H). $^{13}$C-NMR (126 MHz, $CDCl_3$) δ 157.1; 155.8; 147.8; 147.3; 141.9; 141.5; 137.3; 131.3; 131.1; 130.1; 128.5; 128.4; 120.0; 119.5; 25.8; 18.4; −4.2. HRMS (ESI-TOF) $[M + H]^+$ *m*/*z*: Calcd. for $C_{22}H_{22}Cl_4IN_2OSi$ 624.9275, found: 624.9295.

3.1.4. 3,3′,5,5′-Tetrachloro-2-iodo-2′-(4-hydroxyphenyl)-4,4′-bipyridine (**9**)

To a stirred solution of bipyridine **14** (70 mg, 0.11 mmol) in THF (3 mL), under argon and at 0 °C, a TBAF solution (0.016 mL, 1M in THF) was slowly added. After 30 min stirring at 0 °C, the reaction was quenched with $NH_4Cl$ and extracted with dichloromethane (3 × 10 mL). After drying over $Na_2SO_4$, filtration, and concentration, the product was purified by chromatography on silica gel (cyclohexane/ethyl acetate 85/15) to give **9** as a viscous wax (50 mg, 87%). $^{1}$H-NMR (500 MHz, $CDCl_3$) δ 8.72 (s, 1H), 8.48 (s, 1H), 7.69 (d, *J* = 8.7 Hz, 2H), 6.93 (d, *J* = 8.7 Hz, 2H), 5.24 (s, 1H). $^{13}$C- NMR (126 MHz, $CDCl_3$) δ 156.9; 155.6; 147.8; 147.3; 142.0; 141.4; 137.3; 131.4; 131.2; 129.6; 128.6; 128.4; 119.5; 115.3. HRMS (ESI-TOF) $[M + H]^+$ *m*/*z*: Calcd. for $C_{22}H_{22}Cl_4IN_2OSi$ 510.8430, found: 510.8449.

3.1.5. Synthesis of 3,3′,5,5′-Tetrachloro-2-iodo-2′-hydroxymethyl-4,4′-bipyridine (**10**)

Bipyridine **3** (0.458 mmol, 250 mg) was dissolved in toluene (5 mL) and the solution was cooled to −78 °C. *n*-BuLi (1.2 M, 0.458 mmol, 0.38 mL) was added dropwise and the mixture was stirred at −78 °C for 1 h. DMF (0.916 mmol, 71 μL) was added and stirring was continued at the same temperature for 1 h. $NaBH_4$ (1.374 mmol, 52.2 mg) was added followed by methanol (0.5 mL), the cooling bath was removed and stirring was maintained for 1 h. The mixture was hydrolysed at 0 °C and extracted with ethyl acetate. After drying over $Na_2SO_4$, filtration and evaporation, the residue was purified twice by chromatography on silica gel (cyclohexane/ethyl acetate 9/1) to give bipyridine **10** as colourless wax (66 mg, 18%). $^{1}$H-NMR (500 MHz, $CDCl_3$) δ 8.67 (s, 1H); 8.48 (s, 1H); 4.85 (s, 2H), 3.98 (bs, 1H). $^{13}$C-NMR (126 MHz, $CDCl_3$) δ 155.3; 147.8; 146.2; 141.3; 140.3; 137.3; 131.1; 129.6; 128.0; 119.5; 61.9. HRMS (ESI-TOF) $[M + H]^+$ *m*/*z*: Calcd. for $C_{11}H_5Cl_4IN_2O$ 448.8273, found: 448.8281.

3.1.6. Multimilligram Enantioseparation of **7**–**10**

An Agilent Technologies (Waldbronn, Germany) 1100 Series HPLC system (high-pressure binary gradient system equipped with a diode-array detector operating at multiple wavelengths (220, 254, 280, 360 nm), a programmable autosampler with a 20 L loop, and a thermostatted column compartment) was employed for analytical and multimilligram separations. Data acquisition and analysis were carried out with Agilent Technologies ChemStation Version B.04.03 chromatographic data

a possible molecular mechanism for the observed inhibition activity. Both experimental and theoretical results evidenced the importance of HB sites located in the distinctive 2′-substituent and the capability of 2-iodine as XB donor. Despite the fact that some issues such as plasma TTR binding selectivity has still to be tackled and that the new structures need optimization, the present study revealed the potentiality of halogenated 4,4′-bipyridines for the development of new TTR amyloidogenesis inhibitors.

**Supplementary Materials:** The following are available online: Figure S1: $V_S$ molecular isosurfaces (0.002 au) calculated for (*P*) and (*M*) enantiomers of **9**, $T_4$, and Tafamidis, Figure S2: Blind docking poses of compounds (*M*)-**3** and **6** on the whole TTR, Figure S3: Comparison of the docked pose of $T_4$ into TTR (BD:$T_4$ binding pocket) with the crystallographic structure of $T_4$ (released from PDB ID: 1ICT), Figure S4: Linear regression analysis describing the relationships between FF% and calculated EFEB by docking in the $T_4$ pocket (BD), Figures S5-S16: NMR spectra, Figures S17-S20: HPLC chromatograms, Figures S21-S24: ECD spectra, Figures S25-S28: comparison of calculated and experimental ECD spectra, Figure S29: Inhibition of WT-TTR in the presence of (*M*)-**9** and (*P*)-**9** tested at different concentrations, Table S1: Calculated $V_S$ on a 0.002 au isosurface and molecular geometrical parameters for polyhalogenated 4,4′-bipyridines **1–6**, Table S2: Calculated $V_S$ on a 0.002 au isosurface and molecular geometrical parameters for Tafamidis and Thyroxyne ($T_4$) (from crystal structure, PDB ID:1ICT), Table S3: Calculated distribution, pattern and properties of conformations A and B of 4,4′-bipyridines **7–9**, Table S4: Calculated distribution, pattern and properties of conformations A-F of 4,4′-bipyridine **10**, Table S5: Calculated $V_S$ on a 0.002 au isosurface and molecular geometrical parameters for conformations A and B of 2′-aryl-3,3′,5,5′-tetrachloro-2-iodo-4,4′-bipyridines **7–9**, Table S6: Calculated $V_S$ on a 0.002 au isosurface and molecular geometrical parameters for conformations A-F of 4,4′-bipyridine **10**, Table S7: Parameters used for the extra point (ExP) of charge (X = Cl, I), Table S8: Blind docking resultsa targeting poses found in the $T_4$ binding pockets, Table S9: Docking results for 4,4′-bipyridines **1–6** in the $T_4$ binding pocket, Table S10: Optimized multimilligram enantioseparation of 4,4′-bipyridines **7–10**.

**Author Contributions:** Conceptualization, P.P. (Paola Peluso) and V.M.; methodology, P.P. (Paola Peluso), A.D. and G.A.; syntheses, V.M., P.P. (Patrick Pale) and R.W.; HPLC, P.P. (Paola Peluso); X-ray analysis and TD-DFT calculations, E.A.; $V_s$ calculations and docking, P.P. (Paola Peluso), A.D. and R.D.; biological experiments, G.A. and M.A.; data curation, P.P. (Paola Peluso); writing-original draft preparation, P.P (Paola Peluso) and V.M.; writing, review and editing, all authors; funding acquisition, V.M. and S.C. All authors have read and agreed to the published version of the manuscript.

**Funding:** This research was funded by the International Center Frontier Research in Chemistry (icFRC), the LabEx CSC (ANR-10-LABX-0026 CSC) and Venice Ca' Foscari University, Italy (Department of Molecular Science and Nanosystems, DSMN ADIR funds).

**Acknowledgments:** This work has been supported by Università Ca' Foscari Venezia, Italy (Dipartimento di Scienze Molecolari e Nanosistemi, DSMN ADIR funds). We thank the International Center Frontier Research in Chemistry (icFRC) and the Laboratory of Excellence for Complex System Chemistry (LabEx CSC). M.A., PhD program at the DISTABIF, Università degli Studi della Campania "Luigi Vanvitelli", PhD fellowship POR Campania FSE 2014/2020 "Dottorati di Ricerca Con Caratterizzazione Industriale".

**Conflicts of Interest:** The authors declare no conflict of interest.

## References

1. Wojtczak, A.; Cody, V.; Luft, J.R.; Pangborn, W. Structures of human transthyretin complexed with thyroxine at 2.0 Å resolution and 3′,5′-dinitro-*N*-acetyl-*L*-thyronine at 2.2 Å resolution. *Acta Cryst.* **1996**, *52*, 758–765. [CrossRef] [PubMed]
2. Wojtczak, A.; Neumann, P.; Cody, V. Structure of a new polymorphic monoclinic form of human transthyretin at 3 Å resolution reveals a mixed complex between unliganded and $T_4$-bound tetramers of TTR. *Acta Cryst.* **2001**, *57*, 957–967. [CrossRef] [PubMed]
3. Palaninathan, S.K. Nearly 200 X-Ray crystal structures of transthyretin: What do they tell us about this protein and the design of drugs for TTR amyloidosis? *Curr. Med. Chem.* **2012**, *19*, 2324–2342. [CrossRef] [PubMed]
4. Blaney, J.M.; Jorgensen, E.C.; Connolly, M.L.; Ferrin, T.E.; Langridge, R.; Oatley, S.J.; Burridge, J.M.; Blake, C.C.F. Computer graphics in drug design: Molecular modelling of thyroid hormone-prealbumin interactions. *J. Med. Chem.* **1982**, *25*, 785–790. [CrossRef]
5. Khanam, H.; Ali, A.; Asif, M. Shamsuzzaman Neurodegenerative diseases linked to misfolded proteins and their therapeutic approaches: A review. *Eur. J. Med. Chem.* **2016**, *124*, 1121–1141. [CrossRef]
6. Pande, M.; Srivastava, R. Molecular and clinical insights into protein misfolding and associated amyloidosis. *Eur. J. Med. Chem.* **2019**, *184*, 111753. [CrossRef]

7. McCutchen, S.L.; Lai, Z.; Miroy, G.J.; Kelly, J.W.; Colón, W. Comparison of lethal and nonlethal transthyretin variants and their relationship to amyloid disease. *Biochemistry* **1995**, *34*, 13527–13536. [CrossRef]
8. Redondo, C.; Damas, A.M.; Olofsson, A.; Lundgren, E.; Saraiva, M.J.M. Search for intermediate structures in transthyretin fibrillogenesis: Soluble tetrameric TYR78Phe TTR expresses a specific epitope present only in amyloid fibrils. *J. Mol. Biol.* **2000**, *304*, 461–470. [CrossRef]
9. Gimeno, A.; Santos, L.M.; Alemi, M.; Rivas, J.; Blasi, D.; Cotrina, E.Y.; Llop, J.; Valencia, G.; Cardoso, I.; Quintana, J.; et al. Insights on the interaction between transthyretin and Aβ in solution. A saturation transfer difference (STD) NMR analysis of the role of iododiflunisal. *J. Med. Chem.* **2017**, *60*, 5749–5758. [CrossRef]
10. Rios, X.; Gómez-Vallejo, V.; Martín, A.; Cossío, U.; Morcillo, M.A.; Alemi, M.; Cardoso, I.; Quintana, J.; Jimeénez-Barbero, J.; Cotrina, E.Y.; et al. Radiochemical examination of transthyretin (TTR) brain penetration assisted by iododiflunisal, a TTR tetramer stabilizer and a new candidate drug for AD. *Sci. Rep.* **2019**, *9*, 13672. [CrossRef]
11. Miroy, G.J.; Lai, Z.; Lashuel, H.A.; Peterson, S.A.; Strang, C.; Kelly, J.W. Inhibiting transthyretin amyloid fibril formation via protein stabilization. *Proc. Natl. Acad. Sci. USA* **1996**, *93*, 15051–15056. [CrossRef]
12. Hammarström, P.; Wiseman, R.L.; Powers, E.T.; Kelly, J.W. Prevention of transthyretin amyloid disease by changing protein misfolding energetics. *Science* **2003**, *299*, 713–716. [CrossRef]
13. Yee, A.W.; Aldeghi, M.; Blakeley, M.P.; Ostermann, A.; Mas, P.J.; Moulin, M.; de Sanctis, D.; Bowler, M.W.; Mueller-Dieckmann, C.; Mitchell, E.P.; et al. A molecular mechanism for transthyretin amyloidogenesis. *Nat. Commun.* **2019**, *10*, 925. [CrossRef]
14. Rosenblum, H.; Castano, A.; Alvarez, J.; Goldsmith, J.; Helmke, S.; Maurer, M.S. TTR (Transthyretin) stabilizers are associated with improved survival in patients with TTR cardiac amyloidosis. *Circ. Heart Fail.* **2018**, *11*, e004769. [CrossRef]
15. Oza, V.B.; Smith, C.; Raman, P.; Koepf, E.K.; Lashuel, H.A.; Petrassi, H.M.; Chiang, K.P.; Powers, E.T.; Sacchettini, J.C.; Kelly, J.W. Synthesis, structure, and activity of diclofenac analogues as transthyretin amyloid fibril formation inhibitors. *J. Med. Chem.* **2002**, *45*, 321–332. [CrossRef]
16. Adamski-Werner, S.L.; Palaninathan, S.K.; Sacchettini, J.C.; Kelly, J.W. Diflunisal analogues stabilize the native state of transthyretin. Potent inhibition of amyloidogenesis. *J. Med. Chem.* **2004**, *47*, 355–374. [CrossRef]
17. Gales, L.; Macedo-Ribeiro, S.; Arsequell, G.; Valencia, G.; Saraiva, M.J.; Damas, A.M. Human transthyretin in complex with iododiflunisal: Structural features associated with a potent amyloid inhibitor. *Biochem. J.* **2005**, *388*, 615–621. [CrossRef]
18. Johnson, S.M.; Wiseman, R.L.; Sekijima, Y.; Green, N.S.; Adamski-Werner, S.L.; Kelly, J.W. Native state kinetic stabilization as a strategy to ameliorate protein misfolding diseases: A focus on the transthyretin amyloidosis. *Acc. Chem. Res.* **2005**, *38*, 911–921. [CrossRef] [PubMed]
19. Miyata, M.; Sato, T.; Kugimiya, M.; Sho, M.; Nakamura, T.; Ikemizu, S.; Chirifu, M.; Mizuguchi, M.; Nabeshima, Y.; Suwa, Y.; et al. The crystal structure of the green tea polyphenol (-)-epigallocatechin gallate-transthyretin complex reveals a novel binding site distinct from the thyroxine binding site. *Biochemistry* **2010**, *49*, 6104–6114. [CrossRef] [PubMed]
20. Yokoyama, T.; Kosada, Y.; Mizuguchi, M. Inhibitory activities of propolis and its promising component, caffeic acid phenethyl ester, against amyloidogenesis of human transthyretin. *J. Med. Chem.* **2014**, *57*, 8928–8935. [CrossRef] [PubMed]
21. Ortore, G.; Orlandini, E.; Braca, A.; Ciccone, L.; Rossello, A.; Martinelli, A.; Nencetti, S. Targeting different transthyretin binding sites with unusual natural compounds. *ChemMedChem* **2016**, *11*, 1865–1874. [CrossRef] [PubMed]
22. Kim, B.; Park, H.; Lee, S.K.; Park, S.J.; Koo, T.-S.; Kang, N.S.; Hong, K.B.; Choi, S. Systemic optimization and structural evaluation of quinoline derivatives as transthyretin amyloidogenesis inhibitors. *Eur. J. Med. Chem.* **2016**, *123*, 777–787. [CrossRef] [PubMed]
23. Smith, T.P.; Windsor, I.W.; Forest, K.T.; Raines, R.T. Stilbene boronic acids form a covalent bond with human transthyretin and inhibit its aggregation. *J. Med. Chem.* **2017**, *60*, 7820–7834. [CrossRef] [PubMed]
24. Yokoyama, T.; Mizuguchi, M. Inhibition of the amyloidogenesis of transthyretin by natural products and synthetic compounds. *Biol. Pharm. Bull.* **2018**, *41*, 979–984. [CrossRef]
25. Yokoyama, T.; Mizuguchi, M. Crown ethers as transthyretin amyloidogenesis inhibitors. *J. Med. Chem.* **2019**, *62*, 2076–2082. [CrossRef]

26. Green, N.S.; Palaninathan, S.K.; Sacchettini, J.C.; Kelly, J.W. Synthesis and characterization of potent bivalent amyloidosis inhibitors that bind prior to transthyretin tetramerization. *J. Am. Chem. Soc.* **2003**, *125*, 13404–13414. [CrossRef]
27. Corazza, A.; Verona, G.; Waudby, C.A.; Mangione, P.P.; Bingham, R.; Uings, I.; Canetti, D.; Nocerino, P.; Taylor, G.W.; Pepys, M.B.; et al. Binding of monovalent and bivalent ligands by transthyretin causes different short- and long-distance conformational changes. *J. Med. Chem.* **2019**, *62*, 8274–8283. [CrossRef]
28. Inoue, M.; Ueda, M.; Higashi, T.; Anno, T.; Fujisawa, K.; Motoyama, K.; Mizuguchi, M.; Ando, Y.; Jono, H.; Arima, H. Therapeutic potential of polyamidoamine dendrimer for amyloidogenic transthyretin amyloidosis. *ACS Chem. Neurosci.* **2019**, *10*, 2584–2590. [CrossRef]
29. Bulawa, C.E.; Connelly, S.; DeVit, M.; Wang, L.; Weigel, C.; Fleming, J.A.; Packman, J.; Powers, E.T.; Wiseman, R.L.; Foss, T.R.; et al. Tafamidis, a potent and selective transthyretin kinetic stabilizer that inhibits the amyloid cascade. *Proc. Natl. Acad. Sci. USA* **2012**, *109*, 9629–9634. [CrossRef]
30. Zhao, Y.; Xin, Y.; Song, Z.; He, Z.; Hu, W. Tafamidis, a noninvasive therapy for delaying transthyretin familial amyloid polyneuropathy: Systematic review and meta-analysis. *J. Clin. Neurol.* **2019**, *15*, 108–115. [CrossRef]
31. Falk, R.H. Tafamidis for transthyretin amyloid cardiomyopathy: The solution or just the beginning of the end? *Eur. Heart J.* **2019**, *40*, 1009–1012. [CrossRef] [PubMed]
32. Sant'Anna, R.; Gallego, P.; Robinson, L.Z.; Pereira-Henriques, A.; Ferreira, N.; Pinheiro, F.; Esperante, S.; Pallares, I.; Huertas, O.; Rosário Almeida, M.; et al. Repositioning tolcapone as a potent inhibitor of transthyretin amyloidogenesis and associated cellular toxicity. *Nature Commun.* **2016**, *7*, 10787. [CrossRef] [PubMed]
33. Rezania, K.; Saadat, L. Neurological manifestations of transthyretin-related amyloidosis. In *Amyloid Diseases*; Kurouski, D., Ed.; IntechOpen: London, UK, 2019. [CrossRef]
34. Klabunde, T.; Petrassi, H.M.; Oza, V.B.; Raman, P.; Kelly, J.W.; Sacchettini, J.C. Rational design of potent human transthyretin amyloid disease inhibitors. *Nat. Struct. Biol.* **2000**, *7*, 312–321. [CrossRef] [PubMed]
35. Palaninathan, S.K.; Mohamedmohaideed, N.N.; Orlandini, E.; Ortore, G.; Nencetti, S.; Lapucci, A.; Rossello, A.; Freundlich, J.S.; Sacchettini, J.C. Novel transthyretin amyloid fibril formation inhibitors: Synthesis, biological evaluation, and X-ray structural analysis. *PLoS ONE* **2009**, *4*, e6290. [CrossRef]
36. Choi, S.; Reixach, N.; Connelly, S.; Johnson, S.M.; Wilson, I.A.; Kelly, J.W. A substructure combination strategy to create potent and selective transthyretin kinetic stabilizers that prevent amyloidogenesis and cytotoxicity. *J. Am. Chem. Soc.* **2010**, *132*, 1359–1370. [CrossRef] [PubMed]
37. Ciccone, L.; Nencetti, S.; Rossello, A.; Stura, E.A.; Orlandini, E. Synthesis and structural analysis of halogen substituted fibril formation inhibitors of human transthyretin (TTR). *J. Enzyme Inhib. Med. Chem.* **2016**, *31*, 40–51. [CrossRef]
38. Ortore, G.; Martinelli, A. Identification of transthyretin fibril formation inhibitors using structure-based virtual screening. *ChemMedChem* **2017**, *12*, 1327–1334. [CrossRef]
39. Loconte, V.; Menozzi, I.; Ferrari, A.; Folli, C.; Imbimbo, B.P.; Zanotti, G.; Berni, R. Structure-activity relationships of flurbiprofen analogues as stabilizers of the amyloidogenic protein transthyretin. *J. Struct. Biol.* **2019**, *208*, 165–173. [CrossRef]
40. Gales, L.; Almeida, M.R.; Arsequell, G.; Valencia, G.; Saraiva, M.J.; Damas, A.M. Iodination of salicylic acid improves its binding to transthyretin. *Biochim. Biophys. Acta* **2008**, *1784*, 512–517. [CrossRef]
41. Mairal, T.; Nieto, J.; Pinto, M.; Almeida, M.R.; Gales, L.; Ballesteros, A.; Barluenga, J.; Pérez, J.J.; Vázquez, J.T.; Centeno, N.B.; et al. Iodine atoms: A new molecular feature for the design of potent transthyretin fibrillogenesis inhibitors. *PLoS ONE* **2009**, *4*, e4124. [CrossRef]
42. Cotrina, E.Y.; Pinto, M.; Bosch, L.; Vilaà, M.; Blasi, D.; Quintana, J.; Centeno, N.B.; Arsequell, G.; Planas, A.; Valencia, G. Modulation of the fibrillogenesis inhibition properties of two transthyretin ligands by halogenation. *J. Med. Chem.* **2013**, *56*, 9110–9121. [CrossRef] [PubMed]
43. Ribeiro, C.A.; Oliveira, S.M.; Guido, L.F.; Magalhães, A.; Valencia, G.; Arsequell, G.; Saraiva, M.J.; Cardoso, I. Transthyretin stabilization by iododiflunisal promotes amyloid-β peptide clearance, decreases its deposition, and ameliorates cognitive deficits in an Alzheimer's disease mouse model. *J. Alzheimers Dis.* **2014**, *39*, 357–370. [CrossRef] [PubMed]
44. González, A.; Quirante, J.; Nieto, J.; Almeida, M.R.; Saraiva, M.J.; Planas, A.; Arsequell, G.; Valencia, G. Isatin derivatives, a novel class of transthyretin fibrillogenesis inhibitors. *Bioorg. Med. Chem. Lett.* **2009**, *19*, 5270–5273. [CrossRef] [PubMed]

45. Wilcken, R.; Zimmermann, M.O.; Lange, A.; Joerger, A.C.; Boeckler, F.M. Principles and applications of halogen bonding in medicinal chemistry and chemical biology. *J. Med. Chem.* **2013**, *56*, 1363–1388. [CrossRef]
46. Cody, V.; Murray-Rust, P. Iodine···X(O, N, S) intermolecular contacts: Models of thyroid hormone-protein binding interactions using information from the Cambridge Crystallographic Data files. *J. Mol. Struct.* **1984**, *112*, 189–199. [CrossRef]
47. Mamane, V.; Aubert, E.; Peluso, P.; Cossu, S. Lithiation of prochiral 2,2′-dichloro-5,5′-dibromo-4,4′-bipyridine as a tool for the synthesis of chiral polyhalogenated 4,4′-bipyridines. *J. Org. Chem.* **2013**, *78*, 7683–7689. [CrossRef]
48. Mamane, V.; Peluso, P.; Aubert, E.; Cossu, S.; Pale, P. Chiral hexalogenated 4,4′-bipyridines. *J. Org. Chem.* **2016**, *81*, 4576–4587. [CrossRef]
49. Abboud, M.; Mamane, V.; Aubert, E.; Lecomte, C.; Fort, Y. Synthesis of polyhalogenated 4,4′-bipyridines via a simple dimerization procedure. *J. Org. Chem.* **2010**, *75*, 3224–3231. [CrossRef]
50. Mamane, V.; Aubert, E.; Peluso, P.; Cossu, S. Synthesis, resolution, and absolute configuration of chiral 4,4′-bipyridines. *J. Org. Chem.* **2012**, *77*, 2579–2583. [CrossRef]
51. Peluso, P.; Mamane, V.; Aubert, E.; Dessì, A.; Dallocchio, R.; Dore, A.; Pale, P.; Cossu, S. Insights into halogen bond-driven enantioseparations. *J. Chromatogr. A* **2016**, *146*, 228–238. [CrossRef]
52. Dallocchio, R.; Dessì, A.; Solinas, M.; Arras, A.; Cossu, S.; Aubert, E.; Mamane, V.; Peluso, P. Halogen bond in high-performance liquid chromatography enantioseparations: Description, features and modelling. *J. Chromatogr. A* **2018**, *1563*, 71–81. [CrossRef] [PubMed]
53. Connelly, S.; Choi, S.; Johnson, S.M.; Kelly, J.W.; Wilson, I.A. Structure-based design of kinetic stabilizers that ameliorate the transthyretin amyloidosis. *Curr. Opin. Struct. Biol.* **2010**, *20*, 54–62. [CrossRef] [PubMed]
54. Politzer, P.; Murray, J.S.; Clark, T. Halogen bonding and other σ-hole interactions: A perspective. *Phys. Chem. Chem. Phys.* **2013**, *15*, 11178–11189. [CrossRef] [PubMed]
55. Riley, K.E.; Tran, K.-A.; Lane, P.; Murray, J.S.; Politzer, P. Comparative analysis of electrostatic potential maxima and minima on molecular surfaces, as determined by three methods and a variety of basis sets. *J. Comput. Sci.* **2016**, *17*, 273–284. [CrossRef]
56. Lange, A.; Heidrich, J.; Zimmermann, M.O.; Exner, T.E.; Boeckler, F.M. Scaffold effect on halogen bonding strength. *J. Chem. Inf. Model.* **2019**, *59*, 885–894. [CrossRef]
57. Wojtczak, A.; Luft, J.R.; Cody, V. Structural aspects of inotropic bipyridine binding. *J. Biol. Chem.* **1993**, *268*, 6202–6206. [CrossRef]
58. Pennington, L.D.; Moustakas, D.T. The necessary nitrogen atom: A versatile high-impact design element for multiparameter optimization. *J. Med. Chem.* **2017**, *60*, 3552–3579. [CrossRef]
59. Peluso, P.; Mamane, V.; Dallocchio, R.; Dessì, A.; Villano, R.; Sanna, D.; Aubert, E.; Pale, P.; Cossu, S. Polysaccharide-based chiral stationary phases as halogen bond acceptors: A novel strategy for detection of stereoselective σ-hole bonds in solution. *J. Sep. Sci.* **2018**, *41*, 1247–1256. [CrossRef]
60. Wang, Z.; Sun, H.; Yao, X.; Li, D.; Xu, L.; Li, Y.; Tian, S.; Hou, T. Comprehensive evaluation of ten docking programs on a diverse set of protein–ligand complexes: The prediction accuracy of sampling power and scoring power. *Phys. Chem. Chem. Phys.* **2016**, *18*, 12964–12975. [CrossRef]
61. Irwin, J.J.; Shoichet, B.K. Docking screens for novel ligands conferring new biology. *J. Med. Chem.* **2016**, *59*, 4103–4120. [CrossRef]
62. Ferreira, L.G.; dos Santos, R.N.; Oliva, G.; Andricopulo, A.D. Molecular docking and structure-based drug design strategies. *Molecules* **2015**, *20*, 13384–13421. [CrossRef] [PubMed]
63. Adcock, S.A.; McCammon, J.A. Molecular dynamics: Survey of methods for simulating the activity of proteins. *Chem. Rev.* **2006**, *106*, 1589–1615. [CrossRef] [PubMed]
64. De Lima, W.E.A.; Pereira, A.F.; de Castro, A.A.; de Cunha, E.F.F.; Ramalho, T.C. Flexibility in the molecular design of acetylcholinesterase reactivators: Probing representative conformations by chemometric techniques and docking/QM calculations. *Lett. Drug Des. Discov.* **2016**, *13*, 360–371. [CrossRef]
65. Fine, J.; Konc, J.; Samudrala, R.; Chopra, G. CANDOCK: Chemical atomic network-based hierarchical flexible docking algorithm using generalized statistical potentials. *J. Chem. Inf. Model.* **2020**, *60*, 1509–1527. [CrossRef] [PubMed]
66. Zhu, J.; Wu, Y.; Xu, L.; Jin, J. Theoretical studies on the selectivity mechanisms of glycogen synthase kinase 3β (GSK3β) with pyrazine ATP-competitive inhibitors by 3DQSAR, molecular docking, molecular dynamics simulation and free energy calculations. *Curr. Comput.-Aided Drug Des.* **2020**, *16*, 17–30. [CrossRef]

67. Shen, C.; Wang, Z.; Yao, X.; Li, Y.; Lei, T.; Wang, E.; Xu, L.; Zhu, F.; Li, D.; Hou, T. Comprehensive assessment of nine docking programs on type II kinase inhibitors: Prediction accuracy of sampling power, scoring power and screening power. *Brief. Bioinform.* **2020**, *21*, 282–297. [CrossRef]
68. Morris, G.M.; Goodsell, D.S.; Halliday, R.S.; Huey, R.; Hart, W.E.; Belew, R.K.; Olson, A.J. Automated docking using a Lamarckian genetic algorithm and an empirical binding free energy function. *J. Comput. Chem.* **1998**, *19*, 1639–1662. [CrossRef]
69. Huey, R.; Morris, G.M.; Olson, A.J.; Goodsell, D.S. A semiempirical free energy force field with charge-based desolvation. *J. Comput. Chem.* **2007**, *28*, 1145–1152. [CrossRef]
70. Pettersen, E.F.; Goddard, T.D.; Huang, C.C.; Couch, G.S.; Greenblatt, D.M.; Meng, E.C.; Ferrin, T.E. UCSF Chimera - a visualization system for exploratory research and analysis. *J. Comput. Chem.* **2004**, *25*, 1605–1612. [CrossRef]
71. Ibrahim, M.A.A. Molecular mechanical study of halogen bonding in drug discovery. *J. Comput. Chem.* **2011**, *32*, 2564–2574. [CrossRef]
72. Ibrahim, M.A.A. Molecular mechanical perspective on halogen bonding. *J. Mol. Model.* **2012**, *18*, 4625–4638. [CrossRef] [PubMed]
73. Kolář, M.H.; Hobza, P.; Bronowska, K. Plugging the explicit σ-holes in molecular docking. *Chem. Commun.* **2013**, *49*, 981–983. [CrossRef] [PubMed]
74. Kolář, M.H.; Hobza, P. On extension of the current biomolecular empirical force field for the description of halogen bonds. *J. Chem. Theory Comput.* **2012**, *8*, 1325–1333. [CrossRef] [PubMed]
75. Fanfrlík, J.; Ruiz, F.X.; Kadlčíková, A.; Řezáč, J.; Cousido-Siah, A.; Mitschler, A.; Haldar, S.; Lepšík, M.; Kolář, M.H.; Majer, P.; et al. The effect of halogen-to-hydrogen bond substitution on human aldose reductase inhibition. *ACS Chem. Biol.* **2015**, *10*, 1637–1642. [CrossRef]
76. Arsequell, G.; Planas, A. Methods to evaluate the inhibition of TTR fibrillogenesis induced by small ligands. *Curr. Med. Chem.* **2012**, *19*, 2343–2455. [CrossRef]
77. Dolado, I.; Nieto, J.; Saraiva, M.J.; Arsequell, G.; Valencia, G.; Planas, A. Kinetic assay for high-throughput screening of in vitro transthyretin amyloid fibrillogenesis inhibitors. *J. Comb. Chem.* **2005**, *7*, 246–252. [CrossRef]
78. Weiss, R.; Aubert, E.; Peluso, P.; Cossu, S.; Pale, P.; Mamane, V. Chiral chalcogen bond donors based on the 4,4′-bipyridine scaffold. *Molecules* **2019**, *24*, 4484. [CrossRef]
79. Jiang, X.; Buxbaum, J.N.; Kelly, J.W. The V122I cardiomyopathy variant of transthyretin increases the velocity of rate-limiting tetramer dissociation, resulting in accelerated amyloidosis. *Proc. Natl. Acad. Sci. USA* **2001**, *98*, 14943–14948. [CrossRef]
80. Shao, Y.; Molnar, L.F.; Jung, Y.; Kussmann, J.; Ochsenfeld, C.; Brown, S.T.; Gilbert, A.T.B.; Slipchenko, L.V.; Levchenko, S.V.; O'Neil, D.P.; et al. Advances in methods and algorithms in a modern quantum chemistry program package. *Phys. Chem. Chem. Phys.* **2006**, *8*, 3172–3191. [CrossRef]
81. Frisch, M.J.; Trucks, G.W.; Schlegel, H.B.; Scuseria, G.E.; Robb, M.A.; Cheeseman, J.R.; Scalmani, G.; Barone, V.; Mennucci, B.; Petersson, G.A.; et al. *Gaussian 09, Revision B. 01*; Gaussian, Inc.: Wallingford, CT, USA, 2010.
82. Lu, T.; Chen, F. Multiwfn: A multifunctional wavefunction analyser. *J. Comp.Chem.* **2012**, *33*, 580–592. [CrossRef]
83. Lu, T.; Chen, F. Quantitative analysis of molecular surface based on improved marching tetrahedra algorithm. *J. Mol. Graph. Model.* **2012**, *38*, 314–323. [CrossRef] [PubMed]
84. Gasteiger, J.; Marsili, M. Iterative partial equalization of orbital electronegativity -a rapid access to atomic charges. *Tetrahedron* **1980**, *36*, 3219–3228. [CrossRef]
85. Sanner, M.F. Python: A programming language for software integration and development. *J. Mol. Graph. Model.* **1999**, *17*, 57–61. [PubMed]
86. Dennington, R.; Keith, T.; Millam, J. *GaussView Version 5*; Semichem Inc.: Shawnee Mission, KS, USA, 2009.

**Sample Availability:** Samples of the compounds **1–10** are available from the authors.

www.ingramcontent.com/pod-product-compliance
Lightning Source LLC
Chambersburg PA
CBHW061844210926
51850CB00006B/966
*9783725870226*

MDPI AG
Grosspeteranlage 5
4052 Basel
Switzerland
Tel.: +41 61 683 77 34

*Molecules* Editorial Office
E-mail: molecules@mdpi.com
www.mdpi.com/journal/molecules